Hospital Preparation for Bioterror

Hospital Preparation for Bioterror: A Medical and Biomedical Systems Approach

Edited by

Joseph H. McIsaac, III

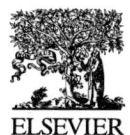

AMSTERDAM • BOSTON • HEIDELBERG • LONDON
NEW YORK • OXFORD • PARIS • SAN DIEGO
SAN FRANCISCO • SINGAPORE • SYDNEY • TOKYO

Academic Press is an imprint of Elsevier

Academic Press is an imprint of Elsevier
30 Corporate Drive, Suite 400, Burlington, MA 01803, USA
525 B Street, Suite 1900, San Diego, California 92101-4495, USA
84 Theobald's Road, London WC1X 8RR, UK

This book is printed on acid-free paper. ∞

Copyright © 2006, Elsevier Inc. All rights reserved.

No part of this publication may be reproduced or transmitted in any form or by any means, electronic or mechanical, including photocopy, recording, or any information storage and retrieval system, without permission in writing from the publisher.

Permissions may be sought directly from Elsevier's Science & Technology Rights Department in Oxford, UK: phone: (+44) 1865 843830, fax: (+44) 1865 853333, E-mail: permissions@elsevier.com. You may also complete your request on-line via the Elsevier homepage (http://elsevier.com), by selecting "Support & Contact" then "Copyright and Permission" and then "Obtaining Permissions."

Library of Congress Cataloging-in-Publication Data
Preparing hospitals for bioterror : a medical and biomedical systems
　approach / Joseph H. McIsaac, III, editor.
　　　p. ; cm.
　Includes bibliographical references and index.
　ISBN-13: 978-0-12-088440-7 (casebound : alk. paper)
　ISBN-10: 0-12-088440-2 (casebound : alk. paper)
　1. Emergency medical services. 2. Hospitals–Emergency service.
　3. Bioterrorism.　I. McIsaac, Joseph H.
　　　[DNLM: 1. Bioterrorism. 2. Emergency Service, Hospital.
　3. Hospital Administration.　WX 185 P927 2006]
　RA645.5.P7365 2006
　362.18—dc22
　　　　　　　　　　　　　　　　　　　　　　　　　　　2006011115

British Library Cataloguing-in-Publication Data
A catalogue record for this book is available from the British Library.

ISBN 13: 978-0-12-088440-7
ISBN 10: 0-12-088440-2

For information on all Academic Press publications
visit our Web site at www.books.elsevier.com

Printed in the United States of America
06　07　08　09　10　　9　8　7　6　5　4　3　2　1

**Working together to grow
libraries in developing countries**

www.elsevier.com　|　www.bookaid.org　|　www.sabre.org

ELSEVIER　　BOOK AID International　　Sabre Foundation

This book is dedicated to
Randi, Ellen, Lauren, and Katie

"Chance favors the prepared mind."—Louis Pasteur

Contents

Contributor list ix

Preface xiii

Acknowledgments xv

1. Recurring Pitfalls in Hospital Preparedness and Response 1
   Jeffrey N. Rubin

2. The History and Threat of Biological Weapons and Bioterrorism 17
   Zygmunt F. Dembek

3. Hospital Syndromic Surveillance 37
   Kathy J. Hurt-Mullen, Howard Burkom, Joe Lombardo, Sheryl Happel Lewis, Nicola Marsden-Haug, and Julie Pavlin

4. Biological Agents, Effects, Treatment, and Differential Diagnosis 49
   Zygmunt F. Dembek and Theodore J. Cieslak

5. Medical Considerations for Radiological Terrorism 61
   James Winkley and Paul D. Mongan

6. Nerve and Chemical Agents 73
   Paul D. Mongan and James Winkley

7. Decontamination and Personal Protection 89
   Joseph H. McIsaac, III

8. EMS Preparation for Terrorist Events 119
   Michael Zachera, III

9. Emergency Department Preparation 135
   Michael Zacchera, III and Michael F. Zanker

10. Pediatrics: Special Considerations for Children 143
    James F. Wiley, II

11. The Role of Psychiatry and Social Services in the Hospital Response to Bioterrorism 157
    Julian D. Ford

12. Bioterrorism and Obstetrics The Exposed Pregnant Patient 177
    Renee A. Bobrowski, John F. Greene, Jr., and Joel Sorosky

13. Operating Room Preparation for Mass Casualties 183
    Joseph H. McIsaac, III

14. Bioterrorism and Implications for Nurses and Nursing 193
    Jacquelyn McQuay

15. The Role of Pharmacy in Emergency Preparedness 201
    Robert S. Guynn

16. The Clinical Engineering Department Role in Emergency Preparedness 207
    Duane Mariotti

17. Amateur Radio Support for Hospitals 219
    Marina Zuetell

18. Hospital Power: Critical Care 229
    James F. Newton, P. E.

19. Electromagnetic Interference 233
    Joseph H. McIsaac, III

20. Chapter for Simulation for Bioterrorism 241
Thomas C. Mort and Stephen Donahue

21. Simulation II: Preparing for Biodisasters 255
Richard R. Kyle, Jr.

22. Hospital Large-Scale Drills 267
Garrett Havican

23. Response to SARS as a prototype for bioterrorism: Lessons in a Regional Hospital in Hong Kong 281
Arthur Chun-Wing Lau, Ida Kam-Siu Yip, Man-Ching Li, Mary Wan, Alfred Wing-Hang Sit, Rodney Allan Lee, Raymond Wai-Hung Yung, and Loretta Yin-Chun Yam

Appendix A: Emergency Preparedness, Response & Recovery Checklist Beyond the Emergency Management Plan 295

Appendix B: Model Hospital Mutual Aid Memorandum of Understanding 333

Appendix C: Protecting Building Environments from Airborne Chemical, Biological, or Radiological Attacks 345

Appendix D: Develop a Mitigation Plan (FEMA) 359

Appendix E: Medical Examiner/Coroner Guide for Mass Fatality Management of Chemically Contaminated Remains 369

Appendix F: Systems and Communications Security During Recovery and Repair 375

Appendix G: Altered Standards of Care in Mass-Casualty Events 383

Appendix H: Surge Hospitals: Providing Safe Care in Emergencies 413

Appendix I: Medical-Surgical Supply Formulary by Disaster Scenario 433

Index 437

Contributor list

Renee A. Bobrowski, MD (12),
Assistant Professor Obstetrics and Gynecology
Maternal Fetal Medicine Department of
Obstetrics and Gynecology,
Hartford, CT.

Howard Burkom, PhD (3),
John Hopkins University
Applied Physics Laboratory,
Laurel, MD.

Theodore J. Cieslak, MD, FAAP (4),
Chairman, San Antonio Military Pediatric
Center and Biodefence Consultant,
Office of the Army Surgeon General,
C/o Dept. of Pediatrics Brooke
Army Medical Center
3851, Roger Brooke Drive,
Ft. Sam Houston, Tx.

Zygmunt Francis Dembek, PhD, MS, MPH (2, 4),
Assistant Clinical Professor,
Masters in Public Health Program,
University of Connecticut Health Center
Farmington, CT.

Stephen Donahue, BS, RRT (20),
Director of the Simulation Center,
Hartford Hospital,
Hartford, CT.

Julian D. Ford, PhD (11),
Department of Psychiatry MC1410,
University of Connecticut Health Center,
Center of Trauma Response,
Recovery and Preparedness, CT.

John F. Greene, Jr., MD (12),
Associate Professor of Obstetrics and Gynecology,
Residency Program Director,
University of Connecticut School of Medicine,
Assistant Director Women's Health,
Hartford Hospital,
Hartford, CT.

Robert S. Guynn, RPb, MBA (15),
Connecticut Commission of Pharmacy,
Department of Pharmacy,
University of Connecticut Health Center,
Farmington, CT.

Garrett Havican, MBA,
EMT-P (22),
Regional Planning Coordinator,
Hartford Hospital.

Kathy J. Hurt-Mullen, MPH (3),
Montgomery County Maryland Department of
Health and Human Services,
Silver Spring, MD.

Richard R. Kyle Jr. (21),
Co-Founder and Operation Director,
Patient Simulation Laboratory,
Uniformed Services University,
Bethesda, MD.

Arthur Chun-Wing Lau,
MBBS MRCP, FHKCP,
FHKAM (Medicine) FCCP (23),
Department of Medicine,
Pamela Youde Nethersole Eastern Hospital,
Hong Kong SAR,
China.

Rodney Allan Lee,
MBBS FRCPA FHKCPath FHKAM (Pathology)
Department of Clinical Microbiology
and Infection,
Pamela Youde Nethersole Eastern Hospital,
Hong Kong SAR, China.

Sheryl Happel Lewis, MPH (3),
John Hopkins University
Applied Physics Laboratory, Laurel, MD.

Man-Ching Li,
MIIE IEng MEM PFM (23),
Health Sector Division,
Electrical and Mechanical Services Department,
Hong Kong SAR, China.

Joe Lombardo, MS (3),
John Hopkins University
Applied Physics Laboratory, Laurel, MD.

Duane Mariotti,
Biomedical Engineering Consultant (16),
Seattle, WA.

Nicola Marsden-Haug, MPH (3),
Walter Reed Army Institute of Research,
Silver Spring MD.

Joseph H. McIsaac, III,
MD MS (7, 13, 19)
Chief of Trauma Anesthesia
Hartford Hospital, Hartford, CT
Assistant Clinical Professor of Anesthesiology,
University of Connecticut School of Medicine,
Associate Adjunct Professor of
Biomedical Engineering,
University of Connecticut Graduate School.

Jacqueline McQuay,
RN, MS, SANE (14),
Trauma Team Coordinator Hartford Hospital,
Hartford, CT.

Paul D. Mongan, MD (5, 6),
COL MC US ARMY,
Director,
National Capital Consortium,
Anesthesiology Residency Program,
Associate Professor and Chair,
Department of Anesthesiology,
The Uniformed Services University,
Bethesda, MD.

Thomas C. Mort, MD (20),
Medical Director,
Simulation Center,
Hartford Hospital,
Hartford, CT.

James F. Newton, P.E. (18),
Mechanical Department Head,
Senior Associate,
TRO/The Ritchie Organization,
Newton, MA.

Julie Pavlin, MD MPH (3),
Walter Reed Army Institute of Research,
Silver Spring, MD.

Jeffrey N. Rubin, PhD (1),
Tualatin Valley Fire & Rescue,
Aloha, OR.

Alfred Wing-Hang Sit,
MBA FPFM FHFKIE MIEE CEng (23),
Health Sector Division,
Electrical and Mechanical Services Department,
Hong Kong SAR,
China.

Joel Sorosky, MD (12),
Professor of Obstetrics and Gynecology,
University of Connecticut School of Medicine,
Director Women's Health,
Hartford Hospital,
Hartford, CT.

Mary Wan,
MHS (NSW) MSc (FM) (23),
Administrative Services,
Pamela Youde Nethersole Eastern Hospital,
Hong Kong SAR,
China.

James F. Wiley, II, MD (10),
Professor of Pediatrics and
Emergency Medicine/Traumatology,
School of Medicine,
University of Connecticut;
Emergency Department,
Connecticut Children's Medical Center,
Hartford, CT.

James Winkley, MD (5, 6),
Associate Program Director,
National Capital Consortium,
Anesthesiology Residency Program,
Assistant Professor,
Department of Anesthesiology,
The Uniformed Services University,
4301 Jones Bridge Road, Bethesda, MD.

Loretta Yin-Chun Yam,
MBBS MRCP FRCP FHKCP FHKAM (Medicine)
FCCP (23),
Department of Medicine,
Pamela Youde Nethersole Eastern Hospital,
Hong Kong SAR,
China.

Ida Kam-Siu Yip,
RN BHSc (23),
Infection Control Unit,
Pamela Youde Nethersole Eastern Hospital,
Hong Kong SAR,
China.

Raymond Wai-Hung Yung,
MBBS FHKAM,
FRCPath (23),
Infection Control Branch,
Center of Health Protection,
Hong Kong SAR, China.

Michael Zachera III,
NREMT-P (8, 9),
EMS educator,
Department of EMS Education,
Hartford Hospital.

Michael F. Zanker, MD (9),
Attending Emergency Physician,
Assistant Professor of
Emergency Medicine,
School of Medicine,
University of Connecticut.

Marina Zuetell, N7LSL (17),
District Emergency Coordinator,
Western Washington,
Medical Services Communications.

Preface

This text is intended to be a guide to those interested in improving the readiness of their hospital or healthcare organization to manage mass casualties resulting from a bioterror incident. It is intended to appeal to three diverse groups: clinicians, administrators, and support personnel. Rather than focus exclusively on the medical treatment of patients exposed to weapons of mass destruction, we have tried to take a more holistic approach. A hospital is a living, breathing entity, much the same as the human body. All parts are interdependent and must function in a tightly coordinated manner to survive and prosper. We have tried to present this organism from a multiple of perspectives, each representing a functional unit of the larger system. The authors are as diverse as the material. They range from nationally recognized authorities to those whose expertise is derived from years of practical experience. Each has a unique orientation that, when added to the whole, gives a result greater than sum of the parts. This book is an attempt to present as many of these views as possible, from individual patient treatment to facilities management, and from simulation to practical advice from a hospital that successfully managed a SARS outbreak.

While the overall theme of the book is response to bioterrorism, the principles and techniques discussed clearly are applicable to all disasters, both large and small. The fundamental message is that preparation, communications, and cooperation, on all scales, will determine the institution's success or failure in managing a mass casualty incident.

In medicine, an expert is an individual who has treated a large number of patients with a particular disease over an extended length of time, and who has published scholarly works on the subject. Thankfully, there are few who meet these criteria in the field of bioterrorism, at this time. Few authors here will represent themselves as true experts, yet each has expertise, often in translation from a related field, which can be of benefit to us all.

Unfortunately, the world is changing rapidly. We cannot continue to sit by unprepared for what many believe is the inevitable proliferation and implementation of these weapons. It is my sincere hope that this book continues to be more theory than reality.

Acknowledgments

I would like to thank all the contributors for their work, but especially Dr. Zygmunt Dembek for his invaluable advice and his tireless effort to recruit authors. Without him, this book would not exist. I would also like to thank my family and my many colleagues at Hartford Hospital, the Connecticut Children's Medical Center, and the University of Connecticut for their support and tolerance.

1 Recurring Pitfalls in Hospital Preparedness and Response

JEFFREY N. RUBIN

Hospitals are an essential component of community preparedness for terrorism and other hazards, both natural and manmade. Despite general preparedness requirements within the industry, hospitals typically are a weak link with respect to community disaster preparedness, particularly for those incidents involving contaminated patients. Significant systemic constraints make most hospitals reluctant partners in preparedness and generate ineffective response; this condition has been highlighted by the antiterrorism training and preparedness programs in the past few years. Results of numerous exercises and actual responses across the United States indicate a predictable list of pitfalls, most of them related to inherent system limitations that continue to hinder effective disaster operations in hospitals:

- Communications
- Hospital security
- Decontamination procedures, equipment, and training
- Hospital staff management
- Exercise realism, content, follow-up

1.1 Introduction

Recent events have focused attention on the ability of communities to respond to acts of terrorism. In addition to intentionally generated incidents, most communities have been struggling with preparedness against a range of natural and technological hazards. Public safety and emergency management personnel have developed and tested response plans, and considerable federal resources have been expended toward the same end—albeit with inconsistent results. With some exceptions, community preparedness efforts have faltered at a common, though not exclusive, point: hospitals. Those involved in preparedness and response recognize the quandary: hospitals are essential, irreplaceable resources for planning, response, and recovery associated with disasters, but they carry a unique set of constraints that makes effective participation in such efforts challenging at best.

1.2 Hospital Challenges and Constraints

Barbera et al. [1] cogently discussed the constraints and challenges facing hospitals, along with public expectations. Hospitals as a whole face difficult financial times: approximately 30% of U.S. hospitals are operating at a financial loss, with many more teetering on the financial brink [2]. Hospitals face increasing operating costs coupled with decreasing reimbursement rates. Emergency departments (EDs) have become primary care intake points for much of the public [3], regardless of their insurance status. Staffing shortages are becoming the rule for most departments across a wide range of skill levels and specialties [4]; loss of experienced staff exacerbates the problem. High staff turnover rates further burden the remaining staff and add overtime and incentive costs to already strained budgets [5].

Costs have not been the only increasing item. Healthcare facilities are hardly exempt from government regulations (a recent example is the Health Insurance Portability and Accountability Act [6]—HIPAA) and are strongly affected by changes in Medicare reimbursement patterns, but accredited hospitals also deal with the non-governmental Joint Commission for the Accreditation of Healthcare Organizations (JCAHO). To achieve and maintain accreditation, hospitals must adhere to JCAHO's consensus standards as demonstrated during periodic onsite and remote surveys. Standards are diverse in scope and generally derived from clinical, ethical, technological, environmental, or occupational indications. Like many government regulations, they tend to add expense and are not accompanied by new revenue streams.

Hospitals rely on public trust as much as on reimbursement revenue. More than most corporations or government agencies, a healthcare facility that suffers a crisis of public confidence stands to lose both funding and patients along with its reputation. Public expectations, commonly in the form of blind assumptions, are that hospitals should be able to handle whatever they receive—and do it right the first time. With respect to disasters, this includes:

- Managing medical assessment, treatment, and continuing care for acute incidents involving large numbers of patients
- Effectively managing contaminated patients
- Recognizing, identifying, and managing consequences of bioterrorism
- Protecting employees, patients and their families, and anyone else within the facility
- Dealing with all of these while continuing to provide everyday emergency care

Public agencies responsible for preparedness and response have little direct control over public hospitals and none over private facilities (which are not accountable to public officials). There is no suitable alternative to engaged hospitals when trying to plan for or manage a mass-casualty incident or other type of large-scale disaster affecting a community. Should the incident be at the hospital itself (such as a fire or hazardous material release) or involve the hospital (for example, a flood or hurricane), a prepared facility and staff may be the difference between minimal loss of life and a true catastrophe.

1.3 Hospital Requirements

Hospitals have been required to have and exercise emergency preparedness plans (formerly known as "disaster plans") for many years. As of January 2001, hospitals wishing to achieve or retain JCAHO accreditation had to have a comprehensive plan in place, covering the four traditional phases of emergency management (mitigation, preparedness, response, and recovery) [7]. A hazard vulnerability analysis, part of the new standards, not only determines both the most likely and the most catastrophic incidents, but also identifies the range of hazards for a given hospital. This all-hazard approach, like municipal emergency operations plans, allows preparedness and a measured, flexible response to a variety of potential incidents. Plans may contain annexes for specific hazards, but an all-hazard plan should obviate a separate plan for each hazard (an "earthquake plan," a "terrorism plan," etc.). Plans are supposed to be tested and updated by at least one tabletop or similar exercise and one full-scale exercise or actual activation per year. The standards also establish requirements for staff training and familiarization with the plan.

The wave of training and other preparedness programs, accompanied by requirements and expectations regarding preparedness for acts of terrorism, has not ignored hospitals. The Defense Department's Domestic Preparedness Program (continued by the Justice Department) in the late 1990s provided basic training on medical management of casualties affected by chemical, biological, and radiological warfare agents. Curriculum and training were limited by design: it was largely military in origin, focused on the response phase, and did not contain much depth in hospital preparedness. The Metropolitan Medical Response System (MMRS) [8], initially overseen by the Department of Health and Human Services and now part of the Department of Homeland Security, was the first large-scale federal program to focus on improving the ability of healthcare systems to detect, identify, and manage incidents involving large numbers of potentially contaminated casualties. The goal of incorporating first responders (public safety agencies), public health agencies, hospitals, and emergency management and linking local, state, and federal agencies was an innovative global approach to a healthcare system that is commonly approached via its components. The challenges faced by MMRS participants and administrators in the program's initial incarnation were less a result of the philosophy than of the style and method of administration. The MMRS is now part of the multi-faceted Homeland Security Grant Program [8A], addressing key issues of medical surge capacity in the community.

Surge capacity, the ability to handle a large influx of ill or injured people beyond standard community resources, is a critical component of hospital preparedness. As additional (i.e., unused) hospital bed-space has dwindled over the years, surge capacity in American hospitals has been allowed to reach an extreme low [9,10]. Even were there significant excess hospital beds, it would be difficult to staff and equip them. Realistically, solutions must involve alternative assessment and treatment centers rather than physically expanding hospitals—and most do (either via adapting existing alternate facilities or setting up temporary ones). Providing adequate staffing for these alternative centers is the greater challenge.

In addition to preparedness requirements, hospitals fall under regulations of the Occupational Safety & Health Administration (OSHA) and the Environmental Protection Agency (EPA). As with many detailed federal standards, OSHA's requirements for hospitals are open to interpretation, with a great deal riding on sources such as OSHA opinions and interpretations: often the closest to a de facto standard. The lack of a clear and consistent application of OSHA regulations has been an obstacle to developing consistency, although progress appears to be in the making when this was written.

Plan development, staff training, and equipment maintenance are non-reimbursable costs in terms of billing, but some financial support has developed. In June 2002, the Healthcare Resources and Services Administration (HRSA) initiated grants to states and a few cities focusing on preparedness for bioterrorism in state and local governments and hospitals [11,12]. The grants were supposed to assist states in achieving "critical benchmarks for bioterrorism preparedness planning," promulgated by the Department of Health and Human Services. Three of the initial benchmarks were to designate a bioterrorism preparedness coordinator, establish a hospital preparedness planning committee to advise the state health department, and develop a plan for managing epidemics, regardless of origin [13]. States have some discretion on disbursement (provided that funds are directed toward fulfillment of primary grant goals), with many aiming for general hospital preparedness as a first step in bioterrorism preparedness. Subsequent and planned grants from HRSA have allowed expansion of preparedness funding from hospitals to health systems and encourage regional and statewide coordination. In combination with public health preparedness grants from the CDC and the MMRS component of the Homeland Security Grant Program, the HRSA National Bioterrorism Hospital Preparedness Program [13A] is addressing local, regional, and state aspects of health-system surge capacity and capability.

Despite requirements, some standards, and best intentions, significant obstacles remain, including the combination of staff and equipment shortages, lack of surge capacity, and minimal funding. Although there have been (and likely will continue to be) substantial improvements, most hospitals are still unprepared to effectively manage the results of a major incident—whether due to mishap, terrorism, natural disaster, or infectious disease outbreak—requiring treatment of mass casualties, staff protection, or facility evacuation [14,15]. An incident contemporaneous with local or regional infrastructure disruption will not only magnify hospital shortcomings, it will further hamper effective hospital response and hospital and community recovery.

1.4 Observations

Milsten [16] surveyed 22 years of incidents in the United States and abroad, identifying a broad list of hospital challenges (communications and power failures, water shortages and contamination, structural damage, hazardous materials exposure, facility evacuation, and resource allocation), accompanied by general suggestions (such as developing plans and procedures for disasters).

The observations on which the discussion and conclusions in this chapter are based on multiple sources:

- Direct personal observation (generally as controller or evaluator) of tabletop, functional, and full-scale exercises, along with actual incidents such as tornadoes, ice storms, floods, hazardous materials spills, and multiple-casualty events.
- Personal communications and written after-action reports from local exercises and actual incidents elsewhere.
- Published observations and after-action reports from three large-scale exercises: TOPOFF (May 2000) [17], Dark Winter (June 2001) [18], and TOPOFF 2 (May 2003) [19–21].

Hospitals consistently encountered challenges in the following areas: communications, security, decontamination, staff training, staff protection, and exercise design and conduct. The most significant aspect of these observations may be their consistency: the challenges and pitfalls encountered by hospitals and the agencies supporting them are definable and reproducible—and thus predictable. As such, there is value in their description, discussion, and analysis.

1.5 Communications

Intrafacility communications during exercises and actual events have been described as "difficult," "inconsistent," "marginal," and "nonexistent." Phones are overloaded, radios—when available—are insufficient in number, range, and frequency options (or a combination of those), and staff commonly lack adequate training in communications procedures or equipment operation. This should come as little surprise, because similar complaints are expressed about everyday operations—that is, a system that does not work well under normal conditions should not be expected to do so under extreme stress. Few facilities devote planning or resources to external communications. Although most acute-care facilities are able to use the Hospital Emergency Area Radio network, it was designed for short communications between EMS providers and EDs as well as limited interfacility traffic; it was not intended for continuous heavy traffic among multiple parties. Many hospitals host licensed amateur radio operators during disasters; the ham networks provide an important communications resource, allowing voice, data, and even video transmissions among incident scenes, hospitals, emergency operations centers, and other critical facilities.

1.6 Security

Security staff in most hospitals that have them are private guards, either hospital or contract employees. Most are unarmed and have no powers of arrest. Although their responsibilities vary considerably, most are there as deterrents and to restrain violent patients or visitors. Hospital security is an important part of JCAHO's "secure environment," protecting patients, staff, visitors, information, and the physical infrastructure [22,23]. Some hospitals, particularly large ones in urban areas, employ sworn law enforcement officers, either on contract or as employees. Regardless of the type and powers of security staff, the trend of minimal staffing applies across the board, commonly resulting in inadequate coverage for most facilities. Recurrent security-related challenges have internal and external foci: lockdown and the role of local law enforcement.

Lockdown is a common constituent of hospital emergency plans, but there is little consistency to its definition, even between facilities in the same community. In its ideal use, lockdown is an incident management tool that allows hospital staff to assert or regain control of a situation that appears or escalates with little warning. Lockdown is analogous to cardiopulmonary resuscitation (CPR): it is a short-term step intended for use early in the incident to buy time for more definitive measures. In securing all or part of the facility against additional entry, staff implementing lockdown can gain some breathing room while providing short-term protection to themselves and their patients. Also, as with CPR, lockdown can make the difference between success and failure in implementation of an emergency plan but is rarely effective on its own; a plan that ends with lockdown is doomed to fail.

In most exercises simulating a terrorist incident, naturally occurring disease outbreak, or unintentional hazardous material release, the hospital in question has been "overrun," meaning that a portion (generally the ED) or all of the facility is no longer able to function cohesively, protect its staff, or provide organized care to current and prospective patients. This can be due to contamination of the area, an unmanageable crush of incoming patients, perceived threat of violence, or loss of infrastructure. In many of these exercises, hospital staff recognized impending failure and requested assistance from law enforcement agencies for facility security and crowd control. With few exceptions these requests were not met (or were met too late), although it eventually became apparent to most participants that these needs were indeed urgent and the loss of hospitals disastrous. Although it is not an exaggeration to say that law enforcement was not an eager player in hospital security, this was not due to laxity on the part of police. As expressed in the first TOPOFF exercise after-action report [24], law enforcement agencies were overrun with urgent requests for multiple types of assistance. As they were given little to no external guidance on how to rank request urgency, they found themselves with too many priorities. This issue offers a compelling example of the need to consider hospital preparedness within the context of *community* resources.

1.7 Decontamination

Mass decontamination has been a common focus since antiterrorism training became a mass-market product in the late 1990s. Considerable sums have been spent on extensive training and equipment designed to decontaminate thousands of people at an incident scene and hundreds at a hospital. Common goals in cities participating in MMRS contracts were for hospitals to be able to decontaminate at least 100 ambulatory patients without relying on external assistance (i.e., a fire service hazmat team). Goals related to HRSA grants focus on 500 per million of population, but do not specify an interval. Both MMRS and HRSA goals represent significant expectations, and to date they have proved largely fanciful. Terrorism aside, all acute-care hospitals should be able to successfully manage a *single* contaminated patient without external resources [25]. A 2002 American Hospital Association survey [26] reported that a majority of hospitals had plans in place for managing chemical and biological attacks; this is a marked increase relative to surveys taken before 11 September 2001 [27]. This encouraging report notwithstanding, most hospital plans likely fall into the category of "fantasy documents" [28]—that is, meeting legal and political requirements but not grounded in realistic capabilities or expectations and not conferring functionality. The great majority still find single-patient decontamination an elusive goal.

1.8 Staff Training

As with the public-safety sector, there is no shortage of training and equipment for hospital preparedness; there is also little in the way of functional standards, guidelines, or quality control among programs and their purveyors. Few hospitals have full-time emergency managers or emergency preparedness coordinators: most commonly those responsibilities fall under "other duties as required" for clinical managers, facilities staff, environmental health and safety officers, or administrative staff. Whether the purview of an individual or committee, the decisions are the same. The lack of standardization and the vast range of executive support almost guarantee that each facility or hospital market will go through its own set of decisions, all driven at least as much by financial considerations as by need.

1.8.1 What Type of Training Should be Provided?

There are many training options, but the most common (and the most applicable) include the HEICS (currently being updated) [29], terrorism and weapons of mass destruction, and general and medical management of hazardous materials. HEICS is a standardized incident management system adapted from incident command system variants used by local, state, and federal public-safety and emergency-management personnel. It is specified in the JCAHO emergency management standards and is one of the few consistencies in hospital preparedness training. Beyond HEICS, options are numerous and unregulated, with varying degrees of standardization. How much training should be provided? What are useful and realistic competencies? What will an individual hospital, hospital group, or regional consortium support? To add to the mix, sweeping (and verging on the arbitrary) training requirements related to compliance with the National Incident Management System and other federal homeland security initiatives consume substantial staff resources while yielding little apparent benefit.

1.8.2 Who Should be Trained?

Principal distinctions include clinical vs. non-clinical, executive vs. managerial vs. labor, determining which departments should be included, the number of trained staff needed to provide adequate coverage on all shifts, frequency of initial and refresher training, and how much effort should be made to include physicians, particularly those who contract with hospitals (a common arrangement, especially in the ED). High turnover rates can quickly deprive a facility of trained employees. Insufficient or ineffective refresher training can produce the same effect as high turnover, as hard-won skills deteriorate due to lack of use. Many preparedness and decontamination training programs are provided in "train-the-trainer" format—that is, a small group of employees is trained and expected to cascade the training down to fellow employees, even though their newly acquired "expertise" is unaccompanied by experience, additional knowledge, or implementation capability. Lack of effective follow-up creates the all-too-common phenomenon of "trainers" who teach few if any classes and soon lose whatever competencies they may have acquired—particularly if there is no executive support for continued training.

1.9 Staff Protection

Essential components of staff protection include personal protective equipment (PPE) for common tasks and decontamination, chemoprophylaxis and immunization, and sufficient training, education, and policy development to ensure that they are available and appropriately used. Common PPE pitfalls include inadequate training for existing equipment, inadequate equipment itself, and ineffective policies and procedures governing PPE use. The SARS outbreak of 2003 and the effect it had on hospitals and EMS staff is an excellent example: insufficient and inappropriate PPE contributed to the disruptive effect on health systems and exposure among healthcare workers [30,31]. The safety net that chemoprophylaxis (for example, antibiotics for possible anthrax exposures) and immunization (for example, smallpox vaccine for healthcare workers) can provide will fail if it is not made available promptly and to all affected and potentially affected employees. Employees who are not confident that their employer will offer appropriate protection are unlikely to show up for work during a crisis. Likewise, employees who are concerned about the health and safety of their families are unlikely to perform their duties well, if at all, if their concerns are not adequately addressed. This is by no means limited to issues of terrorism, but extends to all potentially catastrophic events.

1.10 Exercise Design and Conduct

So far we have examined common pitfalls that relate to staffing, equipment, training, and procedures. One of the mechanisms for determining and evaluating these and other challenges can itself be a challenge: exercises. The purpose of an exercise is to evaluate one or more measurable performance items via objective criteria. Performance items may include use of specific equipment, procedures, emergency plans, communications systems, or a combination of those. Given the longstanding JCAHO requirement of at least two exercises per year, hospitals should house considerable expertise in exercise design, conduct, and evaluation. In fact, a most significant recurring pitfall in hospital exercises is a distorted picture. An exercise, like a written plan, may meet JCAHO standards without conferring significant benefit in terms of actual preparedness or response capability on the hospital(s) in question.

The most common types of exercises (tabletop and functional) do not involve hands-on operations but rather focus on decision making and plan evaluation. Even full-scale exercises, which combine command-level decision making with hands-on tasks, are limited in terms of space, personnel, use of supplies, and the exercise schedule itself. Hospitals must be able to receive and manage actual patients during exercises, requiring either additional staffing to allow exercise operations to go on alongside everyday operations or limiting the scope and duration of play. Additional staffing for exercises means additional cost and staff scheduling challenges.

Because of the need for advance scheduling of personnel and simply having sufficient personnel on hand, two common exercise deficiencies ensue: lack of surprise and preferential testing of the most populated shifts. Lack of surprise may manifest itself in numerous ways, including on-duty staff having recently reviewed emergency procedures (when they otherwise would not have done so), necessary equipment and supplies in unusual states of readiness and/or stocked in unusually high levels, and specialized equipment set up in advance of the exercise, even though there would have been no reason to do so under non-emergency conditions. Examples include ED physicians immediately diagnosing rare conditions that are part of the exercise scenario, with equally rarely used medications being immediately available in the ED or pharmacy and, in more than one exercise, a large ED having a full decontamination station set up, with staff wearing full PPE, before play even began. Any exercise scenario induces a certain degree of artificiality, but effective exercises are designed so that artificiality does not interfere with evaluation of identified objectives. Untoward, artificial, staff preparation for an exercise adds artificiality that directly compromises effective evaluation. In addition, the overwhelming lack of exercises on evening and night shifts tests capabilities only when a hospital is at its highest staffing levels. This not only deprives some staff of exercise experience, but also deprives the facility of evaluating performance during off-shifts.

The combination of insufficient training and ineffective exercises deprives staff of experience in improvisation and decision making, thus increasing the likelihood that a single significant obstacle (for example, difficulty setting up decontamination equipment, or even presentation of a contaminated patient) can derail the exercise or actual response.

1.11 Suggestions

There are multiple potential solutions for the challenges herein identified. Clearly, fundamental changes are needed, either in the expectations of hospitals (unlikely) or the resources made available to them to further the cause of preparedness (more likely and currently improving). The following suggestions are based largely on operational, intrafacility details ("what works"). There is no question that hospital preparedness must be part of a regional approach to health systems and general preparedness across agency, jurisdictional, and corporate boundaries. Hospitals are part of a greater whole, but *each* hospital must also have a degree of self-sufficiency to enable independent operations should regional assistance be unavailable. My suggestions focus on making things work better in individual hospitals; in so doing I temporarily de-emphasize larger-scale financial, political, and legal issues, which I will reexamine at the end of this article.

1.12 Communications

The first step in designing an internal communications system that works in emergencies is to have one that works on an everyday basis. The second step is to realize that any system can be overtaxed and that there will be some incidents in which even the most durable system will fail. Realistic expectations for communications systems in disasters are essential for effective implementation of an emergency operations plan. Redundancy is an obvious and desirable solution; simple low-tech equipment can be effective. Satellite phones and trunked and repeated radios that allow flexible external communications are important, but if the trunking system and/or repeaters are external to the hospital, the most the hospital can do is buy into the system. Likewise, amateur radio offers a vital and achievable link to other hospitals and public-safety providers, but by definition they are *outside* the facility. This is not meant to de-emphasize the importance of being able to communicate with public safety and other agencies, but rather to focus on what can be done internally. A hospital's communication system might be improved by use of the following:

- *Business radios*: Inexpensive handheld radios that do not require a license but will work in multi-storey buildings with reinforced construction and extensive electronic machinery. These are similar to the popular family radios but are intended (and required) for business use.
- *Phone/intercom systems*: An internal communications system that is powered by emergency generators and does not require functioning external equipment (such as remote switching stations). These systems can be surprisingly robust, even if communications into and out of the facility are disrupted. A facility that owns its own phone switch (that is, switching is done by an internal rather than an external computer) is more likely to retain internal function than one relying on a service provider's switch. This is even more important for large campuses comprising multiple buildings.
- *Status boards*: The bane of many a JCAHO survey, further restricted by HIPAA (due to open display of confidential patient information). Simple dry-erase boards in operational areas are an effective way of providing updated information to the staff working there. Most hospitals have such boards in place, but they are not necessarily used during emergency operations. Status boards serve an important function away from patient-care areas as well: information management in hospital emergency operations centers (also known as command centers, coordination centers, and facility command posts). Effective display media in emergency operations centers are essential for managing incoming information, tracking resources and events, and making appropriate resource allocation decisions.
- *Runners*: When all else fails—and even when it does not—runners are commonly employed to carry information between functional areas or groups. Given the universality of this function, it might as well be part of the plan, to be practiced and tested. Combining runners, status boards, and digital cameras creates the opportunity to receive quick, non-intrusive status reports from various parts of a hospital: literally a snapshot of status that may be delivered to the hospital's emergency operations center and displayed there.
- *Self-initiation*: This is more a training than a communications issue, but the point is that the better trained and exercised employees are, the more capable they will be of independent implementation of an emergency operations plan when activation is initiated. If employees can perform critical initial functions without needing centralized communications in place, successful implementation is far more likely.

1.13 Security

Of all the issues related to hospital preparedness, security is one of the most important and one of the least directly controllable by most hospitals. Functional security is an everyday issue that is greatly magnified during disasters; it is part of staff protection and allows implementation of emergency plans. Many potential solutions to security issues require hospitals to increase their level of interaction with local emergency management and public safety agencies and may require substantial revision of those agencies' existing policies, procedures, and mutual aid agreements:

- *Meet with local law enforcement agencies*: Hospitals are essential resources during disasters and may be targets of terrorism. Law enforcement must see protection of hospitals as a high priority. Everyday security resources, where present, are likely to be insufficient during disasters, particularly those involving terrorism. If possible, special units may be identified and preassigned to hospitals; this ideal arrangement removes a decision step during an incident.
- *Consider private security to provide or augment protection*: Although private security guards do not have powers of arrest, they can provide substantial numbers for securing facility access. Some private security companies provide bonded personnel, trained and equipped for use of lethal and non-lethal force, but the presence of a trained, uniformed staff may be the most important. Contrary to popular perception and many exercise scenarios, panicking mobs overrunning hospitals are not a realistic expectation [32–35]. If numerous self-referred patients arrive at a hospital and are met with clear information and directions, they will likely comply. Incorporation of private security personnel into emergency plans should include specifications of available staff, call-up procedures, and consultation with local law enforcement regarding policies and procedures for disasters.
- *Make lockdown a realistic part of the plan*: Facilities in a multi-hospital region should reach consensus on a functional definition and share it with local emergency management and public safety providers. All staff should understand the purpose of lockdown and when and how it is to be implemented. Internal training and resources should include readily understandable designation for building entrances and exits. Prepositioned, or readily available, signage and pre-scripted messages (both for public address systems and local media broadcast as needed) to direct patients and families to appropriate entrances will speed emergency implementation and improve compliance. All doors with outside access should be numbered in a simple, consecutive fashion, so that staff may be sent to secure "door number two" rather than "northwest access 1.4." Once in place, this numbering system can be added to facility floorplans and shared with public safety agencies for routine, emergency, and disaster response.

1.14 Decontamination

Focus on the achievable. The biggest step is to be able to decontaminate a single patient without endangering staff, patients, or visitors and without rendering the ED unavailable to incoming traffic [36]. Only when and if that step is achieved is it appropriate to examine multi-patient scenarios. Industrial incidents can contaminate several patients, making multi-patient capability particularly important for hospitals in industrial areas. Most incidents resulting in contaminated patients occur at fixed facilities or in agricultural applications [37], but they can happen anywhere there is a transportation route; moreover, contaminated patients do not always go to the nearest hospital. The leap from multi-patient to mass decontamination is expensive, requires far more extensive training and drilling, and may be unrealistic (both in capabilities and likelihood) for smaller facilities. For facilities where mass decontamination is considered a legitimate potential need, temporary facilities will likely need to be established; either "dry" decontamination or self-disrobement and decontamination ("strip and shower") [38] should be seriously considered. Whether in the form of trailers, tents, canopies, or large open areas, equipment (and training) must be provided with the foreknowledge that it will be used rarely if at all. This is an important consideration: the greatest likelihood is that employees' only exposure to the knowledge, skills, abilities, and decision-making processes involved in mass decontamination will be gained and applied only in training and exercises.

The Agency for Healthcare Research and Quality (AHRQ) has produced numerous useful references and guidelines for hospital preparedness [38A], including models for decontamination, PPE, and isolation and quarantine [38B], and California's Emergency Medical Services Authority has updated their Patient Decontamination Recommendations for Hospitals [38C]. These and similar references represent substantial resources in planning an training for single-patient and mass decontamination.

1.15 Staff Training

Hospital training staff tend to be overloaded with a wide variety of responsibilities, including clinical competencies, continuing education, community education, and non-clinical staff training. Most hospital staff have little expertise in developing and providing training for disaster procedures, particularly patient and facility decontamination. Although "train-the-trainer" classes are popular and readily available, newly minted trainers commonly find themselves with few resources and little or no experience, with a resultant dearth of cascaded training. The following steps can help compensate:

- *An effective training program requires executive support*: A directive, backed up by appropriate resource allocation, is the basis on which a successful program progresses.
- *Contract for specialized training*: Rather than attempting to develop and maintain such expertise, hospitals, hospital groups, or—even better—communities should strongly consider contracting for expertise. As with any contract service, it is essential to select reputable, competent providers. Contracts should include follow-up services (refresher training and assistance with exercise development as needed) and provide the option of developing internal capability for conducting informal training and drills within individual units. This approach requires the same degree of executive commitment as internally derived training, particularly with respect to initial and recurring expenses. Hick et al. [39] effectively summarized healthcare-specific needs and goals for decontamination training that incorporate recent OSHA interpretations [40–43].
- *Let clinicians be clinicians*: There are a few positions within a HEICS organization that should be filled by physicians, but in general the most important function for physicians in a disaster is that of a clinician. As many hospitals contract with physician groups, particularly for ED coverage, ensuring training is difficult. Therefore, hospitals should include select staff physicians in HEICS and other disaster training and provide brief orientations to the bulk of physicians, so that they understand the roles, responsibilities, and function of the emergency organization.
- *Move some training to the schools*: New guidelines from the Association of American Medical Colleges [44] suggest a *curriculum* for future physicians in medical schools. Several nursing schools have been offering disaster courses for a year or more.

1.16 Staff Protection

No emergency plan can be implemented without staff. The most important provision for staff protection is irrespective of specific issues, procedures, or equipment. *Staff protection must be an executive priority, and it must be communicated as such.* To enable operations to continue under emergency conditions, staff protection measures must be designed with the intent of demonstrating an institutional commitment to employee safety. This is as much an exercise in trust as in deed; facilities with strained labor-management relations will face greater difficulty in this pursuit than those with smooth partnerships.

- *PPE must meet realistic needs*: There is no consistent standard for PPE for incidents involving hazmat or weapons of mass destruction. These incidents would send potentially contaminated patients to hospitals. Personal protection standards defined by OSHA [45] and the National Fire Protection Association [46] are unrealistic for an acute-care environment—and recent OSHA interpretations support this. Level B ensembles (splash protection with self-contained or supplied-air breathing apparatus) offer substantial respiratory protection, but there is little evidence that it is necessary in this setting, and the additional equipment weight, maintenance, and potential claustrophobic reaction of its users may make it deleterious. In addition, regulatory, financial, and training requirements for Level B are likely to render it both prohibitive and ineffective. Self-referring patients arriving at an ED under their own power are likely to have minimal if any contamination (as distinct from exposure) and are well removed from the site of initial contact; effective decontamination training and equipment make Level C (splash protection with air-purifying respirators) appropriate for the great majority of incidents. Clearer guidelines and national consensus standards are essential; the White House's National Strategy for Homeland Security [47] tasked the (EPA) with developing standards for decontamination equipment and procedures, but the EPA's Strategic Plan for Homeland Security [48] does not indicate a focus on hospital activities. Hick et al. [49] lucidly summarized recent interpretations, considerations, and justifications for Level C PPE in healthcare settings until more definitive standards are promulgated. OSHA has issued comprehensive and functional best practices for "first receivers" [49A] (the first hospital providers to make contact with patients from a large-scale external event), but at this writing they have not been formally adopted as standards.

- *Level C is still a step up*: The decision to use Level C protection does not encompass an escape from OSHA standards for respiratory protection; [50] it requires personnel using respirators to undergo medical screening, fit-testing (not necessary if hooded positive air-purifying respirators are used), training, and refreshers. Certain circumstances could justify Level B PPE, but this would be beyond the baseline and would be limited to facilities capable of implementing and maintaining the training and regulatory upkeep.

- *Plan to provide staff with chemoprophylaxis and/or immunizations as indicated*: Whether chemoprophylaxis and/or immunizations come from internal stocks (most likely for initial use), locally cached supplies, or the material from the Strategic National Stockpile (SNS) [51], internal and community plans and policies and must specify priority distribution for critical staff and must include procedures for doing so. Cities participating in a Metropolitan Medical Response System contract are required to incorporate caches and SNS deliveries into their plan, but they must specify priority recipients.

- *Consider staff families in plans*: It is the unusual healthcare employee who will be satisfied with individual protection that does not cover the family. Plans providing for employee chemoprophylaxis and/or immunizations should include distribution to employee families; this will complicate planning and implementation but will help achieve the goal of having staff available to perform critical functions.

1.17 Exercises

Exercises, traditionally (and still) a JCAHO requirement, are now part of the HRSA National Bioterrorism Hospital Preparedness Plan as well. Beyond compliance issues, exercise are an excellent method of testing plans, training, and equipment—but only if the exercises are designed and conducted with that intent. This requires that hospitals:

- *Base exercises on realistic plans and models*: Start at manageable scales and build on demonstrated principles and procedures. An exercise where everything goes great can be just as counterproductive as one where everything *fails*. Exercises should focus on specific measurable objectives and be conducted realistically. Pre-exercise warning should be minimized, and all shifts should be involved as much as possible. External evaluators will enhance objectivity and help keep employees out of difficult situations (such as evaluating their supervisors). Focused exercise design and competent controllers can prevent or minimize distractions arising from obstacles encountered during play. Local and state emergency management and public safety agencies are excellent resources.

- *Use realistic staffing patterns for exercises*: In addition to the need for covering all shifts on training and exercises, it is essential to employ staffing patterns that are likely to be in effect when a real incident happens. Task-based drills may not need scenarios, but larger-scale exercises do. Exercises for off-peak shifts should use off-peak staffing; incidents that would require callbacks to provide additional staffing or specialized skills should not assume that *those assets are present at the outset.*

- *Recognize that success has multiple definitions*: An exercise that evaluates its intended objectives and yields action items is a success, but only if there is action. "Lessons" are not necessarily "learned." It is appropriate to determine whether a plan or procedure was successful, particularly regarding specific tasks or functions. Failure requires corrective action, but the objective determination of success or failure has value as well—not everything is relative. Successes should be publicized, internally and externally. An effective preparedness program can use successes and failures as motivators for continued improvement.

1.18 Critical Steps

To facilitate hospital and community preparedness, there are some essential needs that require action on the federal level (and in some cases require not just a federal but a national approach):

- *Financial incentives and support for hospital preparedness*: As long as preparedness is competing with everyday essential needs, it will fail to thrive. Whether by grant, reimbursement, or other means, hospitals must have some type of dedicated (and internally immutable) funding stream to cover not just equipment but planning, initial training, refresher training, and exercises. Preparedness is an ongoing process and must have ongoing support. The current multi-year cycle of HRSA preparedness grants is an important step in the right direction (albeit already reduced from in its initial funding levels), but it needs to evolve into a secure funding stream and be tied to measurable, sustainable improvements in broad-spectrum (as opposed to bioterrorism-dominant) preparedness. For now and the foreseeable future, NIMS compliance is a necessary price to pay for maintaining access to federal preparedness grants.

- *Realistic consensus standards*: Hospitals and public safety agencies still rely on unproven tenets, many incorporating military models that have little application in the civilian world. In the absence of national standards, states and even localities have been developing their own. In many areas and individual facilities, equipment and training are determined in the absence of standards or even an identified strategy. Such standards are most important with respect to PPE, mass decontamination (including "no decontamination"), and dealing with mass illness. The EMSA and AHRQ best practices and models are substantial resources, but they are not yet standards.

- *Ethics and liability*: As discussed by Pesik et al. [52], triage following use of a weapon of mass destruction on the U.S. civilian population will not fit familiar models. In particular, mass illness related to bioterrorism could create a paradox in which the sickest patients receive palliative care only. Effective, ethical planning is as essential as the legal protection to conduct it. Currently such indemnity from liability does not exist in most states.

References

1. Joseph A. Barbera, Anthony G. Macintyre, and Craig A. DeAtley. Ambulances to nowhere: America's critical shortfall in medical preparedness for catastrophic terrorism. *Journal of Homeland*

Security, March 2002. [This is an excellent treatment not just of the constraints hospitals face, but of the national and local threat the constraints represent.]
2. Hospital Preparedness for Mass Casualties: Summary of an Invitation Forum. Final report, August 2000, summary of an invitational forum convened 8–9 March 2000 by the American Hospital Association with the support of the Office of Emergency Preparedness, U.S. Department of Health and Human Services.
3. S. M. Schneider, M. E. Gallery, R. Schafermeyer, and F. L. Zwemer. Emergency department crowding: a point in time. *Annals of Emergency Medicine*, 42(2):167–172, 2003.
4. "Health Care at the Crossroads: Strategies for Addressing the Evolving Nursing Crisis," Joint Commission on Accreditation of Healthcare Organizations.
5. First Consulting Group. The healthcare workforce shortage and its implications for America's hospitals. 2001.
6. Health Insurance Portability and Accountability Act of 1996.
7. A summary of the new standards, discussion of the underlying philosophy, examples, and resources. *Joint Commission Perspectives*, 21(12), 2001. [Additional information is available at the Joint Commission on Accreditation of Healthcare Organizations website.]
8. Metropolitan Medical Response System website.
8A. Homeland Security Grant Program website.
9. American Hospital Association. Hospital preparedness for mass casualties. August 2000.
10. R. W. Derlet and J. R. Richards. Overcrowding in the nation's emergency departments: complex causes and disturbing effects. *Annals of Emergency Medicine*, 35(1):63–68, 2000.
11. HHS Approves State Bioterrorism Plans so Building Can Begin. Press release, Department of Health and Human Services, 6 June 2002.
12. Bioterrorism preparedness grants. Press release, Department of Health and Human Services, 6 June 2002.
13. 17 Critical Benchmarks for Bioterrorism Preparedness Planning. Press release, Department of Health and Human Services, 6 June 2002.
13A. HRSA National Bioterrorism Hospital Preparedness Program website.
14. Hospital preparedness: most urban hospitals have emergency plans but lack certain capacities for bioterrorism, General Accounting Office Report 03-924, August 2003.
15. Carl H. Schultz, Kristi L. Koenig, and Roger J. Lewis. Implications of hospital evacuation after the northridge, California earthquake. *New England Journal of Medicine*, 348(13):1349–1355, 2003.
16. Andrew Milsten. Hospital responses to acute-onset disasters: a review. *Prehospital and Disaster Medicine*, 15(1):32–45, 2000.
17. Thomas V. Inglesby, Rita Grossman, and Tara O'Toole. A plague on your city: observations from Topoff. *Clinical Infectious Disease*, 32(29):436–445, 2001.
18. Dark winter. ANSER Institute for Homeland Security website.
19. Top Officials (TOPOFF) exercise series: TOPOFF 2 after action summary report for public release. U.S. Department of Homeland Security, 19 December 2003.
20. Robert Block. FEMA points to flaws, flubs in terror drill. *Wall Street Journal*, 31 October 2003.
21. Martha Frase-Blunt. Operation TOPOFF 2' Bioterrorism Exercise Offers Educational Lessons. *AAMC (Association of American Medical Colleges) Reporter*, August 2003.
22. Joint Commission on Accreditation of Healthcare Organizations website.
23. *NFPA (National Fire Protection Association) Journal*, 96(4):44–47, 2002.
24. Presentation by Mark Quick, epidemiologist with Colorado's Department of Public Health and Environment, at the National Environmental Health Association's Bioterrorism Conference in Denver, 18–19 June 2000.
25. Agency for Toxic Substances and Disease Registry. Managing hazardous material incidents, 2001. [An excellent training and reference resource.]
26. Talking with your community about disaster readiness. American Hospital Association Disaster Readiness Advisory #7, 28 August 2002.
27. Kimberly N. Treat, Janet M. Williams, Paul M. Furbee, William G. Manley, Floyd K. Russell, and Clarence D. Stamper, Jr. Hospital preparedness for weapons of mass destruction incidents: an initial assessment. *Annals of Emergency Medicine*, 38(5):562–565, 2001. [The low level of preparedness indicated within is typical of small- and large-scale surveys assessing hospital capabilities for events involving weapons of mass destruction as well as ordinary hazmat incidents. A bright side could be that an institution is better off correctly knowing it is not prepared than erroneously believing it is.]

28. Lee Clarke. *Mission Improbable: Using Fantasy Documents to Tame Disaster*. Chicago, University of Chicago Press, 1999.
29. Hospital Emergency Incident Command System website. [NOTE: the HEICS IV update is currently scheduled for completion and release by April 2006.]
30. Damon C. Scales, Karen Green, Adrienne K. Chan, Susan M. Poutanen, Donna Foster, Kylie Nowak, Janet M. Raboud, Refik Saskin, Stephen E. Lapinsky, and Thomas E. Stewart. Illness in intensive care staff after brief exposure to severe acute respiratory syndrome. *Emerging Infectious Diseases*, 9(10):1205–1210, 2003.
31. Mark A. Rothstein, M. Gabriela Alcalde, Nanette R. Elster, Mary Anderlik Majumder, Larry I. Palmer, T. Howard Stone, and Richard E. Hoffman. Institute for Bioethics, Health Policy and Law, University of Louisville School of Medicine. Quarantine and Isolation: Lessons Learned From SARS. A report to the Centers for Disease Control and Prevention, November 2003.
32. Erik Auf der Heide. *Disaster Response: Principles of Preparation and Coordination*. St. Louis: Mosby, 1989. [Out of print, but available free of charge, through the Center of Excellence in Disaster Management and Humanitarian Assistance.]
33. Joseph Barbera, Anthony McIntyre, Larry Gostin, Tom Inglesby, Tara O'Toole, Craig DeAtley, Kevin Tonat, and Marci Layton. Large-scale quarantine following biological terrorism in the United States. *Journal of the American Medical Association*, 286(21):2711–2717, 2001.
34. Lee Clarke. Panic: myth or reality? *Contexts*, fall:21–26, 2002.
35. Thomas A. Glass and Monica Schoch-Spana. Bioterrorism and the people: how to vaccinate a city against panic. *Clinical Infectious Diseases*, 34(2):271–223, 2002.
36. This is not a new concept. ED physicians and consultants Howard Levitin and Henry Siegelson have been emphasizing this for years, as have the George Washington University trio of Joseph Barbera, M.D. Anthony Mcintyre, M.D. and Craig DeAtley, PA-C.
37. Agency for Toxic Substances and Disease Registry. Hazardous substances emergency events surveillance. Annual report, 1998.
38. K. L. Koenig. Strip and Shower: The Duck and Cover for the 21st Century (editorial). *Annals of Emergency Medicine*, 42(3):391–394, 2003.
38A. Agency for Healthcare Research and Quality. Bioterrorism planning and response resources.
38B. Agency for Healthcare Research and Quality. Development of models for emergency preparedness: personal protective equipment, decontamination, isolation/quarantine, and laboratory capacity, May 2004.
38C. California Emergency Medical Services Authority. Patient decontamination recommendations for hospitals, http://www.emsa.ca.gov/hbppc/hbppc.asp, July 2005.
39. John L. Hick, Paul Penn, Dan Hanfling, Mark A. Lappe, Dan O'Laughlin, and Jonathan L. Burstein. Establishing and training health care facility decontamination teams. *Annals of Emergency Medicine*, 42(3):381–390, 2003.
40. Medical personnel exposed to patients contaminated with hazardous waste. OSHA standard interpretation, 31 March 1992.
41. Training requirements for hospital personnel involved in an emergency response of a hazardous substance. OSHA standard interpretation, 27 October 1992.
42. Emergency response training requirements for hospital staff. OSHA standard interpretation, 25 April 1997.
43. Emergency response training necessary for hospital physicians/nurses that may treat contaminated patients. OSHA standard interpretation, 10 March 1999.
44. Association of American Medical Colleges. Training future physicians about weapons of mass destruction: report of the expert panel on bioterrorism education for medical students. 2003.
45. Hazardous waste operations and emergency response. 29 CFR 1910.120.
46. National Fire Protection Association standards 471—Recommended practice for responding to hazardous materials incidents, 472—Standard for professional competence of responders to hazardous materials incidents, and 473—Standard for competencies for EMS personnel responding to hazardous materials incidents.
47. *National Strategy for Homeland Security*, July 2002.
48. Environmental Protection Agency. *Strategic Plan for Homeland Security*, September 2002.
49. J. L. Hick, D. Hanfling, J. L. Burstein, J. Markham, A. G. McIntyre, and J. A. Barbera. Protective equipment for health care facility decontamination

personnel: regulations, risks, and recommendations. *Annals of Emergency Medicine*, 42(3): 370–380, 2003.

49A. Occupational Safety and Health Administration, Best practices for hospital-based first receivers of victims. Available at http://www.osha-slc.gov/dts/osta/bestpractices/firstreceivers_hospital.html, January 2005.

50. Respirator Fit-Testing. 29 CFR 1910.134.

51. Immediate response 12-hour Push Packages "are caches of pharmaceuticals, antidotes, and medical supplies designed to provide rapid delivery of a broad spectrum of assets for an ill defined threat in the early hours of an event," according to the website of the Centers for Disease Control and Prevention. "These Push Packages are positioned in strategically located, secure warehouses ready for immediate deployment to a designated site within 12 hours."

52. N. Pesik, M. E. Keim, and K. V. Iserson. Terrorism and the Ethics of Emergency Medical Care. *Annals of Emergency Medicine*, 37(6):642–646, August 1999 and June 2001. [Pesik has spoken and written about this topic with great insight; this is one of the major "hidden" issues of preparing for terrorism.]

2 The History and Threat of Biological Weapons and Bioterrorism

ZYGMUNT F. DEMBEK

2.1 Introduction

Modern societies well-understand the potential for catastrophic consequences through use of weapons of mass destruction. Nations have all too often suborned expertise in the biochemical, molecular, and epidemiological sciences to create biological weapons. It cannot be assumed that past cultures did not create and use similar weapons simply through an empirical understanding of their effects. Recognition of the effect of infectious diseases on populations resulted in the use of infected individuals, toxins, human waste, cadavers, and animal carcasses as weapons against armies. Whether by driving infected livestock into an opponent's camp over 3000 years ago, catapulting plague-infested bodies over castle walls during the Middle Ages, or sending anthrax-filled envelopes in the mail during the twenty-first century, the intent of these efforts throughout time has been the same: to cause illness and death among one's enemies. It is encouraging to think that the current age will be one in which biological weapons will no longer be used. However, the study of their use throughout history dictates otherwise, and serves as a warning of our need for coordinated preparations against the next purposeful biological event.

2.2 Biological Weapons in the Ancient World

Cuneiform tablets from 1770 B.C. Sumeria claim details of lethal pathogens. The use of biological toxins extracted from plants and animals on arrowheads or poison darts predates recorded history, and has also been recorded as used in battles in many ancient cultures. Arrows were common weapons in ancient civilizations, and toxic arrows were used. Among the arrow poisons used by ancient cultures were snake toxins, scorpion venom, and various plant toxins, including helleborus from the buttercup *Helleborus orientalis*, aconitine from *Aconitum napellus*, and scopolamine from *Hyoscyamus niger* (henbane). The potential for a current-day threat from these toxins should not be dismissed. During the World War II, Russian scientists isolated aconitine to create poison bullets, which were used as assassination weapons [1].

2.3 Battlefield Use of Infectious Diseases, or "Giving The Gift That Keeps On Giving"

Many ancient commanders had a basic understanding of disease transmission from animal-to-man (zoonoses) and from person-to-person. During the twelfth to fifteenth century BC, the Hittites are known to have driven animals infected with disease and a syphilitic woman into enemy territory with the intent of plague initiation. Since armies were composed of men separated from their loved ones, the allure of "toxic women" may not have easily been overcome. The King of India presented a deadly gift to Alexander the Great in the form of a "poison maiden": a "beautiful maiden whom had fed on poison until she had the nature of a venomous snake" [2]. Thirty centuries later, Spanish forces were "intentionally chasing beautiful, infectious prostitutes into the French army camp" during the Naples Campaign of 1494 [2].

The *Arthashastra*, written in India during the fourth century BC by Kautilya, provides recipes for transmitting infectious disease to enemies [3]. Among the greatest scourges of the ancient world were those diseases of bioterrorism that are feared today for their ability to be transmitted from person-to-person. The Roman historian, Cassius Dio, reported plagues begun by saboteurs in Rome in 90–91 AD, and again in 189 AD. He described deliberate attempts to use smallpox and bubonic plague against enemy troops and cities, in what Roman historians decried as "man-made pestilence" [2].

The spread of plague and its causative agent *Pasteurella pestis* was not well understood in 1346. However, during the fourteenth-century siege of Caffa (now Feodossia, Ukraine), the attacking Tartar force experienced a plague epidemic [4]. The Tatars, led by the Muslim commander De Mussis, attempted to convert their misfortune into a battlefield opportunity by catapulting the cadavers of their deceased into the city in hopes of initiating a plague epidemic. The outbreak of plague in Caffa was soon followed by the retreat of its defending forces and conquest of the city. Since plague-transmitting fleas leave cadavers to parasitize a living host, the corpses catapulted over the walls of Caffa may not have been carrying competent plague vectors [4]. The siege of this city likely had only minimal importance in the spread of plague through Europe [5].

Medieval military commanders paid attention to the "lessons learned" from the siege of Caffa. In 1422, during the Hussite wars in Bohemia, at the siege of Karlstejn (located in the current Czech republic), the invading forces led by Prince Zygmunt Korybutovic (Coribut), hurled corpses of plague-stricken soldiers, dead cows and 2000 cartloads of excrement at the enemy troops [6,7].

In 1650, Polish General Jan Kazimierz Siemienowicz, an expert in artillery and rocketry, fired hollow artillery spheres filled with the saliva from rabid dogs at enemy forces. It is unknown whether General Siemienowicz was successful with this tactical use of animal saliva, but he was prescient in his understanding of the causative agent of rabies. Although rabies transmission results from virus inoculation through the bite of a rabid animal, this was not proven until the early eighteenth century [8].

Smallpox devastated Native Americans in the eighteenth century [9]. Francisco Pizarro's conquest of the Inca empire in South America during the fifteenth century had been aided by the Inca's susceptibility to the virus. Speculation has been raised that he had made gifts of smallpox-contaminated cloth to the Incas [10]. Sir Jeffrey Amherst, commander of British forces in North America during the French and Indian War (1754–1767), may have known those rumors. Amherst recommended the deliberate use of smallpox to "reduce" Native American tribes hostile to the British. An outbreak of smallpox at Fort Pitt resulted in the generation of fomites (an inanimate object contaminated with infectious microorganisms that can serve in disease transmission) and an opportunity to execute Amherst's plan [11]. On June 24, 1763, Captain Simeon Ecuyer, one of Amherst's subordinates, gave blankets and a handkerchief from the smallpox hospital to the Native Americans and recorded in his journal, "I hope it will have the desired effect" [4]. Shortly afterwards, Native Americans defending Fort Carillon sustained epidemic smallpox casualties, which directly contributed to the loss of the Fort to the English, later renamed Fort Ticonderoga [12].

During the Revolutionary War, General George Washington ordered variolation (an early form of smallpox immunization) for the Continental Army in 1777 after the loss of the siege of Quebec. Washington's order was given because of the devastation already rendered on his forces by smallpox, and also to decrease the potential for purposeful spread of smallpox among the Colonials by the British [9].

Perhaps taking a lead from the battle plans of the fourteenth century Tartars, Tunisians in 1785 threw plague-infected clothing into the Christian-held city of La Calle, in hopes of spreading this illness [13]. During 1796–1797, while besieging the Austrian fortress at Mantua, Italy, Napoleon ordered the surrounding land area to be flooded, in an attempt to infect the inhabitants with malaria (then known as "swamp fever") [13].

During the Civil War, Dr. Luke Blackburn, who later became the governor of Kentucky, attempted to infect clothing with smallpox and yellow fever and then sell it to unsuspecting Union troops. His success is unknown, but at least one Union officer's obituary stated that he died of smallpox that could be ascribed to Blackburn's scheme. Although smallpox can be transmitted through contact with fomites, it was not known at the time that yellow fever could only be transmitted to humans from mosquitoes [14].

2.4 Biological Contamination of Water Supplies

The purposeful poisoning of wells and water supplies was a tactic often used during battles. In 590 BC, Solon of Athens used hellebore to poison the water source from the Pleistrus River to the city of Kirrha in Greece. Records indicate that the inhabitants of Kirrha became "violently sick to their stomachs and all lay unable to move. They took the city without opposition." In 350 BC, Aeneas the Tactician wrote in a manual for military commanders the recommendation to "make water undrinkable" by polluting rivers, lakes, springs, wells, and cisterns. In 1155, at the battle of Tortona, Italy, Barbarossa put human corpses in his enemy's water supply, successfully contaminating it. During the eighteenth century, the Iroquois Indians used animal skins to cause illness in the water supply of over 1000 French soldiers in the Americas [2].

In 1861, Union troops advancing south into Maryland and other border states were warned not to eat or drink anything provided by unknown civilians for fear of being poisoned. Despite the warnings, numerous soldiers thought they had been poisoned after eating or drinking. Confederate General Albert Johnston, retreating through Mississippi in 1863, tried to poison water supplies by dumping dead animals into the wells and bodies of water that they passed [15]. The same year, U.S. Army General Order No. 100 stated that "The use of poison in any manner, be it to poison wells, or food, or arms, is wholly excluded from modern warfare" [14].

2.5 Biological Contamination of Food

Purposeful poisoning of food supplies has also long been a tactic of warfare. Wine poisoned with mandrake (*Podophyllum peltatum*) root was used by Julius Caesar to poison Cilician pirates to affect his rescue after they had captured him in about 75 BC. In about 65 BC, Pompey's army approaching Colchis fell victim to toxic honey left for their demise along the rout of attack by the Heptakometes. About 1000 of Pompey's men were slaughtered after they collapsed with vomiting and diarrhea from this toxic meal [2]. How likely is the creation of a toxic honey? If the bees in a hive collected nectar from plants that contained alkaloids toxic to humans, such as ragwort, azaleas, and rhododendrons, poison honey could result. And, in 1485 near Naples, the Spanish supplied their French enemies with wine laced with leprosy patients' blood, hoping to transmit this disease to their enemies [2].

In 946 AD, Olga of Kiev provided poisoned mead (honey wine) to his Russian opponents [2]. It appears that rulers of Russia did not forget the lesson they learned from this event. Over 500 years later, the Russian army slaughtered about 10,000 Tartar soldiers after they had drunk similarly tainted mead in 1489 [2]. It is worth noting that food and water safety threat microorganisms are today considered to be Category B pathogens (second highest priority agents) by the US Centers for Disease Control and Protection (CDC).

2.6 Toxin Weapons

Bees, hornets, and other stinging insects have long been used as weapons. Beehive and hornet nest bombs were among the earliest projectile weapons, and venomous insects are thought to be "important military agents in tactics of ambush." Catapulting beehives at enemy troops was a favorite tactic of the ancient Romans. The Mayan text *Popol Vuh* describes bees used as booby traps against invaders [16]. Henry I catapulted beehives at the Duke of Lorraine's army in the eleventh century. In 1289, this tactic was also used by Hungarian troops against invading Turks [2].

Venomous insects and reptiles have been enlisted during battles. Hannibal catapulted clay jars filled with venomous snakes during the decisive naval battle of Eurymedon against King Eumenes of Pergamum between 190 and 184 BC. During 198–199 AD, the citizens of Hatra (this city's remains are located near Mosul, Iraq) successfully defended their city from a Roman attack by the use of clay pot bombs likely filled with scorpions and other venomous insects gathered from the surrounding desert [2].

No history of ancient toxicological experts would be complete without mentioning perhaps the most notorious, Scythian King Mithridates VI of Pontus [17]. Obsessed with a phobia of assassination by poison (he had murdered family members in this way), Mithridates was accompanied by a team of ancient doctors known for their knowledge of healing potions from various snake venoms. He daily ingested small amounts of various toxins so that he would develop immunity from their effects. He created an elaborate mixture of over 50 ingredients into a single drug for his own protection. Mithridates demise was particularly ironic. While surrounded by his enemies, he chose to commit suicide in 63 BC. He took poison, which was ineffective due to his self-conferred immunity. Mithridates then ordered his bodyguard to run him through with a sword [2].

2.7 World War I—German Saboteurs

Germany used chemical warfare agents such as mustard and chlorine gas extensively during World War I. It is perhaps not as well known that Germany is considered to have developed an ambitious biological warfare program during World War I. German Zeppelins (dirigible airships) were used in bombing raids of England in 1915–1918 [18]. One German plan was to discharge vats of bubonic plague cultures from Zeppelins over English harbors. They hoped to infect rats that would then spread disease among the British population. Fortunately, this was rejected for both moral and practical reasons [19].

Covert biological operations were planned for neutral countries trading with the Allies in order to infect livestock and contaminate animal feed exported to Allied forces. *Bacillus anthracis* and *Burkholderia mallei*, the causative agents of anthrax and glanders, were to be used to infect Romanian sheep for export to Russia. In 1916, cultures confiscated from German diplomats in Romania were identified as *Ba. anthracis* and *Bu. mallei* at the Bucharest Institute of Bacteriology and Pathology. *Bu. mallei* was allegedly used by German saboteurs operating in Mesopotamia to inoculate 4500 mules and in France to infect French cavalry horses. Livestock in Argentina intended for export to Allied forces were infected with *Ba. anthracis* and *Bu. mallei*, resulting in the deaths of more than 200 mules from 1917 to 1918 [19,20].

German operations in the United States included attempts to contaminate animal feed and to infect horses intended for export during World War I [4]. In Chevy Chase, Maryland, Dr. Anton Dilger, a German–American physician, set up a secret biological warfare laboratory. Large quantities of *Ba. anthracis* and *Bu. mallei* were grown in a workshop known to other German agents as "Tony's Lab." Perhaps the largest explosion in New York City until September 11, 2001 occurred when members of this group detonated 2 million pounds of ammunition at the Black Tom freight terminal in New York Harbor on the night of July 29–30, 1916 [21]. Dilger paid Baltimore longshoreman and other dockworkers to spread his cultures among horses that were being shipped to England. He distributed glass bottles, about an inch and a half long with needles protruding from cork stoppers, which were filled with his homemade anthrax and glanders cultures. This group traveled along the East coast, inoculating horses in livestock pens in New York City, Norfolk, and Newport News [19]. They also poured anthrax into the animals' food and water [20].

2.8 World War I—US Research

Although never used, tests conducted in the US during this time revealed that ricin toxin derived from castor beans could have military applications. A 1918 report reads: "These experiments show two important points: (1) easily prepared preparations of ricin can be made to adhere to shrapnel bullets, (2) there is no loss in toxicity of firing and even with the crudest method of coating the bullets, not a very considerable loss of the material itself... It is not unreasonable to suppose that every wound inflicted by a shrapnel bullet coated with ricin would produce a serious casualty... Many wounds which would otherwise be trivial would be fatal." [13].

2.9 World War II—Japan

From 1932–1945, Japan conducted biological warfare research in occupied Manchuria under the direction of Generals Shiro Ishii and Kitano Misaji [22]. Unit 731, a biological warfare research facility located near the town of Pingfan (Harbin), was the center of the Japanese biological weapons development program and contained 150 buildings, five satellite camps, and a staff of more than 3000 scientists and technicians. Additional units were located at Mukden, Changchun, and Nanking. Prisoners at these camps were infected with pathogens including *Ba. anthracis, Neisseria meningitidis, Shigella* sp., *Vibrio cholerae,* and *Yersinia pestis* [23]. The first use of biological weapons by the Japanese was the contamination of the Soviet water supply at the city of Nomonhan along the Mongolian border with typhoid [22]. Eventually, over 3000 prisoners died as a result of experimental infection or subsequent execution during the Japanese program between 1932 and 1945 [22].

During war crimes prosecution, participants in the Japanese program captured by the Soviet Union during World War II admitted to a dozen large-scale field trials of biological weapons. At least 11 Chinese cities were attacked with biological agents. Water supplies and food items were contaminated with cultures of *Ba. anthracis, V. cholerae, Shigella* spp, *Salmonella* spp, and *Y. pestis,* bacterial cultures were thrown directly into homes, and also sprayed from aircraft [22,24]. Plague was developed as a biological weapon through laboratory-bred fleas feeding on plague-infected rats. These infected fleas were then harvested and released from aircraft over Chinese cities. Plague initiation was begun by the release of up to 15 million fleas during aerial attacks, together with rice and wheat [22]. It was hoped that the grain would attract the local rat population, as rats serve as carriers for infected fleas that transmit plague to a human population. Epidemic plague has been attributed to these attacks, but rigorous epidemiological or microbiological verification is not available.

In 1945, General Ishii ordered the labs of Unit 731 burned to the ground. At the end of World War II, the US granted amnesty to those Japanese scientists who had participated in the research on the condition that these scientists disclose all information accumulated during their programs to the US government. This situation likely developed as the US and USSR also competed for German rocket experts. In 1945, 22 former biological weapons scientists in Japan were interviewed. The information they provided was not particularly useful, since the data could not be quantitated [24]. It was discovered that, in 1945, the Japanese BW program at Unit 731 had stockpiled 400 kg of anthrax to be used in a specially designed fragmentation bomb. Unit 731 and its satellite camps may have killed as many as 250,000 Chinese during its existence, but the total number cannot be verified [25,26].

One bizarre anecdote to Unit 731's legacy could have brought biological warfare directly to the US during WWII. From November 1944 to April 1945, during Operation Fugo (wind ship), 9300 balloons were released from Japan to travel the Gulf Stream to the west [27]. They were equipped with incendiary and anti-personnel bombs, and flew as far East as Michigan and Texas. Six people were killed in Oregon [27,28]. There were fears that these balloons could be loaded with biological weapons [29]. During July 1945, Unit 731 was involved in another plan, codenamed Cherry Blossoms at

Night, to use kamikaze pilots to infest California with the plague [28]. A submarine was scheduled to carry the pilots off of Southern California, from which they were to fly to San Diego and release plague-infected fleas. The target date was to be September 22, 1945. Fortunately Japan signed the act of unconditional surrender on September 2 [23,30].

2.10 World War II—Germany

There are claims that Germany continued biological weapons research between the Wars. In the early 1930s, German agents may have used the biological warfare simulant *Serratia marcescens* (then known as *Micrococcus prodigiosus*) to study airflow in ventilating shafts in the London tube railways and Paris Metro. The basis for these studies was to be able to effectively release a biological agent into an area where a large population of the city would take refuge during an air attack [31,32].

Hitler reportedly issued orders prohibiting biological weapons development in Germany. However, supported by high-ranking Nazi officials, German scientists began biological weapons research. At the Raubkammer Proving Ground in Lüneberger Heath, scientists performed research into foot and mouth disease, plague, rinderpest, typhus, yellow fever, potato beetle, and potato blight as biological warfare agents. Their results lagged behind those of other countries, and Nazi offensive biological weapons were never developed [33].

Nazi concentration camp prisoners were purposefully infected with *Rickettsia prowazekii*, *Rickettsia mooseri*, hepatitis A virus, *Plasmodia* spp, and treated with investigational vaccines and drugs. These inhumane experiments may have been done to study pathogenesis, to develop vaccines against rickettsiae, and to develop antimicrobial sulfa drugs rather than to develop biological weapons. As previously mentioned, German researchers attempted to create poison bullets from aconitine, and poison bullets were used on concentration camp prisoners [34]. This work was in direct violation of the 1675 Strasbourg agreement between the France and Germany, which banned the use of poison bullets. The sole known German tactical use of biological warfare was the pollution of a large reservoir in northwestern Bohemia with sewage in May 1945. Ironically, two Polish physicians used a combination of a vaccine and a serologic test as a biological defense against the Nazis. The German army avoided areas of epidemic typhus by using the Weil–Felix reaction as a diagnostic test. Consequently, Drs. Eugene Lazowski and Stanislaw Matulewicz vaccinated about 8000 individuals with formalin-killed *Proteus* OX-19 in order to induce biological false-positive tests for typhus in an area of occupied Poland, thereby protecting residents from deportation to concentration camps [35].

2.11 World War II—United States

In 1941, in response to reports indicating that Germany and Japan might utilize biological weapons, Secretary of War Henry Stimson requested that the National Academy of Sciences appoint a committee to conduct a biological weapon feasibility study. In 1942, this committee concluded that biological weapons might be feasible and recommended US vulnerability to such weapons be reduced. The War Reserve Service was formed under George Merck, of the Merck pharmaceutical company, which concluded that large-scale developmental operations were required. In 1942, an offensive biological weapons research and development program began at Camp Detrick in Frederick, MD [36].

In 1943, Camp Detrick became the parent research and pilot plant center with about 4000 Army, Navy, and civilian personnel. Field-testing facilities were initially established in Mississippi, and then moved to Dugway Proving Grounds in Utah in 1944. A production plant was constructed in Terre Haute, Indiana was never used, since, subsequent to fermentation and processing of the biological agent simulant, *Bacillus globigii*, high levels of spores were found throughout the plant [36].

2.12 Post-WWII to Modern Era

Biological weapons were used for covert assassination during the 1970s. Ricin was concentrated into a weaponized form by Soviet Union's secret service (KGB) and used by the Bulgarian secret service (KDS). Metal pellets 1.7 mm in diameter were filled with ricin and sealed with wax, designed to melt at body temperature. The pellets were discharged from a spring-powered umbrella. In August 1978, this weapon was used in Paris during an unsuccessful assassination attempt against a Bulgarian defector, Vladamir Kostov. That September, another Bulgarian defector living in London, Georgi Markov, was murdered by the KDS, using the same ricin umbrella weapon [37]. Similar weapons may have been used for at least six other assassinations [20].

Planes and helicopters delivering aerosols of several colors (yellow, green, and white) attacked Laos, Kampuchea and Afghanistan during 1975–1983. These attacks became know as "yellow rain." Soon after these attacks, people and livestock became disoriented, sick, and 10–20% of those exposed died [38]. The trichothecene toxins (and most prominently, T-2 mycotoxin) are thought to comprise at least some of these clouds. However, one scientist developed a hypothesis that these chemical attacks were caused by swarms of defecating bees [39]. Irrefutable evidence of a biological attack was never established, although some data suggests that toxins were used, derived from biologically grown microorganisms [40,129].

2.13 Soviet Biological Weapons Program

The Soviets began biological warfare research during the late 1920s to early 1930s [41–43]. Typhus rickettsia were developed for dissemination as an airborne aerosol by this program in the 1930s. By 1941, up to seven Soviet research institutes engaged in the creation of biological warfare agents from anthrax, plague, Q fever, melioidosis, glanders, foot and mouth disease, leprosy and tularemia [40–43]. The Soviets eventually developed a vast complex offensive biological weapons program that continued after their signing the 1972 Biological Weapons Convention. During the 1970s and 1980s, Biopreparat, an organization under the Soviet Ministry of Defense, operated at least six research laboratories and five production facilities and employed over 25,000 scientists and technicians. Biopreparat turned over 50 pathogens into biological weapons [44], including: smallpox, plague, anthrax, Venezuelan equine encephalitis, tularemia, brucellosis, Marburg, Ebola, Machupo viruses, and Bolivian hemorrhagic fever [45]. Russia now controls the extensive scientific programs of the former Soviet Union. Russian President Boris Yeltsin stated in 1992 that he would end further offensive biological research and production [46]. Now privatized under military leadership [47], the extent to which the biological weapons program has been eliminated is unknown. In 2003, Dr. Ken Alibek, a former Deputy Director of Biopreparat, estimated that not more than 10% of his former colleagues were employed, with many unaccounted for, although most do not possess "much direct knowledge" that would permit the manufacture of biological weapons [48].

A recent report revealed that in 1971, a Soviet field-test of smallpox biological weapon caused an outbreak of 10 cases, and three deaths. According to General Pyotr Burgasov, a former official in the Soviet biological weapons program, less than a pound of the aerosolized virus caused the outbreak [42,43]. A crewmember on a research ship contracted the virus when that vessel sailed within 9 miles of Renaissance (Vozrozhdeniye) Island in the Aral Sea in Kazakhstan, the location of the major testing area of the Soviet biological weapons program. The smallpox test is thought to have occurred on July 30, 1971, and the ship sailed nearby between July 29 and July 31. Once a smallpox outbreak began in the port of Aralsk, health officials rushed to control the disease. Nearly 50,000 residents of Aralsk were vaccinated in less than two weeks, and hundreds were placed in isolation in a makeshift facility [42,43,49].

An outbreak of inhalational anthrax occurred in late April 1979 among those who lived or worked within a distance of 4 k downwind of Soviet

Military Compound 19, a microbiology facility in Sverdlovsk (now Ekaterinburg, Russia). Cases of high fever and difficulty in breathing occurred, and about 40 fatalities developed. Autopsies revealed severe pulmonary edema and serious toxemia [50]. Livestock died of anthrax along the extended axis of the epidemic zone out to a distance of 50 km [51]. The military appropriated a local hospital for patient care, and vaccination and antibiotics were provided to area residents. Some Western scientists suspected that Military Compound 19 was a biological warfare research facility, and attributed the epidemic to the accidental airborne release of anthrax spores [51]. The Soviets claimed that the epidemic was caused by ingestion of anthrax-contaminated meat purchased on the black market [52]. Russian president Boris Yeltsin admitted in 1992 that the facility had been part of an offensive biological weapons program and that the epidemic had been caused by an unintentional release of anthrax spores. It was eventually determined that air filters had not been activated early on the morning of April 3. Upon autopsy, inhalation anthrax was identified as the cause of death in victims. At least 77 cases and 66 deaths occurred, constituting the largest documented epidemic of inhalation anthrax [53].

2.14 US Biological Weapons Program

In 1946, a report to Secretary of War Stimson noted that the potential of biological weapons had not been completely assessed, and recommended that the program be continued to provide an adequate defense. From 1947–1949 small scale outdoor testing was conducted at Camp Detrick using two biological simulants, *Bacillus globigii* and *Serratia marscens* [54].

In 1950, the biological weapons program was expanded with efforts to develop retaliatory biological weapons based on the threat of the USSR. In 1951, an anticrop bomb was developed, tested and placed in production for the Air Force. A biological production facility at Pine Bluff Arsenal (PBA) Arkansas began operations in 1954. Further expansion at Camp Detrick occurred in 1953. Data was obtained on personnel protection, decontamination and immunization against biological agents [36]. Anti-personnel biological agent cluster bombs were delivered to PBA for filling with *Brucella suis* in 1954, and large scale production of *Francisella tularemia* was established in 1955. Soviet Marshal Zhukov announced in 1956 that biological and chemical weapons would be used by their armed forces for mass destruction in future wars. Consequently, US efforts to increase military effectiveness were implemented [36].

In 1962, the Desert Test Center was established at Ft. Douglas, Salt Lake City, Utah and had as its mission the testing of biological weapons and defense systems at extra-continental test sites. During 1964–1966, a virus and rickettsiae production plant was built at PBA. Various types of munitions were delivered to PBA, filled and stored there. These munitions were never shipped anywhere except for test purposes [36].

In June 1966, testing of the New York City subway system assessed vulnerability of U.S. cities to covert biological attack. The simulant *B. globigii* was disseminated within the subway tubes and from the street into the subway stations. Simulant data indicated that large numbers of people could be exposed to infectious doses [55]. Also during the 1960s, Project Shipboard Hazard and Defense (SHAD) tested releases of aerosolized biological and chemical simulants in the Pacific Ocean [56]. On November 25, 1969, President Richard M. Nixon visited Fort Detrick and announced a new national policy on biological weapons: "I have decided that the United States of America will renounce the use of any form of deadly biological weapons that either kill or incapacitate" [57].

During 1970–1972, complete destruction was performed of biological weapon stocks and munitions. In January 1975 President Gerald R. Ford signed the Biological Weapons Convention on the prohibition of the development, production and stockpiling of bacteriological (biological) and toxin weapons.

With the de-establishment of the biological warfare laboratories, the U.S. Army Medical Research Institute of Infectious Diseases (USAMRIID) was established at Fort Detrick. Early defensive research products included investigational new drug (IND) submissions for Q fever, tularemia, Venezuelan equine encephalomyelitis (VEE), Eastern (EEE) and Western equine encephalitis (WEE), and Chikungunya vaccines. USAMRIID is a national asset for biological defense and serves as the nation's preeminent biomedical research defense and training facility. Examples of USAMRIID's contribution to the national biomedical defense include:

- Relief efforts for the Rift Valley fever (RVF) outbreaks in Egypt (1977) and Senegal and Mauritania (1988) [58].
- Agreements with the Centers for Disease Control (CDC), Atlanta, Georgia to house and treat any high hazard infections at USAMRIID BSL-4 hospital care.
- Containment of the 1989 outbreak of the Ebola-Reston monkey virus in Virginia, as described in Robert Preston's book *The Hot Zone* [59].
- Field investigation collaboration laboratory support for the hantavirus pulmonary syndrome (HPS) outbreak in the southwestern US, with initial isolation of the responsible hantavirus strain [60].
- Confirmation of a diagnosis of West Nile virus during the 1999 New York City outbreak [61].
- Laboratory and criminal analysis of the anthrax-containing letters during the 2001 bioterrorism incidents [62].
- Biodefense education of tens of thousands of medical professionals through on-site and satellite courses [63].
- Development of a novel anthrax vaccine candidate now undergoing clinical trials after a decade of research and development [64].

2.15 Aum Shinrikyo

In Japan during the 1980s, Shoko Asahara founded the cult Aum Shinrikyo. Its membership grew to about 10,000 with financial assets of at least $300 million. The Aum experimented with botulinum toxin and anthrax, and also was thought to have experimented with Q fever and mushroom spores. In 1992, the cult traveled to Zaire with the intent of obtaining Ebola virus. Their success in this endeavor is unknown.

In April 1990, the Aum Shinrikyo outfitted three vehicles to disseminate botulinum toxin. Their targets were the Diet (Japan's congress), the town of Yokohama, the U.S. Navy base at Yokosuka, and Tokyo's Narita Airport. In June 1993, the cult spread botulinum toxin in downtown Tokyo using a specially equipped automobile, and attempted to spread anthrax in Tokyo using a sprayer system on the roof of a cult-owned building in east Tokyo [65]. In July 1993, an attempt was made to spray the Diet using a truck modified to disseminate anthrax. In the same month, a similar attempt was made to disseminate anthrax near the Imperial Palace in Tokyo. Fortunately, problems with pressurization and clogging of the spray system likely contributed to ineffective spore dispersal [66]. On March 15, 1995, the Aum placed three briefcases designed to release botulinum toxin in the Tokyo subway. The cult member responsible for this attack evidently reconsidered his intentions, and substituted a non-toxic substance for the botulinum toxin. The failure of this attack subsequently led the cult to use sarin in its March 20, 1995 subway attack. The Aum made mistakes either in the way they produced or disseminated biological agents, and all of their attacks failed. They may have relied on a strain of *C. botulinum* that produced little or no toxin, which may have been incapable of producing illness. The quantities of toxin disseminated may have been too small to cause lethal effects. The Aum had also used a vaccine strain of anthrax, Sterne 34F2, which was relatively harmless [66]. As far as is known, no one became ill or died from these bioterrorism attempts by the Aum [20,67].

2.16 Rajneeshees

In September and October 1984, a religious cult, known as the Rajneeshees, intentionally caused illness among the 751 inhabitants of The Dalles, in Oregon. On their Rajneeshpuram Commune, the Rajneeshees had a state-certified clinical laboratory, and purchased seed stock of *Salmonella typhimurium* from a medical supply company.

Ma Anand Sheela, personal secretary to the Bhagwan, leader of the commune, and Ma Anand Puja, a nurse, worked with a trained laboratory technician to culture *Salmonella typhimurium* used to contaminate salad bars throughout the community [20]. They specifically rejected the use of a more dangerous pathogen, *S. typhi*, the causative agent of typhoid fever, due to their concern that an outbreak of typhoid fever would attract too much attention. The Rajneeshees believed that they could accomplish their intended objective, incapacitation, using a generally non-lethal agent, *S. typhimurium*, which causes diarrheal illness, often accompanied by fever, chills, headache, nausea or vomiting [68]. The September and October contamination of salad bars was seen to be practice for incapacitation of the local populace during the November elections, so that the Rajneeshees could influence local elections with their votes. In 1986, Sheela and Puja were sentenced to 24-year prison terms, and served four years in a California prison before parole.

2.17 St. Paul Medical Center, Dallas

On October 29, 1996, twelve people who worked in the laboratory of the St. Paul Medical Center hospital in Dallas, Texas, were deliberately infected with *Shigella dysenteriae* type 2, a rare strain of shigella that causes diarrheal illness. An e-mail message was reportedly sent to laboratory personnel inviting them to eat blueberry muffins and doughnuts available in the laboratory's lunchroom. Everyone who ate a pastry became ill by November 1. Clinical tests revealed that the victims were infected with *S. dysenteriae*, and this pathogen was also found in a saved muffin. Investigators learned that the laboratory had a vial containing beads impregnated with *S. dysenteriae* type 2 of the same strain, and that some of the beads were missing [127]. Police attention was focused on a disgruntled laboratory technician, Diane Thompson, who had access to the laboratory's shigella culture. Thompson was indicted and accused of infecting her co-workers with *Shigella dysenteriae* Type 2, and was sentenced to four concurrent 20-year prison terms in September 1998 [20].

2.18 Other Recent Bioterrorism Incidents

In 1991, a right-wing extremist group, the Minnesota Patriots Council, produced a small quantity of ricin toxin from castor beans, made from a recipe found in a book. They planned to use a mixture of ricin and DMSO, apparently hoping that the DMSO would transport the ricin [128]. In 1994 and 1995, four members of this group were the first to be tried and convicted under the 1989 Biological Weapons Anti-Terrorism Act, for the possession of ricin [69].

In 1995, Larry Wayne Harris, who has been linked to white supremacist groups, was arrested after ordering *C. botulinum* through the mail from a cell culture repository in Maryland. He was later convicted, and re-arrested in 1998 after having possession of *Ba. anthracis* [70].

After terrorist attacks on the World Trade Center and the Pentagon in 2001, envelopes containing *Ba. anthracis* spores were mailed to news media and US government offices [71]. As a result of these exposures, there were 11 cases of inhalation anthrax, 11 cases of cutaneous anthrax, and 5 deaths [72,73]. Public health and law enforcement investigation and response activities across the United States and in other countries occurred as a result of the anthrax mailings. As of October 2004, the perpetrator has still not been apprehended.

In December 2002, six terrorist suspects were arrested in Manchester, England; their apartment was serving as a "ricin laboratory." On January 5, 2003, British police raided two residences near London and found traces of ricin, which led to an investigation of a possible Chechen separatist plan to attack the Russian embassy with the toxin; several arrests were made [74].

Ricin was also found in a South Carolina postal facility in October 2003 [75] and in the mailroom that serves Senate Majority Leader Bill Frist's office in the Dirksen Senate Office Building in Washington, D.C. on February 3, 2004 [76]. Also in February 2004, the Secret Service acknowledged that ricin had also been found at a White House mail-processing center in early November 2003 [77]. Officials suspect that the October and November 2003 ricin attacks are related since both letters were signed "Fallen Angel" and contained ricin of poor quality [78].

2.19 Biological Weapons and Countries Thought to Possess Them

A number of countries with records of supporting terrorist organizations also are believed to have biological weapons programs. The Department of State has named seven countries as state supporters of terrorism: Cuba, Iran, Iraq, Libya, North Korea, Sudan, and Syria [79]. Reports by the Department of Defense and the Arms Control and Disarmament Agency have suggested that Iran, Iraq, Libya, North Korea, and Syria, possess biological warfare programs [80].

Afghanistan. Al Qaeda in Afghanistan was thought to attempt to acquire or manufacture biological weapons [81]. There were several news stories reporting possible chemical labs run by Al-Qaida, but none have been proven [82].

Australia. The Australian Department of Defense formed the New Weapons and Equipment Development Committee at the conclusion of WWII. A recommendation was made to develop biological weapons that would be most effective in tropical Asia without spreading to Australia's temperate cities. During the post-war environment of the 1950s Australian universities were encouraged to research areas of biological science of relevance to biological weapons. This support and activity ended by the 1970s, with the greater inherent global deterrent capabilities of nuclear weapons [83].

Brazil. Although it has the capacity to do so, no evidence exists that Brazil has ever developed or produced biological weapons. Brazil's opposition to biological weapons includes the use of biological agents to control coca production in neighboring Colombia. It is to be noted that Brazil has one of the world's largest crops of the castor bean (which naturally produces the toxin ricin) and has a solid biotechnological infrastructure [84].

Canada. Canada conducted biological weapons research from 1941–1945. Canada weaponized anthrax, and research was conducted into the creation of biological weapons from brucellosis, Rocky Mountain spotted fever, plague, tularemia, typhoid, yellow fever, dysentery, rinderpest, botulinum toxin, and ricin [69].

China. Despite claims to the contrary, China is reported to have active biological and chemical weapons programs, although details are unknown [26]. China has conducted defensive research on potential biological warfare agents, including the causative agents of anthrax, plague, tularemia, Q fever, psitticosis, Eastern equine encephalitis, and others [26]. China has an advanced biotechnology infrastructure as well as the munitions production capabilities necessary to develop, produce and weaponize biological agents [85]. Speculation has occurred that the 1997 outbreak of swine foot and mouth disease on Taiwan in which almost 4 million pigs were destroyed may be attributed to introduction of livestock from China [86].

Cuba. Cuba is thought to have had the technical capability to conduct a biological weapons research program, and its biotechnology industry is among the most advanced of emerging countries (Cuba's Pursuit of Biological Weapons: Fact or Fiction. US Senate, 2002). However, a recent intelligence reassessment concludes that it is unclear whether Cuba now has an active, offensive biological weapons effort [87]. Defectors have claimed that the Center for Genetic Engineering and Biotechnology in Havana is actually a military research center that manufactures anthrax and bubonic plague [88]. In 1997 Fidel Castro compared the US to a dragon and Cuba to a lamb and warned that if the dragon tried to eat the lamb, it would find its meal "poisoned." This led to speculation of Cuba's biological warfare capabilities. Cuba has accused the United States government of a "biological attack" in which the agricultural pest *Thrips palmi* insects (palm or melon thrips) were allegedly dropped from a crop-dusting plane in October 1996. *Thrips palmi* (palm thrips) has been spreading in the Caribbean region since 1985, and has also found in the US in Hawaii and Florida [89].

Egypt. In 1970, Anwar al Sadat reportedly stated that "Egypt has biological weapons stored in refrigerators and could use them against Israel's crowded population" [90]. This statement was understood as warning against a nuclear strike by Israel during the 1973 Yom Kippur War [91]. Allegations have described Egypt as conducting research on anthrax, plague, tularemia, cholera, botulinum toxin, mycotoxins, smallpox, influenza, Japanese B encephalitis, Eastern equine encephalitis, and Rift Valley fever virus for military purposes [69,91]. Egypt has denied these claims, and there is no proof of biological warfare research in Egypt [92].

France. During 1921–1926 and 1935–1940, the French engaged in biological weapons research. This program was continued in 1940–1945 under German occupation [93]. The potato beetle was developed as a biological weapon, and research was conducted upon anthrax, salmonella, cholera, rinderpest, botulinum toxin, and ricin as biological weapons [69,94].

India. Some sources suggest that India possesses biological weapons, but this is unproven. With its' extensive and advanced pharmaceutical industry, India is technically capable of developing biological weapons [95]. The Defense Research and Development Establishment (DRDE) at Gwalior is the primary establishment for biological defense studies for bacterial and viral agents. India has conducted research on countering various diseases, including plague, brucellosis, and smallpox [95].

Iran. Although strongly denied, Iran is suspected of initiating a biological warfare program during the Iran–Iraq War, and to now be in an advanced research and development phase. Iran has skilled scientists, extensive pharmaceutical expertise, and the commercial and military infrastructure to produce biological weapons. Former Russian biological weapons scientists have traveled to Iran, and a combined biological and chemical weapons facility is thought to be located at Damghan, in northern Iran [96]. It has been projected that, within 10 years, Iran's military may have biological weapons [97]. Biological weapons research in Iran is thought to include mycotoxins, ricin, and smallpox virus [98].

Iraq. In 1991, after the Persian Gulf War, UN weapons inspections revealed the Iraqi offensive biological program included basic research on *Ba. anthracis*, rotavirus, camel pox virus, aflatoxin, botulinum toxins, hemorrhagic conjuctivitis virus (Enterovirus 70), rotavirus, mycotoxins, and wheat cover smut [69]. Iraq had research facilities at Salman Pak and other sites, many of which were destroyed during the war. In 1995, further information revealed that field tests were conducted with *B. subtilis* (a simulant for *Ba. anthracis*), botulinum toxin, and aflatoxin. Biological agents were tested in various delivery systems, including rockets, aerial bombs, and spray tanks. In December 1990, the Iraqis filled 100 R400 bombs with botulinum toxin, 50 with anthrax, and 16 with aflatoxin; 13 Al Hussein (SCUD) warheads were filled with botulinum toxin, 10 with anthrax, and two with aflatoxin. These weapons were deployed in January 1991 to four locations. Iraq produced a total of 19,000 liters of concentrated botulinum toxin (nearly 10,000 liters filled into munitions), 8500 liters of concentrated anthrax (6500 liters filled into munitions) and 2200 liters of aflatoxin (1580 liters filled into munitions) [99]. Fortunately, biological weapons were not used during the Persian Gulf War [100]. As of October 2004, it appears that prior to the March 2003 US coalition invasion of Iraq, the biological weapons program was not reinstated other than research interests of the Iraqi Intelligence Service (Mukhabarat) [101].

Israel. Some Arab countries have alleged that Israel has an offensive biological weapons program, but this is unproven. Israeli military personnel reportedly sabotaged wells with typhoid and dysentery in near Haifa and in Gaza during the 1948 war [102]. Reports have been made of a supposed offensive biological weapons program at the Israel Institute of Biological Research (IIBR) in Ness Ziona. Research has been conducted at this Institute on the causative agents of plague, rabies typhus, and many toxins including *Staphycococcus* enterotoxin B [102]. The expansion of this Institute has caused protests due to reports of injuries and deaths within the facility and a near-evacuation of the surrounding area [103].

Kazakhstan. In 1993, Kazakhstan created the National Center for Biotechnology to oversee the administration of former Soviet biological weapons facilities. These include: the Scientific Research Agricultural Institute (SRAI) at Otar, specializing in agricultural and zoonotic diseases; Biokombinat, a small facility in Almaty, now producing vaccines, and the Scientific Center for Quarantine and Zoonotic Infections (SCQZI), now controlled by the Kazakhstan Ministry of Health. Both SCQZI and SRAI have extensive collections of virulent strains, and safety and security have been upgraded at these facilities. Biomedpreparat, a former large-scale anthrax production facility in Stepnogorsk has been dismantled [104].

Libya. Prior to Libya's December 19, 2003 announcement to abandon its WMD programs, Qadhafi was alleged to have attempted to recruit South African scientists to assist in the acquisition of biological weapons [105]. In 2003, Libya admitted past intentions to produce biological weapons. In October and December 2003, American and British scientists toured a number of medical and agricultural research centers that were potentially used for biological weapons research [105].

Democratic People's Republic of North Korea. North Korea has the scientists and facilities for producing biological products and microorganisms, and is thought to have performed biological weapons research and development since the 1960s. North Korea is thought to have increased its development of biological weapons in the 1980s with the assistance of scientists from other countries. In the early 1990s, one source described military biotechnology work at numerous North Korean medical institutes and universities using pathogens that cause anthrax, cholera, plague, yellow fever, typhoid, cholera, tuberculosis, typhus, smallpox, and botulinum toxin. North Korea has a munitions-production infrastructure to weaponize biological agents [69,106–108].

Pakistan. Pakistan has a biotechnology infrastructure that could support work on biological weapons. Pakistan is considered to have the ability to conduct a limited offensive biological warfare research and development effort [109]. One 1996 report stated that Pakistan had been "conducting research and development with potential biological warfare applications" [110]. It is not known whether this is accurate [110].

Saudi Arabia. Six countries that may possess biological or chemical weapons border Saudi Arabia: Egypt, Iran, Iraq, Israel, Sudan, and Syria. There is no credible evidence that Saudi Arabia possesses biological, chemical, or nuclear weapons [111]. However, due to geopolitical incentives, existing scientific expertise, and possession of dual-use technology, one analyst has predicted that Saudi Arabia will seek to produce biological and chemical weapons in the future [112].

South Africa. South Africa developed the ability to produce and to deploy chemical and biological weapons during the mid-1980s. This program included work on *Ba. anthracis*, botulinum toxin, *V. cholerae*, *C. perfringens*, *Yersinia pestis*, *Salmonella* spp., chemical poisoning and large-scale manufacture of drugs of abuse. South Africa may have released cholera into water sources of some South African villages and provided anthrax and cholera to the government troops of Rhodesia (now Zimbabwe) for use in a guerrilla war. The US and Britain notified the South African government on multiple occasions of their concern for transfer of knowledge of biological and chemical weapons to other countries, especially to Libya [113,114]. In 1993, the destruction of remaining chemical and biological substances was ordered [115].

South Korea. South Korea possesses a well-developed pharmaceutical and biotechnology infrastructure. However, there is no evidence that they have an offensive biological weapon program. Citing a biological threat from North Korea, South Korea conducts defensive biological weapons research and development, e.g., development of vaccines against anthrax and smallpox [116].

Sudan. Although alleged to have developed, acquired, and used chemical weapons, there is no confirmed evidence of Sudan having a biological weapons program [117].

30 Preparing Hospitals for Bioterror

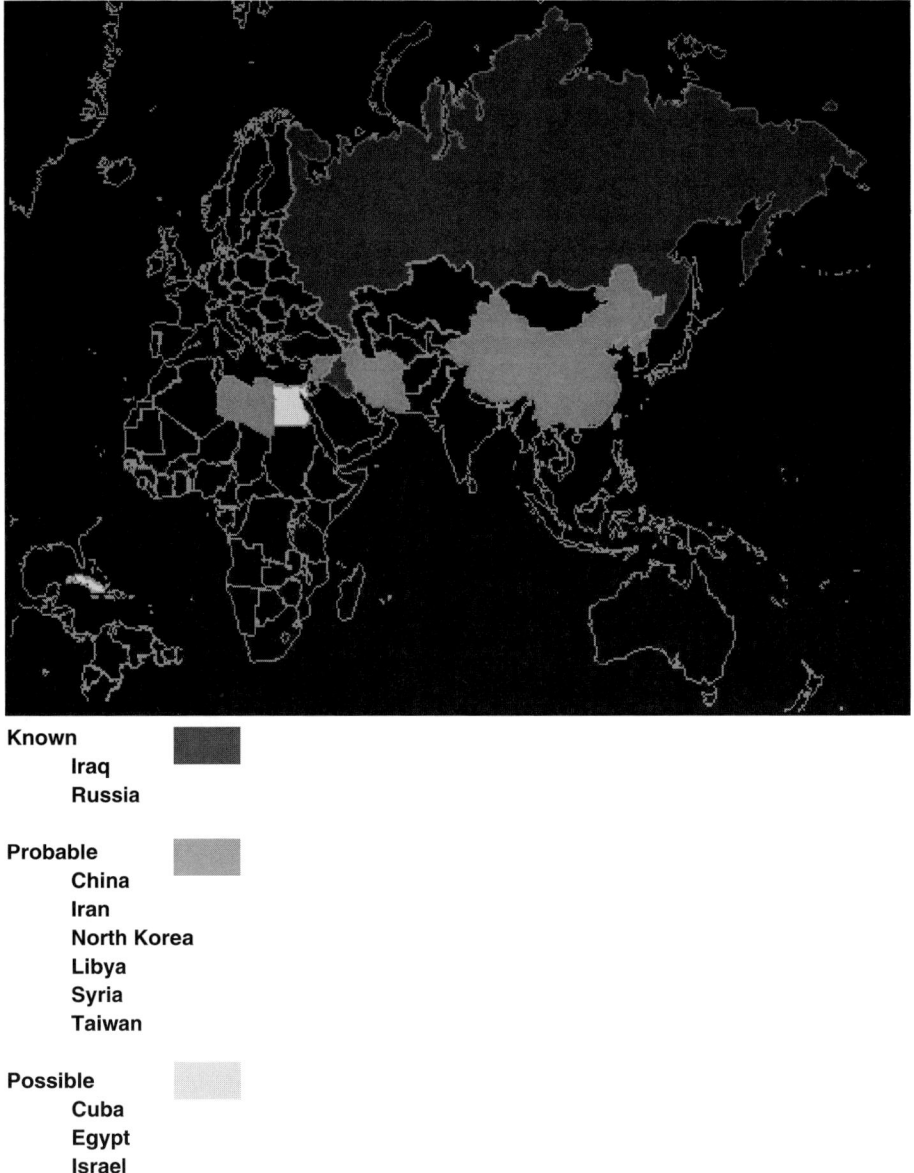

Figure 2.1 Chemical and Biological Weapons Programs. (Source: Committee on Armed Services, House of Representatives. Special Inquiry into the Chemical and Biological Threat. Countering the Chemical and Biological Weapons Threat in the Post-Soviet World. Washington, D.C., U.S. Government Printing Office, 23 Feb 1993. Report to the Congress.)

Syria. Syria has a limited biotechnology infrastructure and some unconfirmed reports assess that Syria is developing an offensive biological weapons capability. Syrian military scientists may have done limited biological weapons research [118]. A facility near Cerin is suspected as used for the development of anthrax, botulinum toxin, and ricin biological agents [119–121].

Taiwan. Despite persistent suspicions of offensive and defensive biological and chemical weapons programs, there is no convincing evidence that Taiwan has developed or deployed chemical or biological weapons [122].

United Kingdom. Britain's biological weapons program was initially developed for potential retaliatory use in response to a German biological attack, and lasted from 1936 to 1956. The British tested *Ba. anthracis* bombs on Gruinard Island near Scotland, resulting in heavy contamination. Viable anthrax spores persisted until the island was decontaminated in 1986. Research had also been conducted into plague, typhoid, and botulinum toxin as biological weapons [4]. Research for plague, brucellosis, tularemia, and Venezuelan equine encephalitis and vaccinia virus also occurred offshore of the northwest Hebrides, the Bahamas, and Antigua [123].

Uzbekistan. Since independence, Uzbekistan has dismantled the Soviet chemical and biological weapons facilities in its territory [124]. The US has assisted Uzbekistan in removing tons of anthrax spores from Renaissance Island in the Aral Sea (the site of the previously mentioned 1971 smallpox outbreak) where they were buried by the former Soviet Union [125]. Anthrax was buried here after the Sverdlovsk anthrax release provoked alarm in the West [51]. In 1997, American survey teams found that anthrax spores in soil samples from 6 of the 11 burial pits were viable. There is great concern that terrorists or rogue states might seek to obtain anthrax spores from the former Soviet biological warfare test site on the island [126]. Ken Alibek, a defector from the Soviet germ warfare program, has stated that the island was used to test tularemia, Q fever, brucellosis, glanders and plague [41].

References

1. The Mazal Library. Trials of War Criminals Before the Nuernberg Military Tribunals Under Control Council Law No. 10. October 1946–May 1949. NMT Vol II, pp. 57–60. http://www.mazal.org/archive/nmt/02/NMT02-T057.htm
2. A. Mayor. *Greek Fire, Poison Arrows & Scorpion Bombs: Biological and Chemical Warfare in the Ancient World*, The Overlook Press, New York, 2003.
3. Swaveda Forum for Indian Studies. Arthashastra. Book XIV. Secret Means. Chapter 1. Means to Injure and Enemy. Kautilya. http://www.swaveda.com/etext.php?title=Arthashastra&page=14
4. G. W. Christopher, et al. Biological warfare: a historical perspective. *JAMA*, 278:412–417, 1997.
5. M. Wheelis. Biological warfare at the 1346 siege of Caffa. *Emerging Infect Dis* 8:971–975, 2002.
6. G. B. Roberts, 2003. Arms Control Without Arms Control: The Failure of the Biological Weapons Protocol and a New Paradigm for Fighting the Threat of Biological Weapons. INSS Occasional Paper 49. USAF Institute for National Security Studies. USAF Academy, CO.
7. WordiQ.com. Definition of Hussite Wars. http://www.wordiq.com/definition/Hussite_Wars#The_First_Anti-Hussite_Crusade
8. U.S. Pharmacist. Rabies: A History and Update on Prophylaxis Regimens in the U.S. http://www.uspharmacist.com/oldformat.asp?url=newlook/files/Feat/aug00rabies.cfm&pub_id=8&article_id=563
9. E. A. Fenn. *Pox Americana: The Great Smallpox Epidemic of 1775–1782*. New York, Hill and Wang, 2001.
10. American Medical Association. Historical postmortem. Old tactics, new threat: what is today's risk of smallpox? http://www.ama-assn.org/ama/pub/category/8755.html
11. NativeWeb.org. Jeffrey Amherst and Smallpox Blankets. http://www.nativeweb.org/pages/legal/amherst/lord_jeff.html
12. R. E. Armstrong and J. B. Warner. Biology and the battlefield. Defense Horizons No. 25, National Defense University, March 2003.
13. K. V. Iserson. Chapter 8: Viruses and vivisections: Japan's inhuman experiments. In *Demon Doctors: Physicians as Serial Killers*. Galen Press, 2002.

14. J. K. Smart. Chapter 2. History of Chemical and Biological Warfare: An American Perspective. In *Medical Aspects of Chemical and Biological Warfare*. Borden Institute. Washington, DC, 1997.
15. Discovery Channel. Bioterror Through Time. http://dsc.discovery.com/anthology/spotlight/bioterror/history/history2.html
16. D. Goetz and S. G. Morley. *The Popul Vuh. The Sacred Book of the Mayas. The Book of the Community*. Tulsa, University of Oklahoma Press, 1950, http://www.geocities.com/athens/academy/7286/popolvuhmain.html
17. Ancient History. Mithridates. http://ancienthistory.about.com/library/bl/bl_mithridates.htm
18. Nationmaster.com.Encyclopedia:Zeppelin. http://www.nationmaster.com/encyclopedia/Zeppelin
19. M. Wheelis. Biological Sabotage in World War I. Chapter 3. In *Biological and Toxin Weapons: Research, Development and Use from the Middle Ages to 1945. SIPRI Chemical & Biological Warfare Studies*, no. 18. Erhard Geissler, John Ellis Van Courtland Moon, eds. Oxford University Press. Oxford, UK, 2000.
20. W. S. Carus. Working Paper: The illicit use of biological agents since 1900. August 1998 (February 2001 Revision). Center for Counterproliferation Research. National Defense University. Washington, DC.
21. J. Witcover, *Sabotage at Black Tom: Imperial Germany's Secret War in America, 1914–1917*. New York, Algonquin Books of Chapel Hill, 1989.
22. S. H. Harris, *Factories of Death: Japanese Biological Warfare, 1932–45 and the American Cover-Up*. New York, NY, Routledge, 1995.
23. World War II in the Pacific. Japanese Unit 731. Biological Warfare Unit. http://www.ww2pacific.com/unit731.html
24. H. Gold, *Unit 731 Testimony*. Tokyo, Yenbooks, 1995.
25. The Associated Press. September 3, 2002. Germ warfare victims file appeal. The New York Times.
26. E. Croddy, China's role in the chemical and biological disarmament regimes. *The Nonproliferation Review*. 9:16–47, 2002.
27. Japanese Fugo Bombing Balloons. Marshall Stelzreide's Wartime Story. http://www.stelzriede.com/ms/html/mshwfugo.htm
28. Fugos: Japanese Balloon Bombs of World War II. http://www.seanet.com/~johnco/fugo.htm
29. INS. Greatest fear about Jap balloons was that they might bear deadly germs. The Seattle Times. February 9, 1946.
30. BBC. On this day: 2 September. http://news.bbc.co.uk/onthisday/hi/dates/stories/september/2/newsid_3582000/3582545.stm
31. H. Liepmann. *Death From the Skies: A Study of Gas and Microbial Warfare*. Martin Secker & Warburg, Ltd. London, 1937.
32. M. Hugh-Jones, Wickham Steed and German biological warfare research. *Intelligence and National Security*, 7:379–402, 1992.
33. E. Geissler, 1999. "Biological warfare activities in Germany, 1923–45," in *Biological and Toxin Weapons: Research, Development and Use from the Middle Ages to 1945*, Erhard Geissler and John Ellis van Courtland Mood, eds. New York: Stockholm International Peace Research Institute.
34. PBS. The Experiments. Peter Tyson. http://www.pbs.org/wgbh/nova/holocaust/experiside.html#pois
35. D. Adams, American Medical Association. Amednews.com. 2 doctors used typhus to save thousands in wartime. July 5, 2004. http://www.ama-assn.org/amednews/2004/07/05/prsb0705.htm
36. Cutting Edge. A History of Fort Detrick, Maryland. October 2000. http://www.detrick.army.mil/cutting_edge/index.cfm?chapter=titlepage
37. Gangsters Incorporated. Puparo's Bulgaria. http://gangstersinc.tripod.com/PupBulgaria.html
38. J. B. Tucker. Center for Nonproliferation Studies. Conflicting Evidence Revives "Yellow Rain" Controversy. August 5, 2002. http://cns.miis.edu/pubs/week/020805.htm
39. F. Pearce. Green rain over India evokes memories of cold war paranoia. *New Scientist*, 174:13, 2002.
40. R. T. Rosen and J. D. Rosen. Presence of four Fusarium mycotoxins and synthetic material in "yellow rain." Evidence for the use of chemical weapons in Laos. *Biomed Mass Spectrom*. 9:443–450, 1982.
41. K. Alibek and S. Handelman, *Biohazard*. New York, Random House, 1999.
42. J. N. Tucker and R. A. Zilinskas. Public Health Experts Comment on Analysis of the 1971 Smallpox Outbreak in the Soviet Union. Center for Nonproliferation Studies. Montery Institute of International Studies, 2002.
43. J. N. Tucker and R. A. Zilinskas, eds. The 1971 Smallpox Epidemic in Aralsk, Kazakhstan, and

44. A. L. Smithson. Keep Soviet bioweaponeers gainfully employed. USA Today. October 31, 2001. http://www.stimson.org/?SN=CB20020111230
45. Fact Index. Biopreparat. http://www.fact-index.com/b/bi/biopreparat.html
46. M. Leitenberg. Biological Weapons Arms Control. Project on Rethinking Arms Control. PRAC Paper No. 16. Center for International and Security Studies at Maryland. University of Maryland at College Park, 1996.
47. Federation of American Scientists. Biopreperat AO. http://www.fas.org/irp/world/russia/fbis/Biopreparat.html
48. The L. Henry Stimson Center. Security for a New Century: A Study Group Report. October 16, 2003. http://www.stimson.org/newcentury/pdf/101603Alibek.pdf
49. W. J. Broad and J. Miller. Report provides new details of Soviet smallpox accident. The New York Times, June 15, 2002.
50. F. A. Abramova, et al. 1993. Pathology of inhalational anthrax in 42 cases from the Sverdlovsk outbreak of 1979. *Proc Natl Acad Sci* USA. 90:2291–2294, 1993.
51. M. Meselson, et al. The Sverdlovsk anthrax outbreak of 1979. *Science*, 266:1202–1208, 1994.
52. I. S. Bezdenezhnykhm, and V. N. Nikiforov. Epidemiologic analysis of anthrax in Sverdlovsk [Article in Russian] *Zh Mikrobiol Epidemiol Immunobiol*. 5:111–113, 1980.
53. J. Guillemin. *Anthrax: The Investigation of a Deadly Outbreak*. Berkeley and Los Angeles, CA, University of California Press, 1999.
54. The L. Henry. Stimson Center. History of the US Offensive Biological Weapons Program (1941–1973). http://www.stimson.org/?SN=CB2001121275
55. L. A. Cole. Confronting the horror of biological warfare. *The Los Angeles Times*, November 30, 1997.
56. Fact Sheets. DTC Test 68-50. DTC Test 69-32. Project Shipboard Hazard and Defense (SHAD). Special Assistant to the Under Secretary of Defense (Personnel and Readiness) for Gulf War Illnesses, Medical Readiness, and Military Deployments.
57. E. Regis. *The Biology of Doom: The History of America's Secret Germ Warfare Project*. New York, Henry Holt and Company, 1999.
58. USAMRIID. USAMRIID Highlights Over The Years. http://www.usamriid.army.mil/highlightspage.htm
59. R. Preston. *The Hot Zone*. New York, Anchor Books, 1994.
60. Y. K. Chu, et al. Serological relationships among viruses in the Hantavirus genus, family Bunyaviridae. *Virology*, 198:196–204, 1994.
61. G. V. Ludwig, et al. An outbreak of West Nile virus in a New York City captive wildlife population. *Am J Trop Med Hyg*. 67:67–75, 2002.
62. Federal Bureau of Investigation. Opening of the Letter. http://www.fbi.gov/anthrax/vanharp/introleahy.htm
63. USAMRIID. Education and Training. http://www.usamriid.army.mil/education/satellite.htm
64. S. Jendrek, et al. Evaluation of the compatibility of a second generation recombinant anthrax vaccine with aluminum-containing adjuvants. *Vaccine*. 21:3011–3018, 2003.
65. S. WuDunn, et al. How Japan germ terror alerted world. *The New York Times*. May 26, 1998.
66. H. Takahashi, et al. *Bacillus anthracis* incident, Kameido, Tokyo, 1993. *Emerging Infect Dis* 10:117–120, 2004.
67. Centers for Disease Control. Emergency Preparedness and Response. Bioterrorism Agents/Diseases. http://www.bt.cdc.gov/agent/agentlist-category.asp#bdef
68. T. Torok, et al. A large community outbreak of Salmonellosis caused by intentional contamination of restaurant salad bars. *JAMA* 278:389–395, 1997.
69. CNS Reports. Ricin found in London: An al-Qa'ida connection? January 23, 2003. http://cns.miis.edu/pubs/reports/ricin.htm
70. A. C. Revkin, February 21, 1998. Arrests highlight growing threat of bioweapons. The New York Times. http://www.nytimes.com/library/national/science/022198anthrax-primer.html
71. Federal Bureau of Investigation. Amerithrax Press Briefing. November 9, 2001. http://www.fbi.gov/anthrax/amerithrax.htm
72. D. B. Jernigan, et al. Investigation of bioterrorism-related anthrax, United States, 2001: Epidemiologic findings. *Emerging Infect Dis* 8:1019–1028, 2002.

73. L. A. Barakat, et al. Fatal inhalational anthrax in a 94-year-old Connecticut woman. *JAMA* 287:863–868, 2002.
74. J. M. Bale, et al. Center for Nonproliferation Studies. CNS Reports. Ricin Found in London: An al-Qa'ida connection? http://cns.miis.edu/iiop/cnsdata?Action=1&Concept=0&Mime=1&collection=CNS+Web+Site&Key=pubs%2Freports%2Fricin%2Ehtm&QueryText=bale&QueryMode=FreeText
75. CDC. Investigation of a ricin-containing envelope at a postal facility—South Carolina, 2003. 52:1129–1131, 2003.
76. CNN.com. Frist: Ricin confirmed, but no illness reported. February 4, 2004. http://www.cnn.com/2004/US/02/03/senate.hazardous/
77. eMedicine.com. Ricin Overview. http://www.emedicinehealth.com/articles/42387-1.asp
78. Federal Bureau of Investigation. Ricin Envelope and Letter. http://www.fbi.gov/ricin/envelopeletter.htm
79. R. Perl. CRS Report for Congress. U.S. State Department. The Department of State's Patterns of Global Terrorism Report: Trends, State Sponsors and Related Issues. June 1, 2004. http://fpc.state.gov/documents/organization/33630.pdf
80. U.S. Arms Control and Disarmament Agency. Biological Weapons. http://dosfan.lib.uic.edu/acda/bw.htm
81. G. Cameron, et al. The 1999 WMD chronology: involving sub-national actors and chemical, biological, radiological, and nuclear materials. *The Nonproliferation Review*, 7:157–174, 2000.
82. GlobalSecurity.org. Afghanistan Special Weapons. http://www.globalsecurity.org/wmd/world/afghanistan/index.html
83. Federation of American Scientists. Australia: Biological Weapons. http://www.fas.org/nuke/guide/australia/bw.html
84. Nuclear Threat Initiative. Brazil Overview: Biological. http://www.nti.org/e_research/profiles/Brazil/index.html
85. Federation of American Scientists. China: Chemical and Biological Weapons. http://www.fas.org/nuke/guide/china/cbw/index.html
86. Antec Biosentry. http://www.antecint.co.uk/main/antectai.htm
87. S. R. Weisman. In stricter study, U.S. scales back claims on Cuba arms. *The New York Times*, September 18, 2004.
88. United States Senate, One Hundred Seventh Congress, Second Session, June 5, 2002. Cuba's Pursuit of Biological Weapons: Fact or Fiction? Hearing before the subcommittee on Western hemisphere, Peace Corps, and narcotics affairs of the Committee on Foreign Relations, US GPO, Washington, 2002. http://www.fas.org/nuke/guide/cuba/sfrc060502.pdf
89. GlobalSecurity.org. Cuba: Biological Weapons. http://www.globalsecurity.org/wmd/world/cuba/bw.htm
90. Federation of American Scientists. Egypt: Biological Weapons Program. http://www.fas.org/nuke/guide/egypt/bw/index.html
91. D. Shoham. Chemical and biological weapons in Egypt. *The Nonproliferation Review*. 5:48–58, 1998.
92. Nuclear Threat Initiative. Egypt Profile: Biological. http://www.nti.org/e_research/profiles/Egypt/index.html
93. Nuclear Threat Initiative. France Overview: Biological. http://www.nti.org/e_research/profiles/France/index.html
94. Federation of American Scientists. France: Chemical and Biological Weapons. http://www.fas.org/nuke/guide/france/cbw/index.html
95. Nuclear Threat Initiative. India Profile: Biological. http://www.nti.org/e_research/profiles/India/index.html
96. GlobalSecurity.org. Iran: Facilities. Damghan. http://www.globalsecurity.org/wmd/world/iran/damghan.htm
97. Federation of American Scientists. Iran: Biological Weapons. http://www.fas.org/nuke/guide/iran/bw/index.html
98. Nuclear Threat Initiative. Iran Profile: Biological. http://www.nti.org/e_research/profiles/Iran/index.html
99. R. A. Zilinskas. Iraq's biological weapons: The past as future? *JAMA* 278:418–424, 1997.
100. M. Leitenberg. Biological weapons in the twentieth century: a review and analysis. Crit Rev Microbiol. 27:267–320, 2001.
101. P. Binder, et al. Commentary: The Kay Report to Congress on the activities of the Iraq survey group: former bioweapons inspectors comment. *Biosecurity and Bioterrorism: Biodefense Strategy, Practice, and Science*. 1:239–246, 2003.
102. A. Cohen. Israel and chemical/biological weapons: history, deterrence and arms control. *The Nonproliferation Review*. 8:27–53, 2001.

103. Nuclear Threat Initiative. Israel Profile: Biological. http://www.nti.org/e_research/profiles/Israel/index.html
104. Nuclear Threat Initiative. Kazakhstan Profile: Biological. http://www.nti.org/e_research/profiles/Kazakhstan/index.html
105. Nuclear Threat Initiative. Libya Profile: Biological. http://www.nti.org/e_research/profiles/Libya/index.html
106. Federation of American Scientists. DPRK: Biological Weapons Program. http://www.fas.org/nuke/guide/dprk/bw/index.html
107. GlobalSecurity.org. DPRK: Biological Weapons Program. http://www.globalsecurity.org/wmd/world/dprk/bw.htm
108. Nuclear Threat Initiative. North Korea Profile: Biological. http://www.nti.org/e_research/profiles/NK/index.html
109. Federation of American Scientists. Pakistan: Biological Weapons. http://www.fas.org/nuke/guide/pakistan/bw/index.html
110. Nuclear Threat Initiative. Pakistan Profile: Biological. http://www.nti.org/e_research/profiles/Pakistan/index.html
111. G. H. W. Bush. President's Statement. April 13, 1989. http://www.findarticles.com/p/articles/mi_m1079/is_n2147_v89/ai_7723219
112. D. Shoham. Does Saudi Arabia have or seek chemical or biological weapons? *The Nonproliferation Review*. 6:122–130, 1999.
113. Nuclear Threat Initiative. South Africa Profile: Biological. http://www.nti.org/e_research/profiles/SAfrica/index.html
114. Federation of American Scientists. South Africa: Chemical and Biological Weapons. http://www.fas.org/nuke/guide/rsa/cbw/index.html
115. C. Gould and P. L. Folb. The South African chemical and biological warfare program: an overview. *The Nonproliferation Review*. 7:10–23, 2000.
116. Nuclear Threat Initiative. South Korea Profile: Biological. http://www.nti.org/e_research/profiles/SKorea/index.html
117. CNS. Weapons of Mass Destruction in the Middle East. http://cns.miis.edu/research/wmdme/sudan.htm
118. M. Z. Diab. Syria's chemical and biological weapons: assessing capabilities and motivations. *The Nonproliferation Review*. 4:104–111, 1997.
119. GlobalSecurity.org. Syria: Biological Weapons. http://www.globalsecurity.org/wmd/world/syria/bw.htm
120. Nuclear Threat Initiative. Syria Profile: Biological Overview. http://www.nti.org/e_research/profiles/Syria/Biological/3338.html#fnB4
121. A. Cordesman. Weapons of Mass Destruction in the Middle East. Regional Trends, National Forces, Warfighting Capabilities, Delivery Options, and Weapons Effects. Center for Strategic and International Studies. Washington, D.C. October 4, 1999. http://www.csis.org/mideast/reports/WMDinMETrends.pdf
122. Nuclear Threat Initiative. Taiwan Overview: Biological. http://www.nti.org/e_research/profiles/Taiwan/index.html
123. E. A. Willis. Seascape with monkeys and guinea pigs: Britain's biological weapons research programme, 1948–1954. *Med Conflict Survival*. 19:285–302, 2003.
124. Nuclear Threat Initiative. Uzbekistan Overview: Biological. http://www.nti.org/e_research/profiles/Uzbekistan/1633.html
125. J. Miller. October 23, U.S. agrees to clean up anthrax site in Uzbekistan. *The New York Times*, 2001.
126. J. B. Tucker, et al., Biological Contamination of Vozrozhdeniye Island: The U.S.-Uzbek Agreement. Center for Nonproliferation Studies. Monterey Institute of International Studies. Briefing Series, 2002.
127. S. A. Kolavic, A. Kimura, S. L. Simons, L. Slutsker, S. Barth, and C. E. Haley. An outbreak of shigella dysenteriae type 2 among laboratory workers due to intentional food contamination. *JAMA*. 278: 396–398, 1997.
128. Center for Nonproliferation Studies. CNS Reports. Chronology of incidents involving ricin. http://cns.miis.edu/pubs/reports/ricin_chron.htm
129. J. B. Tucker. The "Yellow Rain" controversy: lessons for arms control compliance. *The Nonproliferation Review*. 8:25–42, 2001.

3 Hospital Syndromic Surveillance

KATHY J. HURT-MULLEN, HOWARD BURKOM, JOE LOMBARDO, SHERYL HAPPEL LEWIS, NICOLA MARSDEN-HAUG, AND JULIE PAVLIN

Syndromic surveillance systems have been under development in the last several years as an alternative to the types of surveillance systems traditionally used in hospital and public health settings. These systems can be described as the monitoring of available data sources for outbreaks of unspecified disease or of specified disease before the confirmation of identifying symptoms. Its goal is to complement existing sentinel surveillance by identifying outbreaks while keeping false alarm rates acceptable to the public health infrastructure. The goals of these systems is the earliest possible detection of important changes in community health status in order to increase the timeliness of response and limit the morbidity and mortality experience of the community. Furthermore, they can also be useful to track and investigate existing outbreaks as well as provide reassurance of normal rates of illness in a community.

The potential for an intentional release of a pathologic agent into a community for the purpose of causing illness, panic, and terror warrants an assessment of all tools, information and resources available for detection of the diseases that could be caused by such activity. Hospitals have long used many different surveillance systems for a wide variety of purposes, including monitoring of surgical site infections, nosocomial infections, and acquisition of antibiotic resistant infections, among others [1]. These systems are usually designed to capture very specific and well-defined clinical outcomes with the ultimate goal of monitoring and improving patient outcomes. They are not by themselves useful for the purpose of detecting a broad set of important changes in the health status of a patient population that could indicate a community-wide health emergency since there is no way to predict with certainty what pathogens or symptom presentation an unknown exposure may involve.

Public health surveillance is defined traditionally as the ongoing, systematic collection, analysis, interpretation, and dissemination of data regarding a health-related event that enables public health authorities to reduce morbidity and mortality [2]. Such surveillance is conducted for a specified set of diseases, conditions, or laboratory findings in addition to recognized clusters, or outbreaks, of these and yet other health events. Traditional public health surveillance systems yield very specific and reliable information, and hospitals have long been participants in these systems. The major limitations of these traditional systems in detection of a widespread emergency, such as a bioterrorist attack, are comprehensiveness and timeliness [3]. Rather than delaying reporting of illnesses until confirmation of disease is made, syndromic surveillance systems group sets of clinical symptoms or presentations into syndromes that are intended to be representative of the kinds of clinical presentations likely to be manifested by deliberate exposure to pathogens.

The advent of electronic capture of hospital encounter data and the widespread dissemination of computing resources allow for consideration of new methodologies to meet the needs of both hospital institutions and the support of public health organizations' obligation to monitor and protect their communities' health status. So long as pertinent information is captured close to the time of the patient encounter and certain security provisions are followed, it is reasonable and prudent to develop disease detection systems that allow hospitals to monitor their patient populations for important changes that could signal a deliberate exposure to pathogens.

In addition to monitoring counts of syndromic groupings of clinical presentations and diagnoses, these systems also collect non-clinical health-related data such as retail sales of over-the-counter pharmaceutical sales or absentee rates of schools or large employers in an effort to corroborate findings from the clinical data. For the purposes of this discussion, particular emphasis will be placed on the hospital-derived data that may be useful to hospitals and public health organizations as well as the statistical methods that may be employed to detect changes in health status.

3.1 Hospital Inpatient Data

Hospitals routinely collect patient information that could be useful for the detection of an institution-specific or a community-wide health emergency.

Diagnosis codes, such as the International Code of Diseases (ICD) Clinical Modifications, have been used both domestically and internationally to monitor the health of communities, particularly for infectious disease outbreaks [4–9]. Diagnosis codes are usually entered electronically into billing databases and other information resources making them a readily available source for data mining. When assigned early in the patient encounter, diagnosis codes can expedite timely ascertainment of health events. In many hospitals, however, diagnosis codes may not be assigned until the patient is discharged from the hospital, thus limiting their utility for outbreak detection. However, some hospitals do record diagnosis codes early in the patient encounter. To begin designing diagnosis code-based syndromic surveillance systems, it is first necessary to select the syndromes to be monitored and to develop clinical definitions for the syndromes according to the diseases whose presentations they are intended to represent. Recommendations for syndrome groupings have been put forth by a work group that represented federal and local

Table 3.1 Representative ICD-9-CM Code Syndrome Assignment

ICD-9 Code	Diagnosis	Syndrome	Subgroup
001.9	Cholera NOS	Gastrointestinal	Cholera
003.0	Gastroenteritis, salmonella	Gastrointestinal	Salmonella
004.9	Shigellosis NOS	Gastrointestinal	Shigella
005.0	Poisoning, food, staphylococcal	Gastrointestinal	Food poisoning
007.5	Cyclosporiasis	Gastrointestinal	Cyclospora
008.00	Enteritis, E. coli NOS	Gastrointestinal	E coli
787.01	Nausea with vomiting	Gastrointestinal	Gastritis
787.02	Nausea alone	Gastrointestinal	Gastritis
787.03	Vomiting alone	Gastrointestinal	Gastritis
787.91	Diarrhea NOS	Gastrointestinal	Enteritis
382.9	Otitis media NOS	Respiratory	Otitis Media
460	Nasopharyngitis, acute	Respiratory	URI
462	Pharyngitis, acute	Respiratory	URI
463	Tonsillitis, acute	Respiratory	URI
486	Pneumonia, organism NOS	Respiratory	Pneumonia
487.8	Influenza w/ manifestation NEC	Respiratory	Influenza
490	Bronchitis NOS	Respiratory	Bronchitis
784.1	Pain, throat	Respiratory	Sore throat
786.2	Cough	Respiratory	Cough

public health agencies as well as academia [10]. These syndromes represent broad groupings such as gastrointestinal, respiratory, and botulism-like complaints or illnesses. Table 3.1 shows representative assignments of diagnosis codes to syndromes and the potential to break syndromes into smaller subgroups for better understanding of the types of illness driving observed increases.

In developing syndrome coding rules, codes can be initially assigned to syndromic categories on the basis of clinical judgment. However, many coding assignments reflect the lack of firm diagnosis, and codes for symptoms such as "cough," "diarrhea," or "viral syndrome" are commonly used when the complaint or diagnosis is unclear or not completely ascertained. Moreover, variability in coding practices exists among providers; between hospitals serving primarily pediatric versus adult populations; and between inpatient, outpatient, and emergency/urgent care facilities. The frequency with which diagnosis codes are used may also be inadvertently affected by coding practices designed to simplify data entry, such as the use of super-bills or the format of electronic input systems, e.g., having pre-selected subsets of diagnosis codes available in pick lists. For example, experience with the Department of Defense's Electronic Surveillance System for the Early Notification of Community-based Epidemics (ESSENCE) system [11] has shown that the most commonly used code during several Norovirus outbreaks at military treatment facilities is actually a non-infectious gastroenteritis diagnosis. Therefore it is recommended that developers of new systems analyze the data of the institutions to be included in the systems and adopt coding strategies to accommodate those practices.

Another issue for consideration in adopting a diagnosis-coding based syndrome scheme is the sheer number of diagnoses included in a syndrome category. Some diagnosis codes may be used so infrequently that an important increase in their frequency is lost among the background of other more commonly used codes. It is therefore important to examine the frequency of each code in the syndrome group under normal circumstances and to characterize the attributes of the codes as a group in order to determine whether they will be useful in detecting changes in disease incidence. Additionally, when possible, it is valuable to compare diagnosis code groups to a "gold standard" data source that exemplifies the trend for the diseases the syndrome addresses. Figure 3.1 shows an example of a comparison designed to determine which set of ICD-9-CM codes is best able to capture the seasonal influenza trend seen in positive viral respiratory specimens collected in a laboratory-based surveillance system [12]. This analysis shows that manipulating the selection of diagnosis codes can produce more specific syndromes that fit the needs of a particular surveillance program, such as the influenza-like illness (ILI) category used by the ESSENCE system.

Each individual hospital or other care facility should analyze what information is captured in their new patient encounters to determine what information might be useful for surveillance

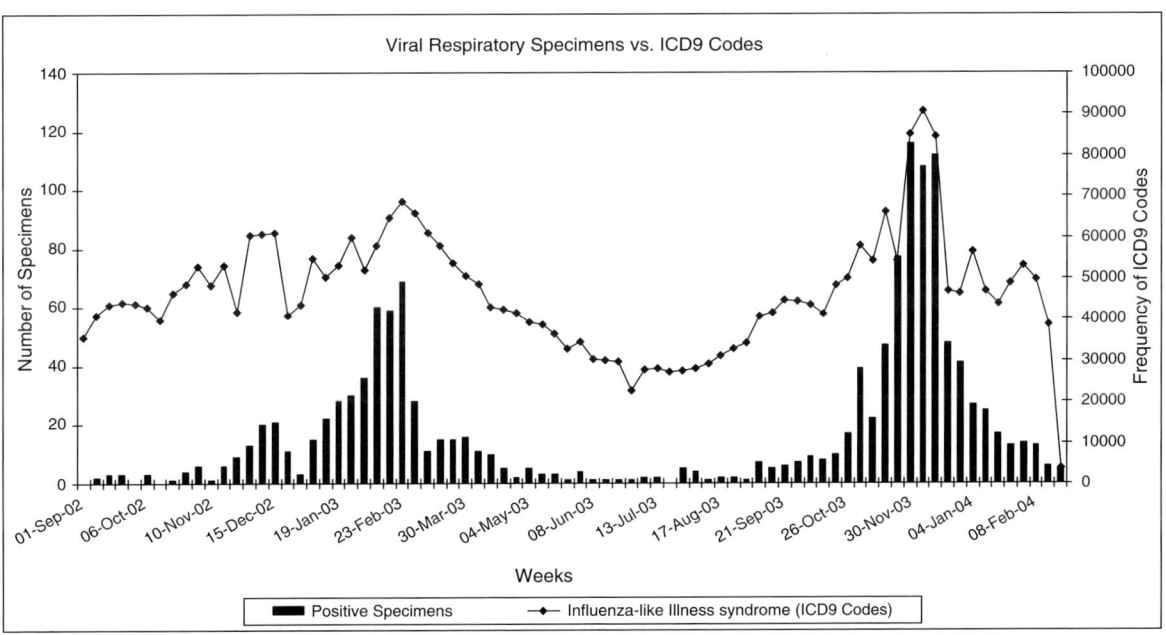

Figure 3.1 Frequency of ICD-9-CM codes grouped as influenza-like illness compared to specimens positive for influenza virus. (Specimen data was provided by the Air Force Institute for Operational Health.)

purposes. When available, diagnosis codes entered for patients who present themselves to acute care clinics or emergency departments and who are subsequently admitted to a hospital can be used to track the types of presenting symptoms or illnesses that are most likely to result in admissions. Other information collected at the time of patient admission, such as text fields containing admitting diagnosis, current procedure terminology (CPT) codes, and even nursing admission orders could be used to categorize patients syndromically.

A second approach to the syndromic coding and evaluation of all admitting diagnosis codes is the tracking of admissions by different wards in the hospital (medical versus surgical), severity of illnesses (e.g., admission to the intensive care unit), age of patients, or even time of day of admissions, as all of these factors may provide an indication that something unusual is occurring in the health of the community. Even if diagnosis codes are not available upon admission, discharge diagnoses can be useful in the development of syndromic systems, although timeliness of event detection would be affected. Evaluation of whether any discharge diagnoses of acute infectious diseases of interest correspond to initial chief complaints may help define which presenting complaints are most important to monitor.

3.2 Hospital Emergency Department Data

Emergency Department (ED) chief complaint data represent a second major source of hospital information that may be useful to hospital institutions and public health officials for routine surveillance. Such efforts began as "drop-in" surveillance systems for focused periods of time such as following major disasters (natural and otherwise) and during high profile sporting and political events [13]. This type of surveillance assumed a high level of visibility and scrutiny immediately following the attacks on New York City's World Trade Center in 2001 [14].

For most of these drop-in surveillance systems, collection and processing of data by hospital staff and public health officials is enormously burdensome. Typically, either the ED staff is required to fax chief complaint logs to public health entities, or public health staff is physically detailed to hospitals to enter data during the surveillance period. When the data collection consists of faxing ED logs, substantial work has to be performed by health department staff upon receipt of the data: Staff is required to review the logs and manually code each patient into the selected syndrome groups and enter the information into computerized databases. Following this data preparation, staff must analyze the data, follow up on important findings, and report the results of their work. This process is difficult to sustain over long periods of time due to the large burden imposed on already resource-limited health departments—particularly given the increased workload brought about by the threat of bioterrorism [15].

However, advances in informatics can expedite the entire process with new capabilities to capture chief complaint data directly from hospital data sources, transmit the information electronically, and automate the coding process. Such automation removes the burden from emergency department staff and dramatically reduces the burden on health department staff. Indeed, a number of jurisdictions have systems in operation with completely automated data transmission, coding and preliminary analyses, and thereby allowing health department staff to focus their efforts on reviewing important findings [3]. The development of chief-complaint based syndromic surveillance has been developed for use in the public health sector. However these systems also provide a valuable resource for hospitals in the absence of any such system by local health authorities. Ideally, however, syndromic surveillance systems can, and should, be developed as a joint endeavor between hospital and public health authorities for coordinated use by both.

Chief-complaint data often provide more timely information than diagnosis-coded information because of the significant delay in many hospitals in classifying complaints into diagnosis coding schemes. Chief complaints, however, are available as free or fixed text at the time of patient registration. The free text data can be transmitted to a surveillance system that will parse it into the syndrome groups that have been adopted for the particular system. There are a number of ways of parsing this free text data into the syndrome groups [16,17]. The parsed data then may be available to the hospital and/or public health staff long before they might be available with manual coding or diagnosis code based systems.

3.3 Other Data Streams

In addition to the coding of diagnoses at admission or discharge and the emergency department chief complaint information, other sources of health indicator data are available for inclusion in syndromic surveillance systems. Three categories of health indicator data are considered here: confirmatory diagnostic data sources, medical encounter data of various types that are pre-diagnostic, and non-traditional indicators.

3.4 Confirmatory Clinical Data

Confirmatory data have been considered the gold standard for public health practice and is the foundation upon which traditional public health surveillance is built. Biological specimens are collected from patients showing signs of illness and analyzed to identify the organism, or the known laboratory characteristics of the organism, causing the illness. Most public health organizations cannot afford to launch a costly investigation or large prophylaxis effort without specific knowledge of the illness and the extent to which it has affected the population. As a result of these constraints, a confirmation of the presence of an infectious organism from a laboratory has been needed, and in the absence of a recognized widespread health emergency, such confirmation remains the most prudent approach to routine disease surveillance. The method used to capture laboratory data is dependent upon the laboratory location and informatics capability. Hospital-based systems should be accessible within the hospital enterprise. Acquiring data from major laboratory chains requires their willingness to provide the data as well as compliance with the Health Insurance Portability and Accountability Act of 1996 (HIPAA) and security requirements.

3.5 Pre-Diagnostic Clinical Data

The pre-diagnostic clinical data category is defined as data that provide an indication of an illness without a confirmed diagnosis based upon the results of laboratory tests. This category includes the experience of trained health care practitioners and can include patient encounter information from different ends of the health delivery system. Initial encounters may occur with phone triage services like a nurse telephone hotline, a Health Maintenance Organization (HMO) appointment service, or even a poison center. If data on the call are recorded in a structured database, then the information can be categorized and included in a surveillance system for analysis. Alternatively, data may be created and be available after a physical encounter with a practitioner. Based on the encounter, there will be some documentation of the encounter, likely a claim for services, possibly requests for laboratory or other clinical tests, and perhaps prescriptions for medication.

Receiving compensation for services can be a lengthy process and varies by the disease or procedure performed. Traditionally this process has been paper-based and not very timely or useful for rapidly identifying an infectious disease outbreak. In recent years the compensation process has been expedited greatly by the increased use of Internet and electronic submission of claims. Many physician offices currently submit their claims immediately after a patient is seen. A National Center for Health Statistics [18] study ascertained that approximately 1.9% of individuals seek emergency room care during the initial phase of their disease while 64% will seek help from their family practice physician. Capturing this information greatly increases the sample size and makes it easier to identify outbreaks earlier while they are in their evolution and case numbers are small. Like diagnosis-coded inpatient visits, this class of health indicator data represents a valuable source of information for surveillance purposes when the data are captured electronically close to the time of encounter.

Many HMOs provide a nurse hot-line or reservation triage service manned by experienced personnel who record chief-complaint descriptions into a database which may then available for surveillance purposes and may be valuable if electronic capture coincides closely with the time of patient interaction. Similarly, data from emergency medical services such as 911 calls and ambulance runs may be valuable for surveillance purposes. However, these encounters are more likely to represent the victims of traumatic injury and careful evaluation of the data is required to determine whether or not increases in non-traumatic events are detectable.

3.6 Non-Traditional Health Indicator Data

Non-traditional health indicator data are typically less specific than the data sources described previously, but can provide earlier indication of an unusual changes in community health status. Two data sources that have been examined are over-the-counter medication sales and school absenteeism reports. Sales of over-the-counter remedies may increase for a variety of reasons. Sales promotions, stockpiling of medications for the winter cold and flu season, and changes in product placement to increase product visibility can all result in increased sales.

Changes in rates of school absenteeism must be interpreted with caution. Absenteeism can vary by location and grade level of the school. Inner city schools typically have the higher absenteeism rates than suburban schools and schools located near military bases typically have even lower rates.

Non-traditional data sources have not been relied upon for primary surveillance due to the difficulty in differentiating between the many possible causes for change in normal rates. However, they do represent a potentially valuable source of information for corroboration of findings from clinical sources.

3.7 Selection of Data Elements

System developers should consider what information is available and would be of greatest value to the institutions that the system is being built to serve. To date, the data elements found to be most useful for the purposes of syndromic surveillance are:

- Patient-Encounter specific index code
- Hospital ID
- Date of visit
- Time of visit
- Patient age
- Patient sex
- Residential zip code
- Chief Complaint
- Discharge diagnosis (where available)
- Discharge disposition (where available)

The data elements chosen, however, may vary depending on the recipient of the data. If the data are being sent directly to a health department with appropriate authority, then fully identifiable information may be transmitted as long as the transmission is secured. Regardless of the data recipient, the epidemiologist or data analyst must have some way to identify particular entries to the hospital for the purposes of disease investigation. Medical record numbers or hospital assigned patient codes are suitable as long as they allow a particular record to be identified for further review if required. The date and time of visit are essential for determining whether cases are related, and the time of visit can possibly provide an indication of the severity of the illness. Age may also be a crucial element in determining whether a chief complaint is related to a particular condition. For example, chest pains in a young adult are more remarkable than in an older adult more prone to a heart attack. Residence and/or employment zip code is essential for the purpose of mapping cases to determine whether an illness is clustering in a particular region. Discharge disposition is useful in determining the severity of the illness, while the discharge diagnosis can also aid in linking or not linking similar cases.

Discharge diagnosis, if readily available, may be of equal or greater value than the chief complaint. However, as mentioned previously, discharge diagnoses are typically not available without substantial delay, usually limiting their utility for a surveillance system designed to minimize reporting time. Additionally, while chief-complaint description may be variable in its accuracy, it remains the most critical data element. While case studies exist for many diseases, no one can know how a weaponized, possibly genetically engineered disease may propagate through a community and what primary symptoms it may cause to the majority of its victims. Capturing the main symptoms that brought a person to the ED is very important for the purpose of trying to link cases. However, studies have shown that the disparity between chief complaint and final diagnosis is relatively minor and does not nullify the timeliness advantage of chief complaint descriptions [15].

3.8 Data Acquisition and Presentation

Within a single hospital enterprise, there are few data acquisition considerations. All desired data should be stored within institutional databases and the task of creating a surveillance dataset should be only a matter of data base administration. However, when creating systems that consolidate data from outside of a single institution it is necessary to consider how information will be transferred from the data owners to end-users. Automation of the process is critical for the success of any syndromic surveillance system as the goals for these systems are rapid detection and access to critical information during emergency situations. Automated, electronic data acquisition and transmission may be conducted using a variety of protocols such as Health Level Seven (HL-7), Simple Mail Transfer Protocol (SMTP) or File Transfer Protocol (FTP) to name but a few. When considering the type of acquisition and transmission routines to implement it is important to simplify the process as much as possible for the data provider. If providing data is cumbersome to the organization then timeliness and completeness of data reporting is very likely to be compromised.

3.9 Data Analysis: Algorithms for Aberration Detection

Aberration detection algorithms have long been used to aid decision-making in the hospital surveillance process. This process includes: (1) Case definition, (2) Data conditioning (tabulation, adjustment), (3) Analysis, (4) Reporting, (5) Investigation if required, and (6) Consequence management if required.

A review article on infection control by Smyth and Emmerson [19] discusses the practical aspects of the implementation of this process. Detection algorithms are more than statistical hypothesis tests; the case definition and data conditioning steps have key roles in determining their utility. The role of these algorithms is to automate the analysis in a uniform, replicable fashion with effective detection performance, measured by sensitivity, specificity and timeliness. The input to an anomaly detection algorithm is typically a time series of counts, proportions, or other functions of a monitored quantity. Examples of such quantities are risk-adjusted surgical site infection rates or counts of diagnoses of ILI. The time series are obtained by aggregating data at some regular time interval. Older surveillance methods [20,21] used longer aggregation time intervals of weeks or months to reduce data noisiness and to get more regular time series distributions. The threat of bioterrorism is increasing the emphasis on rapid alerting and shortening these intervals to days and hours, gradually pushing toward real-time detection [22]. The case definition and data conditioning steps thus determine the inputs, approach, and adaptive tuning of the algorithmic methods.

3.10 Control Chart Usage

Hospital surveillance algorithms have made widespread use of industrial process control chart methods [1]. Control charts provide a graphical, understandable approach for automated anomaly detection with a foundation in probability theory [23]. A process is deemed *in control* if the corresponding monitored quantity varies within confidence limits expected from an underlying statistical distribution and is said to show only *common cause variation*. For an example, an endemic disease process such as the incidence of influenza might be considered in control if the charted daily fraction of hospital admissions diagnosed as ILI lie within control limits, as in Figure 3.2. The process is held *out of control* and suggestive of *special cause variation*, such as a rise in disease incidence to epidemic levels, when the confidence limits are exceeded. Since surveillance applications are usually concerned with unexpected increases, interest is often restricted to upper confidence limits and one-sided tests.

Accounting for common cause variation depends on the type of quantity chosen for monitoring and on its underlying distribution. Several common distributions are associated with canonical chart types. For example, for continuous quantities (e.g., blood pressure and temperature) often considered having a normal distribution, X-bar and S charts are used for the mean and standard deviation, respectively. P-charts, with limits derived from the binomial distribution, are used for proportions such as the fraction of total admissions with gastrointestinal chief complaints. U-charts derived from the Poisson distribution are often used for count data such as the weekly number of admissions for neurological disorders. Numerous other basic and hybrid chart types are available.

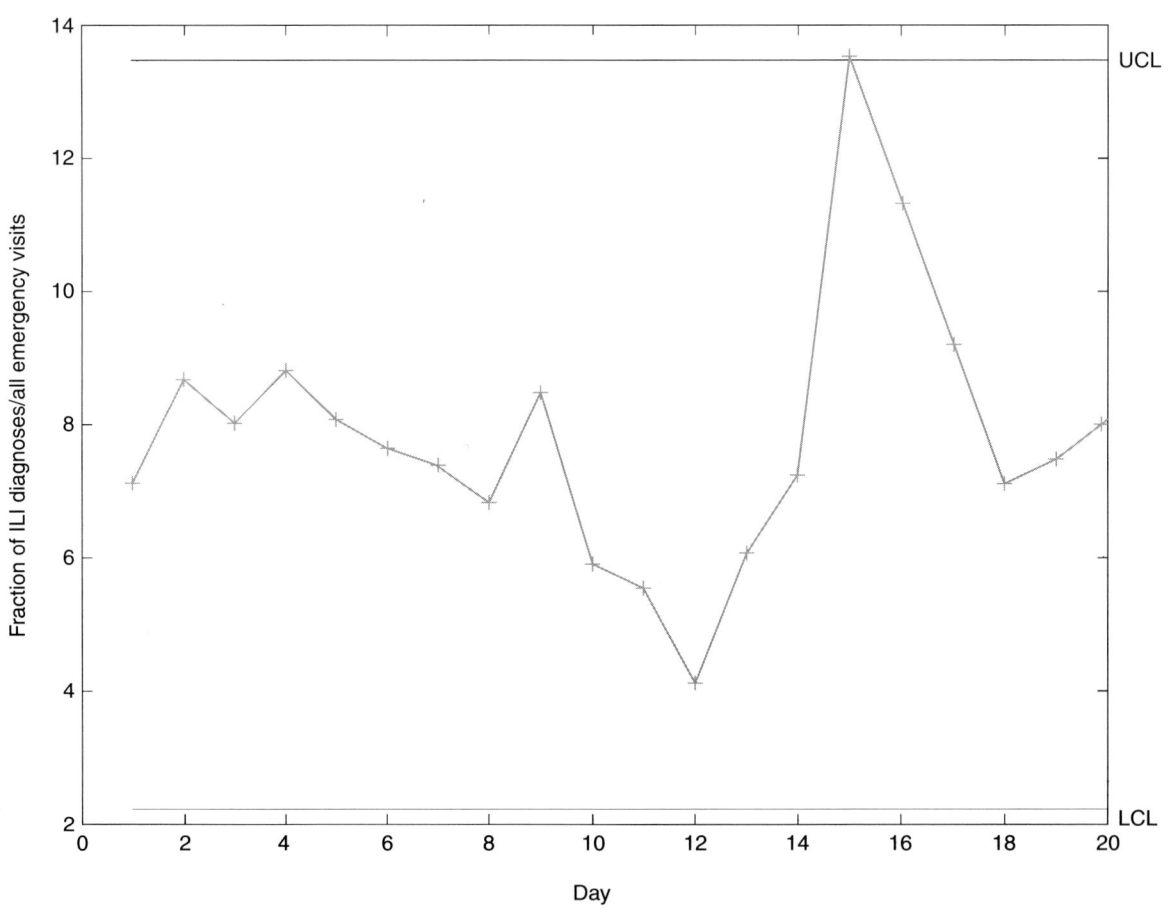

Figure 3.2 Sample control chart.

3.11 Issues in Aberration Detection

The appropriate chart for any particular process depends on both the in-control data behavior and the effect expected from special cause variation. For example, Shewhart charts are most effective for rapidly detecting sudden changes, while Exponentially Weighted Moving Averages (EWMA) and Cumulative Summation (CUSUM) charts are used to detect gradual changes. A thorough discussion of these issues has been presented by Morton et al. [24].

Other data complications, including varying risks, small counts, and lack of data history have been treated successfully in practical contexts [25–28], and the respective adaptations are being evaluated for the detection of outbreaks in syndromic surveillance systems.

The application of these methods to bioterrorism surveillance poses several challenges. Alibek [29] reported biowarfare research aimed at altering disease symptomatology by genetically altering the antigenic presentation in the host. Other sections of this chapter discuss the aggregation of diagnosis-coded and chief-complaint data into syndrome group categories to increase the sensitivity to an unknown data signal. The time series behavior of the counts or rates of these non-specific syndrome groups must be understood in order to manage false alarm rates in routine health monitoring. Mandel observed [30] in 1969 that control chart performance could be improved by replacing monitored quantities by the residuals of regression using independent covariates. Regression modeling has since been applied to reduce the effects of day-of-week, seasonality, late reporting, and other covariates [23,31,32], and research is ongoing to produce optimal combinations of data modeling and control chart methods.

3.12 Upcoming Challenges in Hospital-Based Aberration Detection

Increasing concern over the threat of bioterrorism is driving research for decision-making capability well beyond interest in the change points of a single time series. Multiple hypothesis testing using disparate data streams in multicenter data is a substantial challenge. Marshall et al. [33] considered the problem of assessing control charts applied to multiple care providers or hospitals. They adjusted for several sources of between-unit variation and treated the multiple testing problem using false discovery rate estimates. The search for significant spatiotemporal clusters of cases using multicenter data has generated several algorithmic approaches [34], notably in scan statistics widely used in cancer epidemiology [35]. Kulldorff et al. [36] investigated the power of this approach with syndromic data records from New York City, organized by patient zipcode. Burkom [37] extended the approach to multiple data types, controlling for differences in scale and allowing for different spatial organization between data types.

Aberration detection algorithms have been developed to aid in hospital surveillance. Researchers have adapted process control charts and other tools to solve routine decision problems, and the resulting methods are being applied to monitor for outbreaks of unknown description that could result from a deliberate, covert act of biological warfare. New case definition and data adjustment procedures are producing time series to be monitored for this purpose, and both data modeling and hypothesis testing are being refined to obtain the sensitivity, specificity, and timeliness that bioterrorism surveillance will require. Even so, the resulting algorithms can find only statistical anomalies; follow-up investigation must efficiently explain away irrelevant events that cannot be modeled and examine those that remain for public health significance.

3.13 Summary

Syndromic surveillance is a new and rapidly evolving approach to detecting important changes in community health status as early as possible. It depends upon the identification of opportunities to use data in new ways as well as the identification of novel data sources and statistical methods. It is intended to enhance the traditional surveillance systems already in place, such as traditional notifiable disease surveillance and the anecdotal surveillance carried out by the astute clinician. Such surveillance is valuable at the hospital level but perhaps even more so at the community level. For this reason, now more than ever, it is critical to share this type of information with officials in public health to meet mutually held goals and develop agreements to determine how the information will be shared and utilized.

References

1. J. C. Benneyan. Statistical quality control methods in infection control and hospital epidemiology, part I: introduction and basic theory. *Inf Contr and Hosp Epid*, 19(4):194–214.
2. CDC MMWR 2201; 50(No. RR-13).
3. R. Heffernan, F. Mostashari, D. Das, A. Karpati, M. Kulldorff, and D. Weiss. Syndromic surveillance in public health practice, New York City. *Emerg Infect Dis*, 10:858–864, 2004.
4. R. Lazarus, K. Kleinman, I. Dashevsky, C. Adams, P. Kludt, A. Jr. DeMaria, and R. Platt. Use of automated ambulatory-care encounter records for detection of acute illness clusters, including potential bioterrorism events. *Emerg Infect Dis*, 8:753–760, 2002.
5. A. J. Beitel, K. L. Olson, B. Y. Reis, K. Mandl et al. A comprehensive set of coded chief complaint and diagnostic codes for identifying respiratory illness in a pediatric population. *Pediatr Emerg Care*, 20(6):355–360, 2004.
6. D. M. Fleming, M. A. Barley, R. S. Chapman. Surveillance of the bioterrorist threat: A primary care response. *Commun Dis Public Health*, 7(1):68–72, 2004.
7. N. Jones, Monitoring population health using routinely recorded family practice clinical practice data: Evaluation of a sentinel surveillance system in Auckland, New Zealand [abstract]. National Syndromic Surveillance Conference, Sept 2002, New York, NY.
8. M. D. Lewis, J. A. Pavlin, J. L. Mansfield, S. O'Brien, L. G. Boomsma, Y. Elbert, and P. W. Kelley. Disease outbreak detection system using syndromic data in the greater Washington DC area. *Am J Prev Med*, 23:180–186, 2003.
9. J. A. Fleishman, and F. H. Hellinger. Recent trends in HIV-related inpatient admissions 1996–2000: A 7-state study. *J Acquir Immune Defic Syndr*, 34:102–110, 2003.
10. Centers for Disease Control and Prevention. Syndrome Definitions for Diseases Associated with Critical Bioterrorism-associated Agents. Available at http://www.bt.cdc.gov/surveillance/syndromedef. Accessed Aug 19, 2004.
11. Department of Defense Global Emerging Infection System. Electronic Surveillance System for the Early Notification of Community-based Epidemics (ESSENCE). Available at: http://www.geis.ha.osd.mil/GEIS/SurveillanceActivities/ESSENCE/ESSENCEinstructions.asp.
12. N. Marsden-Haug, V. B. Foster, P. Gould, and J. A. Pavlin. Evaluation of ICD-9 Based Influenza-like Illness Surveillance. Available at http://www.cdc.gov/phin/04conference/05-25-04. Accessed Aug 25, 2004.
13. L. Goss, R. Carrico, C. Hall, and K. Humbaugh. A Day at the Races: Communitywide syndromic surveillance during the 2002 Kentucky Derby Festival. *J Urban Health*, 80(Suppl 1):i124 (abstract), 2003.
14. D. Das, D. Weiss, F. Mostashari, T. Treadwell, J. McQuiston, L. Hutwagner, A. Karpati, K. Bornschlegel, M. Seeman, R. Turcios, P. Terebuh, R. Curtis, R. Heffernan, and S. Balter. *Enhanced Drop-In Syndromic Surveillance in New York City Following September 11, 2001*. J Urban Health, 80(Suppl 1):i76–i88, 2003.
15. E. Begier, D. Sockwell, L. Branch, J. Davies-Cole, L. Jones, L. Edwards, J. Casani, and D. Blythe. The national capitol region's emergency department syndromic surveillance system: Do chief complaint and discharge diagnosis yield different results? *Emerging Infects Dis*, 9(3):393–396, 2003.
16. C. Sniegoski. *Automated Syndromic Classification of Chief Complaint Records*. JHU/APL Technical Digest. 25(1):68–75, 2004.
17. W. Chapman, M. Wagner, O. Ivanov, R. Loszewski, and J. Dowling. Syndromic surveillance from free-text chief complaints. *J Urban Health*, 90(Suppl 1):i120(abstract), 2003.
18. P. F. Adams, G. E. Hendershot, and M. A. Marano. "Current Estimates from the National Health Interview Survey, 1996", National Center for Health Statistics, *Vital Health Stat*, 10(200), 1999.
19. E. T. Smyth, and A. M. Emmerson. Surgical site infection surveillance; *J Hosp Infect*, 45:173–184, 2000.
20. D. F. Stroup, G. D. Williamson, J. L. Herndon, and J. Karon. Detection of aberrations in the occurrence of notifiable diseases surveillance data. *Stat Med*, 8:323–329, 1989.

21. C. P. Farrington, N. J. Andrews, A. D. Beale, and M. A. Catchpole. A statistical Algorithm for the early detection of outbreaks of infectious disease. *J Royal Stat Soc A*, 159:547–563, 1996.
22. H. S. Burkom, and Y. A. Elbert. The role of data aggregation in biosurveillance detection strategies with applications from the electronic surveillance system for the early notification of community-based epidemics. *MMWR*, 53(Suppl), 2004.
23. T. P. Ryan. Statistical methods for quality improvement. New York: John Wiley & Sons; 1989.
24. A. P. Morton, M. Whitby, M-L. McLaws, A. Dobson, S. McElwain, D. Looke, J. Stackelroth, and A. Sartor. The application of statistical process control charts to the detection and monitoring of hospital-acquired infections; *J Qual Clin Prac*, 21:112–117, 2001.
25. J. Lovegrove, O. Valencia, T. Treasure, C. Sherlaw-Johnson and S. Gallivan. Monitoring the results of the cardiac surgery by variable life-adjusted display. *Lancet*, 305:1128–1130, 1997.
26. T. L. Gustafson. Practical risk-adjusted quality control charts for infection control. *Am J Infect Control*, 28:406–414, 2000.
27. C. P. Quesenberry. Statistical process control geometric Q-chart for nosocomial infection surveillance. *Am J Infect Control*, 28(4):314–320, 2000.
28. N. A. Ismail, A. N. Pettitt, and R. A. Webster. "Online" monitoring and retrospective analysis of hospital outcomes based on a scan statistic. *Statistics in Medicine*, 22:2861–2876, 2003.
29. Alibek, Ken, *Biohazard*, Random House, New York, 1999.
30. B. H. Mandel. The regression control chart. *Journal of Quality Technology* 1(1):1–9, 1969.
31. G. D. Williamson and L. VanBrackle. A monitoring system for detecting aberrations in public health surveillance reports. *Statistics in Medicine*, 18(23):3283–3298.
32. B. Y. Reis, and K. D. Mandl. Time series modeling for syndromic surveillance. *BMC Medical Informatics and Decision Making* 3:2, 23 January 2003.
33. C. Marshall, N. Best, A. Bottle, and P. Aylin. Statistical issues in the prospective monitoring of health outcomes across multiple units. *J R Statist Soc A*, 167 n3:541–559, 2004.
34. M. Kulldorff, T. Tango, and P. J. Park. Power comparisons for disease clustering tests. Computational Statistics and Data Analysis, 42:665–684, 2003.
35. M. Kulldorff. Prospective time-periodic geographical disease surveillance using a scan statistic. *Journal of the Royal Statistical Society JR Stat Soc*, A;164:61–72, 2001.
36. M. Kulldorff, Z. Zhang, J. Hartman, R. Heffernan, L. Huang, and F. Mostashari. Benchmark data and power calculations for evaluating disease outbreak detection methods. *MMWR* 53(Suppl), 2004.
37. H. S. Burkom. Biosurveillance applying scan statistics with multiple, disparate data sources. *J Urban Health*, Proceedings of the 2002 National Syndromic Surveillance Conference. 80(2 Suppl 1):i57–i65, 2003.

4 Biological Agents, Effects, Treatment, and Differential Diagnosis

ZYGMUNT F. DEMBEK AND THEODORE J. CIESLAK

4.1 Disease: Anthrax

4.1.1 Causative Agent

Bacillus anthracis is a sporulating Gram-positive rod. Three forms of anthrax are known: inhalational anthrax from inhalation of aerosolized anthrax spores, gastrointestinal anthrax from eating food contaminated with the bacterium, and cutaneous anthrax from skin contact with an item contaminated with anthrax spores [5].

4.1.2 Clinical Description

The incubation period for inhalational anthrax is 1–6 days. Patients with inhalational anthrax typically have a biphasic illness with a nondescript initial phase followed by an acute second phase. Initially, non-specific symptoms appear, similar to a common upper respiratory infection: fever, fatigue, malaise, myalgia, mild chest pain, and a non-productive cough. These initial symptoms are often followed by a brief period of improvement (from hours to 2–3 days) followed by a rapid onset of severe respiratory distress with dyspnea, diaphoresis, stridor, and cyanosis. Chest wall edema may be observed. Without treatment, shock and death follow within 24–36 hours of onset of severe symptoms [5].

4.1.3 Diagnosis

Because of the urgent need to begin therapy, an initial diagnosis of anthrax should be made clinically. A widened mediastinum is the hallmark clinical association in inhalational anthrax. In the absence of an alternative explanation, such a finding in an ill, febrile patient is highly suggestive of a diagnosis of anthrax. Definitive diagnosis may be made by isolating *B. anthracis* from a culture of blood (or spinal fluid, as 50% of inhalational anthrax victims will develop hemorrhagic meningitis) [5].

4.1.4 Differential Diagnosis

The differential diagnosis for inhalational anthrax must include coccidiomycosis, diphtheria, meningitis, pneumonia, aerosol exposure to staphylococcal enterotoxin B (SEB), pneumonic plague or tularemia, invasive group A streptococcal pneumonia, and other forms of severe acute pneumonitis. With SEB, no prodrome would be evident prior to onset of severe respiratory symptoms. Patients with plague, tularemia, or invasive group A streptococcal pneumonia are far more likely than those with anthrax to have pulmonary infiltrates [5].

4.1.5 Medical Management

Inhalational anthrax is almost always fatal if treatment is begun after the patient is symptomatic. Penicillin has been the treatment of choice for naturally occurring strains. Resistant strains do occur; in the absence of sensitivity data, empiric treatment should be instituted with ciprofloxacin 400 mg IV q12h (10–15 mg/kg IV q12h in children) or doxycycline 100 mg IV q12h (2.2 mg/kg IV q12h in children). When clinically appropriate, oral antimicrobials can be given: ciprofloxacin 500 mg po BID (10–15 mg/kg po q12h) or doxycycline 100 mg po BID (2.2 mg/kg po q12h) (adult dose).

Therapy should be continued for 60 days (IV and po combined).

A licensed vaccine is available and is administered as a 0.5 ml SC dose at 0, 2, and 4 weeks and then at 6, 12, and 18 months. Boosters are given yearly to those at ongoing risk of exposure. Anthrax vaccination is not recommended for the general public. Post-exposure prophylaxis (PEP) against inhalational anthrax is accomplished with ciprofloxacin 500 mg (10–15 mg/kg) po bid for 60 days, or doxycycline 100 mg (2.2 mg/kg) po bid. Exposed individuals may receive three doses of vaccine (at 0, 14, and 28 days), potentially enabling a shortened 30-day course of antimicrobials. If penicillin sensitivity is established, PEP can be switched to penicillin V 500 mg po q6h (40–80 mg/kg/day divided q6h in children), or amoxicillin 500 mg po q8h (40–80 mg/kg/day divided q8h in children) [2,3,4,5,9,11,13].

4.2 Disease: Botulism Intoxication

4.2.1 Causative Agent

Clostridium botulinum is an anaerobic Gram-positive sporulating bacillus that may produce any of seven neurotoxins (Types A–G). Illness occurs between 1–5 days following exposure to botulinum toxin, dependent upon the toxin dose and the condition of the individual [5].

4.2.2 Clinical Description

The concurrent inception of cranial nerve palsies and descending paralysis may alert clinicians to the diagnosis of botulism. Fever is absent, neurologic manifestations are symmetric, the patient remains responsive, the heart rate is normal or slow in the absence of hypotension, and sensory deficits are absent, except for diploplia. Inhaled botulinum toxin is clinically similar to foodborne botulism, although the time of onset of paralytic symptoms may be longer than for foodborne cases. Initial symptoms include ptosis, generalized weakness, lassitude, and dizziness. Diminished salivation with extreme mouth dryness may contribute to a sore throat. With the progression of the disease, more severe motor symptoms begin to appear. Diplopia, dysphonia, dysarthria, and dysphagia occur, followed by a symmetric, descending, progressive weakness of the extremities along with weakness of the respiratory muscles. Other symptoms may include nausea and vomiting. The patient is alert, oriented, and afebrile. Additional neurologic findings may include a diminished gag reflex, facial paresis, tongue weakness, and nystagmus. Respiratory failure due to paralysis of respiratory muscles may cause death of the patient [1,5].

4.2.3 Diagnosis

The diagnosis of botulism is largely clinical. A mouse-neutralization assay can provide confirmation [5].

4.2.4 Differential Diagnosis

The differential diagnosis of botulism includes myasthenia gravis and the Lambert–Eaton myasthenic syndrome, but these conditions are rarely fulminant and lack autonomic features. Guillain–Barré syndrome and other acute inflammatory polyneuropathies should also be included among differential diagnostic possibilities, but these entities seldom begin with cranial nerve dysfunction. Polio patients generally present with fever and asymmetric flaccid paralysis. Magnesium intoxication, diphtheria, organophosphate poisoning, and brain stem infarction may be mistaken for botulism intoxication [5].

4.2.5 Medical Management

Supportive care and prolonged nursing may be necessary for treatment. Suspected cases should be monitored for respiratory compromise using forced expiratory volume measurements. Intubation and ventilatory assistance may be required in the event of respiratory failure. Tracheotomy may also be required. A trivalent (types A, B, and E) botulinum antitoxin (of equine origin) is used in the treatment of foodborne botulism. Administration should begin at the first indication of possible intoxication, in the absence of horse serum sensitivity. A botulism toxoid (inactivated toxin) vaccine offering immunity to toxin types A–E is available as an investigational new drug (IND). Stool and serum should be obtained from patients. In cases where botulism factors high among diagnostic possibilities, electromyography, using repetitive stimulation at 40 Hz or greater, may be considered. Moreover, cerebrospinal fluid may be examined for white blood cells and protein, and a Tensilon challenge test can be performed. The patient's vital capacity should be monitored [1,5].

4.3 Disease: Plague

4.3.1 Causative Agent

Yersinia pestis, a Gram-negative bacillus, may be inhaled as an aerosol (pneumonic plague), or contracted by the bite of infected fleas (bubonic plague). The incubation period for pneumonic plague is from 2–3 days, and is 2–10 days for the bubonic form of the disease [5,10].

4.3.2 Clinical Description

In the pneumonic form, the onset of symptoms is acute and fulminant with high fever, chills, headache, malaise, myalgia, and cough. The patients may have lymphadenopathy and blood-tinged sputum. Pneumonia progresses rapidly, resulting in dyspnea, stridor, and cyanosis. Terminal events are respiratory failure, circulatory collapse, and hemorrhage; mortality is 100% in untreated patients. In the bubonic form, initial symptoms include malaise, high fever, and one or more painful swollen lymph nodes ("buboes"). The vast majority of buboes occur in the groin, cervical, and axillary lymph nodes may also be involved. Up to 80% of patients with bubonic plague also become septic ("septicemic plague"); 5–15% develop pneumonia. Circulatory collapse, hemorrhage, and peripheral thrombosis are the terminal events. About half of untreated bubonic cases die [10].

4.3.3 Diagnosis

As prompt therapy is critical to survival for plague victims, an initial diagnosis should be made clinically in patients with severe, rapidly progressive pneumonia accompanied by hemoptysis. Supporting evidence can be obtained by finding "safety-pin"-shaped Gram-negative coccobacillary organisms on stained sputum, lymph node aspirate, blood, or spinal fluid. Confirmation is by culture of these same specimens, which should only be attempted under BSL-3 conditions [5,10].

4.3.4 Differential Diagnosis

The differential diagnosis for the bubonic form includes ulceroglandular tularemia, staphylococcal or streptococcal adenitis, meningococcemia, enteric Gram-negative sepsis, gas gangrene, cat-scratch disease, scarlet fever, Rocky Mountain spotted fever, necrotizing fasciitis, and rickettsioses. In tularemia or cat-scratch disease, the inoculation site is usually more evident than in bubonic plague, and the patient is not usually septic. The differential diagnosis for pneumonic plague includes other etiologies of fulminant pneumonia, tularemia, trench fever, anthrax and staphylococcal enterotoxin B (SEB) inhalation. Continued deterioration without stabilization rules out SEB. Patients with plague have a cough productive of bloody sputum, while those with tularemia generally have a non-productive cough. Secondary spread may occur with pneumonic plague [5,10].

4.3.5 Medical Management

For pneumonic plague, streptomycin 30 mg/kg/day IM in 2 divided doses for 10 days or gentamicin 2.0 mg/kg IV loading dose, then 1.7 mg/kg IV q8h or 5 mg/kg once daily (in children, 2.5 mg/kg IV q8h is recommended). Alternate treatments are doxycycline 200 mg IV initially, then 100 mg q12h IV (2.2 mg/kg IV q12h in children) for 10–14 days; or chloramphenicol 1000 mg qid IV (25 mg/kg IV q6h in children) for 10–14 days (preferred for plague meningitis). Supportive therapy is provided as required.

Plague prophylaxis is achieved with tetracycline 500 mg qid po or doxycycline 100 mg bid po (2.2 mg/kg po q12h in children) for 7 days or duration of exposure, whichever is longer. Ciprofloxacin 500 mg bid po (20 mg/kg po q12h in children) for seven days may also be used. Alternatives include ofloxacin, levofloxacin, chloramphenicol, and TMP-SMX.

Hospital infection control measures are an important component of management of plague patients. The incision and drainage of buboes may pose a hazard to medical personnel, although buboes may be aspirated for diagnostic purposes. Droplet precautions should be strictly enforced for at least 72 hours after the initiation of effective therapy. Surface decontamination can be performed with 0.5% sodium hypochlorite solution (1 part household bleach added to nine parts water) [3,5,8,10,11,13].

4.4 Disease: Smallpox

4.4.1 Causative Agent

Variola (smallpox) virus could be used as a biological weapon in aerosol form or inoculated onto fomites. The virus is usually spread by the respiratory route, is environmentally stable, and may also be spread through direct contact [5,7].

4.4.2 Clinical Description

The incubation period for smallpox is between 7–17 days. Smallpox is an illness with acute onset of fever of 101 °F or more followed by a rash characterized by vesicles or firm pustules. Lesions are classically synchronous in nature. The prodrome lasts 2–4 days and includes malaise, fever, rigors, headache, and backache. This is followed by a typical skin eruption (from macules to papules to vesicles to pustules, and then scabs over 7–14 days). Fever may reappear 7 days after the onset of the rash. Smallpox has had a 20–50% mortality rate. Flat-type smallpox, characterized by slow evolution of flat, soft, focal skin lesions, and severe systemic toxicity has been noted in 2–5% of patients. Mortality for flat-type smallpox was 66% in vaccinated patients and 95% in unvaccinated. Hemorrhagic-type smallpox is characterized by the appearance of extensive petechiae and mucosal hemorrhage, is seen in about 3% of patients, and usually results in death [5,7].

4.4.3 Diagnosis

As with other BT threat diseases, a preliminary diagnosis should be based upon clinical findings. Supporting evidence may be gained by demonstrating classic poxviruses on material from lesions. Culture should only be attempted in a qualified BSL-4 laboratory at the CDC or USAMRIID [5,7].

4.4.4 Differential Diagnosis

The differential diagnosis for smallpox includes chickenpox and monkeypox, allergic contact dermatitis, erythema multiforme with bullae, orf, disseminated herpes zoster, impetigo, coxsackievirus, secondary syphilis, atypical measles, and adverse drug eruptions. Smallpox cases often present with a rash that is centrifugal in distribution, or most dense on the face and extremities. The lesions appear at a 1–2 day period, evolve at the same rate, and are generally at the same stage of development (i.e., vesicles, pustules, or scabs). In varicella (chicken pox), new lesions appear in groups every few days, and lesions at different stages of maturation are found in adjacent dermal areas. Varicella lesions are distributed centripedally, with a greater concentration on the trunk than the extremities; and are superficial, not occurring on the palms and soles, unlike variola. Monkeypox is more difficult to distinguish from smallpox, although generalized lymphadenopathy is a common feature of monkeypox, the lesions are not as numerous, nor is the disease as severe. Person-to-person spread of monkeypox is rare [5,7].

4.4.5 Medical Management

Antivirals for use against smallpox (e.g., cidofovir) are under investigation. Supportive treatment should be given [5,7].

4.4.6 Vaccine/Prophylaxis

Wyeth Calf Lymph Vaccine and DOD cell-culture-derived Vaccinia must be given by scarification. Smallpox vaccination should be given to all contacts and healthcare workers caring for suspect smallpox patients, irrespective of prior vaccination status. With the exception of significant impairment of systemic immunity, there are no contraindications to post-exposure vaccination of a person who experiences bona-fide exposure to variola. However, concomitant administration simultaneously with vaccinia immune globulin (VIG) 0.3–0.6 ml/kg IM is recommended for pregnant and eczematous persons in such circumstances [5,7,11].

4.5 Disease: Tularemia

4.5.1 Causative Agent
Francisella tularensis is a small Gram-negative coccobacillus. Two main serotypes exist (A and B), with A the more virulent form and is endemic in the US [5,6].

4.5.2 Clinical Description
The incubation period for tularemia can range from 1–21 days, with an average of 3–5 days. The primary clinical signs and symptoms of tularemia vary in severity according to virulence of the infecting strain, dose, and site of inoculum. Acute onset usually occurs after a dose-dependent incubation period of 1–21 days (average 3–5 days). Various schemes have been proposed to classify clinical manifestations of tularemia; tularemia is best described as two syndromes: ulceroglandular and typhoidal. Tularemia can be thought of as a plague-like illness, with ulceroglandular disease exhibiting characteristics like bubonic plague, and typhoidal disease similar to pneumonic/septicemic plague.

In ulceroglandular tularemia (approximately 75% of naturally occurring cases) patients have ulcers on the skin or mucous membranes, and tender lymph nodes (typically larger than 1 cm in diameter) in the lymphatic distribution of the skin lesion. The pathogen exhibits a vigorous inflammatory reaction, pneumonia is less common, and the patient's prognosis is good. Ulceroglandular tularemia is characterized by fever, chills, headache, malaise, an ulcerated skin lesion, and painful regional lymphadenopathy. A pulse–temperature disassociation (i.e., the pulse increases less than 10 beats per min per 1°F increase in temperature above normal) often accompanies the fever.

Patients with typhoidal tularemia (about 25% of naturally occurring cases) present with lymph nodes smaller than 1 cm in diameter, and without skin or mucous membrane lesions. The lower respiratory tract is often involved with either syndrome. Approximately 30% of patients with ulceroglandular tularemia and 80% of patients with typhoidal tularemia have pneumonia. The higher incidence of pneumonia in patients with typhoidal tularemia likely accounts for the associated higher mortality. Pneumonic tularemia is a severe atypical pneumonia that can be fulminant with a high case fatality rate if untreated, and may be the primary manifestation after inhalation of organisms [5,6].

4.5.3 Diagnosis
Definitive diagnosis can be made by culture of *F. tularensis* from blood, skin lesions, conjunctival exudates, sputum, and other appropriate body fluids. Culture should only be attempted in a qualified BSL-3 laboratory. ELISA-based serologic assays are available, but are often negative early in the course of illness [5,6].

4.5.4 Differential Diagnosis
The illness, while often severe, is generally nonspecific. Typhoidal syndromes such as salmonellosis or rickettsial infections are included in the differential diagnosis. Other causes of pneumonia (such as infection with *Mycoplasma pneumoniae*, *Chlamydia pneumoniae*, *Legionella pneumophila*, *Coxiella burnetii*, *Chlamydia psittaci*, or various viruses), lymphogranuloma venerum, malaria, mononucleosis, mumps, pharyngitis, and other tick-borne diseases, as well as exposure to staphylococcal enterotoxin B should be considered. Large numbers of patients presenting with similar systemic illnesses, a portion having pneumonia with non-productive cough, may be indicative of tularemia. In fulminant pneumonias, plague and inhalational anthrax should also be included in the differential diagnosis. Diagnosis is generally based on clinical suspicion, and can be made

with serologic evidence of infection in a patient with a compatible clinical syndrome. Tularemia can be diagnosed by recovery of *F. tularensis* from clinical specimens, although cultivation is difficult and slow. Blood smears can be stained with specific fluorescent antibody. Hemagglutinins appear in 10–12 days; a rising titer is diagnostic [5,6].

4.5.5 Medical Management

Patients with tularemia who do not receive appropriate antibiotic treatment may have a prolonged illness characterized by malaise, weakness, weight loss, and other symptoms that last for months. Streptomycin 15 mg/kg IM q12h for 10–14 days, or gentamicin 3–5 mg/kg IV qd (2.5 mg/kg IV q8h in children) for 10–14 days are generally considered the treatments of choice. Doxycycline and ciprofloxacin may also be used in doses equal to those given for plague. Doxycycline 100 mg po q12h (2.2 mg/kg po q12h in children) for 14 days, or tetracycline 500 mg po qid for 14 days may be given as PEP [5,6,10,11].

4.6 Disease: Viral Hemorrhagic Fever

4.6.1 Causative Agent

The viral hemorrhagic fever (VHF) viruses include filoviruses [e.g., Ebola, Marburg], arenaviruses [e.g., Lassa, Machupo], bunyaviruses [e.g., Hantaviruses], and flaviviruses [e.g., Dengue and Yellow Fever]. They may cause clinical hemorrhagic fever, where the target organ is the vascular bed, and the dominant clinical features are often due to microvascular damage and changes in vascular permeability [5,14].

4.6.2 Clinical Description

These viruses cause febrile illnesses that can feature flushing of the face and chest, petechiae, bleeding, edema, hypotension, and shock. Malaise, myalgia, headache, vomiting and diarrhea may also occur. Disseminated intravascular coagulation and coagulopathy occur to varying degrees with various VHFs. Common symptoms include fever, myalgia, and prostration. Physical examination may reveal conjunctival injection, mild hypotension, flushing, and petechial hemorrhages. Illness may progress to shock, with generalized mucous membrane hemorrhage, and is often accompanied by neurological, pulmonary, and hematopoietic involvement. Renal insufficiency is usually proportional to cardiovascular compromise. Mortality can be substantial (50–90% among Ebola victims) [5,14].

4.6.3 Diagnosis

A general clinical diagnosis of "viral hemorrhagic fever" can be made in febrile patients with a bleeding diathesis. Definitive diagnosis relies on viral isolation or on the detection of viral antigen in acute phase serum by immunoassay [5].

4.6.4 Differential Diagnosis

VHF can be suspected in any patient presenting with a severe febrile illness and evidence of vascular involvement (postural hypotension, petechiae, easy bleeding, flushing of the face or chest, non-dependent edema) who has traveled to an area where the virus is known to occur, or a bioterrorism threat is suspected. Signs and symptoms suggesting additional organ system involvement are common (headache, photophobia, pharyngitis, cough, nausea or vomiting, diarrhea, constipation, abdominal pain, hyperesthesia, dizziness, confusion, tremor).

Definitive diagnosis is made by specific viral identification. Other clinical tests can be useful, e.g., thrombocytopenia and leukopenia will be seen in the filoviruses, but not with Lassa virus; proteinuria and/or hematuria are common. Malaria is the major disease to be considered in the differential diagnosis of naturally acquired VHF. Others include typhoid fever, non-typhoidal salmonellosis, leptospirosis, rickettsial infections, shigellosis, relapsing fever, fulminant hepatitis, meningococcemia, acute leukemia, lupus erythematosus, idiopathic or thrombotic thrombocytopenic purpura, hemolytic uremic syndrome, and the many other causes of disseminated intravascular coagulation [5].

4.6.5 Medical Management

Supportive care should be applied to the hemodynamic, hematologic, pulmonary, and neurologic manifestations of VHF. Intensive care is the sole measure that can salvage severely ill patients. Consideration of fluid resuscitation of hypotensive patients must be tempered when pulmonary capillary leakage occurs. Pressor agents are frequently required. Risk of hemorrhage must be considered when intravascular devices and invasive hemodynamic monitoring are employed. Analgesics and sedatives may be judiciously employed for management of restlessness, confusion, myalgia and hyperesthesia. Secondary infections may occur. Management of clinical bleeding follows the same principles as for any patient with systemic coagulopathy, assisted by coagulation studies. Intramuscular injections, aspirin, and anticoagulants should be avoided. Antiviral drugs (e.g., ribavirin) may have compassionate use protocols for therapy, and the hospital pharmacist should be consulted for approved use [5].

4.7 Disease: Brucellosis

4.7.1 Causative Agent

Brucella species are Gram-negative coccobacillary organisms, of which four are pathogenic in humans (*Brucella melitensis*, *B. abortus*, *B. canis* and *B. suis*) [5].

4.7.2 Clinical Symptoms

Brucellosis normally presents as a non-specific febrile illness with a long and variable incubation period (3–60 days). Characteristic "undulant" fever, headache, chills, myalgias, arthralgias, weakness, and malaise are the most common complaints. Gastrointestinal symptoms can occur with ingestion or inhalation; symptoms include constipation, anorexia, nausea, and diarrhea. One or both sacroiliac joints may become infected causing low-back and buttock pain that is intensified by stressing the sacroiliac joints on physical exam. Peripheral joint involvement may occur and vary from pain on range of motion testing to joint immobility and effusion. Hepatomegaly or splenomegaly may occur in up to 45–63% of cases. Meningitis occurs occasionally (<5% of cases). Symptoms may persist from 3–6 months and sometimes for over a year [5,11].

4.7.3 Diagnosis

Definitive diagnosis is by the isolation of *Brucellae* from blood or bone marrow. Culture should only be attempted under BSL-3 conditions. Antibody detection via a serum agglutination method is an alternative means of diagnosis [5].

4.7.4 Differential Diagnosis

A very broad differential diagnosis is necessary due to the non-specific symptoms and include bacterial, viral, and mycoplasmal infections. The symptoms of viral and mycoplasmal infections are usually present for a few days, while in brucellosis they persist longer. Typhoidal tularemia and typhoid fever may be indistinguishable clinically from brucellosis. Radiographic findings similar to those in tuberculosis infection may occur, including disk space narrowing and epiphysitis. Unequivocal diagnosis requires isolation of the organism. Blood culture is the method of choice but specimens need to be obtained early in the disease and cultures may need to be incubated for up to four weeks. Failure to grow the organism is common, and isolation rates of only 20–50% are reported even from experienced laboratories [5,11].

4.7.5 Treatment

Doxycycline 100 mg bid po plus rifampin 600 mg qd po for a minimum of six weeks. Ofloxacin 400 mg qd po plus rifampin 600 mg qd po for 6 weeks is also effective [5,11].

4.8 Disease: Glanders

4.8.1 Causative Agent

Burkholderia mallei, a Gram-negative bacilli, exists in nature only in infected hosts (horses, mules, and donkeys). The organism spreads to man by invading the nasal, oral, and conjunctival mucous membranes, inhalation into the lungs, or by invading abraded or lacerated skin. There is neither available vaccine nor dependable therapy [5,11].

4.8.2 Clinical Features

Glanders may occur in an acute localized form, as a septicemic rapidly fatal illness, or as an acute pulmonary infection. Combinations of these syndromes commonly occur in human cases. A chronic cutaneous form with lymphangitis and regional adenopathy is also frequent. Aerosol infection produced by a *B. mallei* could produce any of these syndromes. The incubation period ranges from 10–14 days, depending on the inhaled dose and agent virulence. The septicemic form begins rapidly with fever, rigors, sweats, myalgia, pleuritic chest pain, photophobia, lacrimation, and diarrhea. Physical examination may reveal fever, tachycardia, cervical adenopathy, and mild splenomegaly. Blood cultures are usually negative until the patient is moribund. Mild leukocytosis with a shift to the left or leukopenia may occur.

The pulmonary form may follow inhalation or occur by hematogenous spread. Systemic symptoms as described for the septicemic form occur. Chest radiographs may show miliary nodules (0.5–1.0 cm) and/or a bilateral bronchopneumonia, segmental, or lobar pneumonia and necrotizing nodular lesions.

Acute infection of the oral, nasal and/or conjunctival mucosa can cause mucopurulent, blood-streaked discharge from the nose, associated with septal and turbinate nodules and ulcerations. If systemic invasion occurs from mucosal or cutaneous lesions then a papular and/ or pustular rash may occur that can be mistaken for smallpox (another possible BW agent).

The chronic form is unlikely to be present within 14 days after an aerosol exposure, and is characterized by cutaneous and intramuscular abscesses on the legs and arms. These lesions are associated with enlargement and induration of the regional lymph channels and nodes. Recovery from chronic glanders may occur or the disease may erupt into an acute septicemic illness. Nasal discharge and ulceration are present in 50% of chronic cases [5,11].

4.8.3 Diagnosis

Gram stain of lesion exudates reveals small Gram-negative bacteria. *B. mallei* grows slowly on ordinary nutrient agar, and special growth media may be used to enhance isolation. Agglutination tests are not positive for 7–10 days, and a high background titer in normal sera (1:320 to 1:640) makes interpretation difficult. Complement fixation tests are more specific and are considered positive if the titer is equal to, or exceeds 1:20. Cultures of autopsy nodules in septicemic cases will usually establish the presence of *B. mallei* [5,11].

4.8.4 Medical Management

Standard Precautions should be used to prevent person-to-person transmission in proven or suspected cases. Sulfadiazine 100 mg/kg per day in divided doses for 3 weeks has been found to be effective. Various isolates have markedly different antibiotic sensitivities, so that each isolate should be tested for its own individual resistance pattern [5,11].

4.8.5 Prophylaxis

There is no vaccine available for human use. PEP may be tried with TMP–SMX [5,11].

4.9 Disease: Q Fever

4.9.1 Causative Agent

Coxiella burnetii, the causative agent of Q fever, is a Gram-negative coccobacillus, is resistant to heat and desiccation and is highly infectious by aerosol exposure [5].

4.9.2 Clinical Description

The incubation period for Q fever is between 10–40 days. There are a variety of Q Fever clinical syndromes. Flu-like symptoms occur as soon as 10 days after exposure. Q fever is usually a self-limiting febrile illness lasting 2–14 days. Patients usually present with headaches, fatigue, chills, sweats, and myalgias. Infections range from asymptomatic to severe. Severe headache is present in about 75% of patients. Pneumonia occurs in about half of all patients. There are three presentations of Q fever pneumonia: pneumonia presenting as a fever with no pulmonary symptoms, atypical pneumonia, and rapidly progressive pneumonia.

Cough, usually non-productive, is present in 25–50% of those with radiographically confirmed Q fever pneumonia. Pleuritic chest pain may also occur. Rales are probably the most common physical finding. Patients with rapidly progressing pneumonia often have signs of pulmonary consolidation. Q fever infections are rarely fatal. Q fever hepatitis occurs in about a third of all cases. Q fever endocarditis is a rare complication, very difficult to treat, and may require valve replacement. Person-to-person transmission is rare, but has been reported via tissue transplantation and sexual contact. There are also psychological effects to chronic Q fever infection, including depression and mental status changes [5].

4.9.3 Diagnosis

Culture of *C. burnetii* is difficult. Diagnosis is typically made by antibody detection using any of a variety of serologic means [5,11].

4.9.4 Differential Diagnosis

Q fever is not a clinically distinct illness. The atypical pneumonia may resemble a viral illness or pneumonia caused by *Mycoplasma pneumoniae*, *Legionella pneumophila*, *Chlamydia psittaci*, and *Chlamydia pneumoniae*. All causes of rapidly progressive pneumonia would enter the differential diagnosis. Rapidly progressing pneumonia mimics bacterial pneumonias due to atypical agents such as *Yersinia pestis* and *Francisella tularensis*. Endocarditis, hepatitis, mononucleosis, ornithosis, and tick-borne diseases may be part of the differential diagnosis [5].

4.9.5 Treatment

Most cases of acute Q fever will resolve without antibiotic treatment. Tetracycline, 500 mg q6h po × 5–7 days or doxycycline 100 mg q12h × 5–7 days are the treatments of choice. A combination of erythromycin 500 mg q6h and rifampin 600 mg qd is also effective. Chronic infection, especially involving endocarditis, often requires extended treatment and should involve appropriate specialists [5].

4.9.6 Prophylaxis

Tetracycline 500 mg q6h po × 5 days or doxycycline 100 mg q12h po × 5 days started 8–12 days post exposure. Antibiotic prophylaxis must be timed properly. Antibiotics given within the first week following exposure will delay but not prevent onset of illness [5].

4.10 Disease: Ricin Intoxication

4.10.1 Causative Agent

Ricin, a glycoprotein toxin derived from castor plant beans, has great potential as a biological agent due to its wide availability. Ricin produces its damage by inhibiting cellular protein synthesis [5].

4.10.2 Clinical Description

The incubation period for ricin intoxication is 4–8 hours. Symptoms will depend on the dose and route of exposure. Initial symptoms following inhalation include weakness, fever, cough, dyspnea, nausea, chest tightness, and arthralgia. Sweating, pulmonary edema, and cyanosis usually follow. Necrotizing, suppurative airway lesions may be noted in conjunction with rhinitis and laryngitis. If left untreated, respiratory failure and cardiovascular collapse due to inhalation of the agent can lead to death after 36–72 hours. Ingestion will be followed by rapid onset of nausea, vomiting, abdominal cramps, and severe diarrhea. Other symptoms include fever, thirst, headache, sore throat, and dilation of the pupils. Death may occur on the third day or later and is usually due to vascular collapse [5].

4.10.3 Diagnosis

A diagnosis may be made by the detection of antibodies via an ELISA assay. PCR may be helpful in demonstrating the presence of toxin in environmental specimens [5].

4.10.4 Differential Diagnosis

For inhalational exposure, similar symptoms in large numbers of patients might suggest several respiratory pathogens. Influenza, Q fever, tularemia, plague, and respiratory illnesses due to exposure to SEB and chemical agents such as phosgene should be included in the differential diagnosis. SEB intoxication would likely have a more rapid onset and lower mortality. Acute lung injury induced by phosgene would progress much faster than that caused by ricin. Nerve agent intoxication would be characterized by acute onset of cholinergic crisis with dyspnea and profuse secretions. The differential diagnosis for patients who have ingested ricin would include disease due to all the major enteric pathogens. These should be ruled out with culture [5].

4.10.5 Treatment

Management of patients is supportive. Acetaminophen for fever, and cough suppressants may make the patient more comfortable. Management of ricin-intoxicated patients depends on the route of exposure. Patients with pulmonary intoxication are managed by appropriate treatment for pulmonary edema and respiratory support as indicated. Gastrointestinal intoxication is best managed by vigorous gastric decontamination with super-activated charcoal, followed by use of cathartics such as magnesium citrate. Volume replacement of GI fluid losses is important [5,12].

4.11 Disease: Staphylococcal Enterotoxin B Intoxication

4.11.1 Causative Agent

Staphylococcal enterotoxin B (SEB) is one of several exotoxins produced by the Gram-positive bacilli *Staphylococcus aureus* [5].

4.11.2 Clinical Description

From 3–12 hours after aerosol exposure, fever, chills, headache, myalgia and non-productive cough may appear. Shortness of breath and retrosternal chest pain may develop. If the patient develops pulmonary edema or adult respiratory distress syndrome (ARDS), there may be a cough with frothy sputum. Fever may last 2–5 days, and cough may persist for up to 4 weeks. Toxin ingestion leads to acute salivation, nausea, and vomiting followed by abdominal cramps and diarrhea. Fever and respiratory involvement are not seen in foodborne SEB intoxication. Higher exposure can lead to septic shock and death if left untreated. Physical examination is often unremarkable. Postural hypotension may be present, particularly with ingestion of SEB, due to fluid loss. Conjunctivitis and rales may be present [5].

4.11.3 Diagnosis

A diagnosis may be made by the detection of antibodies via an ELISA assay. Toxin accumulates in urine and may be detected via ELISA for several hours after exposure. PCR may be helpful in demonstrating the presence of toxin in environmental specimens [5].

4.11.4 Differential Diagnosis

Influenza, adenovirus, parainfluenza, or mycoplasma infection could cause fever, non-productive cough, myalgias, and headache in large numbers of people in a short time. Early clinical manifestations of SEB may be similar to those of inhalation anthrax, tularemia, plague, or Q fever. However, the rapid progression of respiratory signs and symptoms to a stable state differentiates SEB intoxication. Chemical agents, such as mustard gas, would show marked vessiculation of the skin as well as pulmonary injury. During 6–12 hours following exposure, clinical tests may detect toxin, including blood samples, urine nasal swabs, and induced respiratory secretions. Most patients develop a significant antibody response after 6 days following exposure. Acute and convalescent sera should be drawn for immunological testing [5,12].

4.11.5 Medical Management

Supportive care with close attention to oxygenation and hydration. In severe cases, ventilation is provided, with positive-end-expiratory pressure and diuretics. Acetaminophen and cough suppressants may make the patient more comfortable [5].

4.12 Disease: Trichothecene Mycotoxin (T2) Intoxication

4.12.1 Causative Agent

Trichothecene mycotoxin (T2) can theoretically be used in aerosol to form "yellow rain" which produces casualties. T2 can enter the body through the skin and aero-digestive epithelium, and quickly inhibit protein and nucleic acid synthesis. These mycotoxins are low molecular weight compounds produced by filamentous fungi of the genera *Fusarium*, *Myrotecium*, *Trichoderma*, *Stachybotrys* and others [5].

4.12.2 Clinical Description

Time to onset of symptoms is from minutes to hours from exposure. T2 exposure causes pruritis, redness, vesicles, necrosis, epidermal sloughing, dysesthesias, nausea, weight loss, vomiting, and diarrhea. Effects on the airway include nose and throat pain, nasal discharge, itching and sneezing, cough, dyspnea, wheezing, chest pain, and hemoptysis. T2 also produces effects after ingestion or eye contact. Severe poisoning results in prostration, weakness, ataxia, collapse, reduced cardiac output, shock, and death [5].

4.12.3 Diagnosis

Specific identification of the various mycotoxins is by chromatography and/or mass spectrometry performed on clinical or environmental samples [5].

4.12.4 Differential Diagnosis

Mycotoxin poisoning should be considered especially when multiple patients present with similar clinical syndromes, particularly if victims report a "yellow rain" or if droplets of yellow fluid contaminate clothing or the environment. Radiation, chemical, or plant toxicity are other diagnoses to consider [5,12].

4.12.5 Treatment

Outer clothing should be removed and exposed skin should be decontaminated with soap and water. Super-activated charcoal should be given orally if toxin is swallowed. Eye exposure should be treated with copious saline irrigation. Supportive therapy should be provided as needed [5].

References

1. S. S. Arnon, R. Schechter, T. V. Inglesby, D. A. Henderson, J. G. Bartlett, M. S. Ascher, E. Eitzen, A. D. Fine, J. Hauer, M. Layton, S. Lillibridge, M. T. Osterholm, T. O'Toole, G. Parker, T. M. Perl, P. K. Russell, D. L. Swerdlow, and K. Tonat. Working Group on Civilian Biodefense. Botulinum toxin as a biological weapon: medical and public health management. *JAMA*, 285:2081, 2001.
2. T. J. Cieslak and E. M. Eitzen. Anthrax. In: *Conn's Current Therapy 2004* (R. E. Rakel and E. T. Bope, eds.) and Elsevier, Philadelphia, PA, 2004.
3. T. J. Cieslak and F. M. Henretig. Biological and chemical terrorism. In: *Nelson Textbook of Pediatrics*, 17th Edition [Chapter 706] (R. E. Behrman, R. M. Kliegman and H. B. Jensen, eds.) W. B. Saunders, Philadelphia, PA, 2003.
4. R. G. Darling, E. M. Eitzen, J. F. Waeckerle, and J. L. Mothershead, Eds. Bioterrorism. *Emergency Medicine Clinics of North America*. May, 2002.
5. R. G. Darling, J. B. Woods, Z. F. Dembek, B. K. Carr, T. J. Cieslak, A. C. Littrell, M. G. Kortepeter, N. W. Rebert, S. A. Stanek and J. W. Martin, Eds. USAMRIID's *Medical Management of Biological Casualties Handbook*. 5th Edition. USAMRIID, Frederick MD, 2004.
6. D. T. Dennis, T. V. Inglesby, D. A. Henderson, J. G. Bartlett, M. S. Ascher, E. Eitzen, A. D. Fine, A. M. Friedlander, J. Hauer, M. Layton, S. R. Lillibridge, J. E. McDade, M. T. Osterholm, T. O'Toole, G. Parker, T. M. Perl, P. K. Russell, and K. Tonat. Working Group on Civilian Biodefense. Tularemia as a biological weapon: medical and public health management. *JAMA*, 285:2763–2773, 2001.
7. D. A. Henderson, T. V. Inglesby, J. G. Bartlett, M. S. Ascher, E. Eitzen, P. B. Jahrling, J. Hauer, M. Layton, J. McDade, M. T. Osterholm, T. O'Toole, G. Parker, T. Perl, P. K. Russell, K. Tonat. Working Group on Civilian

Biodefense. Smallpox as a biological weapon: medical and public health management. *JAMA*, 281:2127–2137, 1999.
8. F. M. Henretig, T. J. Cieslak, and E. M. Eitzen. Biological and chemical terrorism. *Journal of Pediatrics*, 141:311–326, 2002.
9. T. V. Inglesby, T. O'Toole, D. A. Henderson, J. G. Bartlett, M. S. Ascher, E. Eitzen, A. M. Friedlander, J. Gerberding, J. Hauer, J. Hughes, J. McDade, M. T. Osterholm, G. Parker, T. M. Perl, P. K. Russell, and K. Tonat. Working Group on Civilian Biodefense. Anthrax as a biological weapon: updated recommendations for management. *JAMA*, 287:2236–2252, 2002.
10. T. V. Inglesby, D. T. Dennis, D. A. Henderson, J. G. Bartlett, M. S. Ascher, E. Eitzen, A. D. Fine, A. M. Friedlander, J. Hauer, J. F. Koerner, M. Layton, J. McDade, M. T. Osterholm, T. O'Toole, G. Parker, T. M. Perl, P. K. Russell, M. Schoch-Spana, and K. Tonat. Plague as a biological weapon: medical and public health management. Working Group on Civilian Biodefense. *JAMA*, 83:2281–2290, 2000.
11. L. E. Lindler, F. J. Lebeda, and G. Korch, Eds. *Biological Weapons Defense: Infectious Disease and Counterbioterrorism*. Human Press. Totowa, NJ. December, 2004.
12. J. M. Madsen. Toxins as weapons of mass destruction. A comparison and contrast with biological-warfare and chemical-warfare agents. *Clin Lab Med* 21:593–605, 2001.
13. National Center for Disaster Preparedness. Pediatric preparedness for disasters and terrorism: a national consensus conference. Executive summary. Columbia University 2003.
14. R. F. Pilch and R. A. Zilinskas, Eds. *Encyclopedia of Bioterrorism Defense*. Wiley, NY. January, 2005.

5 Medical Considerations for Radiological Terrorism

JAMES WINKLEY AND PAUL D. MONGAN

Disclaimer

All statements and opinions are the author's, and are not official positions or policies of the Uniformed Services University, the Department of Defense, or the US federal government.

5.1 Introduction

Since September 11, U.S. intelligence agencies have issued alerts that Islamic terrorists continue to plan for further terror attacks. U.S. intelligence agencies have uncovered plans of U.S. nuclear power plants at terrorist bases in Afghanistan. There is also evidence of plans designed to cause mass casualties and spread deadly radiological debris by a bombing or airline attack on a U.S. nuclear power plant or one of the Energy Department's nuclear facilities. This type of attack, known as radiological warfare (RW) is the deliberate use of radiological materials to produce injury and death. The explosion of a radiological weapon, similar to that of an ordinary bomb, causes damage by the heat and blast liberated at the time of detonation. While such attacks have not occurred, many experts agree that it is a matter of "when" and not "if" such an event will occur. Unfortunately, the proliferation of nuclear material and technology has made the acquisition and terrorist use of ionizing radiation more probable than ever. Fortunately, the treatment of most radiation casualties is both effective and practical to decrease the morbidity and mortality from the use of nuclear and radiological weapons.

Currently there are three threat scenarios for radiological terrorism. The most probable scenario for the near future would be a radiological dispersion device. Such a weapon can be developed and used by any terrorist with conventional weapons and access to radionuclides. This is an expedient weapon, in that radioactive waste material is relatively easy to obtain from any location that uses radioactive sources. These sites could be a nuclear waste processor, a nuclear power plant, a university research facility, a medical radiotherapy clinic, or an industrial complex. The radioactive source is disseminated by using conventional explosives and the debris is subsequently is scattered across the targeted area. In 1996, Islamic rebels from Chechnya planted, but did not detonate a device packed with Cesium 137, one of the most highly radioactive by-products of nuclear fission, in a Moscow park. Depending on the size of the explosive and the surrounding population density, the medical effects of the explosion could have produced a significant number of deaths, while many thousands would have suffered from radiation exposure.

A terrorist attack could also be made on a nuclear power plant using a commercial jet, heavy munitions or internal sabotage. This type of attack would have a similar effect to a radiological bomb and could cause far greater casualties. If such an attack were to cause either a meltdown of the reactor core or a dispersal of the spent fuel waste, extensive casualties could be expected. To date, the significant medical effects of the radiological accident at Chernobyl is the model for this type of radiological event and the possibility that terrorists may attempt to attack such facilities has led to the implementation of more stringent security measures at nuclear facilities.

While the traumatic effects of blast and thermal injury are visible and tangible, the effects of radiation are not directly apparent and can only be discerned by the secondary effects. This is evident in the aftermath of the effects of the nuclear accident that took place in Chernobyl on 26 April 1986. On that day, an explosion secondary to loss of cooling capacity destroyed the nuclear reactor at Chernobyl. This explosion sent a cloud of radioactive material and gases 1 km high. Two workers died as a direct effect of the explosion. Those that remained in shielded areas of the plant survived while some of those that went to fight the fires died of radiation effects. Sources of radiation exposure in this catastrophe came from the short-term gamma/beta emissions in the explosion and the subsequent gamma/beta radiation from the reactor core debris. Because of a lack of waterproof protective clothing and respirators, another principal source of radiation was from the deposition of particulate matter on the skin and mucous membranes of personnel in the area. The primary sources of residual radiation were due to iodine 131, strontium 90, and cesium 137 [1,2]. During the acute event in this low population density area, 29 casualties were evaluated in the first 30 minutes. In the next 24 hours, 140,000 people were evacuated from the 30 km surrounding Chernobyl and potassium iodate tablets distributed. Over the next few weeks 230 patients were hospitalized with priority given to those with early onset of nausea and vomiting, skin and mucous membrane radiation burns and a decrease in the lymphocyte count to less than $1000/mm^3$. Infectious disease therapy consisted of standard regimens for the neutropenic patients. Bone marrow transplantation was attempted in 19 patients receiving >6Gy irradiation. However, this did not seem promising, as 17 of 19 died due to the associated radiation burns. All told, radiation burns (40–90% BSA) contributed to the deaths of 21 patients. In addition, 82 patients had respiratory difficulty secondary to oropharyngeal radiation burns. Over the next 4 years, the average radiation exposure around Chernobyl was 4 times the normal. This was primarily due to residual ground contamination with cesium 137. Despite the relatively low number of acute casualties given the magnitude of the accident, the long-term impact predicts an additional 24,000 cancers in Europe and 280 in the region around Chernobyl [3–5].

The worst scenario, and the least likely, is a terrorist organization diverting an existing nuclear device or procuring enough material and expertise to manufacture a nuclear device. In this scenario a terrorist group could try to purchase a nuclear weapon, as the Japanese Aum Shinrikyo cult tried to do in Russia, or build a crude device on its own and utilize ground or ship transport to deliver the weapon to the point of detonation. Evidence suggests that some groups, including the Al-Qaeda network, have attempted to obtain weapons grade nuclear material. Since 1993, there have been 175 cases of trafficking in nuclear material; 18 of which involved substantial quantities of weapons grade material. After acquiring fissionable nuclear material, sophisticated terrorists could design and fabricate a workable atomic bomb. The wake of a nuclear terror attack would be large numbers of casualties with combined injuries generated from the periphery of the lethal zone. Infrastructure, economic centers, and communications would be destroyed or disrupted by the electromagnetic pulse. The large numbers of fatalities and casualties in conjunction with the psychological effects and long-term radiation effects would impose a massive burden on available medical facilities. For example, a relatively small nuclear device of 15-kilotons detonated in Manhattan could immediately kill upwards of 100,000 inhabitants, followed by a similar number of deaths afterward. In addition, advanced medical care would be available only outside the area of immediate destruction and contamination. Consequently, the primary management importance would be placed on early evacuation of casualties to other available medical centers throughout the United States.

Because of the unique nature of radiological injury, the theory and treatment of radiological casualties is taught in the Medical Effects of Ionizing Radiation Course offered by the Armed Forces Radiobiology Research Institute at Bethesda, Maryland. In addition, the course content is published in *The medical management of radiological casualties*, which is available at http://www.afrri.usuhs.mil.

5.2 Physics

A basic discussion on atomic structure helps one to appreciate what occurs with radiation exposure. All matter is composed of atoms, which are themselves composed of protons (positively charged), neutrons (no charge), and electrons (negatively charged) held together by highly energetic atomic forces. When atoms split, either naturally (radioactive decay) or with the assistance of man (fission), energy is released from the atomic bonds (Figure 5.1). This energy is in the form of heat, high energy gamma rays, similar to X-rays, X-rays and atomic particles: alpha and beta particles, and neutrons. Neutrons are similar to protons except they have no charge. Gamma and X rays are high energy electromagnetic waves. Beta particles are free electrons which have a negative charge, low mass and a high reactivity. Alpha particles are helium nuclei (two protons and two neutrons) stripped of electrons; they are largest of atomic particles. When highly radioactive material is brought together in sufficient quantity and force, i.e., nuclear bomb, an atomic chain reaction takes place causing a rapid splitting of atoms and an exponential release of the atomic energy: nuclear explosion. When these materials are brought together in a controlled fashion, i.e., nuclear reactor, then the energy is released slowly preventing the explosive release of energy. Certain man made and naturally occurring atomic material such as uranium and plutonium, spontaneously decay giving off radioactive energy and particles, which can be harnessed for various useful purposes. When humans are exposed to gamma rays and atomic particles interactions occur between the radioactive particles and DNA, proteins, enzymes, and cell membranes causing damage to the cells and organs. These particles collide with atoms and molecules in the cells stripping electrons, changing the surface charge of enzymes and cell membranes and breaking strands of DNA and RNA. It is this interaction that causes acute radiation sickness (ARS).

The key principles in managing radiation casualties are understanding the sources and effects of radiation exposure. Radiation exposure can be broken down into 2 categories: irradiation and contamination. Irradiation occurs when radiation from an external source interacts with an organism, usually occurring in the first minute after a nuclear accident, explosion or exposure to a radioactive source. During a nuclear detonation, gamma and neutron irradiation are the most serious radiation threats (neutron damage was not detected after the Chernobyl incident). While the residual gamma radiation, which is similar to X-rays, is much less intense than that emitted during the first minute after a nuclear explosion, it is highly energetic, passes through matter easily, and causes whole-body exposure (Figure 5.2). Though exposure to gamma irradiation may be short lived, if a significant dose is absorbed it can be rapidly fatal. Radiation exposure may also come from external and/or internalized radiation sources, such as dust and fallout that is ingested, inhaled or deposited on skin or clothes. Dust and weapons fragments from a nuclear explosion or radiation dispersal device constitute the most significant sources of contamination as they continue to emit alpha, beta, and gamma radiation. Contamination can lead to on going radiation poisoning if decontamination is not undertaken in a timely manner. Alpha particles are a negligible external hazard,

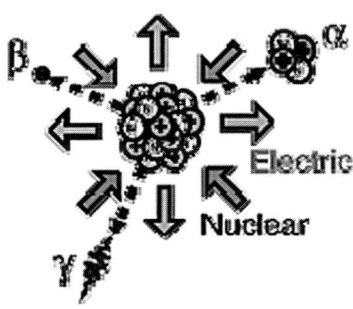

Figure 5.1 Types of radiation released from atomic decay.

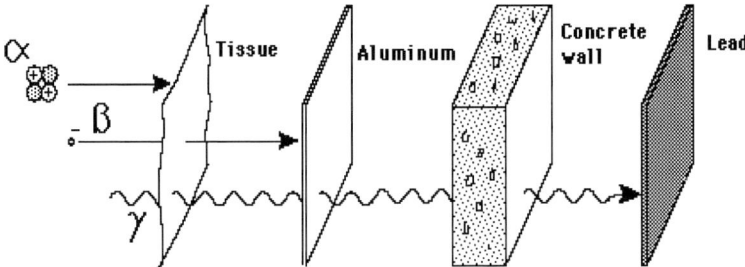

Figure 5.2 Radioactivity penetration.

but as an internalized radionuclide source, they can cause significant local damage. Beta particles are very light, charged particles that are primarily found in radiation fallout. These particles travel a short distance in tissue; but if large quantities are involved, they can produce radiation burns that are similar to a thermal burn. Sources of internal radiation contamination come from radioactive particles absorbed through open contaminated wounds or by inhaled and ingested radioactive material. Once internalized radioactive contaminates will cause ongoing radioactive exposure and radiations poisoning.

After exposure, the radiation effects can be grouped into acute and latent effects and are dependant on the radiation dose (Table 5.1). In the United States, the *radiation absorbed dose* (rad) is the measure of absorbed radiation. However, this is being replaced by the International System unit for radiation absorbed dose, the gray (Gy) (1 joule per kilogram); 1 Gy = 100 rad; 1 centigray (cGy) = 1 rad (Table 5.2). The earliest effects of radiation exposure are limited to early transient incapacitation (ETI) during extensive exposure and nausea and vomiting during lesser exposures. ETI is associated with very high acute doses of radiation (20–40 Gy) and has only occurred during fuel reprocessing accidents. This level of exposure is unlikely in a terror attack. After an initial brief loss of consciousness during ETI the patient lapses into coma within 1–3 days and dies from central nervous system dysfunction and vascular instability. The severity and onset of the other effects after radiation exposure is predictable. The three most significant radiosensitive organ systems in the body are the skin and mucosa, hematopoietic and the gastrointestinal systems. The specific effects that occur after a variable latent phase of days to weeks are (1) thermal burn-like effects to skin and mucosa, (2) gastrointestinal enteritis, (3) bone marrow suppression with immunological dysfunction and subsequent secondary infections, and, (4) hemorrhagic complications from thrombocytopenia.

5.3 Decontamination, Diagnosis, and Management

5.3.1 External Contamination and Injury

While information regarding the comprehensive medical management of radiation injury is extensive, there are general guidelines that apply to decontamination, diagnosis and management of radiological and combined injuries (Table 5.1). Ideally, decontamination should be preformed outside the hospital. Since this will not always be possible, decontamination procedures should be part of the operational plans of any treatment facility. A radiologic survey with an appropriate radioactivity detector (RADIAC, Geiger) should be systematically performed on all patients before and after decontamination (Figure 5.3). Decontamination consideration for non-injured casualties requires standard universal precaution and removal of patient clothing. Contaminated clothing should be carefully removed, placed in marked plastic bags, and removed to a secure location within a contaminated area. Removal of clothing can reduce radiological contaminants by as much as 90%.

Table 5.1 Acute Radiation Syndrome (1 Gray (Gy) = 100 rads; 1 centiGray (cGy) = 1 rad)

Phase of Syndrome	Feature	Whole body radiation from external radiation or internal absorption				
		Subclinical range		Sublethal range		Lethal range
		0–100 rad or cGy	100–200 rad 1–2 Gy	200–600 rad 2–6 Gy	600–800 rad 6–8 Gy	800–3000 rad 8–30 Gy	>3000 rad >30 Gy
Prodromal Phase	Nausea, vomiting	None	5–50%	50–100%	75–100%	90–100%	100%
	Time of onset		3–6 hrs	2–4 hrs	1–2 hrs	<1 hr	Minutes
	Duration		<24 hrs	<24 hrs	<48 hrs	<48 hrs	N/A
	Lymphocyte count	Unaffected	Minimally decreased	<1000 at 24 hr	<500 at 24hr	Decreases within hours	Decreases within hours
	CNS function	No impairment	No impairment	Routine task performance Cognitive impairment for 6–20 hrs	Simple and routine task performance Cognitive impairment for >24 hrs	Rapid incapacitation, may have a lucid interval of several hours	
Latent Phase (subclinical)	Absence of Symptoms	>2 wks	7–15 days	0–7 days	0–2 days	None	
Acute Radiation Illness or "Manifest illness" phase	Signs and symptoms	None	Moderate leukopenia	Severe leukopenia, purpura, hemorrhage Pneumonia Hair loss after 300 rad/3 Gy		Diarrhea Fever Electrolyte disturbance	Convulsions, Ataxia, Tremor, Lethargy
	Time of onset		>2 wks	2 days to 2 wks		1–3 days	
	Critical period		None	4–6 wks – Most potential for effective medical intervention		2–14 days	1–48 hrs
	Organ system	None		Hematopoietic and respiratory (mucosal) systems		GI tract Mucosal systems	CNS
Hospitalization	% Duration	0	<5% 45–60 days	90% 60–90 days	100% 90+ days	100% weeks to months	100% days to weeks
Mortality		None	Minimal	Low with aggressive therapy	High	Very high, significant neurological symptoms indicate lethal dose	

Table 5.2 Radioactivity Nomenclature

	Radio-activity	Absorbed dose	Dose equivalent	Exposure
Common units	Curie (Ci)	Rad	Rem	Roentgen (R)
SI units	Becquerel (Bq)	Gray (Gy)	Sievert (Sv)	Coulomb/kilogram (C/kg)

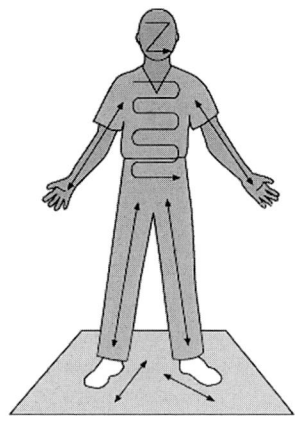

Figure 5.3 Systematic survey for radiologic contamination AFRR1.

Passing a radiation detector over the entire body can readily assess the presence of radiological contamination. The goal should be less than 1 mrem per hour of beta and 1000 disintegrations per min alpha radiation. If present, decontamination of the skin and hair is accomplished by washing. However, open wounds should be covered before decontamination to prevent further contamination. Care should be taken to avoid scrubbing or abrading the skin as this can break the protective barrier of the skin and introduce contaminates. If practical, the decontamination effluent should be sequestered and disposed of appropriately. For all patients with confirmed or suspected exposure, a complete blood count should be obtained on presentation and after 24 hours to determine the absolute lymphocyte count. At 24 hours, an absolute lymphocyte count $<1000/mm^3$ suggests moderate exposure and $<500/mm^3$ suggests severe exposure. All body orifices (each nostril, ears, mouth, and rectum) should be swabbed and a 24-hour stool and urine collection should be done if internal contamination is considered. The swabs and 24-hour collections should be assayed for radioactivity. This information will help determine the extent of the exposure, need for internal decontamination, and prognosis (Table 5.1).

In the case of injury and radiological exposure, aggressive therapy will be required to allow survival. Surgical priorities for acute or life-threatening injury must precede any treatment priority for associated radiation injury. Because radiologic contamination poses little risk to health care providers, these patients are prioritized by standard trauma protocols. In the presence of traumatic injury, hypotension must be considered to be due to hypovolemia and not radiological injury. While the skin is impermeable to most radionuclides, particles can be absorbed through wounds. Therefore, contaminated wounds should be decontaminated with copious irrigation. It should be noted that any residual fluid in the wound might hide weak beta and alpha emissions from detectors. Because wound healing is markedly compromised by radiation injury, open wounds that are allowed to heal by secondary intention will serve as a potentially fatal nidus of infection in the radiologically injured patient. If possible, all wounds should be extensively debrided and closed as soon as possible.

Patients with combined trauma and radiological contamination pose a significant challenge to the medical system. Given the immunosuppressive effects of radiation exposure and associated delayed wound healing, there is a narrow time window for accomplishing definitive and reconstructive surgical care (Figure 5.4). The surgical correction of injuries must be done within 36–48 hours post injury or delayed 6–8 weeks. The surgical system maybe faced with a large number of patients who need surgical correction of wounds within a narrow window of time. This differs from the normal time course of routine trauma and could put a large burden on the medical system caring for these patients while they recover from their radiation illness with untreated wounds.

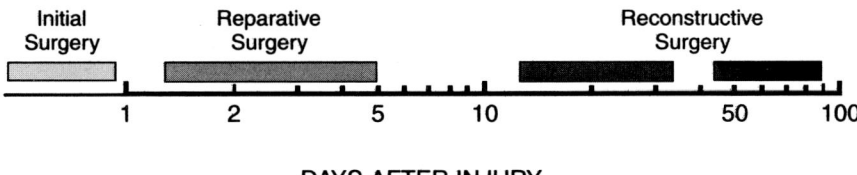
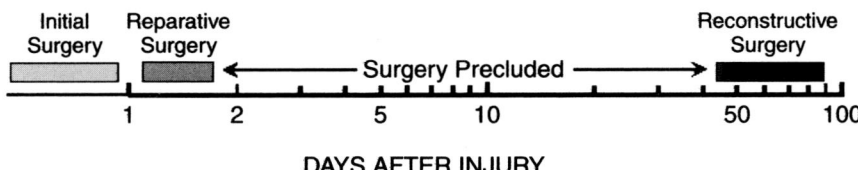

Figure 5.4 Trauma timecourse.

5.3.2 Internal Contamination

After inhalation, particles less than 5 μm in diameter can be deposited in the alveoli. Larger particles will be limited to the mucociliary apparatus of the tracheobronchial tree or the oropharynx. In either area, soluble particles will be absorbed into the blood stream via the lymphatic system. Insoluble particles will continue to irradiate surrounding tissues until cleared from the respiratory tract. This will cause inflammation and result in fibrosis and scarring. Absorption of ingested radioactive particles depends on the solubility of the contaminant. Iodine 131 and cesium 127 are rapidly absorbed by the gut while plutonium, radium, and strontium are not. The lower GI tract is the target organ for insoluble particles that pass unchanged in the feces.

For internal contamination, decontamination is also indicated. This will reduce the ongoing radioactive injury. Recommendations can be obtained by a Radiation Safety Officer or Nuclear Medicine Physician. There are several medications and chemicals that can be used for internal decontamination.

Prussian or Berlin blue is ferric ferrocyanide. This chemical is not absorbed by the gastrointestinal (GI) tract and works through two modes of action. It decreases the absorption of many radionuclides from the GI tract and removes some radionuclides from the capillary bed surrounding the intestine and prevents their reabsorption. Prussian blue is effective in removing cesium, thallium, and rubidium by the fecal route. It has been used, without serious side effects, outside the United States to treat humans for cesium 137 internal contamination. Main side effects are nausea, vomiting, constipation and staining. Prussian blue decreases the biological half-life of cesium 137 to 30 per cent of the original 100 days. Prussian blue is approved as an investigational new drug; Radiation Emergency Assistance Center/Training Site (REAC/TS) has the license for research use.

If radioiodine (reactor accident) is considered, prophylactic potassium iodide (Lugol's Solution) should be administered within the first 24 hours to be efficacious. If given within 30 minutes of exposure to iodine-131, potassium iodide prevents the uptake of iodine-131 by the thyroid gland. Potassium iodide should be given for 7–14 days to prevent the uptake of recycled iodine-131. The recommended daily dose of iodide is 300 mg given as 390 mg of potassium iodide. Any readily available soluble form of iodine with equivalent iodide content is suitable. Potassium perchlorate (200 mg by mouth daily) may be given to individuals who are sensitive to iodine.

5.3.3 Mobilizing Agents

Mobilizing agents are compounds that increase the metabolic rate of internal contaminants, resulting in an increase in elimination. Examples of mobilizing agents are the anti-thyroid medications propylthiouracil, methimazole, and potassium thiocyanate. These medications reduce the manufacture of thyroid hormone (T3 and T4) reduce the presence of radioactive iodine in this critical organ. Iodine, which has not been oxidized and incorporated into thyroid hormone, is excreted at a much faster rate. However, the toxicity of these three anti-thyroid drugs and the relative ineffectiveness make them less appealing for use than potassium iodide.

Ammonium chloride, an acidifying salt given orally, mobilizes strontium from body tissues and, if given with calcium gluconate intravenously, causes a 40–75 per cent decrease in body stores of strontium over a period of 3–6 days. The combined treatment is most effective if given early after strontium deposition, but some effectiveness is still demonstrated if given as late as 2 weeks after deposition.

Diuretics are known to decrease sodium, potassium, and chloride serum levels. In theory, diuretics may be useful in reducing sodium-22, sodium-24, potassium-42, and tritium levels.

Chelators are mobilizing agents that enhance the elimination of metals from critical organs. Chelators are organic compounds (ligands) that exchange less firmly bonded ions for metal ions. The kidney then excretes the stable chelator-metal complex. Chelation therapy has been used for lead, mercury, arsenic, and other heavy metals. New chelators, including DMSA (meso-2,3,-dimercaptosurrinic acid) for lead toxicity and DMPS (2,3 dimercapto-1-propanesulfonic acid) for mercury toxicity, have not been used for metals, including plutonium and americium.

One of the older chelators, CaEDTA (calcium ethylenediaminetetraacetate), was used extensively in the past to treat lead intoxication, and it has been used to treat plutonium and americium toxicity. Given intravenously or intramuscularly, it has significant side effects, including gastrointestinal upset, pain at the injection site, bone marrow depression, and nephrotoxicity.

The chelator DTPA (diethylenetriaminepentaacetic acid), in the zinc (Zn) or calcium (Ca) salt state, can form stable soluble complexes with a large number of metal ions. When DTPA releases its calcium or zinc, it binds to soluble plutonium, americium, or curium and carries it to the kidneys where it is then excreted in the urine. The plasma half-life of CaDTPA is 20–60 minutes. No accumulation of DTPA occurs in tissues or specific organs. CaDTPA is approximately 10 times more effective than ZnDTPA for initial chelation of transuranics. Therefore, CaDTPA should be used whenever larger body burdens of transuranics are involved. DTPA has been shown to greatly reduce the uptake of absorbed plutonium-239 if given within an hour of contamination. The most effective dose schedules have not been determined. As with most chelators, it is more effective when it is given earlier. Both salts can be given intravenously or as a nasal inhalant. Dose recommendations are, for adults, 1 g in 100–250 cc of normal saline infused intravenously over 3–4 minutes and repeated on 5 successive days per week. Given through the aerosolized route, 1 g in a 4 cc vial is placed in a nebulizer, and the entire volume is inhaled over 3–4 minutes and repeated daily. DTPA is distributed by Oak Ridge Associate Universities under contract with the U.S. Department of Energy as an investigational new drug.

The initial care of radiologic casualties with moderate and severe radiation exposure should include early measures to reduce pathogen acquisition. These could include low-microbial-content food, clean water supplies, frequent hand washing, and air filtration. When possible, oral feeding is preferred to intravenous feeding to maintain the immunologic and physiologic integrity of the gut.

During the neutropenic phase of the radiation syndrome, the prevention and management of infection is the mainstay of therapy. These patients should be treated with a hospitals standard regimen for neutropenic patients [6–8]. Empirical antibiotic regimens should be selected based on the pattern of bacterial susceptibility and nosocomial infections in each institution. In addition, hematopoietic growth factors, such as filgrastim (Neupogen®), a granulocyte colony-stimulating factor (G-CSF), and sargramostim (Leukine®), a granulocyte-macrophage colony-stimulating factor (GM-CSF), are potent stimulators of hematopoiesis and may shorten the duration of neutropenia and thus reduce morbidity and mortality [9–11]. As with all neutropenic patients, blood products administered should be fresh, irradiated and CMV negative.

In summary, it is obvious that terrorist groups have investigated actions using radiological material or nuclear devices. If such an attack were to occur, the strain on medical resources will be significant due to the severity of bone marrow suppression that occurs after even moderate exposure to radioactive substances and delayed wound healing that accompanies radiological contamination of wounds. However, the relatively slow onset of the syndromes and the advances in medical care will dramatically improve the survivability of such injuries.

References

1. V. A. Kashparov, D. H. Oughton, S. I. Zvarich, V. P. Protsak, and S. E. Levchuk. Kinetics of fuel particle weathering and 90Sr mobility in the Chernobyl 30-km exclusion zone. *Health Phys* 76:251–259, 1999.
2. T. Takatsuji, H. Sato, J. Takada, S. Endo, M. Hoshi, V. F. Sharifov, I. I. Veselkina, I. V. Pilenko, W. A. Kalimullin, V. B. Masyakin, A. I. Kovalev, I. Yoshikawa, and S. Okajima. Relationship between the 137Cs whole-body counting results and soil and food contamination in farms near Chernobyl. *Health Phys* 78:86–89, 2000.
3. A. Abbott and S. Barker. Chernobyl damage "underestimated". *Nature* 380:658, 1996.
4. V. K. Ivanov, A. I. Gorski, M. A. Maksioutov, A. F. Tsyb, and G. N. Souchkevitch. Mortality among the Chernobyl emergency workers: estimation of radiation risks (preliminary analysis). *Health Phys* 81:514–521, 2001.
5. F. H. Mettler, D. V. Becker, B. W. Wachholz, and A. C. Bouville. Chernobyl: 10 years later. *J Nucl Med* 37:24N, 26N–27N, 1996.
6. J. N. Greene, D. C. Linch, and C. B. Miller. Current treatments for infection in neutropenic patients with hematologic malignancy. *Oncology (Huntingt)* 14:31–34, 2000.
7. J. Klastersky. Empirical treatment of sepsis in neutropenic patients. *Hosp Med* 62:101–103, 2001.
8. G. I. Reeves. Radiation injuries. *Crit Care Clin* 15:457–473, 1999.
9. G. Freyer, B. Ligneau, and V. Trillet-Lenoir. Colony-stimulating factors in the prevention of solid tumors induced by chemotherapy in patients with febrile neutropenia. *Int J Antimicrob Agents* 10:3–9, 1998.
10. E. B. Rubenstein. Colony stimulating factors in patients with fever and neutropenia. *Int J Antimicrob Agents* 16:117–121, 2000.
11. S. Serke. Hematopoietic growth factors as an adjunct for neutropenic patients in the ICU: still a controversial issue. *Intensive Care Med* 25:901–902, 1999.

Radiological Casualty Related Websites

1. www.afrri.usuhs.mil
2. www.orau.gov/reacts/default.htm
3. www. radefx.bcm.tmc.edu/ionizing/ionizing.htm
4. http://www.epa.gov/radiation/rert/
5. http://www.doctrine.usmc.mil/mcrp/view/mcr4111b/mcr4111b.pdf
6. http://www.fema.gov/pte/rep/

Appendix   Terrorism with Ionizing Radiation General Guidance Pocket Guide

Diagnosis: Be Alert to the Following

- Acute radiation syndrome (Table 5.1) follows a predictable pattern after substantial exposure or catastrophic events
- Victims may also present individually, as described in Table 5.3, over a longer period

of time after exposure to contaminated sources hidden in the community
- Specific syndromes of concern, especially with a 2–3 week prior history of nausea and vomiting, are
  - thermal burn-like skin lesions without documented heat exposure
  - immunological dysfunction with secondary infections
  - a tendency to bleed (epistaxis, gingival bleeding, and petechiae)
  - marrow suppression (neutropenia, lymphonenia, and thrombocytopenia)
  - epilation (hair loss)

Understanding Exposure
- Exposure may be known and recognized or clandestine through
  - large radiation exposures, such as a nuclear bomb or catastrophic damage to a nuclear power station
  - small radiation source emitting continuous gamma radiation producing chronic intermittent exposures (such as radiological sources from medical treatment or industrial devices.)
- Exposure to RADIATION may result from any one or combination of the following
  - external sources (such as radiation from an uncontrolled nuclear reaction or radioisotope outside the body)
  - skin contamination with radioactive material ("external contamination")
  - internal radiation from absorbed, inhaled, or ingested radioactive material ("internal contamination")

Confirmation of Cases
- Contact radiation safety officer (RSO) for help
- For help in projecting clinical effects, contact
  - nuclear medicine physician
  - Medical Radiological Advisory Team (MRAT) at Armed Forces Radiobiology Research Institute (AFRRI) 301-295-0530
- Obtain complete blood count
  - absolute lymphocyte count $< 1000\,mm^3$ suggests moderate exposure
  - absolute lymphocyte count $< 500\,mm^3$ suggests severe exposure
  - Acute, short-term rise in neutrophil count
- Swab both nares
- Collect 24 hour stool if GI contamination is possible
- Collect 24 hour urine if internal contamination with radionuclides is possible

Decontamination Considerations
- Externally irradiated patients are not contaminated
- Treating contaminated patients before decontamination may contaminate the facility: plan for decontamination before arrival
- Exposure without contamination requires no decontamination (RSO measurement)
- Exposure with contamination requires Universal Precautions, removal of patient clothing, and decontamination with soap and water
- For internal contamination, contact the RSO and/or Nuclear Medicine Physician
- Patient with life-threatening condition: treat, then decontaminate Patient with non-life-threatening condition: decontaminate, then treat

Treatment Considerations
- If life-threatening conditions are present, treat them first
- If external radioactive contaminants are present, decontaminate
- If radioiodine (reactor accident) is present, consider protecting the thyroid gland with prophylactic potassium iodide if within first few hours only (ineffective later) (Table 5.4)

- Review http://www.afrri.usuhs.mil or http://www.orau.gov/reacts/guidance.htm

Institutional Reporting

- If reasonable suspicion of a radiation event, contact hospital leadership (Chief of Staff, Hospital Director, etc)
- Immediately discuss hospital emergency planning implications

Public Health Reporting

- Contact local public health office (city, county or State)
- If needed, contact the FBI (for location of nearest office, see http://www.fbi.gov/contact/fo/info.htm)

Produced by the Employee Education System for the Office of Public Health and Environmental Hazards, Department of Veterans Affairs.

Table 5.3 Symptom Clusters as Delayed Effects after Radiation Exposures

Headache	Partial and full thickness
Fatigue	skin damage
Weakness	Epilation (hair loss)
	Ulceration
Anorexia	Lymphopenia
Nausea	Neutropenia
Vomiting	Thrombopenia
Diarrhea	Purpura
	Opportunistic infections

Table 5.4 Potassium Iodide Dosages

Age group	Dosage* (mg)
Infants <1 month	16
Children 1 months to 3 yrs	32
Children 3–18 yrs	65
Adults	130

*The information in this card is not meant to be complete but to be a quick guide; please consult other references and expert opinion, and check drug dosages particularly for pregnancy and children.

6 Nerve and Chemical Agents

PAUL D. MONGAN AND JAMES WINKLEY

Disclaimer

All statements and opinions are the author's, and are not official positions or policies of the Uniformed Services University, the Department of Defense, or the US federal government.

6.1 Introduction

Chemical warfare agents have been used by armies and for hundreds of years. In the twentieth century chemical engineering and technological advances improved the variety, delivery, and lethality of these agents. Many agents were used in the early 1900s during World War I and since then more have been discovered and tons stockpiled. Fortunately, excluding World War I, their use has been limited to a few short military conflicts and small radical terrorist group activities.

Offensive use of chemical agents continues to be attractive to some nations and terrorist organizations. Chemical agents can be dispersed over large areas, penetrate structures, kill or sicken entire populations, and overwhelm medical resources. They can be employed against specific targets, including headquarters and control centers and, depending on the chemical agent or combination of agents, the effects can be immediate or delayed incapacitation, disorientation, or death. The psychological impact is ever-present as troops, public servants and populations can be turned to chaos just from a perceived threat. Many of the more common classic chemical agents can be produced inexpensively and quietly, and stored indefinitely. Their minimal cost has earned chemical warfare agents the appellation "the poor man's atomic bomb."

Although treaties dealing with control or elimination of classic chemical weapons may reduce the danger that chemical warfare agents will ever be used, enforcing these treaties is difficult. Controlling the manufacturing, acquisition, and storage of precursor chemicals make chemical war and terrorism a continuing concern for the U.S. government.

Threat of chemical agent proliferation and use has not decreased. Saddam Hussein's use of chemical warfare against the Kurds in 1988 demonstrates how readily such weapons can be used, even within the confines of one's own country. The 1994 and 1995 incidents involving the Aum Shinrikyo cult use of the nerve agent sarin to cause fatalities and disruption in Matsumoto and in the Tokyo subway system demonstrate how easily a terrorist organization can quietly produce and use a classic chemical warfare agent.

6.2 Nerve Agents

6.2.1 History

Nerve agents are extremely toxic chemicals that were developed in Germany for military use before and during World War II. By the end of World War II Germany had produced and weaponized approximately 25,000 tons of tabun and sarin [1]. While the use of these weapons would have probably altered the outcome of the war, German scientists had tested nerve agents on inmates of concentration camps to determine their lethality and to aid in the development of antidotes [2]. Near the end of World War II, United States and the United Kingdom troops captured some of these munitions at a German testing facility in Raubkammer. The munitions were taken to the United Kingdom Chemical Defense Establishment for examination and a group of scientists determined the pharmacology and toxicity of tabun and documented the antidotal activity of atropine after the miosis caused by accidental exposure to vaporized Tabun [3].

While many countries developed and weaponized nerve agents it was not until March 1984 when Iraq used tabun filled aerial bombs against Iranian soldiers in the Iran–Iraq War. The Iraqis continued to use tabun in addition to sarin until the end of the war in August 1988. In addition to the use of nerve agents against Iranian soldiers, in March of 1988 Iraq soldiers killed hundreds of Iraqi Kurds in the town of Halabja (population 80,000) during aerial bombing raids a day after troops from the Kurdish Patriotic Union of Kurdistan (PUK) entered the town. These attacks involved multiple chemical agents—including mustard gas, and the nerve agents SARIN, TABUN and VX, and possibly cyanide [4].

In June 1994, members of Aum Shinrikyo, a Japanese cult, released sarin in an apartment complex in Matsumoto, Japan. In this attack there were almost 300 casualties, including 7 dead [5]. This cult followed with another attack in March 1995 when five two-man teams released nerve gas in Tokyo's subway cars by puncturing liquid sarin-filled plastic bags (30% full strength). This resulted in over 5500 "casualties" seeking medical attention of which 984 were moderately poisoned and held for observation or treatment. Fifty-four were severely poisoned; of which 12 died [6]. While much attention is given to nerve agents the potential enormity of the chemical threat to civilian population was fully displayed in the 1984 industrial accident that released methylisocyanate and chlorine gas over Indian city of Bhopal. Of the estimated 38,000 immediate inhalation casualties, some 8000 eventually died [7].

While industrial terrorism remains a reality, the pragmatic choice for small-unit terrorist action for chemical weapon deployment is the highly vaporizable G-series of nerve agents.

6.2.2 Physical Characteristics

The three G agents, GA (tabun), GB (sarin), and GD (soman), are moderately volatile liquids at normal temperatures (Table 6.1). Though all the nerve agents can be absorbed through the skin, because the G agents are volatile they require larger topical doses for toxicity. Thus, the primary risk of these agents is by inhaling the vapor or aerosol. While vapor or aerosol effects occur within minutes the risk of injury after dermal exposure is prolonged because, even if skin decontamination occurs, continued absorption from the inner layers of the skin can result in a delayed onset of symptoms for as long as 18 hours.

The highly volatile G-agent (sarin) stands out as a terrorist weapon because of it is the most volatile at room temperature and the toxicity of the resultant vapor is quite high. Because of the small amount required for toxic effects it can be transported covertly as clear liquid sealed in a container that can be vaporized when exposed to air. In addition, because of the volatility a small amount of sarin

Table 6.1 Nerve agent toxicological and physical properties

Agent	Volatility[a]	Boiling point °C	Vapor density[b]	Vapor toxicity Ct_{50} (mg min m^{-3})[c]		Skin toxicity	
				Miosis	Death	Death LD_{50} (mg)[d]	Aging
Tabun (GA)	610	240	5.6	2–3	400	1000	Hours
Sarin (GB)	22,000	158	4.7	3–5	100	1700	Hours
Soman (GD)	3900	198	6.3	2–3	70	350	2 min
VX	10.5	298	9.2		50	10	Hours

Information consolidated from text and tables in unclassified military and civilian sources
[a] Volatility is the amount (mg) of agent in 1 m^3 at 25°C.
[b] Vapor Density is compared to air.
[c] Ct_{50}—the product of concentration [C] of the nerve agent over time t[t] o produce effects in 50% of those exposed to vapor or aerosol.
[d] LD_{50}—Dose of liquid nerve gas placed on the skin that will cause death in one half of exposed subjects.

on clothing or skin rapidly evaporates. This eases the work of resource intensive decontamination that is required for the agents with lesser volatility.

Compared to the volatile nerve agents the oily consistency of VX requires cutaneous absorption for toxic effects. Though VX is an extremely lethal the onset is slow. Because the agent that clings to skin and clothing it requires total body protection for rescuers and exhaustive decontamination of victims and environment. As a terrorist weapon however, the necessity for a liquid dispersion system makes VX an unlikely candidate for inflicting casualties.

6.2.3 Mechanism of Toxicity

Nerve agents are organophosphate cholinesterase inhibitors that inhibit cholinesterase enzymes (butyrylcholinesterase in the plasma, acetylcholinesterase on the red cell, and acetylcholinesterase at cholinergic receptor sites in tissue). The primary clinical effect of nerve agents is to inhibit acetylcholinesterase in the cholinergic nervous system so that the neurotransmitter acetylcholine cannot be hydrolyzed. Acetylcholine is the neurotransmitter of the neurons to skeletal muscle (nicotinic receptors), of the pre-ganglionic autonomic nerves (nicotinic receptors), and of the post-ganglionic parasympathetic nerves (muscarinic receptors). Due to blockade of acetylcholinesterase, acetylcholine cannot be metabolized and continues to stimulate the receptors. The clinical effects from nerve agent exposure are caused by excess acetylcholine causing the signs and symptoms of poisoning (Table 6.2).

Nerve agents combine with cholinesterase at the esteratic site, and the stability of the bond depends on the structure of the nerve agent. Cleavage of the nerve agent with reactivated enzyme can only be achieved by administration of an oxime therapeutic agent. Oximes are the most effective agents for reactivation of enzymatic activity. If oximes are not administered within a defined period of time the nerve agent–enzyme complex becomes refractory to oxime reactivation of the enzyme. This process is known as aging. Thus, the enzyme may remain indefinitely inhibited and return of enzymatic activity occurs only with the synthesis of new enzyme. For most nerve agents, the aging time is longer than the time within which acute casualties will be seen.

Table 6.2 Receptor related effects of nerve agent poisoning

Peripheral Nervous System		Central Nervous System
Muscarinic	Nicotinic	
Diarrhea	Mydriasis	Confusion
Urination	Tachycardia	Convulsions
Miosis	Weakness	Coma
Bradycardia	Hypertension	
Bronchorrhea, bronchospasm	Hyperglycemia	
Emesis	Fasciculations	
Lacrimation		
Salivation, secretion, sweating		

The initial effects of nerve agent exposure depends on the dose (Table 6.1) and route of exposure with the initial effects of differing vastly from vapor exposure and exposure to liquid agent on the skin (Tables 6.3 and 6.4).

Initial exposure to low concentrations of nerve agent vapor produces local effects in the eyes, nose, and airways and does not necessarily indicate systemic absorption of the agent. These effects start seconds to minutes after exposure and maximal effects peak within minutes after exposure. However, a small amount of liquid agent on the skin causes localized sweating, blanching, and fasciculations. The onset of gastrointestinal systems indicates systemic effects after dermal exposure. Regardless of the route of exposure lethal systemic absorption of vapor or liquid causes a rapid cascade of events that result in loss of consciousness and convulsive activity, followed by apnea and muscular flaccidity within several minutes.

6.2.4 Signs, Symptoms and Severity of Exposure

6.2.4.1 Ocular, Nasal and Airway effects

The characteristic signs of exposure to nerve agent vapor is miosis that can be accompanied

Table 6.3 Nerve agent effects—vapor exposure

Severity	Symptoms		Onset	Treatment
Mild/moderate	Eyes	Miosis	Seconds to minutes	Atropine eye drops
		Dim vision		Atropine (IV or IM)
		Headache		Oximes (IV or IM)
	Nose	Rhinorrhea		
	Mouth	Salivation		
	Lungs	Dyspnea		
Severe	Severe difficulty breathing or apnea		Seconds to minutes	Atropine (IV)
	Generalized muscle twitching, weakness			Oximes (IV)
	or paralysis Loss of bowel or bladder control			Diazepam (IV)
	Convulsions Loss of consciousness			

Table 6.4 Nerve agent effects—liquid exposure

Severity	Symptoms	Onset	Treatment
Mild/moderate	Muscle fasciculations and sweating at exposure site	Minutes to 18 hours	Atropine (IV or IM)
	Nausea and vomiting		Oximes (IV or IM)
	Weakness		
Severe	Difficulty breathing or apnea	Minutes to 1 hours	Atropine (IV)
	Muscle twitching, weakness or paralysis		Oximes (IV)
	Loss of bowel or bladder control		Diazepam (IV)
	Convulsions		
	Loss of consciousness		

by complaints of pain, dim and/or blurred vision. Miosis will begin within seconds or minutes after the onset of exposure to agent vapor, but it may not be complete for many minutes if the vapor concentration is low. Very low levels of nerve agent can cause these effects, as observed after the 1995 nerve agent attack on the subway system in Tokyo. In that disaster a small number of health care workers at the hospital exhibited these ocular signs secondary to vapor release from patient clothing [8,9]. In contrast, liquid agent exposure to the skin will not cause miosis if the amount of liquid is small unless it is in or near the eye. Only moderate to large amounts of systemically absorbed nerve agent will also result in miosis. Topical homatropine or atropine in the eye can relieve the miosis, pain, and dim vision.

Vapor exposure to nerve agent vapor also increases secretions from exocrine glands, such as the lacrimal, nasal, salivary, and bronchial glands. Rhinorrhea is also an early indication of vapor exposure to nerve agents. If sufficient vapor is inhaled bronchoconstriction and increased airway secretions will present in a dose-related manner. Subjectively the patient may complain of chest tightness and possibly trouble breathing. Apnea can occur within minutes after the exposure to a large amount of nerve agent and is primarily centrally mediated though muscle weakness can play a significant contributing role.

6.2.4.2 Gastrointestinal effects

After exposure to a large dose of nerve agent there is an increase in gastrointestinal motility and secretions along with nausea and vomiting. In the absence of ocular and airway complaints these are the earliest findings of systemic absorption after liquid exposure on the skin. If the absorbed dose in large enough diarrhea may occur with large amounts.

6.2.4.3 Dermal and skeletal muscle effects

Generalized sweating after a large liquid or vapor exposure is common. The first effect on skeletal muscle is muscular fasciculations and twitching. After a large exposure, systemic absorption results in fatigue and weakness of muscles that is rapidly followed by flaccid paralysis.

6.2.4.4 Central nervous system (CNS)

The CNS signs after nerve agent exposure are due to neurotransmitter accumulation and a large exposure will rapidly cause loss of consciousness, seizure activity, and apnea. However, they may be preceded by an asymptomatic period of 1–30 minutes after contact of small amounts of liquid nerve agent with the skin. Prolonged CNS effects (weeks to months) after nerve agent exposure are variable and nonspecific. They may include forgetfulness, an inability to concentrate fully, insomnia, nightmares, impaired judgment, and depression. Confusion and hallucinations are not a part of this symptom cluster.

6.2.4.5 Cardiovascular effects

Cardiovascular effects after nerve agent exposure are variable and often not present. Parasympathetic tone and a slow heart rate may be present and bradyarrhythmias (first-, second-, or third-degree heart block) may occur. However, other factors such as fright, hypoxia, and adrenergic stimulation may cause the heart rate may be high, low, or in the normal range. The blood pressure may be in the normal range or elevated from adrenergic factors.

6.2.4.6 Minimal to mild vapor exposure

Patients in this category present with any or all of miosis, rhinorrhea, dim vision, and moderate eye or head pain. This can occur during primary exposure or as a secondary exposure to improperly decontaminated casualties. This occurred in the Tokyo subway attack when healthcare workers secondarily exposed to sarin vapors from victims reported dim vision and miosis. The important decision in this group is that the exposure was terminated by evacuation from the contaminated area. While exposed the care required is minimal and can easily be treated with eye drops. The goal is to provide the necessary decontamination (removal of clothing) and minimal care to enable others with more serious injuries to receive therapy. Because of the small quantity necessary to cause injury from liquid exposure any localized dermal effects should be considered a potential moderate casualty and observed for further symptoms.

6.2.4.7 Moderate vapor or liquid exposure

Patients in this category may be able to ambulate with assistance because of visual disturbance, muscle weakness, or both and may complain of dyspnea, chest pain, or both. Nausea is frequent and vomiting common after moderate exposure. Localized muscle groups may fasciculate and heart rate and blood pressure are unpredictable with bradycardia being a rare finding. Thorough decontamination and intramuscular or intravenous atropine and oximes are appropriate for this group.

6.2.4.8 Severe vapor or liquid exposure

Casualties experience pronounced respiratory difficulty with drooling, miosis, rhinorrhea, and asthma-like wheezing. The upper and lower airway secretions severely impair gas flow and oxygen exchange and the skin is damp, pale, and dusky. Airway resistance can be as high as 50–60 cm of water due to bronchoconstriction and secretions. Heart rate and blood pressure are unpredictable. Patients may be unresponsive, convulsing intermittently, and apnea may be imminent. After the onset of flaccid muscle paralysis ongoing convulsive activity is no longer observed. If resources are available, airway control, positive pressure ventilation along with intravenous atropine, diazepam and oximes may be life saving.

6.2.5 Medical Management

Complete management of a person exposed to nerve agent requires any or all of the following: decontamination, administration of the antidotes, ventilation, and other supportive therapy. The condition of the patient dictates the need for each of these and the order in which they are done. Complete information on skin decontamination is described elsewhere. However, as observed in treatment of the Tokyo subway victims, after vapor exposure clothing should be removed because it may contain "trapped" vapor. The need for ventilation will depend on the severity of pulmonary symptoms [10].

Three drugs are used to treat nerve agent exposure; atropine, pralidoxime chloride (oxime), and diazepam.

6.2.5.1 *Atropine*

Atropine is a cholinergic blocking agent. It is extremely effective in blocking the effects of excess acetylcholine at peripheral muscarinic sites. The end point of therapy is a reduction in symptoms. In mild cases that only have ocular symptoms this may require atropine (or homatropine) eye drops. However, a severe injury from nerve agent vapor exposure will have copious secretions from the nose, mouth and lungs with severe difficulty breathing and or apnea. Advanced cases be unconscious and have flaccid or convulsive activity. Atropine, 2 mg, should be repeated at 5–10 minute intervals and should be titrated to pulmonary symptoms (Table 6.5). The adequacy of atropine dosing is gauged by improvement in ventilation with suctioning of secretions and the reduction in bronchoconstriction. Because of the short half-life, atropine should be re-administered every few hours and can easily total 20–50 mg/d in severely injured adults with ventilation being required from 30 minutes to hours. A moderately exposed patient will need to be administered atropine until breathing comfortably. The preferred route of atropine administration for severe exposure is intravenous as therapeutic blood levels of atropine appear within minutes in healthy volunteers with intramuscular injection. However, intramuscular absorption is unpredictable when muscle perfusion declines as circulation fails in severe exposure.

6.2.5.2 *Pralidoxime chloride*

Pralidoxime chloride (Protopam chloride) is an oxime with dosing recommendations listed in Table 6.6. It attaches to the nerve agent that is inhibiting the cholinesterase and breaks the agent–enzyme bond to restore the normal activity of the enzyme. This uncoupling of the nerve agent–enzyme bond regenerates the esterase to resume hydrolysis of acetylcholine at the neuromuscular junction, effectively reversing the nicotinic crisis with a decrease in abnormal activity in skeletal muscle and return of normal strength. Since the effects of an oxime are not apparent in organs with muscarinic receptors, oximes do not cause a decrease in secretions, it is necessary to co-administer oximes with atropine to reduce secretions. Oxines also are less useful after aging occurs (nerve agent de-alkylates to form an irreversible covalent bond). Sarin (GA) and tabun (GB) age slowly and pralidoxime may still be effective when supplies eventually catch up with demand. Soman (GD), conversely, ages within minutes. However, Soman (GD) is an unlikely terrorist agent due to its low volatility.

Pralidoxime chloride should be mixed in normal saline over 20–30 minutes as more rapid administration will cause hypertension.

Table 6.5 Atropine dosing

Patient	Dosing recommendation
Adults	2 mg intravenous every 5–10 min (every 20 minutes for IM dosing) until decrease in symptoms
Adolescent	2.0 mg maximum single dose intravenous every 5–10 min (every 20 minutes for IM dosing) until decrease in symptoms
Child (2–10 years old)	1 mg intravenous dose every 5–10 min until decrease in symptoms mg/kg
Infant (<2 years old)	0.5 mg maximum single dose intravenous every 5–10 min (every 20 minutes for IM dosing) until decrease in symptoms repeated as clinically indicated

6.2.5.3 Diazepam

Diazepam is a benzodiazepine used to decrease convulsive activity and reduce the brain damage caused by prolonged seizure activity. The adult and adolescent dose is 10 mg and the dose for children is 0.05–0.3 mg/kg with a maximum single dose of 5 mg. Diazepam may be repeated every 15–30 minutes to control the seizure activity. After the onset of paralysis electrical seizure bursts continue even though the skeletal muscle activity is not apparent.

6.2.5.4 Supportive care

Severely exposed patients may require up to several days of assisted or controlled ventilation in addition to treatment for residual muscarinism (sweating, wheezing, or salivation) and neuromuscular dysfunction. The experience in Japan shows that partial acetylcholinestrase regeneration sufficed to restore neuromuscular transmission within days. Nerve agents can also affect the circulation adversely through vagal stimulation and the loss of substantial quantities of fluids and electrolytes from exocrine gland secretions, vomitus, and diarrhea. IV fluids readily restore circulating volume and atropine promptly reverses the muscarinic crisis. Thus circulatory collapse is of less concern in managing nerve agent casualties than respiratory impairment.

6.3 Cyanide

6.3.1 History

Cyanide is ubiquitous in nature and nearly all living organisms have enzymes to detoxify it. The fruits and seeds, especially pits, of many plants, such as cherries, peaches, almonds, and lima beans contain cyanogens capable of releasing free cyanide following enzymatic degradation [11]. The edible portion (the roots) of the cassava plant (widely used as a food staple in many parts of the world) is also cyanogenic [12]. Still cyanide has been used through out history as a poison. Nero of Rome used cherry laurel water to poison members of his family and others who displeased him. Napoleon III proposed the use of cyanide on soldier's bayonets to enhance effectiveness. Cyanides are also called "blood agents," an antiquated term of military classification from World War I. At the time of the introduction of cyanide in World War I, the other chemical agents in use caused mainly local effects. In contrast, inhaled cyanide produces systemic effects and was thought to be carried in the blood; hence the term "blood agent." The French used about 4000 tons of cyanide in World War I without notable military success because the small one- to two-pound munitions used could not deliver the large amounts needed to cause biological effects. During World War II the Nazi's used Zyklon B, a cyanide based rodentcide, to kill millions of prisoners of war and Jews. In the late 1980s cyanide-like agents may have been used against the inhabitants of the Syrian city of Hama and the Kurdish city of Halabja, Iraq, and Shahabad, Iran during the Iran–Iraq War. In 1978 the followers of the reverend Jim Jones committed mass suicide by drinking cyanide laced Kool-Aid, and cyanide laced Tylenol was responsible for multiple deaths in Washington State in

Table 6.6 Pralidoxime chloride dosing

Patient	Dosing Recommendation
Adults	1–2 g intravenously (severe exposure) or intramuscular (mild to moderate exposure) repeated hourly for two or three additional doses
Adolescent	1–2 g intravenously (severe exposure) or intramuscular (mild to moderate exposure) repeated hourly for two or three additional doses
Child (2–10 yrs old)	25–50 mg/kg intravenously (severe exposure) or intramuscular (mild to moderate exposure) repeated hourly for two or three additional doses
Infant (<2 yrs old)	25–50 mg/kg intravenously (severe exposure) or intramuscular (mild to moderate exposure) repeated hourly for two or three additional doses

Table 6.7 Chemical agents and lethality

Agent	Class	C_{50}^t (mg min m^{-3}) (Death)[a]
CS	Choking agent (tear gas)	60,000
Cyanogen Chloride	Blood agent	1000
Hydrogen Cyanide	Blood agent	2500–5000
Sulfur mustard	Vessicant	1500
Tabun	Nerve agent	400
VX	Nerve agent	50

[a] Information consolidated from text and tables in unclassified military and civilian sources
C_{50}^t the product of concentration [C] of the nerve agent over time [t] to produce effects (death) in 50% of those exposed to vapor or aerosol. Relationship between dose time and concentration:

Delivered dose = Concentration (mg/m^3) × time(min)
10 (mg/m^3) × 10 minutes = 100 (mg/m^3) × 1 minute

1982. In 1995 the Japanese doomsday cult Aum Shinrikyo was believed to have placed cyanide salts and acid in subway restrooms in Tokyo [13]. Cyanide is also the primary agent used in gas chambers for death sentences in the penal system. Cyanide poisoning is believed to be a large factor in smoke inhalation injuries, especial where plastics are burning [14].

Compared to other chemical agents, though cyanide can cause death within six to eight minutes it has had limited military usefulness because of its high Ct_{50} and volatility (Table 6.7). However, despite its limitations of high volatility, low persistence and a high Ct_{50}, cyanide remains a potential threat as an industrial hazard, accidental poison and a chemical terror agent. The combustion of any material containing carbon and nitrogen has the potential to form cyanide; some plastics (particularly acrylonitriles) predictably release clinically significant amounts when burned. Industrial concerns in the U.S. are the manufacture of over 300,000 tons of hydrogen cyanide annually. Cyanides find widespread use in chemical syntheses, electroplating, mineral extraction, dyeing, printing, photography, and agriculture, and in the manufacture of paper, textiles, and plastics.

6.3.2 Physical Characteristics

The term cyanide refers to the anion CN$^-$, or to its acidic form, hydrocyanic acid (HCN). Though a cyanogen (C_2N_2) is the oxidized form of cyanide ions; however, the term cyanogen commonly refers to a substance that forms cyanide upon metabolism and produces the biological effects. Cyanogens may be simple (cyanogen chloride) or complex (sodium nitroprusside). Materials of interest as chemical agents are hydrogen cyanide (hydrocyanic acid, AC) and the simple cyanogen, cyanogen chloride (CK).

Hydrogen cyanide is a colorless, highly volatile liquid and represents a non-persistent hazard. The vapor is less dense than air and has a faint odor of bitter almonds, although 25–50% of the population is missing the gene to be able to smell it. It is highly soluble and stable in water. Cyanogen chloride on the other hand is an irritating colorless gas that is more volatile and dense than hydrogen cyanide (Table 6.8).

6.3.3 Mechanism of Toxicity

Cyanide affects virtually all body tissues by binding to metalloenzymes rendering them inactive. In particular the cyanide ion forms a reversible complex with the respiratory cytochrome oxidase a3 enzyme system, an enzyme system essential for oxidative processes within cells. This results in impairment of cellular oxygen utilization,

Table 6.8 Physical characteristics of cyanogen agents

Property	Hydrogen cyanide	Cyanogen chloride
Appearance	colorless liquid and gas	irritating colorless gas
Chemical formula	HCN	CNCl
Molecular weight	27.02	61.48
Melting point	−13.3 °C	−6.9 °C
Boiling point	25.7 °C	12.8 °C
Vapor density[a]	0.93	2.1
Volatility[b]	1,080,000 (25 °C)	6,132,000 (20 °C)

[a] Vapor density is compared to air.
[b] Volatility is the amount (mg) of agent in 1 m^3.

the cessation of aerobic respiration and cellular hypoxia. The central nervous system, particularly the respiratory center, is especially susceptible to this effect and respiratory failure is the usual cause of death. Tissues with the highest oxygen requirements are also susceptible to cyanide toxicity: brain, liver, heart [15].

6.3.4 Signs, Symptoms and Severity of Exposure

The more rapidly the tissue cyanide levels build up, the more acute the signs and symptoms of poisoning and the smaller the total absorbed dose required to produce a given effect. Hydrogen cyanide causes no distinguishable external effects because it is colorless and a non-irritant. Because cyanogen chloride causes irritation of mucous membranes it produces similar effects as riot-control, mustard and nerve agents with irritation of the eyes, nose, and airways, as well as marked lacrimation, rhinorrhea, and bronchosecretions.

6.3.4.1 *Minimal to mild cyanide exposure*

The onset and progression of signs and symptoms after ingestion of cyanide or after inhalation of a low concentration of vapor are slow. The first effects may not occur until several minutes after exposure, and the time course of these effects depends on the amount absorbed and the rate of absorption. With exposure to low concentrations, after an initial transient hyperpnea, the early symptoms are weakness of the legs, vertigo, nausea and headache for several hours before complete recovery. Later, consciousness is lost, respiration decreases in rate and depth, and convulsions, apnea, and cardiac dysrhythmias and cardiac arrest follows. If exposure is terminated before death it may still be followed by convulsions and coma which may last for hours or days depending on the duration of exposure to the agent. If coma is prolonged, recovery may disclose residual damage to the central nervous system manifested by irrationality, altered reflexes and unsteady gait which may last for several weeks or longer. Permanent deafness (neural damage) has also been described. Because this cascade of events is prolonged with exposure to low concentration, diagnosis, eliminating further exposure and successful treatment are possible.

6.3.4.2 *Severe cyanide exposure*

In high concentrations there is a transient increase in the depth and rate of respiration within a few seconds. This stimulation may be so powerful that a casualty cannot voluntarily hold his or her breath. Violent convulsions occur after 20–30 s with cessation of respiration within 1–2 minutes. Cardiac failure follows 3–4 minutes later.

6.3.5 Medical Management

Successful treatment for acute cyanide poisoning depends upon removal of the casualty from cyanide exposure and rapid fixation of the cyanide ion, either by methemoglobin (metHB) formation or by fixation with cobalt compounds. Management of cyanide gas poisoning begins with removal of the patient to fresh air. Dermal decontamination is unnecessary if exposure has been only to vapor, but wet clothing should be removed and the underlying skin should be washed with soap and water or water alone if liquid on the skin is a possibility. Since cyanide is rapidly detoxified by the body, any casualty who is fully conscious and breathing normally more than 5 minutes after presumed exposure has ceased will likely recover spontaneously and will not require treatment. Artificial resuscitation, though possible, is not likely to be helpful in the absence of drug treatment.

Attention to the basics of intensive supportive care is critical and includes mechanical ventilation as needed, circulatory support with crystalloids and vasopressors, correction of metabolic acidosis with IV sodium bicarbonate, and seizure control with benzodiazepine administration. Because cyanide reversibly inhibits cellular utilization of oxygen the administration of 100% oxygen has been found empirically to exert a beneficial effect and should be a part of general supportive care for every cyanide-poisoned patient.

Severe exposure and those that are symptomatic after cessation of exposure may further benefit from specific antidotal therapy. This is provided in a two-step process. First, a methemoglobin-forming agent such as amyl (inhalant use) or sodium nitrite (for IV use) is administered. The ferric ion (Fe^{3+}) in methemoglobin has a higher affinity for cyanide than cytochrome a_3. The equilibrium of this reaction causes dissociation of bound cyanide from cytochrome a3 and frees the enzyme to produce ATP. The orthostatic hypotension produced by nitrite administration is not usually a concern in a severely intoxicated and prostrate cyanide casualty, but overproduction of methemoglobin may compromise oxygen-carrying capacity. Thus, nitrite therapy is relatively contraindicated in smoke-inhalation victims. The initial adult dose, equivalent to one of the two sodium nitrite vials in the standard Pasadena (formerly Lilly) Cyanide Antidote Kit (Table 6.9). In an average adult one vial will attain a circulating methemoglobin level of about 20%, is 10 ml. Pediatric dosing is dependent on body weight (Table 6.9).

The second step is provision of a sulfur donor, typically sodium thiosulfate, which is utilized as a substrate by the liver enzyme rhodanase for conversion of cyanide to thiocyanate. Sodium thiosulfate itself is efficacious, relatively benign, and also synergistic with oxygen administration and thus may be used without nitrites in situations such as smoke inhalation with high carboxyhemoglobin levels. The initial adult dose, equivalent to one of the two large bottles in the Pasadena Kit, is 50 ml (Table 6.9). The initial thiosulfate dose for pediatric patients is 1.65 ml/kg of the standard 25%

solution, IV (Table 6.9). Second treatments with each of the two antidotes may be given at up to half the original dose if needed [15,16].

It is important to realize that, although the combination of sodium nitrite and sodium thiosulfate may save victims exposed to 10–20 lethal doses of cyanide and are effective even after breathing has stopped, many patients will recover even without specific antidotal treatment if vigorous general supportive care is administered. Lack of availability of antidotes is therefore not a reason to consider even apneic cyanide casualties expectant. It is also important to realize that administration of antidotes, if administered to fast or in extremely large doses, are also associated with morbidity and even mortality.

Several alternative therapies and experimental antidotes are used in other countries. Germany uses dimethylaminophenol (DMAP), a rapid methemoglobin former developed for intramuscular (IM) use. However, muscle necrosis at the site of injection occurs, and only the IV route of administration is recommended [17].

Certain cobalt compounds directly combine with cyanide to reduce its toxicity. Because cobalt compounds do not depend upon the formation of methemoglobin, they may exert their antidotal activity more quickly than do methemoglobin formers. Great Britain and France use cobalt edetate (Kelocyanor), but clear superiority to the methemoglobin formers has not been demonstrated, and cobalt toxicity is occasionally seen, particularly if the patient has only a mild exposure. The other cobalt compound sometimes used in France is hydroxycobalamin (vitamin B_{12a}), which complexes with cyanide on a molar basis forming cyanocobalamine. Clinical trials of this compound are underway in the U.S. [18].

6.4 Vesicants

Vesicant (blister) agents, specifically sulfur mustard (H, HD), have been major military threat agents since their introduction in World War I. They constitute both a vapor and a liquid threat to all exposed skin and mucous membranes. The vesicant agents include sulfur mustard (HD), nitrogen

Table 6.9 Cyanide therapy

Drug	Dosing recommendation
Oxygen	100% for all victims
Sodium nitrate (methemoglobin former)	Adult—300 mg IV over 5–10 minutes
	Pediatric—0.33 ml/kg IV of a 10% solution
Sodium thiosulfate (thiocyanate former)	Adult—12.5 grams IV (25% solution) over 10 minutes
	Pediatric—1.65 ml/kg IV of a 25% solution

Both antidotes may be repeated at half the initial dose if signs/symptoms recur.

mustard (HN), the arsenical vesicants such as lewisite (L) which may be mixed with HD. Vesicants burn and blister the skin or any other part of the body they contact. They act on the eyes, mucous membranes, lungs, skin and bone marrow. They damage the respiratory tract when inhaled and cause vomiting and diarrhea when ingested. Mustard's effects are delayed, appearing hours after exposure. There is no specific antidote, immediate decontamination is the only way to reduce damage and management consists of symptomatic therapy [19–21].

6.4.1 History

Sulfur mustard was first synthesized in the early 1800s and was first used on the battlefield during World War I by Germany in July 1917. Despite its introduction late in that conflict, mustard produced more chemical casualties than all of the other chemical agents combined. However, less than 5% of the mustard casualties who reached medical treatment facilities died. Italy allegedly used mustard against Abyssinia in the 1930s. In the 1960s Egypt apparently employed mustard against Yemen, and Iraq used mustard in the 1980s against Iran and the Kurds. Mustard is still considered a major threat agent of former Warsaw Pact countries and third world countries [20].

The nitrogen mustards (HN1, HN2, and HN3) were synthesized in the 1930s, but were not produced in large amounts for warfare and Mechlorethamine (HN2, Mustargen) became the prototypical cancer chemotherapeutic compound and has remained the standard part of chemotherapy for many years.

Lewisite (L) was synthesized during the late stages of World War I, but probably has not been used on a battlefield. The Lewisite antidote, British-Anti-Lewisite (BAL), finds medicinal use today as a heavy-metal chelator. Although classified as a vesicant, phosgene oxime (CX) is a corrosive urticant that also has not seen battlefield use.

6.4.2 Physical Characteristics

Mustard is an oily liquid with a color ranging from light yellow to brown. Its odor is that of garlic, onion, or mustard, hence its name. However, because of the rapid accommodation to smell, odor should not be relied on for detection. Under temperate conditions, mustard evaporates slowly and thus is primarily a liquid hazard. However, its vapor hazard increases with increasing temperature. At 100°F or above, it is a definite vapor hazard. Of the three vesicant agents, mustard is the only one that does not cause immediate pain. The patient is asymptomatic until the lesion becomes apparent hours later. Lewisite and phosgene oxime, in contrast, cause immediate pain or irritation to the eye, skin, or respiratory tract.

$$S\begin{matrix}\diagup CH_2CH_2-Cl \\ \diagdown CH_2CH_2-Cl\end{matrix}$$
HD

6.4.3 Mechanism of Toxicity

Mustard has many biological actions and the exact mechanism by which it produces tissue injury is not known. According to one prominent hypothesis, biological damage from mustard results from DNA alkylation, crosslinking and strand breakage in rapidly dividing cells, such as basal keratinocytes, mucosal epithelium, and bone marrow precursor cells. This leads to cellular death, an inflammatory reaction, and, in the skin, protease digestion of anchoring filaments at the epidermal–dermal junction and the formation of blisters.

Mustard vapor and liquid readily penetrate thin layers of most fabrics reaching underlying skin where the lipophilicity of mustard guarantees effective absorption through even intact skin. Penetration is rapid (1–4 mcg min cm^{-2}). Approximately 10% of the amount of mustard that begins to penetrate the skin will bind to the skin as "fixed" (reacted) mustard; the remaining 90% of the dose reaches the circulation and is systemically distributed as "free," unreacted and hydrolyzed mustard. However, mustard penetrates the skin without causing any acute concomitant clinical effects, e.g., burning or erythema. Because of the lack of immediate effects, the contaminated person is often unaware of the exposure. Ocular and respiratory routes of entry are also important, as is parenteral absorption in casualties with conventional wounds. Still, late decontamination may prevent further damage, absorption, or spread of the agent [22].

The lethal Ct_{50} of sulfur mustard dispersed as a vapor is 1500 mg min m^{-3} in an unprotected group and 10,000 mg min m^{-3} in a group with respiratory protection. This demonstrates that sufficient concentrations of vapor and sufficient exposure times render mustard vapor lethal, even in masked individuals. The LD_{50} of liquid mustard on the skin is 100 mg/kg. Thus, administration of 7 g, about a teaspoon, of liquid mustard to each member of a group of individuals weighing 70 kg would be expected to cause the death of half of those exposed.

6.4.4 Signs, Symptoms and Severity of Exposure

Signs and symptoms may appear as early as 2 hours after a high-dose exposure, whereas following a low-dose vapor exposure, the latent or asymptomatic period may extend to 48 hours. There are several reports of individuals exposed to very large amounts who died within hours; this type of occurrence is extremely rare. The typical onset time is between four and eight hours. Topical effects of mustard occur in the eye, airways, and skin (Table 6.10). Systemically absorbed mustard may produce effects in the bone marrow, GI tract, and CNS. Direct injury to the GI tract may also occur following ingestion of the compound. The concentration (C) of the mustard vapor, time (t) of exposure, ambient weather, and body site exposed are factors in the onset time. Combined data from the United States forces in World War I and Iranians in the Iraq–Iran conflict suggest a high incidence of eye, airway, and skin involvement (25% and 40% for each) [23]. However, there were higher incidences of eye and lung damage in Iranian casualties than in World War I casualties, probably because of the larger amount of evaporation of the agent in the hot climate.

Table 6.10 Clinical effects from mustard exposure

Organ	Severity	Effects	Onset of t effect
Eyes	Mild	Tearing Itching Burning Gritty sensation	4–12 hours
	Moderate	Above effects plus Reddening Lid edema Moderate pain	3–6 hours
	Severe	Marked lid edema Possible corneal damage Sever pain	1–2 hours
Airways	Mild	Rhinorrhea Sneezing Epistaxis Hoarseness Hacking cough	6–24 hours
	Severe	Above effects plus Productive cough Mild-to-severe dyspnea	2–6 hours
Skin	Mild	Erythema	2–24 hours
	Severe	Vesication	

6.4.4.1 Eyes

The eyes are the organs most sensitive to mustard vapor injury. The latent period is shorter for eye injury than for skin injury. After low-dose vapor exposure reddening of the eyes may be the only effect. As the dose increases, the spectrum of injury includes progressively more severe conjunctivitis, photophobia, blepharospasm, pain, and corneal damage. Miosis noted after mustard exposure in both humans and experimental animals is probably from the cholinomimetic activity of mustard [24].

Blisters do not normally form in the eyes. Instead, swelling and loosening of corneal epithelial cells lead to corneal edema and clouding with leukocytes with decreased visual acuity. Corneal vascularization with secondary edema may last for weeks. Scarring between the iris and lens may follow severe effects; this scarring may restrict pupillary movements and may predispose victims to glaucoma. The most severe damage is caused by liquid mustard from airborne droplets or by self-contamination. After extensive eye exposure, severe corneal damage with possible perforation of the cornea and loss of the eye can occur. Eye loss also results from panophthalmitis.

During World War I, mild conjunctivitis accounted for 75% of eye injuries, with recovery in one to two weeks. Moderate conjunctivitis with minimal corneal involvement, blepharospasm, edema of the lids and conjunctivae, and orange-peel roughening of the cornea accounted for 15% of the cases, with recovery in four to six weeks. Severe corneal involvement accounted for 10% of the cases. Those with permanent corneal damage accounted for less than 1% of cases. About 0.1% of these severe casualties would meet the criteria for legal blindness today.

6.4.4.2 Skin

Erythema is the mildest and earliest form of skin injury after exposure to mustard. It begins to appear in 2–48 hours after vapor exposure and resembles sunburn and is associated with pruritus or a burning, stinging pain. The skin sites most sensitive are the warm, moist locations with thinner skin such as the perineum, external genitalia, axillae, antecubital fossae, and neck. Within the erythematous areas, small vesicles can develop which may later coalesce to form bullae. The typical bulla, or blister, is large, dome-shaped, thin-walled, translucent, yellowish, and surrounded by erythema. The blister fluid is clear, at first thin and straw-colored, but later yellowish and tending to coagulate. The fluid does not contain mustard and is not a vesicant.

At extremely high doses such as those from liquid exposure, lesions may develop a central zone of coagulation necrosis with blister formation at the periphery. These lesions take longer to heal and are more prone to secondary infection than the uncomplicated lesions seen at lower exposure levels.

6.4.4.3 Airways

The primary airway lesion from mustard is necrosis of the mucosa with later damage to the musculature of the airways if exposure is large. The earliest effects involve the nose, sinuses, and pharynx. There may be irritation or burning of the nares, epistaxis, sinus pain or irritation, and irritation or soreness of the pharynx. The damage begins in the upper airways and descends to the lower airways in a dose-dependent manner. Lower airway involvement causes dyspnea and an increasingly severe cough with increased quantities of sputum. Usually the terminal airways and alveoli are unaffected only as a terminal event. Pulmonary edema is not usually present unless the damage is very severe, and then usually it is hemorrhagic.

Necrosis of the airway mucosa with resulting inflammation can cause pseudomembrane formation. Local airway obstruction due to psuedomembrane detachment may lead to obstruction of lower airways. The cause of death in mustard poisoning is commonly respiratory failure. Mechanical obstruction by pseudomembranes and agent-induced laryngospasm are the most common causes of death in the first 24 hours. Deaths occurring from the third to the sixth day after exposure result from secondary bacterial pneumonia caused by bacterial invasion of denuded respiratory mucosa and necrotic debris. Agent-induced bone marrow suppression is a contributory factor in later, septic deaths from pneumonia.

6.4.4.4 Gastrointestinal (GI) tract

The mucosa of the GI tract is very susceptible to mustard damage, either from systemic absorption or ingestion of the agent. Even exposure to a small amount, will often cause nausea, with or without vomiting, lasting 24 hours or less. Diarrhea has been reported; constipation is equally common. Diarrhea and vomiting beginning days after a high-dose exposure imply a poor prognosis.

6.4.4.5 Central nervous system (CNS)

The CNS effects of mustard remain poorly defined. Animal work demonstrated that mustards (particularly the nitrogen mustards) are convulsants, and there are several human case reports describing victims who were exposed to very large amounts and had neurological effects (obtundation, ataxia, convulsions) within several hours after exposure just prior to death. Reports from World War I and Iran described people exposed to small amounts of mustard that appeared sluggish, apathetic, and lethargic. These reports suggest that minor psychological problems could linger for a year or longer.

6.4.4.6 Bone marrow
Significant exposure to mustard will cause damage to precursor cells in the bone marrow causing pancytopenia and immunosuppression similar to chemotherapy or radiation treatment patients. Severity of blisters does not predict marrow involvement as 90% of mustard passes through the skin and is absorbed systemically.

6.4.4.7 Death
Most casualties die of massive pulmonary damage complicated by infection, bronchopneumonia, and sepsis from immune suppression. When exposure is not by inhalation, the mechanism of death is less clear. In studies with animals in which mustard was administered via routes other than inhalational, the animals died from 3 to 7 days after the exposure; they had no signs of pulmonary damage and often had no signs of sepsis. The mechanism of death was not clear, but autopsy findings resembled those seen after radiation. Mustard is considered to be a radiomimetic because it causes tissue damage similar to that seen after radiation.

6.4.5 Medical Management
The management of a patient exposed to mustard may be simple, as in the provision of symptomatic care for a sunburn-like erythema, or extremely complex, as providing total management for a severely ill patient with burns, immunosuppression, and multi-system involvement. Suggested therapeutic measures for each organ system are provided below. Guidelines for general patient care are not intended to take the place of sound clinical judgment, especially in the management of complicated cases [19,21].

6.4.5.1 Eyes
Preventing infection and scarring is the treatment goal for mustard injury of the eyes. Conjunctival irritation will respond to any of a number of available ophthalmic solutions after the eyes are thoroughly irrigated. Regular application of homatropine (or other anticholinergic drug) ophthalmic ointment will reduce or prevent future synechiae formation. A topical antibiotic applied several times a day will reduce the incidence and severity of infection. Vaseline or a similar substance should be applied to the edges of the lids regularly to prevent them from sticking together. This permits drainage of any underlying infection and prevents adhesions and scarring during healing. Topical analgesics may be useful initially if blepharospasm is too severe to permit an adequate examination, but topical analgesics should otherwise be avoided and systemic analgesics should be given for eye pain. Topical steroids are not of proven value, but their use during the first day or two might reduce inflammation. Sunglasses may reduce discomfort from photophobia. For suspected severe exposure early consultation with an ophthalmologist is prudent [24].

6.4.5.2 Skin
Treatment priorities are keeping the patient comfortable, the skin lesion clean and preventing infection. Erythema can be treated with calamine or other soothing lotion or cream (e.g., 0.25% camphor and menthol) to reduce burning and itching. Small blisters (under 1–2 cm) should be left intact. Because larger ones will eventually break they should be carefully unroofed. Denuded areas should be irrigated 3–4 times daily with saline, other sterile solution, or soapy water. Modified Dakins solution (sodium hypochlorite) was used in World War I and in Iranian casualties for irrigation and as an antiseptic. After irrigation the open blisters are liberally covered with a topical antibiotic such as silver sulfadiazine or mafenide acetate to a thickness of 1–2 mm. If an antibiotic cream is not available, sterile petrolatum will be useful. Multiple or large areas of blistering suggest the need for hospitalization and whirlpool bath irrigation. Systemic analgesics should be used liberally, particularly before manipulation of the patient or irrigation of the burn

areas. Systemic antipruritics such as trimeprazine or benadryl may also provide some symptomatic relief. While mustard injuries resemble thermal burns they do not have the associated fluid requirements of thermal burns [22].

6.4.5.3 Pulmonary

Upper airway symptoms such as a sore throat, non-productive cough, and hoarseness; may respond to steam inhalation and cough suppressants. Sterile bronchitis or pneumonitis manifested by productive cough, dyspnea, fever, and leukocytosis often occurs 12–24 hours after exposure. Infection often occurs on or about the third day. Its presence is signaled by an increased fever, increased pulmonary infiltrate by X-ray, and increased sputum production and character. Appropriate antibiotic therapy should be guided by positive sputum Gram stain and culture. Intubation should be performed early before laryngeal spasm or edema makes it difficult or impossible. Intubation permits better ventilation and facilitates suction of the necrotic and inflammatory debris. Oxygen may be needed, and early use of PEEP or CPAP may be of benefit. If there is a suggestion of pseudomembrane formation, bronchoscopy should be done to permit suctioning of the necrotic debris by direct vision. Bronchodilators may be of benefit for bronchospasm. If they fail, steroids may be used. There is little evidence that the routine use of steroids is beneficial. The need for continuous use of assisted or controlled ventilation suggests a poor prognosis. Death often occurs between the fifth and tenth day after exposure because of pulmonary insufficiency and infection complicated by immunosuppression from mustard induced bone marrow damage [25].

6.4.5.4 Gastrointestinal

Antiemetics and anticholinergic drugs should control early nausea and vomiting. Prolonged vomiting or voluminous diarrhea beginning days after exposure suggests severe systemic poisoning which is a poor prognostic sign. Intravenous fluids to maintain intravascular volume are indicated.

6.4.5.5 Bone marrow

Sterilization of the gut by non-absorbable antibiotics should be considered to reduce the possibility of sepsis from enteric organisms. If the patient is neutropenic all transfusion therapy should be irradiated and CMV negative. In addition, hematopoietic growth factors, granulocyte colony-stimulating factors, and granulocyte-macrophage colony-stimulating factor, are potent stimulators of hematopoiesis and may shorten the duration of neutropenia and thus reduce morbidity and mortality. The role of bone marrow transplantation is unclear.

6.4.5.6 Other

Sulfur donors such as sodium thiosulfate decreased systemic effects and elevated the LD_{50} when given before exposure or within 20 minutes after exposure in experimental animals. Activated charcoal given orally to casualties was of no value.

References

1. J. Robinson. *The Rise of CB Weapons The Problem of Chemical and Biological Warfare*, p. 71. New York, NY, Humanities Press, 1971; 71.
2. J. H. Wills and I. A. DeArmon. A Statistical Study of the Adamek Report Medical Laboratory Special Report 54: Army Chemical Center, MD: Medical Laboratories, 1954.
3. K. Wilson. Directorate of Medical Research, Edgewood Arsenal, Md, mid to late 1960's.
4. C. M. Gosden. *Chemical and biological weapons threats to America: are we prepared?* Congressional Hearings Intelligence and Security Committee, 1998.
5. H. Morita, N. Yanagisawa, T. Nakajima, et al. Sarin poisoning in Matsumoto, Japan. *Lancet* 346:290–293, 1995.
6. Y. Asai and J. Arnold. Terrorism in Japan. *Prehospital Disaster Med* 18, 2003.
7. E. Broughton. The Bhopal disaster and its aftermath: a review. *Environ Health* 10:6–12, 2005.
8. H. Nozaki, S. Hori, Y. Shinozawa, et al. Secondary exposure of medical staff to sarin vapor in the emergency room. *Intensive Care Med* 21:1032–1035, 1995.

9. T. Kato and T. Hamanaka. Ocular signs and symptoms caused by exposure to sarin gas. *Am J Ophthalmol* 121:209–210, 1996.
10. A. P. Volans. Sarin: guidelines on the management of victims of a nerve gas attack. *J Accid Emerg Med* 13:202–206, 1996.
11. F. Dicenta, P. Martinez-Gomez, N. Grane, et al. Relationship between cyanogenic compounds in kernels, leaves, and roots of sweet and bitter kernelled almonds. *J Agric Food Chem* 50:2149–2152, 2002.
12. D. D. Ngudi, Y. H. Kuo, and F. Lambein. Cassava cyanogens and free amino acids in raw and cooked leaves. *Food Chem Toxicol* 41:1193–1197, 2003.
13. T. Okumura, N. Ninomiya, and M. Ohta. The chemical disaster response system in Japan. *Prehospital Disaster Med* 18:189–192, 2003.
14. D. W. Walsh and M. Eckstein. Hydrogen cyanide in fire smoke: an underappreciated threat. *Emerg Med Serv* 33:160–163, 2004.
15. A. P. Morocco. Cyanides. *Crit Care Clin* 21:691–705, vi, 2005.
16. R. Gracia and G. Shepherd. Cyanide poisoning and its treatment. *Pharmacotherapy* 24:1358–1365, 2004.
17. H. Kerger, P. Dodidou, D. Passani-Kruppa, et al. Excessive methaemoglobinaemia and multi-organ failure following 4-DMAP antidote therapy. *Resuscitation* 66:231–235, 2005.
18. D. M. Beasley and W. I. Glass. Cyanide poisoning: pathophysiology and treatment recommendations. *Occup Med (Lond)* 48:427–431, 1998.
19. M. Balali-Mood and M. Hefazi. The pharmacology, toxicology, and medical treatment of sulphur mustard poisoning. *Fundam Clin Pharmacol* 19:297–315, 2005.
20. J. McManus and K. Huebner. Vesicants. *Crit Care Clin* 21:707–718, vi, 2005.
21. K. Kehe and L. Szinicz. Medical aspects of sulphur mustard poisoning. *Toxicology* 214:198–209, 2005.
22. K. J. Smith, C. G. Hurst, R. B. Moeller, et al. Sulfur mustard: its continuing threat as a chemical warfare agent, the cutaneous lesions induced, progress in understanding its mechanism of action, its long-term health effects, and new developments for protection and therapy. *J Am Acad Dermatol* 32:765–776, 1995.
23. S. Khateri, M. Ghanei, S. Keshavarz, et al. Incidence of lung, eye, and skin lesions as late complications in 34,000 Iranians with wartime exposure to mustard agent. *J Occup Environ Med* 45:1136–1143, 2003.
24. Y. Solberg, M. Alcalay, and M. Belkin. Ocular injury by mustard gas. *Surv Ophthalmol* 41:461–466, 1997.
25. M. Hefazi, D. Attaran, M. Mahmoudi, and M. Balali-Mood. Late respiratory complications of mustard gas poisoning in Iranian veterans. *Inhal Toxicol* 17:587–592, 2005.

Suggested Comprehensive Resources

Office of the Surgeon General, United States Army. Medical Aspects of Chemical and Biological Warfare. *Textbook of Military Medicine* (B. G. Russ Zajtchuk, ed.). 1997.

Field Management of Chemical Casualties Handbook. 2nd edition. Chemical Casualty Care Division, USAMRICD, MCMR-UV-ZM, 3100 Ricketts Point Rd., Aberdeen Proving Ground, MD 21010-5400, July 2000.

7 Decontamination and Personal Protection

JOSEPH H. McISAAC, III

Decontamination is the most fundamental and potentially the most difficult step in the management of mass casualties. Successful decontamination limits the extent of toxic exposure and converts the contaminated casualty from a hazard to a more manageable patient. Large scale implementation demands considerable resources. This enormous task requires both large numbers of personnel and large amounts of time.[1]

Three levels of decontamination are recognized: personal, casualty, and personnel. Personal refers to self-removal of the offending agent. This is most effective if performed within 1–2 minutes of exposure. The advantage of self-decon methods is the non-specificity, effective equally on agents regardless of chemical structure or knowledge of specific agent, and the timeliness of the procedure [1]. It can make the difference between minimal or no injury and severe toxicity or death. Casualty decontamination refers to the treatment of contaminated patients, whether ambulatory or non-ambulatory. Personnel decontamination refers to those who are considered non-casualties—usually those who are wearing Personal Protective Equipment (PPE).

Decontamination is defined as the reduction, neutralization, or removal of external radiological, chemical, or biological agents to the extent that they are no longer a hazard to the patient or the caregiver [1]. This process consists of either physical removal through mechanical abrasion, solvation and dilution (i.e., washing ± detergent action), and chemical neutralization (detoxification).

7.1 Removal of Clothing

The greatest reduction in agent burden is accomplished by removal of clothing. Complete disrobement is ideal, but in civilian situations, there may be considerable resistance by those who are questionably exposed. A reasonable accommodation for ambulatory patients when expected contamination is minimal and privacy is lacking would be removal of all outer clothing; retaining undergarments into and through the shower should provide a reasonable level of modesty preservation without greatly inhibiting reduction in contamination (Figure 7.1).

7.2 Skin Contamination

The primary concern should be elimination of skin contamination, taking care to include the eyes, ears, hair, and any wounds. Any means possible to mechanically remove the substance, such as scraping or adsorption is acceptable for liquids and solids on skin. "Adsorption refers to the formation and maintenance of a condensed layer of a substance, such as a chemical agent, on the surface of a decontaminant" [1]. Sand, oatmeal, "kitty litter," diatomaceous earth, or other porous/particulate matter will serve as a field

---

Clothing Removal
Washing Skin with Soap and Water
Skin Detoxification (optional depending on agent)

Figure 7.1 Critical Decontamination Steps.

expedient. If available, military M291 Resin is an effective alternative. This material consists of activated charcoal, polystyrene polymer, and ion-exchange resins. This is a single-step, non-toxic, non-irritating decontamination—safe for the skin—including the face and around wounds. "Each packet contains a nonwoven, fiberfill laminated pad impregnated with the decontamination compounds." [1]. Standard soap or detergent and warm water will easily remove the majority of non-persistent contaminants. Both seawater and fresh water are equally suitable. Eyes and hair can be cleaned with non-tearing baby shampoo. Radiological contamination is also effectively reduced through simple washing. Surface contamination with biologicals is equally well-managed. Most biologicals are not surface active, especially if rapidly removed. Deep wound cavities should be lavaged only; thorough debridement should be delayed until proper surgical conditions can be instituted.

In general, timely, copious flushing with water produces better results than high concentrations of hypochlorite solutions. However, gross contamination with persistent military agents of a sticky or oily nature (VX, thickened Soman, mustard) is a more difficult situation. These substances are designed to be retained on the skin, potentiating their toxic action. They may require chemical inactivation to be effectively removed. Chemical detoxification is not an instantaneous process—the larger the quantity of contaminant, the longer the time necessary for the chemical reaction to occur. Dilute (0.5%) sodium or calcium hypochlorite solution (bleach) is considered the "universal decontaminant" by most authorities. It can be made by adding 6 ounces of calcium hypochlorite to 5 gallons of water [1]. Hypochlorite acts by alkaline hydrolysis, breaking chemical bonds and converting the offending substance into a less toxic byproduct. It is equally effective against organophosphates and vesicants. The reaction rate is dependent on the chemical structure, pH, temperature, solvent (usually water), and presence of catalytic reagents. The reaction half-time for VX at pH 10 is 1.5 minutes. The reaction rate for "other agents, such as mustard, are much longer" [1].

Agent	0.5% Bleach	2.5% Bleach	5% Bleach
GB	85%	99%	99%
GF	69%	70%	91%
HD	67%	78%	79%

Percent Agent Detoxified in 15 Minutes.

Figure 7.2 Hypochlorite reaction rates for chemical agents. (USAMRICD, 1998)

Hypochlorite is also is an extremely effective biocide, killing the vast majority of organisms quickly (see Figure 7.2).

Reactive Skin Decontamination Lotion (RSDL) [2] was FDA approved in 2003. It is easy to apply lotion (containing DeKon139) which will decontaminate a broad range of agents. RSDL has "... no significant effect on the normal response of epidermal tissue with respect to the processes leading to repair of skin defects and the process of re-epithelialization" [3]. Thus, RDSL is presumably safe to use in the presence of open wounds.

Alternative chemical detoxificants, effective on equipment but *not for use on skin*, include strongly basic solutions of sodium and potassium hydroxide and DS-2 (diethylenetriamine, ethylene glycol monomethyl ether, and sodium hydroxide mixture). There are also recently marketed decontaminating agents developed at Sandia National Laboratories [4] such as EasyDECON™ [5], MDF-200™ [6], and ALL-CLEAR™ [7]. These foams consist of a complex mixture of quarternary ammonium salts with surfactant properties, a water soluble polymer, a corrosion inhibitor, a fatty alcohol, and a reactive peroxide compound at an alkaline pH. They are capable of rapidly hydrolyzing chemical agents and reducing spores by up to 7 logs in 15 minutes (see Figure 7.3).

This formulation is both non-toxic to animals, including humans, generally non-corrosive and can be used for neutralization of many toxants, both chemical and biological. The formulation allows decontamination of areas populated with both people and sensitive equipment; [it] works on all currently anticipated material surfaces and can be incorporated into a wide

Agent	% Decontamination		
	1 Minute	15 Minutes	60 Minutes
Mustard	95	100	100
VX	60	98	100
G-Series	100	100	100
Bacillus Globigii	NM	100	100
Aflatoxin Mycotoxin	NM	100	100
Bacillus Anthracis AMES-RIID	NM	7-log	7-log
Bacillus Subtillus (19659)	NM	NM	7-log
Bacillus Anthracis ANR-1	NM	7-log	7-log
Yersinia Pestis	NM	7-log	7-log

Figure 7.3 Sandia decontamination foam efficacy [14].

variety of carriers (foams, gels, fogs, aerosols) that satisfy a wide variety of operational objectives...

This technology was demonstrated at the Fixed Site Decon Trials at the Edgewood Chemical Biological Center (ECBC) where the foam successfully neutralized TGD (thickened soman), VX, and HD and at the U.S. Army Dugway Proving Grounds where the formulation successfully killed *Bacillus globigii* spores (an anthrax simulant) on common office materials. [8]

7.3 Training

Good training is paramount to good execution. There is no substitute for intensive, frequent, and repetitive training. People inherently will revert, under stressful circumstances, to whatever they have internalized in their training. Compulsive, detail oriented individuals are ideal to supervise decontamination training as well as actual implementation. Consider enlisting a senior operating room (OR) nurse as a decontamination section trainer. The system employed for HAZMAT decon is very similar to the high level sterile technique utilized in the OR. Training with surrogate agents to continually assess effectiveness is an excellent way to emphasize the need for precision and to instill confidence in the team.

7.4 Surgical Wound Decontamination

"All casualties, ... after a chemical, [nuclear, or biological attack], are considered contaminated unless there is a certification of noncontamination" [1]. Bandages, tourniquets and splints are removed and decontaminated and wounds are flushed with copious amounts of sterile irrigants. Once external decontamination has been achieved, wounds can be safely treated in the operating room if proper safeguards are enforced.

Chemical agents in penetrating wounds are usually rapidly absorbed or buffered by the tissues and present little hazard to treating medical personnel. Once clothing is removed and the skin is cleansed, there is little risk of off-gassing of toxic vapor. Thickened agents, however, by their very nature, require special care. They can remain in a wound for prolonged periods and produce delayed effects to both the patient as well as the care giver. Patients internally contaminated with large quantities of military grade agents are unlikely to survive to reach surgery [1].

There is, likewise, minimal risk of "secondary aerosolization of biological agents" as long as standard barrier protection is used. The exceptions are "plague, smallpox, and viral hemorrhagic fevers" [1]. Under these conditions, the use of HEPA filtered respirators is indicated.

Radiological contamination of wounds usually consists of foreign body material which can be débrided using standard irrigation and surgical technique. Instruments should be utilized to minimize radiation exposure from large, highly radioactive material embedded from detonation of Radiological Dispersion Devices (RDDs). All contaminated dressings and wound material should be double bagged and properly processed (5% hypochlorite for chemical and biologicals; segregation and shielding for radiological).

When available, wounds should be assessed with monitoring equipment appropriate to the type of agent present. The Chemical Agent Monitor (CAM) can be used to detect chemical agents. Irrigation of a wound with 0.5% hypochlorite will virtually eliminate any chance of residual chemical agent presence. It is, however, very damaging to tissue. It should not be used in the eye, on neurological tissue, or in the abdomen or chest cavity. Dakin's solution (pH 4–8) may cause less tissue injury but will hydrolyze agent at a much slower rate and may not be worth the risk to tissue. High volume irrigation with standard irrigants is probably preferable. Waste irrigants should be considered contaminated. A radiologic survey meter can be used to detect radiation. Team members should wear monitoring badges.

Surgical team members should wear a pair of well-fitting (thin) butyl rubber gloves or double latex surgical gloves and to change them often until all potential contaminates are removed from wound. Thin butyl rubber gloves will last 60+ min in an aqueous base. Double latex gloves last 29 min. Wound should be explored with instruments not fingers [1].

7.5 Site Security

Physical security of the decontamination site is critical. Advanced planning and participation of trained security officers is an obvious prerequisite. Crowd control, protection of patient valuables, and maintenance of the integrity of hot vs. cold zones are paramount. Training for security officers should include testing for vulnerability.

7.6 Site Layout

A decontamination site is best placed a distance from the emergency department. It should be accessible to staff but not so close as to obstruct entrances or threaten the hospital by a shift in wind or from contaminated runoff water. Site selection involves a series of trade-offs and is entirely hospital specific. Some hospitals prefer to have their own, self-designed, self-run systems. Others prefer preconfigured portable or mobile systems operated by local fire personnel. Access to water, drainage, power, shelter, storage of supplies (clothing, personal effects, emergency treatment supplies), privacy considerations, security, and a means of identifying patients are all necessary considerations. The expected need to manage large

```
Water (± soap/detergent)
Absorbent Particulates (Sand, etc.)
Hypochlorite (Bleach)
M291 Resin
Reactive Skin Decontamination Lotion (RSDL)
Foams
```

Figure 7.4 Skin Decontamination Agents.

numbers of ambulatory patients who are lightly or minimally exposed should not be underestimated.

Wind direction, Hot, Warm, and Cold zones, water availability, weather (warm vs. cold), and drainage all will impact planning and implementation. The decontamination facilities will require adequate supplies of towels, alternative clothing, soap, shampoo, a contaminated clothing disposal method as well as a means of preserving questionably contaminated items of value (Figure 7.4). The wearer of a $1500 designer suit would be expected to be somewhat reluctant to part with his apparel if he is being processed only as a precaution.

Advanced medical care (life saving interventions) should be available in the hot zone. This requires the presence of a physician, physician's assistant, or advanced practice nurse together with appropriate equipment and supplies (see Figures 7.5, 7.6, and 7.7).

7.7 Patient Identification

The traditional hospital wrist band continues to be the favored system in mass-casualty scenarios. Infant ID bands are especially useful since they come as sets of identically numbered bracelets. Patient valuables can be accounted for and secured with a higher degree of surety if labeled with the identical system (Figures 7.8 and 7.9). Personal property control is likely to be a major source of strife among minimally contaminated ambulatory patients. Wallets and purses, money, watches and jewelry, shoes and clothing are likely to be surrendered only upon assurances that they will be secured and returned promptly. A clearly organized, visibly secure system of labeling and physical security by trusted personnel is essential. The huge potential for theft during mass-casualty operations will not be lost on the public.

Decontamination and Personal Protection   93

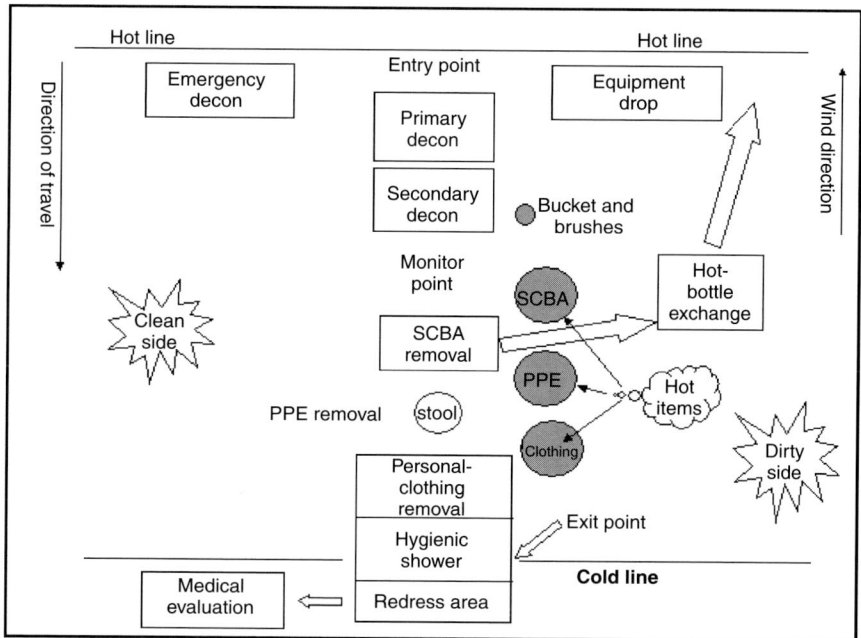

Figure 7.5 Field Decontamination Station.

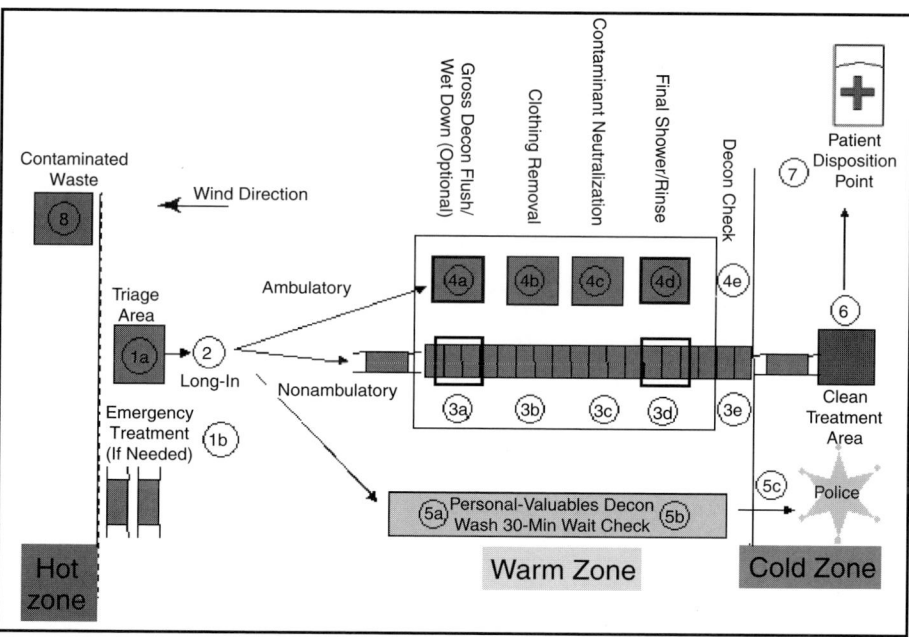

Figure 7.6 Decontamination Unit Schematic.

CPC material	GB-S	VX-S	MAL	Blister-S
PVC/nylon/PV	10 min	4 min	3 min	4 min
Playtex-g	45 min	15 min	10 min	10 min
Tyvek saranex	30 min	50 min	12 min	90 min
Duct tape	210 min	210 min	>24h	>24h
Butyl/nylon/butyl	>24h	>24h	>24h	>24h
Teflon	>100h	>100h	>100h	>100h

Figure 7.7 Time to Penetration for Various Protective Clothing [13].

7.8 Certification of Decontamination

There currently exists, no universally recognized standard for certifying decontamination. Few standards exist for safe levels of many agents. Rabner discusses occupational limit values for time-weighted-average exposures to various war gasses for the general public, taken from multiple sources [9]. Quantitative measurement is, unfortunately, not a practical option for most civilian hospitals receiving mass casualties, even when the offending agent is identified.

Multiple methods of detecting known chemical agents exist, including military M8 and M9 paper, the M256A1 ticket, and the CAM. If available, these will give reasonable assurance of the absence of clinically relevant toxic concentrations. Radiological survey meters can readily assess residual radiation. Rapid biological identification systems are being deployed but are not universally available. Most likely, early in an event, the offending agent will be unknown. An easy to use alternative, useful whether or not the nature of

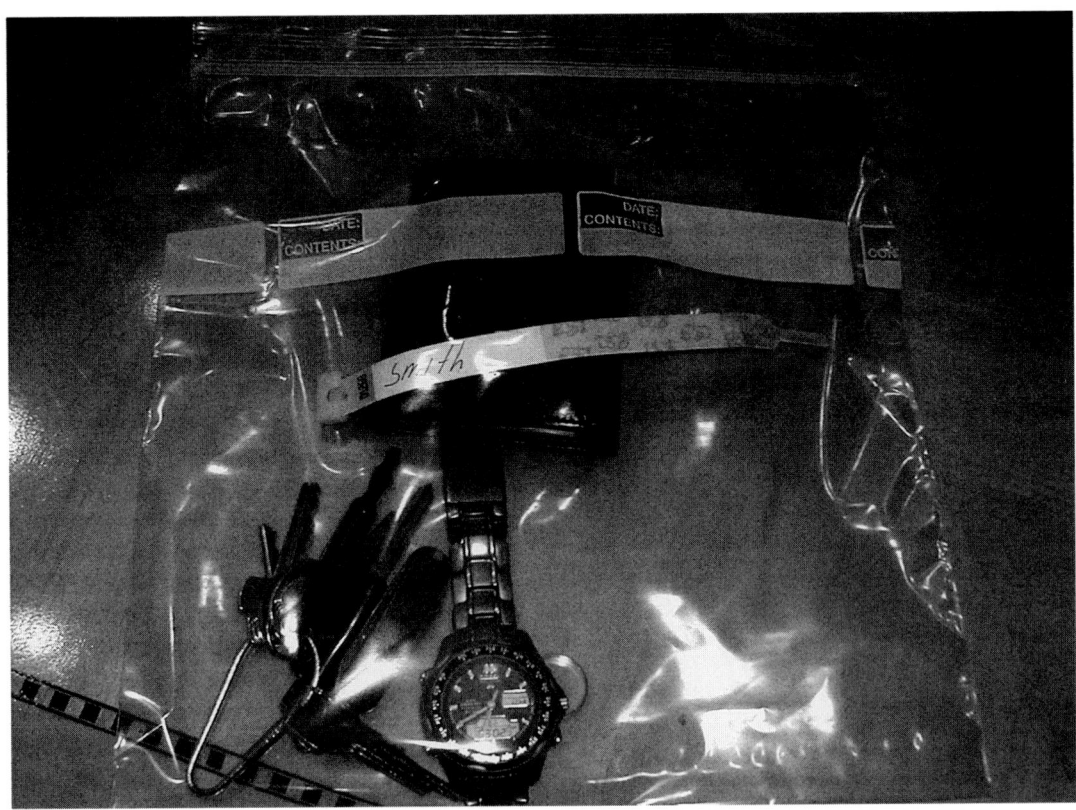

Figure 7.8 Personal effects labled and stored for proper disposition. (Photo courtesy of Cynthia Shields, MD.)

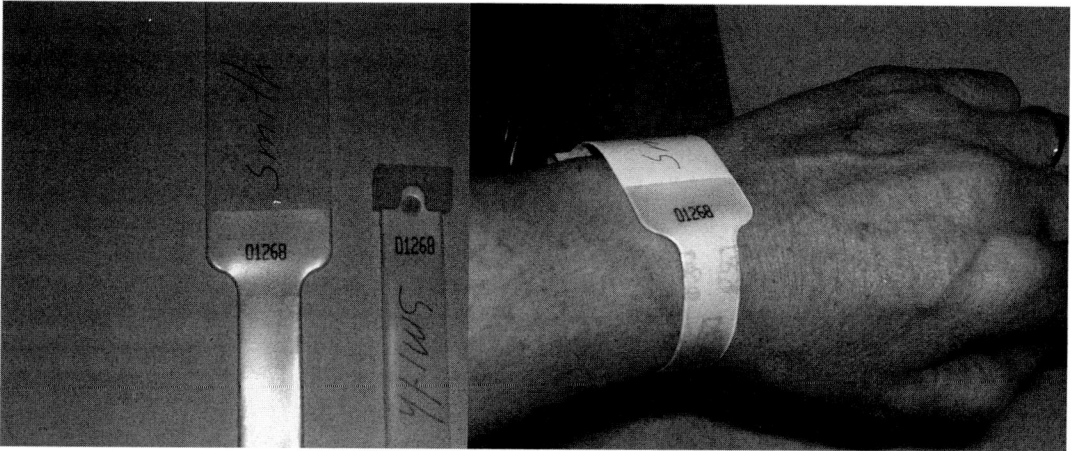

Figure 7.9 Patient identification. (Photo courtesy of Cynthia Shields, MD.)

the contaminant is known, is the introduction of a surrogate marker onto casualties as they enter the system. The simulant should be either visible to the unaided eye, such as food coloring, or detectable with routinely available means, such as with a Wood's ultraviolet lamp (fluorescein injectable USP, or fluorescein, alcohol soluble, USP). The marker can be diluted and mixed with a suitable carrier (mineral oil, vegetable oil, and vegetable fat) to simulate the consistency of a persistent chemical agent. The marker should be non-toxic, hypoallergenic, and not permanently stain the skin. Neither should it be removable by a cursory rinsing of the skin. Total removal of a moderately adherent, poorly soluble simulant is a reliable way to assure adequate decontamination of virtually any foreign substance. This technique, not only allows a continuous quality indicator at the decontamination site, it provides assurance to those further down stream in the chain of casualty care.

An evaluation in Sweden [10] of a three chamber decontamination system using ethyl lactate, a water-soluble simulant for sarin, and methyl salicylate, a poorly soluble simulant of sulfur mustard, was performed on volunteers. Volunteers were showered for 3 minutes with 30 °C water then thoroughly washed twice with soap and water in a second chamber. Vapor measurements were reduced by as much as 10^4 fold by the third chamber. The levels abruptly increased when staff members, who had self-decontaminated, entered the room. This emphasizes the need to assess the thoroughness of staff decon in a similar manner to patients. All staff should always be assisted when removing PPE and undergoing decontamination by a trained individual (also wearing PPE) who can prevent recontamination. Special attention should be paid to footwear.

Along with a physical method of measurement, there should be a written record of decon certification to accompany each patient. This can consist of bracelets, tags, or be as simple as indelible ink marking on the forearm, forehead, or chest. Critical to the success of this technique is the acceptance of the method used throughout the affected region and across all appropriate jurisdictions (fire, EMS, hospitals). Potentially infectious patients should be labeled as such and segregated to isolation units. If proper procedure is followed, the risk of contaminating a medical treatment facility is then extremely low [10].

7.9 Personal Protection Equipment

Chemical and biological threats can be vapor, liquid, or aerosol. Radiological contamination is most commonly solid or particulate. These substances can enter the oral and respiratory tracts or penetrate through the skin, depending upon the specific agent. The Environmental Protection Agency (EPA) defines four levels of personal protection, designated levels A, B, C, and D. These are detailed in [10] (see Figure 7.10).

Level A consists of complete encapsulation against gas, vapors, liquids, and aerosols. It consists of a self-contained breathing apparatus and can be used in oxygen deficient atmospheres. It is not generally indicated for frontline healthcare workers (ECRI, 2002).

Level B consists of a splash protective chemical suit (e.g., Saranex®), and a positive pressure supplied respirator (airline or self-contained). Level B is recommended if the agent concentrations or agents are unknown. The military Mission Oriented Protective Posture (MOPP) suit is a modified level B (ECRI, 2002).

Level C protection utilizes full- or half-face purifying respirator (Powered Air Purifying

---

EPA LEVELS OF PROTECTION

LEVEL A:

Vapor protective suit (meets NFPA 1991)
Pressure-demand, full-face SCBA
Inner chemical-resistant gloves, chemical-resistant safety boots, two-way radio communication

OPTIONAL: Cooling system, outer gloves, hard hat

Protection Provided: Highest available level of respiratory, skin, and eye protection from solid, liquid and gaseous chemicals.

Used When: The chemical(s) have been identified and have high level of hazards to respiratory system, skin and eyes. Substances are present with known or suspected skin toxicity or carcinogenity. Operations must be conducted in confined or poorly ventilated areas.

Limitations: Protective clothing must resist permeation by the chemical or mixtures present. Ensemble items must allow integration without loss of performance.

LEVEL B:

Liquid splash-protective suit (meets NFPA 1992)
Pressure-demand, full-facepiece SCBA
Inner chemical-resistant gloves, chemical-resistant safety boots, two-way radio communications
Hard hat.

OPTIONAL: Cooling system, outer gloves

Protection Provided: Provides same level of respiratory protection as Level A, but less skin protection. Liquid splash protection, but no protection against chemical vapors or gases.

Used When: The chemical(s) have been identified but do not require a high level of skin protection. Initial site surveys are required until higher levels of hazards are identified. The primary hazards associated with site entry are from liquid and not vapor contact.

Limitations: Protective clothing items must resist penetration by the chemicals or mixtures present. Ensemble items must allow integration without loss of performance.

Figure 7.10 OSHA Recommended PPE Levels. (From OSHA.)

LEVEL C:

Support Function Protective Garment (meets NFPA 1993)
Full-facepiece, air-purifying, canister-equipped respirator
Chemical resistant gloves and safety boots
Two-way communications system, hard hat

OPTIONAL: Faceshield, escape SCBA

Protection Provided: The same level of skin protection as Level B, but a lower level of respiratory protection. Liquid splash protection but no protection to chemical vapors or gases.

Used When: Contact with site chemical(s) will not affect the skin. Air contaminants have been identified and concentrations measured. A canister is available which can remove the contaminant. The site and its hazards have been completely characterized.

Limitations: Protective clothing items must resist penetration by the chemical or mixtures present. Chemical airborne concentration must be less than IDLH levels. The atmosphere must contain at least 19.5% oxygen.

Not Acceptable for Chemical Emergency Response

LEVEL D:

Coveralls, safety boots/shoes, safety glasses or chemical splash goggles

OPTIONAL: Gloves, escape SCBA, face-shield

Protection Provided: No respiratory protection, minimal skin protection.

Used When: The atmosphere contains no known hazard. Work functions preclude splashes, immersion, potential for inhalation, or direct contact with hazard chemicals.

Limitations: This level should not be worn in the Hot Zone. The atmosphere must contain at least 19.5% oxygen.

Not Acceptable for Chemical Emergency Response

Figure 7.10 Continued.

Respirator, PAPR, N95 mask, or High-Efficiency Particulate Aerosol, HEPA-filter mask) in addition to a splash resistant, hooded chemical suit.

Level D consists of standard barrier nursing garb.

7.10 Skin Protection

A key factor supporting OSHA's PPE best practices is the limited amount of toxic substance to which first receivers might be exposed. Many recent sources note that the quantity of contaminant on victims is restricted. For example, OSHA has made a clear distinction between the site where a hazardous substance was released and hospital-based decontamination facilities... This distinction is important because it helps define the maximum amount of contaminant to which healthcare workers might be exposed (i.e., the quantity of material on living victims and their possessions when they arrive at the hospital). Horton et al. (2003) stated that, during victim decontamination procedures, the hazard to healthcare workers is strictly from secondary exposure and "depends largely on the toxicity of the substance on the victims' hair, skin, and clothing; the concentration of the substance; and the duration of contact [first receivers have] with the victim". [10]

Butyl rubber gloves are the standard for protection for hands advocated my military

Glove Type	HD Breakthrough time, minutes	GB Breakthrough time, minutes
Best Butyl 878-10, 30 mil	810	>1440
Ansell Edmont Thermaprene, 9-024	119	298
Bayside Latex Examination Glove	23	83
Safety Zone Gloves, GL1-NPFL	54	114
MAPA Neoprene, PN1-N450	298	>1440
Ansell Edmont TNT Nitrile, 92-500	20	106
Ansell Edmont PVA, 15-554	577	110
Hahn Fat, PVC, GL1-VC7714R	97	161
Safety 4H Glove	>1440	>1440
Ansell Edmont Sol-Vex, 37-155	109	>1440
Best Viton 890-10, 30 mil	638	>1440

Figure 7.11 Swatch test results for gloves [12].

authorities. They are available in three thicknesses: 7, 14, and 25 mm. While they offer the best resistance to chemical agent penetration, they are quite difficult to use when performing fine motor tasks. Double latex gloves are adequate if changed frequently or until the patient is decontaminated. They should be changed at least every 20 minutes. Nitrile gloves also may be used if frequently changed. Swatch tests results by the US Army SBCCOM (Figure 7.11) show the wide variation in permeability of various types of gloves. Consideration should be given to wearing two gloves of different composition since each material will have different characteristics with different substances [10].

Likewise, chemical resistant, splash-proof clothing and shoe covers are necessary in the decontamination area. They are available from a wide variety of manufacturers. Figure 7.12 illustrates the chemical permeability for several different products. The Demron™ suit [12] offers a light weight garment for attenuation of low and medium energy radiation exposure for both first responders and medical personnel. They come in a wide variety of styles and are suitable for everyday wear in routine

Test Item	Breakthrough time, minutes GB	Breakthrough time, minutes HD
Lakeland Deluxe Level A 10640	>522	177
Lakeland Economy Level A 10660	128	124
Mar Mac Commander 9400FB	597	216
Giat UNISCAPH Gas Tight Suit	416	180

Figure 7.12 Swatch test results for chemical protection suits [14]. Levels of personal protection.

radiological procedures. Individuals handling contaminated materials (clothing) or sorting patients pre-decontamination for a prolonged period might consider this product useful (see Figure 7.13).

The powered air-purifying respirator (PAPR), equipped with both particulate and chemical filters should serve most hospital based scenarios (OSHA, 2005) (see Figure 7.14). Critical to successful

Decontamination and Personal Protection 99

PAPR use is prior training. A formalized training process with periodic refresher training is recommended, including instruction in donning and removal, and several hours of clinical simulation.

7.11 Conclusion

Respiratory protection equipment is recommended at Level B when substances are unknown or potentially in high concentration, and Level C when lesser threats are present. Studies have demonstrated large reductions in particulate levels and chemical off-gassing, once outer clothing is removed; especially after washing with soap and tepid water [10]. Patients decontaminated pre-hospital should pose minimal risk to hospital workers assuming clothes are removed and skin is washed. The major exception to this rule occurs when highly persistent military chemical agents are employed. Residual agent may continue to pose a small threat to hospital personnel until a more thorough process is completed. The powered air-purifying respirator (PAPR), equipped with both particulate and chemical filters should serve most hospital based scenarios.

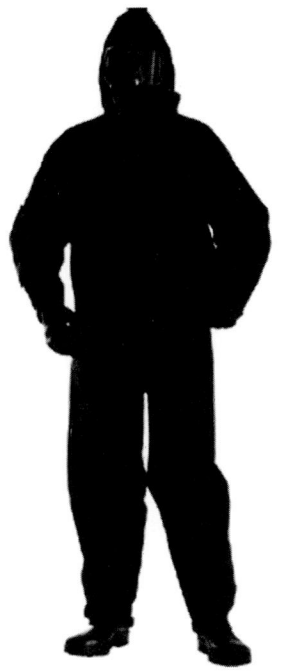

Figure 7.13 Demron™ Radiation Protection Suit [12].

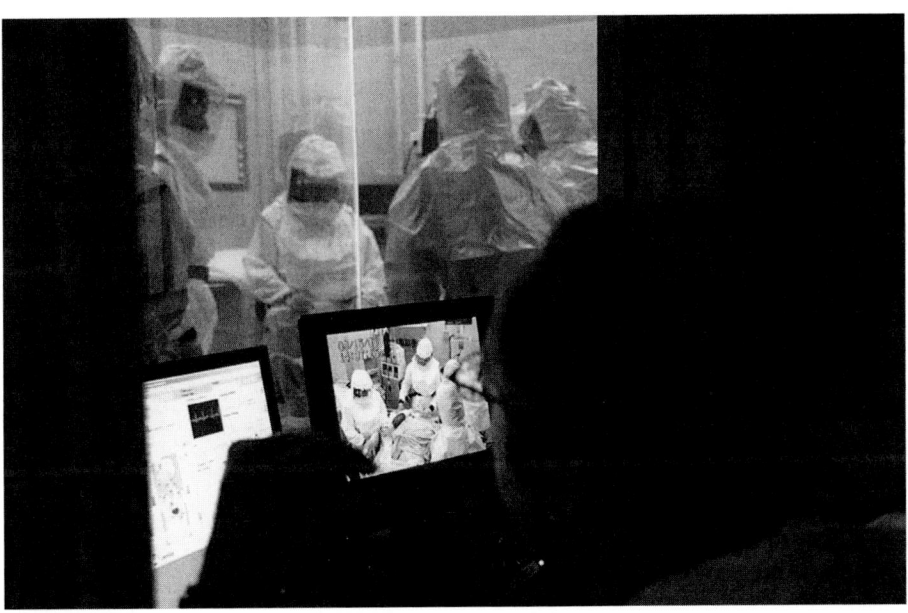

Figure 7.14 Powered Air Purifying Respirator (PAPR) Training in the Operating Room Simulator at Hartford Hospital.

Appendix 7.1 Example 1. Vital Signs and PPE Checklist

(Source: Central Arkansas Veterans Healthcare System.) Force.

NAME_____

DATE_____

(INSPECT condition of ALL PPE prior to use)

*Medical Exclusion INNER SHROUD TUCKED INSIDE **TIME OUT:**

_____ PRE POST **BLOOD PRESSURE: HEART RATE:** * > []

RESPIRATION: TEMPERATURE: SKIN: *Open sore, large rash or **Prior heat stress or exhaustion_____ PAPR–COMBINATION CARTRIDGES.........PAPR FLOW CHECKED...............REMOVED SHOES, JEWELRY, ETC...............INNER NITRILE GLOVES...................................INNER SUIT...................................GLOVES & NECK TAPED..OUTER SUIT..BUTYL HOOD.............................GLOVES & NECK TAPED.............................OUTER GLOVES.........BOOTS.........SUIT TAPED OVER BOOTS...........................**CHECKED BY:**_____ **TIME IN SUIT:**_____ **Employee ID#:** *Diastolic > 105 70% (220 – Age)*Any irregular rate or rhythm * >24/ min* >99.5 F oral **WEIGHT:** sunburn **HYDRATION:**

MENTAL STATUS: Alert; oriented to time & place; clear speech; normal gait **MEDICAL HISTORY:** *Any meds last 72 hours _____ *Alcohol past 24 hours_____ *New meds Rx/diagnosis last 2 weeks _____

Symptoms fever, NV, diarrhea, cough in past 72 hours_____ *Pregnant _____ **NOTES: CHECKED BY:**_____

Example 2. Vital Signs Monitoring Checklist

(Source: U.S. Coast Guard National Strike Force)

ON-SITE MEDICAL MONITORING (ENTRY TEAM)

NAME: _____

CASE: _____

CASE NO.: _____

DATE: _____ EXPOSURE RISK: HIGH/MED/LOW

PROTECTIVE EQUIPMENT: _____

SUBSTANCE(S) INVOLVED: _____

CONCENTRATION/LENGTH OF EXPOSURE: _____

MEDICAL TESTING: _____

COMMENTS:

* *

PRE-ENTRY MEDICAL MONITORING: WEIGHT: _____

TEMPERATURE: _____ METHOD: _____

PULSE: _____ BP:SYSTOLIC _____ /DIASTOLIC _____

METHOD: _____

MONITORING CONDUCTED BY: _____

* *

POST-ENTRY MEDICAL MONITORING:

WEIGHT: _____ TEMPERATURE: _____

METHOD: _____ PULSE: _____ BP:

SYSTOLIC _____ /DIASTOLIC _____ METHOD: _____

MONITORING CONDUCTED BY: _____

* *

SUPERVISOR (RO/RS) VERIFICATION:

NAME: _____

COMMENTS:

Appendix 7.2 Example of Patient Decontamination Procedure

[Source: Northern Virginia Emergency Response Coalition. Available at: http://www.hazmatforhealthcare.org/download/doc/misc/Patient_Decontamination_Procedure-complete.doc (Accessed September 2, 2003).]

Ambulatory Patients

1. Direct patient to decon sector.
2. Children should be kept with their parents if at all possible; if no parent or older sibling is available then a Decon Team member should provide needed assistance to a child.
3. Patient should be given Personal Decon set as soon as it is available and be given rapid instructions on its use—Play the tape recorded set of instructions, if available. The kit stays with you as you proceed through the process. Open up the bag—it has three parts. Take out the plastic bags now.
4. Patient should quickly remove all clothing, putting valuables into the clear plastic bag and clothing into the large bag, then put both bags into the 3rd bag and cinch tight with tag number in pack. Patient should put numbered tag around their neck and wear it through decon and treatment.
5. The clothing bag should be set aside in a secure area.
6. If staff is available, patient's name and number should be recorded on the Patient Decon Record.
7. Patient should continue forward into the decon sector with remaining part of Personal Decon Kit.
8. Patient should quickly rinse themselves from head to toe with water using either the hand held sprayer, garden hose, or shower head.
9. Patient should next wash with soap and wash cloth or brush from the kit in a systematic fashion, cleaning open wounds first and then in a head-to-toe fashion for 5 minutes when the agent is non-persistent and 8 minutes when a persistent or unknown agent is involved. Discourage the patient from rubbing too vigorously while washing. Eye irritation may require the use of a topical anesthetic first before irrigating.
10. The Decon Team should closely observe each victim to ensure they are thorough in washing themselves. Particular attention should be made to ensure they wash the axilla, creases, folds, and hair. Help should be offered as necessary.
11. Once the washing is completed, each patient should thoroughly rinse themselves (this should require about a minute to complete).
12. Decon soap, wash cloths, brushes, and sponges should be put into a nearby trash can and NOT carried into the Cold Zone.
13. After the rinse/wash/rinse cycle is complete the patient should next proceed to the towel off area and complete drying off and leave the towel in the trash can.
14. Following drying off, the patient should put on the patient gown and proceed to the Triage Officer for rapid assessment and assignment to a Treatment Sector.
15. Additional treatment will be limited only to those interventions deemed life saving by the Decon Officer. Antidote administration should be done *via* the intramuscular (IM) route after cleaning the affected area first.
16. Decon Team members should be alert to the possibility that an ambulatory patient may clinically deteriorate and require immediate removal to the Non-Ambulatory Sector *via* backboard, stretcher, or wheelchair.

Non-Ambulatory Patients

1. Patient should be brought to the Decon Sector and tended to by a minimum of four decon personnel.
2. Each patient should be put onto a backboard or EMS stretcher with the pad removed.

3. All patient clothing should be removed and valuables put into the clear plastic bag and clothing into the large bag, then put both bags into the 3rd bag and cinch tight with tag number in pack. Clothing should be cut away where necessary.
4. Attention should be paid to minimizing the aerosolization spread of particulate matter by folding clothing inside out as removal is being done and dabbing the skin with sticky tape and or vacuuming.
5. Patient should have their clothing bag tag around their neck and wear it through decon and treatment.
6. The clothing bag should be set aside in a secure area. If staff is available, the patient's name and number should be recorded on the Patient Decon Record.
7. While resting the backboard on saw horses or other device or with the patient on an EMS stretcher, the patient should quickly be rinsed from head to toe with water using either the hand held sprayer, garden hose, or shower head; protection from aspiration of the rinse water should be ensured.
8. Next the patient should be washed with soap and either a brush or wash cloth in a systematic fashion, cleaning airway first followed by open wounds then in a head to toe fashion for 5 minutes when the agent is non-persistent and 8 minutes when a persistent or unknown agent is involved. Avoid rubbing too vigorously.
9. The patient should be rolled on their side for washing of the posterior head, neck, back, buttocks and lower extremities by 2–4 personnel; attention to a possible neck injury should be given.
10. Careful attention should be given to washing the voids and creases such as the ears, eyes, axilla, and groin.
11. Topical eye anesthetic may be required for effective eye irrigation to be done.
12. The patient should then be rinsed in a head to toe fashion that minimizes contamination spread for about one minute. Overspray or holding the rinsing devise too close so as to irritate the skin should be avoided.
13. Decon Team members should be alert to the probability that the non-ambulatory patient may require ABC's support (airway positioning, suctioning, O_2 administration, spinal stabilization, etc.) and administration of life saving antidote administration by IM injection. If IV therapy is needed the extremity site for the IV should be deconned quickly before the IV is started. If IV therapy is needed the patient should be pulled out of line in the Decon Corridor but remain in the Decon Sector.
14. The patient should be dried off, put into a hospital gown, and transferred to a clean backboard (or clean off and dry the board they are on if additional boards are not available). Patients on an EMS stretcher should be transferred to a clean backboard.
15. Decon soap, brushes and sponges should be put into a trash can and not carried into the Cold Zone. O_2 material should remain in the Decon Sector.
16. The patient should be taken to the Triage Officer for rapid assessment and assignment to area in the Treatment Sector.

Patients with Special Needs
Glasses/Contact Lenses
1. Patients with glasses should keep them if they cannot see without them. They must be washed and rinsed thoroughly during the decon process before being worn. Otherwise, the glasses should be placed in the valuables portion of the clothing bag.
2. Contact lenses should be removed and placed in the valuables portion of the clothing bag.

Canes/Walkers
1. Patients who use walking assist devices may retain them, but the device must be washed with soap and water during the decon process before being allowed into the Treatment Sector.

2. Patients who are unsteady standing and/or walking should be given a walker upon entry into the Decon Corridor. The walker should be used to assist with ambulation until they get to the end of the line when it should be retrieved, deconned, and returned to the front of the Decon Corridor for the next patient who needs it.

Percutaneous Lines/Saline Locks

1. Unless contaminated, percutaneous lines and saline locks should be covered with Tegoderm or Saran wrap before the area is decontaminated.
2. Contaminated percutaneous lines or saline locks should be removed before being decontaminated. After the area is cleaned, a dressing should be applied until in the Treatment Sector where antibiotic ointment and a new bandage should be applied.

Hearing Aids

Hearing aids CANNOT be immersed or otherwise be soaked with water. Thus, they should either be removed and placed in the valuables portion of the patient's clothing bag or if they must be used by the patient because there is no hearing without them, they should be carefully wiped off with a slightly saline moistened 4×4 gauze, dried off, put into a clear plastic bag, and handed to the patient. The cleaned hearing aid is NOT to be worn until the patient has completed the decon process (including washing the ears) and is in the Treatment Sector.

Dentures

1. Unless the oral cavity is contaminated dentures should remain in place and no decontamination is necessary.
2. If the oral cavity is contaminated, then the dentures should be removed, placed in a clear plastic bag with the patient's name or clothing identification number placed on it. The dentures should later be decontaminated in accordance with instructions received from the Poison Center and/or a dentist. The patient's mouth should be decontaminated with mouthwash or saline that is gargled and safely spit out into a bio-hazard bag. Note that, depending on the contaminant, it may not be possible to decontaminate plastic items, such as dentures.

Law Enforcement Officers with Weapons

1. In most cases law enforcement personnel who have been injured on the scene will have had their gun(s) removed before arrival and given to a fellow officer. However, if that is not the case, the weapon should be left in the holster and the gun belt removed by a Decon Team member and placed in a clear plastic bag labeled with the patient's name and/or clothing number. The bag should then be passed to the Treatment Sector where it should be given to a fellow officer or hospital Security Officer for safe keeping until it can be given to a representative of the injured officers department. *The gun should be left in the holster if at all possible.* If the gun must be removed, it should be handled by a Decon Team member familiar with firearms, rendered safe, placed in a clear plastic bag marked with the patient's name and/or clothing identification number, and given to a fellow officer or hospital Security Officer in the Treatment Sector.
2. Decon Team personnel should be aware that oftentimes an officer may have a backup weapon usually found in a holster near the ankle, in their pocket, in a ballistic vest, or near an armpit. The holster with the weapon in place should be removed and secured as described above.
3. An officer's gun belt may also contain items that could prove dangerous if allowed to get in the wrong hands. Thus, the belt should be collected and separately bagged ASAP and passed to a fellow officer or hospital Security Officer in the Treatment Sector.

DECONNING OF AN OFFICER'S WEAPON AND/OR GUN BELT WILL BE THE RESPONSIBILITY OF THE POLICE DEPARTMENT.

4. If the officer is wearing a ballistic vest it must be removed prior to undergoing decon. The vest is usually easily removed by loosening the Velcro straps and then pulling the vest apart and off the patient. It should then be placed in a large plastic bag identified with the patient's name and/or clothing number on it and passed to a fellow officer or Hospital Security Officer in the Treatment Sector.

(Prepared by: Northern Virginia Emergency Response Coalition.)

Appendix 7.3 PPE Donning and Doffing Sequence

(Source: Central Arkansas Veterans Healthcare System.)

PPE Donning Sequence

(*Note*: The following sequence outlines the *order* in which one hospital's employees find it efficient to put on their specific first receiver PPE. The list is not intended to provide detailed step-by-step instructions for putting on the PPE.)

1. Test PAPR flow rate to be sure it meets rate specified by the manufacturer.
2. Remove jewelry and clothing.
3. Put on inner nitrile gloves.
4. In *cold weather*: Put on inner suit. Tape gloves at wrist and zipper at neck.
5. In *warm weather*: Put on scrubs.
6. Put on outer chemical protective suit to waist. Put on boots and outer chemical protective gloves.
7. Connect PAPR to hood with hose; turn airflow on. Put on butyl hood (position the inside shroud between suits). Pull chemical protective suit up and on.
8. Ensure zipper is covered and secured, put tape on top.
9. Belt PAPR to waist.
10. Put outer butyl hood shroud over suit.
11. Stretch arms, pull suit sleeves *over* gloves, tape in place.
12. Pull suit cuff over boot top, tape in place.
13. Place a piece of tape on the hood exterior and label with the employee's name & time that employee is entering Hospital Decontamination Zone.

PPE Decontamination and Doffing Sequence

(*Note*: The following sequence outlines the *order* in which one hospital's employees find it effective to decontaminate themselves and their PPE as one procedure, to minimize the chance of contaminating their skin while removing their first receiver PPE. The list is not intended to provide detailed step-by-step instructions.)

1. Wash hands thoroughly.
2. Still wearing PPE, wash self, starting at the top of the head and working down to the bottom of the boots. Have a partner wash your back.
3. Untape boots and gloves, but do not remove them.
4. Unlock PAPR and place it on chair/gurney/floor, etc.
5. Remove the outer suit—roll the suit away from you, inside out (with help from a partner). Remove outer gloves along with the outer suit.
6. Remove PAPR hood, place in waste.
7. Step out of boots and suit into final rinse area (keep inner gloves and clothing on). Wash and rinse thoroughly (with partner's help).
8. In *cold weather*: Remove (inner) suit, place in waste.
9. Remove nitrile gloves: first pinch one glove and roll it down partially, then place thumb in other glove and remove both gloves simultaneously.
10. Wash again, removing inner clothing, then step out of decontamination shower and into towels/blankets.

Appendix 7.4 Example of Technical Decontamination Process for Hospital Personnel

[Source: *Managing Hazardous Materials Incidents. Hospital Emergency Departments: A Planning Guide for the Management of Contaminated Patients.* Volume II. U.S. Department of Health and Human Services. Public Health Service. Agency for Toxic Substances and Disease Registry (Revised 2000), www.atsdr.cdc.gov.]

Personnel should remove protective clothing in the following sequence.

1. Remove tape (if used), securing gloves and boots to suit.
2. Remove outer gloves, turning them inside out as they are removed.
3. Remove suit, turning it inside out and folding downward (first loosen and secure PAPR belt). Avoid shaking.
4. Remove boot/shoe cover from one foot and step over the clean line. Remove other boot/shoe cover and put that foot over the clean line.
5. Remove respirator. The last person removing his/her respirator may first wash all other respirator hoods or facepieces with soapy water and thoroughly wipe PAPR fan housing, then clean his/her own equipment before removing his/her suit and gloves. Place the masks in plastic bag and hand the bag over the clean line for placement in second bag held by another staff member. Send bag for decontamination. Discard items that cannot be effectively cleaned (e.g., it may not be possible to completely remove persistent contaminants from PAPR belts).
6. Remove inner gloves and discard them in a drum inside the dirty area.
7. Secure the dirty area until the level of contamination is established and the area is properly cleaned.
8. Personnel should then move to a shower area, remove undergarments and place them in a plastic bag. Double-bag all clothing and label bags appropriately.
9. Personnel should shower and redress in normal working attire and then report for medical surveillance.

Appendix 7.5 Example of Integrated Procedures for First Receivers

Note: The *Emergency Management and Disaster Preparedness Plan—Chemically contaminated patient care protocol* included in this appendix was developed by the INOVA Health System (Virginia) for use in INOVA facilities. The INOVA Health System uses powered air-purifying respirators (PAPRs). However, in cases where information is adequate to determine that an air-purifying respirator (APR) would provide adequate protection against the hazard, APRs might be used in place of PAPRs. At INOVA facilities, a specific, designated individual (the *Charge MD*) is responsible for determining the appropriate PPE for the decontamination team and for making appropriate adjustments as the situation evolves.

This example plan represents a portion of the emergency management plan used by one healthcare organization. Based on their individual circumstances, other organizations will have different procedures, terminology, and division of responsibilities.

INOVA HEALTH SYSTEM Emergency Management & Disaster Preparedness Plan

Subject: ANNEX C- Chemically Contaminated Patient Care Protocol

Written: August 5, 2002 Revision:

Emergency Management and Disaster Preparedness Task Force

Purpose

To establish a policy for providing care to victims of hazardous materials and/or chemical terrorism incidents while ensuring the safety of the emergency department (ED) personnel and hospital environment.

Background

The potential for hazardous materials exposure requires specific procedures for the protection of the patient, staff, and the environment. It differs from the other emergency situations because of that added risk of contamination to staff and facility. Worker safety and training are key factors in the management of these medical emergencies. Often these patients may arrive at the hospital unannounced. Patients being transported by EMS may not have been fully decontaminated prior to their arrival to the hospital.

Toxicological principles

A. Exposure to hazardous materials may produce a wide range of adverse health effects. The likelihood of an adverse health effect occurring, and the severity of the effects, are dependent upon:
   a. The toxicity of the agent or pathogen;
   b. Route of exposure;
   c. The nature and extent of exposure to that substance.
B. Toxic chemical effects may be localized at the site of exposure, or may result in systemic symptomatology after absorption into the blood stream.
C. The three main routes of exposure are:
   a. *Inhalation* resulting in the introduction of toxic chemicals, radioisotopes, or pathogens via the respiratory tract. Most of the compounds that are inhaled are gases or vapors of volatile liquids. However, solids and liquids can be inhaled as dusts or aerosols. Inhalation of chemical agents generally result in a rapid absorption into the bloodstream because of the large surface and vascularity of the lungs. The signs and symptoms of pathologic exposure will usually occur 1–10 days after exposure.
   b. *Skin contact* or absorption via mucous membranes is usually not as rapid as inhalation. Exposure can be through the mucus membranes (including conjunctiva) and open wounds.
   c. *Ingestion* is a less common route of exposure. It can be the result of unintentional hand to mouth contamination or swallowing of saliva with trapped airborne particles. Or it may also be intentional, such as an oral ingestion for a suicide attempt.
D. In addition to the route of exposure, the amount of compound absorbed by the body depends upon the:
   a. Duration of exposure
   b. Concentration of contaminant
   c. Time of exposure
   d. Environmental factors
E. Response to toxic chemicals radiological agents and pathogens may differ among individuals because of the physiological variability present in the population.
   a. Age
   b. Pre-existing medical conditions
   c. Prior exposure
   d. Medications
   e. Concurrent injury
   f. Pregnancy

Notification

A. *Unannounced Arrival* refers to a patient that presents to the ED Triage Nurse or other healthcare provider. Once the healthcare provider determines a hazardous materials incident has occurred and contamination may be present he/she should:
   a. Direct the patient outside the ED lobby entrance and proceed to the entryway of the decon room. Confine the patient in this location and remain with them.
   b. Notify the charge nurse.
   c. Notify security at Triage to secure the area.
   d. Any persons the victim came in contact with, including the initial healthcare provider contact, should also be directed to the decon room until the extent of contact and the need for care can be determined.
   e. If there are multiple patients affected, prepare to implement the mass decontamination procedure utilizing identified

areas outside of the hospital facility but contiguous to the ED.

B. *Announced Arrival* is a patient already entered into the EMS system that arrives by ambulance. The major advantage created by pre-hospital notification is the provision of preparatory time and available clinical data and incident information from the field as well as initial intervention by EMS personnel. The arriving patient should be kept with the pre-hospital EMS personnel outside of the ED until the "decontamination team" is prepared to assume patient care.

Consultation with the referring agency as to the decontamination, if any, performed at the incident scene must occur prior to admitting these patients directly into the ED. This should depend on the nature of the agent, degree of decontamination provided in the field, and suspicion of potential contamination upon visual inspection of the patient. If in doubt, have the patient go through decontamination at the hospital.

Emergency Department Responsibilities

A. Communication Nurse
   a. Obtain information from caller.
      Determine caller's ID and telephone number.
      Type and nature of incident
      Number of victims
      Signs and symptoms being experienced by victim
      Nature of injuries
      Prior medical history of victim—meds and allergies
      Name of chemical involved and what information is readily available on product container if present
      Name of facility involved and/or type of contaminants found at facility
      Extent of victim decontamination in field
      Other medical interventions completed
      Estimated time of arrival (ETA)
   b. Notify charge nurse.
   c. Notify EMS Public Safety Communications Center (PSCC) of incident and request redirection of other ambulance traffic to ED lobby entrance.
   d. If incident involves multiple patients, request that ED be placed on "reroute" status.

B. Charge Nurse
   a. Consult with charge MD and assess the present patient capacity and acuity. If incident involves multiple patients, implement *"Disaster Plan—Annex C."*
   b. Expedite movement of "admitted" patients to assigned beds.
   c. Notify the ED Patient Care Director and Administrative Director as to the status of incoming contaminated patients. Consider the need for additional staff and resources and initiate response, if warranted.
   d. Initially assign 2 nurses and 2 technicians to the decontamination team.
   e. Notify ED registration, triage nurse, and security.
   f. Notify respiratory therapy and determine the number of adult/pediatric ventilators.
   g. Determine number of available adult/pediatric beds.

C. Administrative Director
   a. Notify security officers to redirect ED traffic and ambulances.
   b. Notify physical plant staff.
   c. Notify environmental services.
   d. Notify Personal Health for follow up on staff involved.
   e. Notify Media Relations to be available for purpose of public information if needed.
   f. Notify Administrator-on-call that *"Disaster Plan – Annex C"* is being implemented.

D. Charge MD
   a. Confer with ED Charge Nurse regarding the immediate need to implement the *"Disaster Plan – Annex C"* and assess the disposition status of existing patients in the ED.

b. Notify ED Chairman.
   c. Notify Poison Control—obtaining available product information to decontaminate and care for patient(s), when available.
   d. Notify critical care pharmacist with product information for anticipated antidote. Obtain inventory of available antidotes.
   e. Determine appropriate level of Personal Protective Equipment (PPE) for Decon Team.
   f. Assign MD and/or PA to Decon Team.
   g. Direct 1–2 personnel to set up decon area and 1–2 persons to assist decon team with dress out procedures
E. Security
   a. Secure entrances and exits to the ED.
   b. Assist with traffic and crowd control around the ED
   c. Will be responsible for maintaining "chain of custody" of personal belongings of patients undergoing decontamination. These items will NOT be individually cataloged, but rather placed in red biohazard plastic bags that will be tagged, numbered, and recorded.

Decontamination

Purpose

To remove or neutralize harmful materials that have gathered on personnel and/or equipment and to prevent secondary contamination to healthcare workers and the facility. Decontamination is a systematic process that is determined by the nature and degree of contamination. Effective decontamination consists of making the patient as clean as possible, meaning that the contamination has been reduced to a level that is no longer a threat to the patient or healthcare provider.

Decon Setup

In a "traditional" HAZMAT incident involving known exposure to chemical agents involving less than three patients simultaneously, consideration can be given to using the existing Emergency Department Decontamination Room, if available.

A. Decon room preparation technician shall be assigned to:
   a. Remove all non-essential and non-disposable equipment and items from established Hazmat/Decon wash room.
   b. Activate drain switch to contain runoff, if available.
   c. Obtain decon cart with necessary stocked items.
   d. Obtain crash cart and place contiguous to Decon wash room.
   e. Place D or E size O_2 tank with regulator.
   f. Place clean stretcher in Hazmat/Decon wash room with additional O_2 tank, BVM, and non-rebreather mask.
   g. Place stretcher outside of decon room on plastic ground cloth to receive non-ambulatory patient from ambulance.
   h. Place bucket for soiled items used in wash room for technical decon.
   i. Placed lined trash baskets in decon area for Biowaste.
   j. Place Personal Decon Kits (PDK) in decon area.
B. Mass decontamination setup
   In the event that the chemical exposure incident involves more than three people requiring decontamination simultaneously, or incident information suggests the arrival of large numbers of patients requiring decontamination as a result of a mass exposure, the preparation for mass decontamination should commence.
   The following materials have been identified as basic prerequisites for Mass Decontamination set up and preparation:
   a. A hose bib splitter for each bib within 100 feet (within range) of the proposed decontamination area.
   b. Two 100-foot hoses for each hose bib within range of the proposed decontamination area.
   c. Four (2 sets) sawhorses to hold litter bound patients within the decontamination area and set of C-clamps.
   d. Two backpack sprayers per facility.
   e. Two baby pools per facility.

f. Four buckets for each hose bib within range of the proposed decontamination area.
g. Four scrub brushes for each hose bib within range of the decontamination area.
h. Duct tape, flashlights, permanent markers, soap, large trash cans, red biohazard bags, and towels.
i. One blood pressure cuff, stethoscope, and set of trauma scissors per litter decontamination station.
j. Towels and redress kits.
k. Two Geiger counters per facility (Reference "*Disaster Plan – Annex R*").
l. Two Bull horns per facility.
m. Polaroid camera with film or digital camera for later use in identification of moribund patients.
n. A locked, centrally located storage mechanism (cart, closet, etc.) for storage of the aforementioned items.

Included in this Annex is a schematic diagram for use in establishing a Mass Decontamination procedure that details the process flow of patients. This should be adapted to each individual healthcare facility.

Level C Personal Protective Equipment
Decon team preparation

1. Obtain appropriate personal protective equipment (PPE) as recommended by ED charge physician.
2. A minimum of four persons should done PPE.
3. Decon team personnel should undergo pre-entry medical monitoring as soon as possible. Only personnel meeting inclusion criteria, and having met the required training standards will be allowed to dress in PPE.
4. The Inova Health System has elected to use Level C respiratory protection and chemical protective clothing as the highest level of protection available. Level C respiratory protection is comprised of:

   Powered Air Purifying Respirator (PAPR): This provides air that is drawn through organic/HEPA filter cartridges affixed to a battery powered unit worn by the decon team personnel on a belt around their waist. It is worn as a hood placed over the head, with the inner sleeve tucked into the chemical protective clothing suit.

   Air Purifying Respirator (APR): This provides air that is filtered through organic/HEPA filter cartridges dependent on the negative inspiration created by the work of breathing. This is worn as a full-face mask with the cartridges affixed to the mask. (caution: These respiratory protective equipment contain LATEX products and are not to be worn by LATEX-allergic individuals).

Level C chemical protective clothing is contained in the Tri-con PPE packs that include:
   2 layers of gloves,
   chemical resistant suit (check for appropriate sizing), and
   chemical resistant boots.

Note: Some Tri–Con PPE packs will also contain an APR mask. Consult with the ED physician in charge with regards to selection of APR or PAPR. Persons needing to use glasses, or those with beards or full moustaches, are NOT to use a face mask device.

A Decon team member should double check to assure all personnel have donned their PPE properly. Special attention should be paid to proper seal of mask/face and proper occlusion at wrists and ankles. Particular attention must be made to ensure all "pull tabs" are removed from respiratory cartridge filters prior to use.

Immediately evaluate the available information and confirm/re-confirm (as more information becomes available) that your key *operational* planning assumptions for Level C PPE are valid:

Incident location (including area of significant downwind contamination) does not include your facility.

Agent characteristics: Known or suspected agent does not require higher level of PPE (example: high-grade plutonium or other very rare agents).

Event characteristics: Your facility is not being "overrun" by casualties.

Adjust the planned operations as indicated by the evolving circumstances. Possible adjustments include:

Upgrading plan: more personnel protected, shorter rotation periods for PPE personnel, longer soap and wash cycles for victims, obtaining assistance from other hospitals or from emergency response resources.

Evacuating or closing the facility to "shelter in place" if the hospital is in the zone of contamination.

"Lock-down" of facility if agent, agent concentration, or the number of patients exceeds the safe operation of the plan or compromises the hospital integrity.

Any need to isolate the decontamination wastewater (notify authorities to remove it per prior arrangement). Otherwise, notify "downstream" water authorities that decontamination wastewater is entering the sewer system.

Downgrade the plan (lesser protective clothing and/or respiratory protection if agent is identified as non-threatening). This should be a high priority if possible, since safely downgrading the level of PPE will enhance the efficiency of the decontamination process.

A. Donning Procedures

Staff medical monitoring to be completed by assigned Registered Nurse (RN) or MD (use designated medical monitoring form included in this Annex). Use a room with privacy and plenty of sitting space to facilitate donning of PPE.

1. It is preferable that a scrub suit be worn in lieu of regular street clothes. Clothing should be suitable for preserving comfortable body temperature.
2. Remove all jewelry and leather material and place in plastic bag with your name on it—place it in a secure location for the Security to maintain. Persons needing to wear glasses or with beards or mustaches are NOT to use a face mask device.
3. Persons with long hair should apply a hairnet or place-up in a braid.
4. Hydrate with 8–16 ounces of fluid.
5. If time allows have blood pressure (BP), pulse, respiration rate, and temperature taken and recorded on Medical Surveillance form.
6. Obtain appropriate sized PPE ensemble pack or individual pieces, APR/ PAPR, battery, and appropriate cartridges (2–3 depending on APR/PAPR being used).
7. Layout PPE pieces and confirm they are right size and in working order.
8. Apply appropriate type of cartridges (most incidents will require HEPA/organic vapor cartridge set) and remove all pull-tabs. DO NOT OVERTIGHTEN the cartridges on the mask.
9. Put on latex or plastic inner glove—consider placing light circular band around top of glove to lessen chance of premature removal during doffing.
10. While sitting, remove shoes and place on foot covers (foot protection should not present tear risk to the suit nor be heelless).
11. Pull on chemical/biological protective suit to waist.
12. Place outer booties/boots on over the foot portion of the suit.
13. Using duct tape, seal top of booties to protective coverall (use a flap of tape at the end and place facing front to ease removal).
14. For chemical incident, place one set of nitrile gloves and one set of butyl rubber gloves on hands. For biological incident, use double plastic/latex gloves or plastic/latex and nitrile gloves.
15. Seal seam of protective suit and gloves with duct tape (use a flap of tape at the end and on the front of the wrist area to ease removal of tape).
16. Zip up protective suit to neck and close zipper securing and covering zipper seal.
17. If using PAPR, put on vest. Cinch up vest to snug fitting around with motor unit riding above the buttocks. Secure battery to the belt

(side of the dominant hand is suggested) and plug in the PAPR. The air hose should come over the shoulder not under the arm.

18. Position APR/PAPR facepiece to ensure full visibility and comfortable fit. Tighten all bands in pairs by pulling them backwards and not up. Confirm tight seal by covering cartridge opening with hand and taking deep breaths—face shield should pull tight against face. If faulty seal is found, then re-tighten all bands and repeat seal test. If tight seal cannot be obtained, then seek second provider assistance or use hooded devise.
19. Pull suit hood up and over the head maximizing the coverage of the head, neck, and ears and covering the APR/PAPR seal edge around the face—ensure the suit is pulled up and fully under the chin and zipper is closed and covered. There should be *no exposed skin.*
20. Turn PAPR on, also making sure that all cartridge tabs are removed to allow airflow.
21. Have someone place a 3 in. piece of Velcro or tape across shoulders with staff member's last name and function (e.g., Jones RN) written with magic marker.
22. Have second person perform safety check before proceeding to assigned work area.
23. Note time personnel left the dress out area.

B. Ambulatory Patient Decontamination
Children should be kept with their parents if at all possible; if no parent or older sibling is available then a Decon Team member should provide needed assistance to a child.

Patient should be given Personal Decon kit as soon as it is available and be given rapid instructions on its use.

The ambulatory patient may be directed by the decon nurse and technician to self-decon in the Emergency Department Decontamination Room thereby sparing additional staff from involvement (though the full decon team should remain dressed and ready in an adjacent room if intervention is needed). If the situation involves multiple patients requiring simultaneous decontamination, this process will occur using the Mass Decontamination set up.

1. If dry contaminant, remove first by using tape or dust off clothing or skin before wetting.
2. Have patient remove all valuables and place in the small plastic bag.
3. Clothing is removed and placed in the larger plastic bag. Place both bags into the red biohazard plastic bag. Place identifying tag with unique patient number on bag and seal off top. Place outside on ramp area for future disposition by Safety and Security.
4. Patient will do head-to-toe gross decontamination wash using mild soap and water. Have patient place ID band around wrist. This ID band will have the same identifying number that has been placed on the red biohazard plastic bag holding the patient's personal effects.
5. Special attention should be paid in the washing process to hair and all body crevices. Wash time cycle should be five (5) minutes per person under a single stream of water.
6. Water temperature should be tepid.
7. Washing should be gentle to avoid abrading skin.
8. Open wounds should be washed first with sterile water and covered with occlusive dressing prior to remainder of body decontamination.
9. Upon completion of wash cycle, patient should step away from the immediate wash area, towel dry, and put on a supplied Tyvek® gown from the Patient Redress Kit.
10. All ED towels and wash cloths used by patients in the showering process should be placed in a marked contaminated container for later clean up and decontamination.
11. Patient may then enter the ED, where the receiving RN can obtain vital signs, complete secondary triage, complete decon paperwork, and transport to an assigned bed in ED.

12. Decon team personnel should be decontaminated prior to entering the ED as described in Personnel (Technical) Decon section.
13. Soap should be changed out every five patients or whenever needed.

C. Non-Ambulatory Patients

In a mass exposure to chemical agents, non-ambulatory patients will most likely arrive after the initial arrival of ambulatory patients exposed in the same geographic location. Because of the trimodal distribution of injuries, non-ambulatory patients are likely to be more significantly exposed to the contaminating agent. Those who are most severely affected will be in the expectant category at the incident scene, and those who are least affected or only "potentially exposed" will arrive as ambulatory patients.

The non-ambulatory patient decontamination should be performed simultaneously with patient stabilization. Basic life support (ABC's) will be maintained, but definitive intervention should be delayed until the patient is decontaminated, to a degree that ensures staff safety and that invasive procedures will not increase the patient's risk of systemic toxic absorption. If large numbers of non-ambulatory patients are delivered for decontamination and treatment simultaneously, the ED Charge Physician will be required to make urgent triage decisions.

1. Patient should be received on a backboard and stretcher by EMS staff. If incident involves a single non-ambulatory patient, utilization of the Emergency Department Decon Room may be considered. If multiple patients are expected, set up of the non-ambulatory mass decontamination corridor should commence.
   a. Placement of sawhorses with available C-clamps in order to secure backboards to the sawhorses.
   b. Availability of water source for adequate decontamination, including use of back-pack sprayers.
2. The Decon team for non-ambulatory patients must include a minimum of four (4) providers, two of whom will be responsible for turning the patient on the backboard and one who will be responsible for maintaining cervical spine precautions.
3. If the patient has not had a primary gross decon in the field (defined as the removal of clothing and first wash), visible particulate matter should be removed by gently brushing or dusting, and clothing should be cut and rolled away from the center of body, in order to contain the contaminants on the clothing.
4. Follow procedure for removal and bagging of personal valuables.
5. Follow procedure for head-to-toe decontamination wash cycle.
6. Irrigate open wounds with irrigation syringe and copious amounts of saline and cover with occlusive dressings. Any existing dressing must be removed and placed in a biohazard trash container.
7. Eye irrigation may be done with Morgans lens and NS and/or IV tubing alone, if gross contaminants on the face are suspected. Otherwise, perform manual irrigation with copious fluids.
8. Gentle ear and nasal irrigation with frequent suctioning from portable suction may be done if such contamination is suspected.
9. C-collars as well as backboards must be washed or changed if they are still required for patient immobilization.
10. Patient should be transferred to a clean stretcher for entry into the ED.

D. Personnel (Technical) Decon

Prior to leaving the decon room the decontamination team must undergo decontamination.

1. All equipment used by the decon staff must be placed in appropriate receptacles or in bins designated for equipment which can be cleaned and reused. Refer to clean-up and recovery protocol for direction on rehabilitation of used equipment.

2. Decon staff will undergo a technical decontamination wash from head-to-toe involving the outer garments, gloves, and boots.
3. After the wash is complete, personnel should remove protective clothing in the following sequence:
   a. Remove outer gloves, turning them inside out as they are removed and place in biohazard trash container.
   b. Remove tape from wrist and boot tops.
   c. Remove boots.
   d. Remove suit, turning inside out and avoid shaking.
   e. Remove APR mask or PAPR hood. The last member removing his/her respiratory protective equipment may take responsibility for washing all masks in soapy water. Refer to clean-up and recovery protocol.
   f. Remove inner glove and discard into biohazard trash container.
   g. Isolate all potentially contaminated materials until level of contamination is established and arrangements for cleaning and handling of trash and equipment can be determined.
   h. Post-exposure medical monitoring should be initiated and new data recorded on the primary form.
   i. Personnel should then remove scrub wear and shower and dress in replacement scrubs.

E. Emergency Decon

Staff member distress is recognized.
Staff member PPE immediately decontaminated with soap and water.
PPE removed quickly in head to toe fashion in cold zone area. Medical care rendered as warranted.

Key Resources/Points of Contact

Notifications of appropriate authorities:

Law Enforcement-
Local Police Department
Federal Bureau of Investigation/DC [202-324-3000]
Fire/Rescue Department
Local Health Department
State Health Department Emergency Epidemiology After Hours [1-866-820-9611]
National Capital Region Poison Control Center [202-625-3333]
Agency for Toxic Substances and Disease Registry (ATSDR) [1-404-498-0120]
National Response Center [1-800-424-8802]

In-hospital HAZMAT Incident

A. Contain victims in area of incident until contamination is confirmed.
B. Administrative Director to be notified by area supervisor of incident site and specifics.
C. Hospital operator, notified by area supervisor, shall page ED charge nurse with HAZMAT location.
D. Hospital operator shall page Safety and Security to restrict access to the site.
E. ED charge nurse and ED charge physician assign HAZMAT team for response to site *ONLY* if patients are identified to be immediately in danger of exposure.
F. If Emergency Department HAZMAT team required to respond within facility have the communication nurse call PSCC to request ED "reroute" status and request Fire Department HAZMAT response per facility protocol.
G. The HAZMAT team should then dress in appropriate level of PPE for the given response. If unknown contaminant, dress in highest level of protection available.
H. The HAZMAT team responds to site bringing portable decontamination equipment for decontamination at a safe area closest to the site of incident.
   1. Single patient—non-ambulatory bring two stretchers, one with containment cover and hose and container for runoff collection.
   2. Ambulatory—bring kiddy pools (2) and backpack sprayers or large irrigation bottles for decon wash.
I. Decon shall be completed at site (as in previously described manner) until patient is clean

enough for transport to ED for more definitive decon.
J. Transport to ED shall be on the clean stretcher with a clean transport team.
K. ED HAZMAT team to complete personal decon at the incident site prior to return to ED.

Medical Monitoring

The need to perform ongoing medical monitoring of those healthcare personnel participating in the decontamination procedure is *MANDATORY*. This entails a systematic evaluation of all participants, focusing particular attention to the risk of suffering adverse reactions from heat, stress or hazardous materials exposure. This is performed for the purpose of prevention or early recognition of such symptoms, and in compliance with federal regulations.

1. Medical monitoring is performed prior to donning PPE in order to:
   a. Ascertain baseline vital signs.
   b. Identify staff who will be disqualified from donning PPE and participating in the decontamination process due to pre-existing medical conditions.
   c. Identify staff who may be at a higher risk for potential adverse effects while working in this environment.
2. Pre-entry physicals are required on all individuals in protective clothing and performing hazardous material operations. This is to be completed within one hour prior to entry, when possible.

Pre-entrance Exam Components

1. Vital signs
   a. Blood pressure, pulse, respiration rate, and temperature
   b. Weight (estimated)
2. Skin evaluation for presence of
   a. Rashes
   b. Lesions
   c. Open wounds
3. Mental status evaluation, including assessment of psychological stressors.
4. Medical History
   a. Chronic illnesses
   b. Recent illnesses
   c. Medications, including OTC taken within past the 72 hours
   d. Current symptoms of fever, nausea, diarrhea, vomiting, coughing, wheezing, or recent alcohol consumption.
5. Exclusion criteria
   a. Blood pressure: diastolic over 95
   b. Pulse: greater that 70% maximum heart rate (220 age) $\times$ 0.7 irregular rhythm not previously documented
   c. Respiratory rate: greater than 24 per minute
   d. Temperature: less than 97 or greater that 99.5
   e. Weight or Size: inability to fit in available suit without causing undue strain on seams
   f. Skin evaluation: open sores, large areas of rash, or significant sunburn
   g. Mental status: any alteration
   h. Recent medical history: nausea, vomiting, diarrhea within the past 72 hours, recent heat related injury, new prescriptions started within the past 72 hours.
   i. Pregnancy

All staff must be cleared for participation by the ED charge physician prior to participation.

6. Entry Medical Monitoring
   a. Performed before donning PPE.
   b. Based on buddy evaluation by team member.
   c. Observe for changes in gait, speech, or behavior.
   d. Any complaints of chest pain, dizziness, SOB, weakness, headache, nausea or vomiting should be reported.
   e. Reporting of symptoms requires immediate personnel decon and removal from the decon site.

f. Personnel data should be recorded on HAZMAT Medical Monitor form (see attached).
7. Post-entry Medical Monitoring
   a. Vital signs repeated every 10 minutes until return to less that 85% of maximum pulse rate.
   b. Oral rehydration started immediately upon completion of personal decon.
   c. IV hydration and more aggressive medical evaluation shall be initiated for victims displaying medical illness and/or unstable vital signs.
8. The completed Hazmat Medical Monitoring form shall be forwarded to Employee Health for review and decision, if further evaluation is needed. The assessment form is to become part of the individual's occupational health file.

Equipment/Supply Acquisition

If needed equipment and supplies are not available in the ED, the ED charge physician should be notified immediately. This information should be immediately forwarded to the *disaster support center*, which can help procure needed materials. If all on-site resources have been exhausted, the Inova Health System *disaster command center* will be contacted by the hospital Disaster Support Center in order to identify location of needed supplies and additional logistical support.

Clean-up and Recovery

Upon completion of the decontamination process, immediate consideration must be given to the following issues:

- Personal belongings and valuables of patients
  These items will be in tagged, sealed red biohazard bags kept outside of the healthcare facility under the direct supervision of the hospital Safety and Security staff, or local law enforcement personnel. These items may not be returned until they are deemed safe for handling and their evidentiary content has been evaluated.

- Bio-hazard trash can contents
  These trash cans will contain soaps, sponges, scrub brushes, towels, and other items used by patients during the decontamination process. These bags must be sealed and segregated for later removal by contract waste haulers.

- Towel discard bins
  These bins will hold the towels discarded by patients who have completed the decontamination process just prior to their entry into the healthcare facility. These bags must be segregated for possible laundering or later removal by contract waste haulers.

- Wastewater effluent
  In the event that mass decontamination efforts are required, the importance of life safety concerns supercedes the potential environmental impact of contaminated effluent. Every attempt should be made to direct this effluent into the sanitary sewer, with immediate notification of the proper municipal agencies. In those cases in which only limited numbers of patients are involved, every attempt should be made to contain this effluent using "baby pools" or similar methods. Such collected water must then be properly disposed of under the direction and supervision of the appropriate municipal agencies and contract waste haulers.

Any area outside of the healthcare facility that was used in the mass decontamination process and was inside of the warm or hot zones must be cordoned off until such time as it is verified by hazardous materials experts that no risk of contamination exists.

References

1. C. G. Hurst. Decontamination, in *Textbook of Military Medicine: Medical Aspects of Chemical and Biological Warfare*, Office of the Surgeon General, Department of the Army, 1997.
2. www.ezem.com.
3. M. G. Hamilton, J. Conley, and N. Nation. Effect of the Canadian Reactive Skin Decontamination Lotion on Non-occluded Porcine Epidermal Wounds.

4. M. E. Tadros and M. D. Tucker. United States Patent, 6,566,574, Formulations for neutralization of chemical and biological toxants, May 20, 2003.
5. www.envirofoam.com.
6. www.deconsolutions.com.
7. www.usgn.com.
8. Modec, Inc., Technical Report, MOD2003-1012-G, Formulations for the Decontamination and Mitigation of CB Warfare Agents, Toxic Hazardous Materials, Viruses, Bacteria and Bacterial Spores, February, 2003.
9. E. Rabner, et al. Decontamination issues for chemical and biological warfare agents: how clean is clean enough?, International Journal of Environmental Health Research, 11, 128–148, 2001.
10. OSHA, Best Practices for Hospital-Based First Receivers of Victims from Mass Casualty Incidents involving Release of Hazardous Substances, January, 2005.
11. S. Törngren, et al. Personal decontamination after exposure to simulated liquid phase contaminants: Functional assessment of a new unit, *Clinical Toxicology*, 36(6):567–573, 1998.
12. R. S. Lindsay. Swatch Test Results of Commercial Chemical Protective Gloves to Challenge by Chemical Warfare Agents. Executive Summary, Soldier and Biological Chemical Command, Department of the Army, AMSSB-REN, Aberdeen Proving Ground, MD, 2002.
13. www.radshield.com.
14. R. S. Lindsay and A. G. Pappas. Test Results of Phase 3 Level A Suits to Challenge by Chemical and Biological Warfare Agents and Similants: Executive Summary, Soldier and Biological Chemical Command, Department of the Army, AMSSB-REN, Aberdeen Proving Ground, MD, 2002.
15. Pal, et al. *Journal of Hazardous Materials*, 33:123–141, 1993.
16. Sandia National Laboratories, 2003 and Modec, Inc., http://www.deconsolutions.com/TIMS.htm United States Army Medical Research Institute of Chemical Defense, Bioscience 98, 1998.

8 EMS Preparation for Terrorist Events

MICHAEL ZACHERA, III

8.1 Introduction

Terrorist events can happen anywhere. Commonly, the high value targets that everyone thinks of are in the large cities: Office buildings in New York City, bridges in San Francisco, government offices in Washington, DC are all examples of the "classic" urban terrorist target. But we cannot forget that there are plenty of targets of opportunity in rural America. Nuclear power plants, airports, shopping malls, prisons, and drinking water reservoirs are examples.

Preparing for a terrorist event is everyone's responsibility from the medical control physician to the service chief, to the individual crew members. Areas of focus may change but we all share the overall responsibility of planning for terrorism.

8.2 Preparation

The fire service has an excellent concept that EMS can adapt for preparation of terrorist events. It is the process of pre-planning.

A fire department will look at a building/location and plan on how to fight a fire or perform a rescue that may occur there, prior to any emergency happening. The process of pre-planning includes such things as the position of units, the location of the water supply and the presence of hazardous materials and any other hazards that may be present. The need for specialized resources is also identified in this process. After planning is completed, the fire service will then practice the plan to identify weaknesses and go back and make changes to the plan from those identified weaknesses.

An excellent acronym to remember when it comes to disaster/terrorist events is the "6 Ps" (Proper Pre-Planning Prevents Poor Performance). The more we plan, practice and make changes to the plan, the greater the likelihood that should a terrorist event happen we will be able to organized a smooth operation.

8.3 Urban vs. Rural Preparation

Many of us traditionally think of terrorist attacks in an urban environment; Tokyo, New York City, Baghdad, London, Belfast and Madrid are all cities that have had high profile terrorist events. But these events have also happened in Shanksville, PA and in Beslan, Russia; rural America is just as likely to be attacked as urban America.

Differences in preparation should be in scale and not content. Certainly New York City, with a population of 7 million will need to have more supplies, larger shelters and more locations that will need pre-planning. The Town of Chaplin, CT with a population of 2000 will need far fewer supplies, smaller shelters, and fewer pre-planned locations. Both areas should be planning for biological, chemical, nuclear, radiological, and explosive terrorist events (Table 8.1). Again, our differences are in scale, not content.

A sense of safety and complacency can come over the rural provider. As such it is that much more important for rural areas to plan ahead.

Consider where we locate our nuclear power plants. Many are near large urban areas, but are

Table 8.1 Potential targets of terrorist events

Urban	Rural
Water Supply	Water Supply (typically to urban areas)
Electrical Generation	Electrical Generation
Stadiums	Stadiums
Entertainment venues	Entertainment venues
Airports (smaller municipal airports)	Airports (many times larger airports)
Monuments	Monuments
Government Offices	Government Offices
Schools	Schools
Hospitals	Hospitals
Mass Transit	
Internet Hubs	
Communications grids	

actually located in rural communities. For example, Shippingport, PA, population 237, is about 40 miles from Pittsburgh and is home to a nuclear power plant. Our newer, larger airports that serve urban areas are also commonly located outside of city limits in a suburban or rural environment.

8.4 Personnel and Training

The Occupational Health and Safety Administration has rules and regulations regarding training for personnel who respond to Hazardous Materials Incidents (Table 8.2) [1]. A weapons of mass destruction (WMD) event can be thought of a hazardous material incident. Using the same terminology as haz-mat regulations, staff can be thought of as having the following levels of training: Awareness, Operations, Technician, Specialist and Incident Commander.

The National Fire Protection Administration also has guidelines that address the training of staff for response to Hazardous Materials Incidents (NFPA 427). In addition to training staff to the appropriate level, realistic drills are needed to reinforce the training. These drills should be done frequently to keep responders skills sharp.

Drills can be run in a variety of ways. They can be as simple as playing the "Mass-Casualty Board Game" to as complex as a full-fledged exercise with a live burn, explosions, moulaged patients, transporting units and hospital, Emergency Department, Police and Fire Departments as well as Federal assets (Such as a TopOff exercise).

Remember that drills and exercises are meant to be a practice for the real event. The more realistic and stressful the environment for the drill the better. When responders are faced with a real situation they will fall back on what they have practiced. This is a level of skill called "accommodation" by educators. This is when responders know what the appropriate intervention is for the patient, and do not have to think about performing the intervention, they can just do it with minimal direction. It is also referred to "tacit knowledge" or "muscle memory." This level of knowledge and skill comes from hands on, emotional, and realistic practice. These frequent drills are for experience and will help the rescuers to approach a true WMD scenario with confidence. If a responder has never practiced a WMD scenario, then they will be approaching the scene as a novice rather than as a practiced veteran. If we want EMS staff to respond properly, this is the level of knowledge we need to attain.

Besides being practice for street personnel, drills also allow for supervisory and executive personnel to practice their roles in a WMD event. Not having leadership experience in an emergency situation can have poor outcomes, even with experienced street personnel.

Often we promote our experienced street level providers to supervisory positions, without adequate training. Leadership training is important. Practice in the leadership role is important. Remember, changing your normal role is difficult. How many times has second and third arriving units assumed the role of incident commander because the first arriving unit did not? Many times this has happened because the initial responder was unfamiliar with the leadership role that he or she was supposed to assume.

Leaders and managers are trained and just like anyone else when confronted with extraordinary circumstances they may not always rise to the challenge. Some people may say that it is impossible to train someone to that level. But we regularly train street level providers to go into burning buildings, hazardous material incidents and other

Table 8.2 Levels of training for personnel

Awareness (29 CFR 1910.120(q)(6)(i))	At a minimum all responding staff should be trained at the haz-mat awareness level and WMD awareness level. First responders at the awareness level are individuals who are likely to witness or discover a hazardous substance release and who have been trained to initiate an emergency response sequence by notifying the proper authorities of the release. They would take no further action beyond notifying the authorities of the release.
Operations (29 CFR 1910.120(q)(6)(ii))	First responders at the operations level are individuals who respond to releases or potential releases of hazardous substances as part of the initial response to the site for the purpose of protecting nearby persons, property, or the environment from the effects of the release. They are trained to respond in a defensive fashion without actually trying to stop the release. Their function is to contain the release from a safe distance, keep it from spreading, and prevent exposures.
Technician (29 CFR 1910.120(q)(6)(iii))	Hazardous materials technicians are individuals who respond to releases or potential releases for the purpose of stopping the release. They assume a more aggressive role than a first responder at the operations level in that they will approach the point of release to plug, patch, or otherwise stop the release of a hazardous substance.
Specialist (29 CFR 1910.120(q)(6)(iv))	Hazardous materials specialists are individuals who respond with and provide support to hazardous materials technicians. Their duties parallel those of the hazardous materials technician, however, those duties require a more directed or specific knowledge of the various substances they may be called upon to contain. The hazardous materials specialist would also act as the site liason with Federal, state, local, and other government authorities in regards to site activities.
Incident Commander (29 CFR 1910.120(q)(6)(v))	Incident commanders, who will assume control of the incident scene beyond the first responder awareness level, shall receive at least 24 hours of training equal to the first responder operations level and in addition have competency in the following areas: Know and be able to implement the employer's incident command system. Know how to implement the employer's emergency response plan. Know and understand the hazards and risks associated with employees working in chemical protective clothing. Know how to implement the local emergency response plan. Know of the state emergency response plan and of the Federal Regional Response Team. Know and understand the importance of decontamination procedures.

dangerous environments. A leader's response to a crisis can define his career (e.g., former FEMA Director Michael Brown during Hurricaine Katrina in 2005). A good lesson for EMS leaders and elected leaders is to remember that one of the most important roles of a leader is to lead during times of crisis (One of the most important roles of any leader is crisis manager). This includes the ability to make decisions in the heat of battle.

8.5 Treatment Protocols

Part of pre-planning for a WMD event includes the formation of treatment protocols. Examples are attached in the appendix to this chapter.

Besides treatment protocols, appropriate medications need to be stockpiled and EMS responders need to be trained in their use. Specific examples include auto-injectors of 2-pam chloride, atropine, and diazepam for nerve agents. As well as amyl nitrate, sodium nitrite, sodium thiosulfate for cyanide poisoning.

Questions abound regarding where these medications should be stored, who should have access to them and when. Different EMS systems have come to varying conclusions regarding the storage location of the WMD medications. Some services store them at a local hospital, others at the service headquarters. Still others store them in each individual EMS unit or in a supervisor's unit.

For immediate use, they should be stored in each responding EMS unit. This type of preparation comes with a price. The majority of these medications will be wasted, as they are not used frequently (if at all, in your typical EMS service). But to truly be available to those who would have need for them, they should be stored in each unit.

The other consideration with medications is quantity. How much should be stored in an individual unit? Perhaps enough for each crew member and maybe one patient? Ten patients? Physical space becomes an issue here. Some systems stock their supervisory vehicles with larger amounts of WMD medications. Others keep them stocked in a local hospital pharmacy.

8.6 Patient Decontamination

Before any treatment of the patient can happen, decontamination must occur. (see Chapter 7).

Upon recognition of a potential WMD event, creation of a perimeter and denying entry to civilian personnel should become a priority. Normally this is a job for law enforcement, however EMS providers must realize that on many occasions they may arrive prior to many law enforcement officers and that civilians may turn to them for direction. That being the case, a basic knowledge of creating a perimeter for a hazardous material incident should be understood by responding EMS personnel.

EMS and responding personnel also need to realize that by creating a perimeter we are keeping people safe from the agent involved and therefore attempting to keep casualties low. What we may not be able to do is keep people safe from themselves. Remember that in many circumstances we will be splitting up friends, co-workers, and family members who end up on opposite sides of the perimeter. These "halves" of families/friends will work very hard to get back together. Taking time (if it is possible) to explain the circumstances to these "halves" may help to prevent creating more victims. An example of one way to address this issue is to ask that those looking for family members in an affected area to congregate in one place where a liaison between them and the responding agencies can be established (e.g., a briefing area).

8.6.1 Establishing a Perimeter and Treatment Zones

Upon recognition of a terror event, EMS should establish a perimeter around the area. The process for establishing a perimeter at an emergency scene should be similar to the following:

1. If possible, identify the substance involved. Using the North American Emergency Response Guidebook, look up its ID number from its name in the blue pages (if there). If you do not know the exact name of the agent, or its name is not listed, use the agent class. For example, for nerve agents, use ID 2810. For the blood agents use ID 1051. For the blister agents, use ID 2810.

2. Look up the ID number in the green pages, and read across to the initial *isolate* distance and *protect* distance. You will need to know if you are dealing with a *small* incident (less than 55 gallons) or a *large* one (larger than 55 gallons), and if it is *day* (between sunrise and sunset) or *night* (Figure 8.1).

ID	Name	Small spills			Large spills		
		Isolate	Protect		Isolate	Protect	
			Day	Night		Day	Night
1017	Chlorine	200 ft	0.2 mi	0.5 mi	600 ft	0.5 mi	1.9 mi

Figure 8.1 Isolation and protection distances.

3. On a map of the incident area, draw (to scale) a circle with the radius of the initial *isolate* distance, with its center at the center of the incident site. Mark which way the wind is blowing at the site. Then, through the center of this circle, place the upwind edge of a square box which is the *protect* distance on each side. This edge is perpendicular to the wind direction. For practical purposes, you have defined the potential hazard area. The toxic plume should pass somewhere within this area. If you know the approximate wind speed, you can also have an idea of where the leading edge of the cloud might be (wind speed × time = distance) (Figure 8.2).

Once the area of the perimeter is established, EMS providers can assist with the formation of zones. There are three zones for WMD scene management. The first is the Hot Zone (or Red Zone), the next is the Warm Zone (or Yellow Zone) and last is the Cold Zone (or Green Zone).

The significance of the zones is as follows:

The *Hot Zone* (also called the exclusion zone or inner zone, or red zone) is the area that the incident occurred in and that contamination exists in. All individuals entering the hot zone must wear the appropriate levels of personal protective equipment (PPE) and be decontaminated before leaving. Entry and exit points will be established at the outer boundary of the hot zone to regulate the entry and exit of personnel and equipment into and out of the hot zone. The outer boundary of the hot zone is initially established by visually surveying the immediate area and determining where the hazardous materials involved are located. Monitoring equipment may also be used to define this area. The North American Emergency Response Guidebook (NAERG) is also useful in establishing this area, using the isolate and protect guides in the green pages.

The *Warm Zone* (also called the contamination reduction zone, or yellow zone, or middle zone) is the transitional are between the hot zone and the cold zone. This zone usually contains the decontamination area and access control points through which personnel enter and exit the hot zone. This zone is less dangerous than the hot zone and personnel can wear lower levels of PPE than those in the hot zone.

The *Cold Zone* is the outermost part of the scene and is considered to be not contaminated. This is where the command post is located along with support equipment, including ambulances and EMS providers. Normal work clothes are

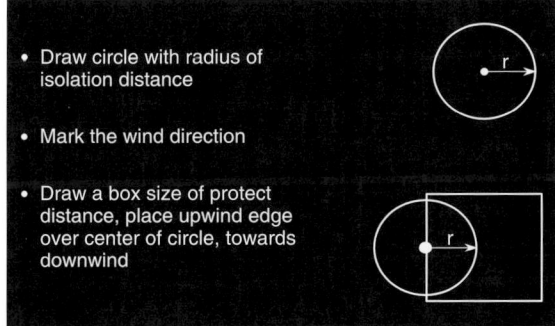

Figure 8.2 Isolation and protection zones.

acceptable PPE in this zone. The press, treatment area, and responder rehabilitation area are located in this zone as well [2]. The size of the zones and the distances between them should be based on conditions specific to each incident, the material involved and the judgement of the incident commander. The following criteria should be used when considering establishing zone boundaries:

Table 8.3 RI DEM ERP 3-1 p1-. 2 Checklist of response issues [2]

Physical and topographical features of the site
Weather conditions and wind direction
Field measurements of air contaminants
Air dispersion models of the chemicals involved
Physical, toxicological, chemical and other characteristics of the agents involved.
Cleanup activities
Potential for fire and/or explosions
Access to roads, power sources and water

The value of quick reference material, such as the NAERG [3], local Standard Operating Procedures (SOPs), pre-plans and treatment protocols cannot be downplayed. These are all tools that every EMS provider should be intimately familiar with. When possible, copies of this material should be in every EMS vehicle for reference. Options include using three ring binders or storing the information electronically in Pesonal Digital Assistants (PDAs), or other "electronic clipboards."

8.7 Planning

Preparation also includes planning. Planning includes sitting down with all responders and agencies that are likely to be involved in a terrorist event. The idea is to establish written response guidelines and create intra-agency agreements and a network whereby individual department heads know each other, as well as what each agency's role is and what their needs and expectations would be during a terror event.

This planning process can lessen tensions and stress when faced with a real scenario. Local planning bodies include Local Emergency Planning Committees (LEPCs) and regional councils of governments. Using these resources terrorist events can be planned for and more importantly can be reviewed post event.

This pre-event planning and post event reviewing is a concept borrowed from the military. Before a standard military operation, a mission briefing is conducted reviewing the mission goals and objectives. After the operation everyone attends a debriefing which among other things looks at lessons learned from the event.

Examples of emergency plans include local EMS service plans, regional disaster plans and state emergency response plans. An example of a regional emergency response plan by the Connecticut Capitol Region Council of Governments appears in the appendix.

Using realistic scenarios with "live" patient actors, EMS, and hospital resources is the only way to truly test any plan prior to it being needed. It is important to be certain that high-level operational management takes part in these drills, as these people are likely to be the ones looked upon to control the situation. Conversely it is equally important for street level providers, including supervisors, crew chiefs, and the greenest of new recruits to know the roles they may play and how to organize the scene. Almost all the time the street level provider will be on scene well before senior officers are. So the initial organization of the scene is many times left to those with the least experience or training with large scene management. This initial organization is one of the most important times during the incident, indeed, it sets the stage for all later operations.

When practicing the plan, there are two options for the practice session. One is to have a table top exercise. Traditionally table top exercises are attended by senior EMS officers and city/town officials. They have the opportunity to practice making difficult decisions. A well-thought out, well-planned table top exercise can be an eye opening experience, especially to those who have never attended one. But one of the major drawbacks to this type of exercise is the lack of participation (at least commonly) by street level providers. Also the feedback that can be brought about by real world problems are not necessarily encountered either. There is less realism in the scenario.

As an example; one area that is often overlooked during this table top type of exercise is the transport and turnaround time of ambulances used to transport casualties from the scene to the hospitals.

The second option to practice the plan is to have a full scale drill with live patients and involving EMS providers, Fire Service, Law Enforcement and Hospitals. Actually handling patients, packaging them and transporting them can be an eye opening experience for management, hospital, and street level personnel. A paper drill may have one ambulance crew transport three critical patients, the real drill may have the paramedic balk at taking more than one critical patient.

Unforeseen difficulties that only come about because of the live drill are also found. For example, many disaster plans call for closing local highways to all but emergency traffic. When put into practice you may find that natural choke points develop on the highway on-ramps, and the roads that lead to them. What happens then is that ambulances find it easy to transport patients into the hospitals, but they are unable to easily get back on the highways when the leave the hospital to return to the incident site. Grid-lock can occur from the hospital to the highway and therefore the plan should allow for such blocks, e.g., the access to the emergency scene was blocked by the plan that meant to allow for clear traffic patterns (Downtown Pittsburgh during the crash of flight 411 in September 1995 is a good example of this happening).

Of course, with any large exercise like this there are difficulties. This includes having active participation by as many providers as possible. This may mean overtime costs for many municipal departments. Cooperation with other public safety services as well as that of the various hospitals that may or may not wish to be involved in the exercise can be a difficult job to coordinate. Also the job of making up and programming of the multiple patients that are needed to truly tax the system.

8.8 Patient Transportation

When it is time to transport, there is little information available as to the recommended number of ambulances to be used. As a rule, patients triaged in the lowest category could be transported en masse by bus or other modes of transport, with an appropriate number of EMS providers who are properly equipped. It is probably a good idea to have at least 1 EMS provider for every 5–7 non-urgent patients.

Dead patients will often be left for placement in a temporary morgue for the local coroner or medical examiner.

This will then leave the urgent and critical patients to be transported by ambulance. While our first instinct often is to transport as many critical patients as possible, providers who have actually been in this situation will tell you that actively caring for more than one critical patient at a time properly is difficult at best.

An example of a good solution to this dilemma is to transport only a single critical patient or a single critical patient with a single moderate/urgent patient per ambulance. Establishing and staffing a treatment area on scene in the green zone can help to organize the effective transportation of patients by providing on scene care until transportation is available.

Another reason to have an organized transportation system is the danger of contamination of the ambulances involved in transporting the patients. While decontamination should be (and is) done on the scene prior to transport, with a large number of patients and a large number of "walking wounded" it is possible and likely that at least one will be transported by ambulance prior to being decontaminated.

The best defense against this will be the establishment of strong perimeters and making certain that all patients are decontaminated before being placed in a transporting unit.

Should an ambulance or other transporting unit become contaminated, three issues become important. First the patient must be decontaminated prior to entering the hospital. Second, the crew may need to be decontaminated depending on the type of contaminant. Third no further "clean" patients should be placed in the contaminated ambulance, and further contaminated patients should be transported by that "dirty" unit.

Aeromedical transport can also be considered for patients involved in terrorist events. In this event, making certain that the patient has been decontaminated first is even more important. Contaminating a $200,000 ambulance is one thing, contaminating a $10 million dollar aircraft is another. It should be noted that immediately after the attacks on September 11, 2001, all aircraft in the country were grounded, including aeromedical flights. So depending on the event, helicopter transport may not be available.

Besides the obvious quick transport ability of aeromedical services, they can also assist in effectively spreading patients to hospitals and facilities further from the scene in a quick fashion.

While transportation is arranged, receiving facilities need to be notified. All hospitals have emergency plans and decontamination facilities and protocols for their implementation and use. Knowing the decontamination process at the receiving hospitals is important, in order to keep from contaminating the hospital. This starts with an early notification to the receiving facility that potential victims of terrorism are enroute to their location. This notification allow for multiple things to happen at the hospital. First, it gives the hospital the opportunity to lockdown and deny access to non-decontaminated patients. Second, it gives them time to set up their decontamination systems. Thirty minutes is about as quick as many hospitals can prepare to decon patients. Remember that not all patients will arrive by EMS. Many will self transport. Japanese hospitals had about 5500 casualties from the release of Sarin gas in the Tokyo subway system in 1995. About 4700 of them were not at the actual site of the gas release. Some only saw it on TV and went to the hospital. Last, early notification by field personnel allows the hospital to recall or hold over staff to properly care for the large influx of patients.

When designating a receiving hospital to a transporting ambulance, common sense should prevail when it comes to choosing the destination. Imagine a scenario where the local civic center is five blocks from the nearest hospital. A terrorist has exploded a bomb and there are a large number of walking wounded and about 30 critical and urgent patients. The first reaction might be to transport all of the critical patients to the local hospital. The problem with this is that that hospital is most likely where all of the walking wounded have gone. If the hospital is within a short distance of the event it is likely these patients will get in before decontamination can be established. Therefore it is likely that this hospital has become contaminated if WMD were involved in the bombing. This hospital may become unavailable to EMS providers when they get control of the scene and begin transporting patients. Transporting to the more distant hospitals might be a better solution as it is likely fewer patients will have arrived there and they will be less likely to be contaminated.

Early contact with all of the hospitals will allow them the time they need to prepare for the influx of patients. It is the key to successful patient flow and transportation.

8.9 Return to Service

Once a terrorist event is contained and the response phase for EMS providers has been completed, the process of taking the system out of emergency response mode and putting it back into day to day operations starts.

Critical Incident Stress Debriefing (CISD) should be required of all responding personnel prior to their being allowed to return to normal operations/shift work. Early integration of mental health teams can head-off feelings of guilt, helplessness, frustration, and anxiety by EMS providers after a terrorist event (see Chapter 11).

CISDs can be career and life saving for the providers involved. Providers needing professional follow-up care can be identified at an early stage and be assisted with putting their lives back into perspective and order after these events.

During CISD debriefings, EMS providers are given the opportunity to discuss the events that they were involved in, including areas that did not go as planned or that did not end with good results. The environment is one of support and no assignation of blame is placed on any provider. A responsible service chief would arrange for mutual aid coverage of district while he stands his crew down for debriefing (both for CISD and normal debriefing) and rest and relaxation. For many services this may be accomplished in as little as a single day or two. For larger services a more thought out and organized approach may be needed. This process can be planned for, just like the rest of the disaster plan.

Long term psychological evaluation need to be made available to staff, many times the effects of a terrorist attack do not manifest until days, weeks or more after the event. Some of these manifestations may need long term psychological care and this should be provided to any EMS provider who needs it.

Last, a final event debriefing should occur, separate from the CISD debriefing. This debriefing should include reviewing lessons learned from the event and the plan for applying those lessons to future EMS responses and into the overall emergency response plan. By reflecting on all the information gathered at an incident, from patients, providers, department heads and municipal leaders, we can learn about areas of the response that went well and areas that did not work well. Considering that knowledge we can make changes plan to address the shortcomings of the original plan. This is not done to assign blame, but to prevent loss of life decrease suffering in the future and to learn from the experience.

Department of EMS Education, Hartford Hospital—Terrorism Protocols

Draft—General Information

When dispatched to a call EMS providers should have a high index of suspicion for terrorist events [4]. When responding to the scene EMS providers should ask the following, if any are present the consider terrorism as a possible cause:

I. Assess security
   a. Is the call at a target hazard (high profile target) or a target event (mass gathering of people).
   b. Has there been a threat?
   c. Is the caller anonymous?
   d. Is the problem not well defined (i.e., Multiple people feeling ill, but no obvious cause).
   e. Are there multiple, non-trauma related victims?
   f. Are hazardous materials involved?
   g. Are responders victims?
   h. Has there been a secondary attack or explosion?
      - *If one of the answers to the above is "Yes"—respond with heightened awareness*
      - *If multiple answers are "Yes"—this may be a terrorist incident*

II. Make contact with law enforcement and the fire department for coordination
   a. Remember that scenes of terrorism are federal crime scenes under the control of the FBI

III. When approaching the scene:
   a. Approach the scene cautiously, from uphill, upwind, and upstream if possible.
   b. Consider law enforcement escort.
   c. Avoid choke points.
   d. Designate escape routes.
   e. Designate regrouping area.
      - A place for crews to meet if they get separated.
   f. Identify staging area

IV. Command considerations
   a. Implement incident command system, assume command until relieved
   b. Isolate the area and deny entry
      i. This is one of the most important things you can do to protect yourself and the public. Do not allow anyone other public safety access to the scene.
   c. Identify/isolate/coral the victims
      i. This is another of the most important things you can do to protect yourself and the public. Isolating the victims will prevent them from contaminating other people and

from going to the hospital without decontamination.
    d. Manage as a Hazardous Material Incident scene
        i. Terrorist events with Biological, Chemical and Nuclear devices are Hazardous Materials Incidents and should be treated as such. "All anthrax is, is a HAZMAT with an attitude" [5].
    e. Manage as a potential crime scene
    f. Ensure scene security
        i. Be alert for possible secondary devices/attacks
        ii. Be alert for chemical dispersal devices
    g. Initiate scene size-up and hazard/risk assessment
        i. Review dispatch information
        ii. Look for physical indicators and outward warning signs
            1. Debris field
            2. Mass casualty with minimal or no trauma
            3. Responder casualties
            4. Severe structural damage
            5. Dead animals
            6. Unusual odors, color of smoke or vapor clouds
            7. Systems disruptions (utilities, transportation, and communications)
        iii. Victims signs and symptoms
            1. Unconscious victims with little or no trauma
            2. Multiple victims with the same or similar complaints
            3. Victims with seizures
            4. Victims with difficulty breathing
            5. Victims with blistering, skin redness, discoloration or irritation
        iv. Make appropriate notifications
            1. Dispatch center
            2. Law enforcement
            3. Department of environmental protection
            4. Local public health department
            5. CMED
        v. Ensure coordination of communications and identify needs
        vi. Ensure personnel accountability
            1. Leave the scene with the same personnel you entered with, know where they are at all times.
        vii. Ensure use of personnel protective measures
        viii. Designate incident safety officer
        ix. Designate an emergency evacuation signal (usually a long blast of horn, or three blasts of horn)
        x. Designate a scribe to record incident
        xi. Assess command post security
            1. Remember that the first WTC command post was destroyed when the first building collapsed.
        xii. Prepare for transition to unified command
    h. Secondary size-up/intelligence
        i. Determine number of victims
            1. Ambulatory
            2. Non-ambulatory
        ii. Identify common signs/symptoms
        iii. Interview victims and witnesses, if possible
            1. Is everyone accounted for?
            2. Was there a threat made?
            3. What happened?
            4. When did it happen?
            5. Where did it happen?
            6. Who was involved?
            7. Did they smell, taste, hear, or feel anything unusual?
        iv. Identify potential type of event
            1. Armed assault
            2. Explosive, incendiary
            3. Chemical
            4. Biological
            5. Radiological
        v. Determine life safety threats
            1. To self, responders
            2. To victims
            3. To general public
    i. Weather—current and forecast
    j. Identify needed resources
    k. Implement EMS sector under ICS/unified command
V. Tactical considerations
    a. Keep yourself alive
    b. Commit only essential personnel/ minimize exposure

c. Decontaminate victims before care
   i. Hasty Decon = remove clothing, rinse thoroughly with water *(this removes 85–95% of contaminates)*
   ii. Do NOT TRANSPORT contaminated victims
   iii. Do NOT TRANSPORT contaminated victim belongings/clothing

Biological Agents
Suspicious Package/Letter
I. Do not shake or empty the contents of any suspicious package or letter [6].
II. Have the victim place the envelope or package in a plastic bag or some other type of container to prevent leakage of contents.
   a. The reason for having the victim move the envelope or package is they are already contaminated. Remember to keep contamination to as few people as possible.
III. If you do not have a container, then cover the envelope or package with anything (e.g., clothing, paper, trash can, etc.) and do not remove this cover.
IV. Leave the room and close the door and windows, or section off the area to prevent others from entering. (i.e., keep others away).
V. Wash your hands with soap and water to prevent spreading any powder to your face
VI. List all people who were in the room or area when the suspicious letter/package was recognized. Give this list to both law enforcement and public health authorities.

Envelope with powder, Powder Spills out onto Surface
I. Do NOT try to clean up the powder. Cover the spilled contents immediately with anything (clothing, trashcan, paper). Do not remove the cover.
II. Leave the room and close the door and windows, or section off the area to prevent others from entering (keep others away).
III. Wash your hands with soap and water as soon as possible. Do not use bleach or other disinfectant on your skin.
IV. Remove heavily contaminated clothing as soon as possible and place in a plastic bag, or some container that can be sealed. DO NOT Transport this with you.
V. Shower with soap and water as soon as possible.
VI. List all people who were in the room or area when the suspicious spill was recognized. Give this list to both law enforcement and public health authorities.

Question of Room Contamination by Aerosolization
(Examples include, small device triggered, warning that air handling system is contaminated or warning that a biological agent is released in a public space.)
I. Have the victims turn off local fans or ventilation units in the area.
II. Have the victims LEAVE the area immediately
III. Close the door or section off the area to prevent others from entering.
IV. Have the victims shut down the air handling system for the building if possible.
V. List all people who were in the room or area. Give this list to both law enforcement and public health authorities.

Management
Precise diagnosis of biologic agent casualties is likely to be difficult [7]. Signs and symptoms of biological agent infection are common to many diseases. The treatment required for biological weapons casualties will not differ in basic principle from that in patients suffering from the same disease incurred by natural means.

I. Primary Contamination—Dermal exposure from a suspected biological weapons attack should be managed by decontamination *at the earliest opportunity* and **before treatment and transportation starts**. Exposed areas should be cleansed using an appropriately diluted hypochlorite solution (0.5%) or copious amounts of plain soap and water. Potentially contaminated clothing should be removed by personnel with PPE, away from non-contaminated patients.

II. Principles of Treatment
   a. General supportive measures
      i. ABCs
      ii. Maintain respirations and hearbeat
      iii. Lowering temperature (for patients with fever)
      iv. Relieve pain
      v. Secure IV access
   b. Use of barrier techniques
      i. Surgical masks
      ii. Gowns
      iii. Goggles
      iv. Gloves
      v. Observe body substance isolation
   c. Antibiotic therapy—most bacterial, chlamydial and rickettsial diseases respond well to antibiotic therapy. The choice of antibiotic will depend on many factors including specific threat, evidence or suspicion of antibiotic resistance, ease in which drug can be manufactured.

III. These are patients who are ill. Treat them as you would any other patient with an illness, with a large emphasis on decontamination and prevention of cross contamination. As a general rule, there will not be an antidote available for field use.

Chemical Agents

There are five types of chemical agents: nerve agents, vesicants, cyanide, pulmonary agents and riot control agents [8,9].

They are each discussed in more detail below.

Nerve Agents

Nerve agents are the most toxic of all chemical agents. Examples of nerve agents are Sarin, Tabun, VX, and Soman. They are stored and transported in a liquid state but are usually released as a gas. They are toxic in either form. All nerve agents act in the same manner, they block the re-uptake of acetylcholine by the nerve endings, thereby creating an endless "stimulation" of the nervous system. Nerve agents are organophosphates and are closely related to insecticides.

Signs and Symptoms of Nerve Agent Poisoning

Vapor small exposure: Miosis, rhinorrhea, mild difficulty in breathing

Vapor large exposure: Sudden loss of consciousness, seizures, apnea, flaccid paralysis, copious secretions, miosis

Liquid on skin, small to moderate exposure: Localized sweating, nausea, vomiting, feeling of weakness.

Liquid on skin, large exposure: Sudden loss of consciousness, seizures, convulsions, apnea, flaccid paralysis, copious secretions.

Patients may complain of dim vision and or eye pain (due to miosis) a mnemonic device to remember is SLUDGE for Salivation, Lacrimation, Urination, Defecation, GI Motility and Eyes (Miosis).

Decontamination of Nerve Agent Poisoning

The patient should be washed with large amounts of water and clothing removed. The patient needs to be decontaminated before treatment and transport can begin. Do NOT transport contaminated patients to the hospital.

Protocol for Management of Nerve Agent Poisoning

I. Assure your own safety
II. Maintain adequate airway control
   a. These patients may need aggressive airway and ventilation control due to bronchoconstriction and secretions
   b. Ventilation of these patients may be difficult prior to the administration of the antidotes.
III. Maintain patient's respirations as needed
IV. Maintain patient's circulation as needed

V. Establish IV access (normal saline, KVO)
VI. Administer Mark I kits as outlined below:
   a. Vapor exposure
      i. Mild (Miosis, dim vision, headache, rhinorrhea, salivation, dyspnea)
         1. 1 Mark I kit
            a. 2 mg of atropine
            b. 600 mg of pralidoxime chloride (2-Pam)
      ii. Severe (all of the above plus severe dyspnea or apnea, muscular twitching, seizures or paralysis, loss of consciousness, loss of bladder or bowel control)
         1. 3 Mark I kits
            a. 6 mg atropine
            b. 1800 mg pralidoxime chloride (2-Pam)
         2. Diazepam (Valium) 10 mg
   b. Liquid on skin exposure
      i. Mild/moderate (muscle twitching at site of exposure, sweating at site of exposure, nausea, vomiting, and weakness)
         1. 1 to 2 Mark I kits (depending on severity of symptoms)
            a. 2–4 mg atropine
            b. 600–1200 mg pralidoxime chloride (2-Pam)
      ii. Severe (All of the above plus, severe dyspnea, apnea, muscular twitching, seizures, loss of consciousness, paralysis, loss of bowel or bladder control)
         1. 3 Mark I kits
            a. 6 mg atropine
            b. 1800 mg pralidoxime chloride (2-Pam)
         2. Diazepam (valium) 10 mg

Vesicants/Blister Agents

Vesicants or blister agents include Mustard Gas, Lewisite and Phosgene Oxime (CX gas). Mustard has a latent period of up to several hours, while Lewisite and Phosgene exposures show immediate signs and symptoms. Regardless of the agent involved, treatment is aimed at supportive therapy and immediate decontamination.

Decontamination of Vesicant Agents

The patient should be washed with large amounts of water and clothing removed. The patient needs to be decontaminated *before treatment and transport* can begin. Do *NOT* transport contaminated patients to the hospital.

Immediate decontamination after exposure is the only way to prevent symptoms.

Protocol for Treatment of Vesicant Agent Exposure

I. Assure your own safety (the patient must be decontaminated prior to treatment)
II. Maintain adequate airway control
   a. Administer high flow oxygen (15 lpm)
III. Maintain patient's respirations as needed
IV. Maintain patient's circulation as needed
V. Establish IV access (normal saline, KVO)
VI. Bandage blisters as needed.

Cyanide

Cyanide is a rapid acting lethal agent, it is however, limited in its military usefulness due to the high amounts needed for lethal doses and its high volatility. Death can occur in 6–8 minutes after exposure to high amounts of cyanide.

Signs and Symptoms of Cyanide Poisoning

Moderate—transient increase in rate and depth of breathing, Dizziness, Nausea, Vomiting and Headache.

Severe—transient increase in rate and depth of breathing within 15 seconds, Convulsions within 30 seconds, Apnea within 2–4 minutes, cardiac arrest within 4–8 minutes, also intense irritation of the eyes, nose, and airways.

Cyanide Decontamination

Skin decontamination is not usually necessary, as the liquid is extremely volatile (evaporates easily). However, wet clothing should be removed and underlying skin should be decontaminated with large amounts of water.

Protocol for Cyanide Poisoning
I. Assure your own safety
II. Maintain adequate airway control
   a. Administer high flow oxygen (15 lpm)
III. Maintain patient's respirations as needed
IV. Maintain patient's circulation as needed
V. Establish IV access (normal saline, KVO)
VI. Administer amyl nitrite (1–2 pearls, crushed and inhaled)
VII. Administer 300 mg of sodium nitrite IV, slowly over 2–4 minutes.
VIII. Administer 12.5 g of sodium thiosulfate (after sodium nitrite).
IX. Sodium nitrite and sodium thiosulfate can be repeated at half of the original dose if symptoms persist (15 mg sodium nitrite, 6.25 g of Sodium Thiosulfate).

Pulmonary Agents

Inhalation of pulmonary agents leads to varying degrees of pulmonary edema, which usually presents after a latent period that varies in length depending on the amount of the agent the patient is exposed to. The principle pulmonary agent is Phosgene Gas.

Signs and Symptoms of Pulmonary Agent Exposure
Eye and airway irritation, dyspnea, chest tightness and delayed pulmonary edema. Phosgene smells like newly mowed hay, cut grass or corn.

Decontamination of Pulmonary Agents
Exposure to Vapor—fresh air
Exposure to Liquid—Large amounts of water

Protocol for Pulmonary Agent Exposure
I. Assure your own safety
   a. Remove patient and self from immediate area to fresh air
II. Maintain adequate airway control
III. Maintain patient's respirations as needed
IV. Maintain patient's circulation as needed
V. Establish IV access (normal saline, KVO)
VI. Prepare to treat Pulmonary Edema, Hypoxia and Hypotension

Riot Control Agents

Riot control agents are designed to produce eye irritation and closure and produce transient discomfort in order to make the recipient temporarily incapable. Their major effect is to cause pain, burning and discomfort on exposed mucous membranes and exposed skin. The effects occur within seconds and seldom persist more than several minutes after exposure has ended. Examples include CS gas.

Signs and Symptoms of Riot Control Agent Exposure
Burning and pain on exposed mucous membranes and skin, eye pain and burning, pain in nostrils, respiratory discomfort and tingling of the exposed skin.

Decontamination of Riot Control Agents
Eyes—Thoroughly flush with water, saline or similar substance
Skin—Flush with large amounts of water

Protocol for Riot Control Agent Exposure
I. Assure your own safety
II. Maintain adequate airway control
III. Maintain patient's respirations as needed
IV. Maintain patient's circulation as needed
V. Establish IV access (normal saline, KVO)
VI. Remainder of treatment is supportive and focused on decontamination, signs and symptoms should be limited after decontamination

Nuclear Agents

The types of ionizing radiation that EMS providers need to be concerned about are alpha particles, beta particles, and gamma particles [10–12]. Alpha particles do not penetrate the skin and are stopped easily by cover such as paper. Our concern is when alpha particles become inhaled or embedded in wounds. Beta particles are somewhat stronger and usually require some type of PPE to stop them. They can penetrate the outer layer of skin to the germinal layer where new cells are made. If allowed to stay on the skin for a prolonged period of time, beta particles can cause skin injury. Again the main concern is internal contamination by inhalation or wound contamination. Gamma particles are much more powerful and require heavy shielding to prevent penetration. Gamma particles are usually accompanied by alpha and beta particles.

Various methods might be used to deploy nuclear agents. They are:

A. Simple radiological device—the act of placing nuclear materials without using an explosion, i.e., Placing radioactive material in a cafeteria.
B. Radiological dispersal device—radioactive material is dispersed via an explosion, however a nuclear reaction does not take place (radioactive material is attached to TNT).
C. Reactor—sabotage to a nuclear reactor site, this is regarded as being highly unlikely.
D. Improvised nuclear device—A "home made" nuclear weapon.
E. Nuclear weapon—a weapon designed to create a nuclear reaction. At least one Russian State has stated that it is missing 50–100 one kiloton "suitcase bombs." Assuming a one kiloton blast:
   1. Blast range would reach a distance of approximately 400 yards.
   2. Thermal radiation would reach the same distance as the blast.
   3. Nuclear radiation (i.e., gamma and neutron) would reach approximately half a mile.
   4. The radioactive fallout could produce very high exposure rates, up to half a mile.
   5. The added factor of the electromagnetic pulse, which only applies to high aerial bursts (several kilometers), would result in damage to electronic equipment.

As the size of the weapon increases, the effects encompass a greater distance.

Decontamination of Patients with Radiologic Contamination

Removal of clothing and rapid washing of exposed skin and hair will remove up to 95% of contamination. The 0.5% hypochlorite solution used for chemical decontamination will also remove radiological contaminants. Care must be taken not to irritate the skin. If the skin is damaged radiological components can be absorbed directly through the skin. Wounds should be irrigated with large amounts of water or saline. *Remember the patient must be decontaminated prior to transport. The receiving hospital must be notified prior to transport.*

The patient should be checked after decontamination with devices that measure radiologic activity to "certify" that the patient has been decontaminated (*Treatment of life threatening injuries may begin before the patient is decontaminated*).

Protocol for Patients Exposed to Radiological Materials

I. Assure your own safety
II. Maintain adequate airway control
III. Maintain patient's respirations as needed
IV. Maintain patient's circulation as needed
V. Establish IV access (normal saline, KVO)
VI. Remainder of treatment is supportive and focused on decontamination. These patients will probably present with traumatic injuries, burns and/or acute radiation sickness.

References

1. (CFR 1910.120(q)(6)(i)).
2. Rhode Island Department Emergency Management. ERP P1-2. Checklist of Response Issues, www.dem.ri.gov/erp/3.pdf/
3. North American Emergency Response Guide, http://hazmat.dot.gov/enforce/forms/ohmforms.htm/
4. State of Connecticut, Department of Public Health, Office of Emergency Medical Services. *Job Aid for Emergency Medical Service Providers: Emergency Response to Terrorism.* (Hartford: State of

Connecticut, Department of Public Health, Office of Emergency Medical Services, October 17, 2001) pp. 2–4 [Their source was "Emergency Response to Terrorism Job Aid, Edition 1.0, FEMA/DOJ May 2000]
5. Centrella, Carmine. October 17, 2001.
6. Centers for Disease Control and Prevention. *CDC Health Advisory: How to Handle Anthrax and Other Biological Agent Threats.* Atlanta, Centers for Disease Control and Prevention, October 12, pp. 1–4, 2001.
7. Departments of the Army, the Navy and the Air Force. *NATO Handbook on the Medical Aspects of NBC Defensive Operations AmedP-6(B) Part II Biological.* Washington, DC, Departments of the Army, the Navy and the Air Force, 4-1 to 4-5, 1996.
8. Suter, Robert, DO, MHA, FACEP. *Treatment of Biological Agent Exposure, a Special Supplement to Emergency Medicine Alert.* Atlanta, Emergency Medicine Alert, Supplement, 2001.
9. Medical Research Institute of Chemical Defense. *Medical Management of Chemical Casualties Handbook.* Aberdeen, MD, Medical Research Institute of Chemical Defense, 17–116, 1995.
10. Lab Safety Supply, *Disaster Preparedness & Response.* Janesville, WI, Lab Safety Supply, 54, 2001.
11. David G. Jarrett. *Medical Management of Radiological Casualties Handbook, First Edition.* Bethesda, Department of the Army, 1–76, 1999.
12. National Domestic Preparedness Office. *EMS Technician: Nuclear Casualties.* Washington, DC, National Domestic Preparedness Office, 1–44, 1998.

9 Emergency Department Preparation

MICHAEL ZACCHERA, III AND MICHAEL F. ZANKER

9.1 Introduction

Preparing a hospital emergency department for the influx of patients from a terrorist attack can be a daunting task. Many hospitals take a "it won't happen here" approach or the equally short-sighted thought of "we are a small community hospital, we'll only accept five or six patients and forward the rest to the larger hospitals."

The first position is untrue. Rural areas are just as likely to be affected by terrorism as the urban areas. The second position will most likely be ignored. The patients will show up at the door regardless of the number of patients you wish to accept.[1]

All hospital emergency departments and their staff, great and small, need to address the training, planning, and practice needed to prepare for terror attacks.

In this chapter, we will discuss preparation and planning, operations during terrorist attacks and post incident activities.

9.2 Preparation

Preparation for terrorism is both an individual and a group responsibility. Individual preparation is the responsibility of every healthcare provider. Physicians and midlevel practitioners, Physician Assistants (PAs) and Advanced Practice Registered Nurses (APRNs), may need different training than general nursing staff who will be different than Patient Care Assistants (PCAs) and aides. The need does exist however, for an awareness of the training, knowledge, and expertise of the others. This will allow for each role to know whom to ask for help when something he is not trained in presents itself.

Physicians obviously need to be trained at recognizing and treating the effects of biological, chemical, radiological, and incendiary attacks. They should also be involved in the systematic planning for the hospital and their department. Physicians have a responsibility to provide leadership and to become advocates for training and preparation.

Physician level training includes short Continuing Medical Education activities (CMEs) to multi-day conferences. Advantages to the training include the ability to recognize the first signs of a biological terrorist attack, appropriate treatment of patients and use of PPE (personal protective equipment). All physicians should practice treating patients while wearing PPE, such as Purified Air Powered Respirator (PAPR) devices. This is important because, while it is likely that most patients will arrive at the hospital decontaminated, there is always the chance that one will slip through and there may be a need for a physician within the decontamination room.

The PCA's and aide level staff need to be trained in a variety of tasks. These include proper decontamination procedures, appropriate disposal of patient belongings and the additional logistics involved in a terror attack.

Decontamination in the hospital setting should be performed either outside of the hospital itself or

---

[1] Remember that at such instances, there is no disaster exemption to EMTALA (Emergency Medical Treatment and Active Labor Act).

in a specially designed room within the hospital. Frequently this task is relegated to the PCA and aide staff, perhaps under the supervision of a nurse or physician. It is likely that the PCA will have the closest contact with the contaminated patient. Appropriate training in various types of PPE and the equipment used in decontamination are important. The skill needed to decontaminate patients while dressed in PPE needs to be practiced frequently if they are expected to be proficient at it. The need for realistic drills with live patients who "get wet" is invaluable.

Besides the decontamination aspect of their job, the PCA/aide staff are the support staff that make the emergency department work. Training in the use and location of specialized equipment that is used in the event of a terror attack (where the disaster cache is located) and how it should be distributed are all-important aspects of this role. Knowing where the cyanide antidote kit, or where the multi-port oxygen regulator is and how to set it up can be lifesaving.

The PCA and aide staff while the lowest level of healthcare providers can often be essential to emergency department operations during a disaster.

The group of emergency department healthcare providers likely to be the group that will be expected to have the most varied training are nurses and paramedics. From a patient care standpoint they will need to know the presentations and treatments of the patients they will receive. From a logistics perspective, they will need to receive training to make those treatments happen. The decontamination procedures and PPE use will also have to be practiced and learned. Commonly nurses and paramedics will assist both physicians in the treatment of the patient and the PCAs and aides with logistics and patient decontamination.

As a hospital, training should consist of the Hospital Emergency Incident Command course for those expected to be in leadership positions. Practice realistic drills and making changes to the emergency plan after the drill to accommodate weaknesses identified. After a terror attack, civilians will be in a state fear. They will look for leadership and structure, and they will expect it from the hospital staff. The best way to have structure is to function under a well-practiced plan. Many hospitals fail to have realistic drills. This in turn may lead to the assumption that all is well with the plan until an actual event occurs and the opposite is learned. There is no substitute for a well planned drill with live patients.

9.3 Planning

When planning for a emergency department response to a terror attack, some basic concepts will need to be addressed. These include the flow of patient traffic into and through the emergency department, security of the emergency department, establishing decontamination and accessing specialized equipment caches. Other items to consider include staff call back and supplementation, research on the type of incident and parking.

When a hospital compiles its plan, consideration must be given to planning with and around the hospital as a whole. Plans should be focused as "all-hazards" with annexes based upon threat/incident. Early integration of the hospital plan with the local city, county and statewide plan will need to be taken into consideration. Planning by hospitals is all too often done in a vacuum. Partnering with outside agencies during the planning phase will prevent unexpected surprises when a disaster strikes.

A good example here is planning on the police to be able to lockdown the facility, without first checking with them. There is a great likelihood that they will not be available.

9.4 Patient Flow

How many entrances are there to the Emergency Department? Most have an ambulance entrance, a walk-in entrance and one or more entrances from the main hospital. How will you receive patients during a terror attack? Will it make a difference which entrance they use?

By limiting access to the Emergency Department, you can control the areas that are potentially contaminated by patients. (While many hospitals have decontamination showers that can be set up outside of the hospital entrance, most do not have enough to cover every entrance. Imagine a contaminated patient entering the Emergency Department via another hospital entrance on the other side of the building).

Limiting access may cause a backlog of patients, but it will allow for better triage as there will be less of a chance of missing a patient. This process can also allow for better patient tracking, especially when paired with only a single, controlled exit from the department. Identifying patients is also another issue, to which various solutions are available. The standard hospital bracelet is a tried and true system. Additional support can come from the use of triage tags, bar codes on patient ID or the potential use of radio frequency identification tags (RFID) to track patients.

Emergency Department directors and their staff need to be prepared for a potentially massive influx of patients. During the Sarin gas attacks on Tokyo's subway, there were thousands of patients who reported to the emergency departments who had no direct exposure to the event. They saw what happened on television and then went to the hospital, fearing they had been exposed. Consideration should be given to how to corral these "worried well" patients. Use of an off-site (not in the emergency department) location may be useful for these pseudo-patients. Critical Incident Stress Debriefing (CISD) may be useful for them as sometimes the "worried well" may need this type treatment.

9.5 Security

Implementing a patient flow plan should be just a small part of the overall plan for securing the Emergency Department. The importance of controlling access cannot be overstated. A contaminated patient could theoretically cause the death of Emergency Department staff members. As an example, at a large urban hospital in Hartford, CT, a mock disaster victim in a drill was placed across the street from the Emergency Department and given directions to "get in." He managed to enter the hospital on the opposite side of the building, walk through the hospital and into the Emergency Department where he ran up to the director, grabbed him and begged him not to let him die. The mock patient managed to contaminate the physician and everything else he touched in the hospital.

The plan for securing the ED should include a definition of "lockdown." Surprisingly, many people think closing some doors is enough. It is not as easy as you would think. Hospitals are not designed to be "locked down", but rather have more points of acces than one might imagine. You may also need to consider "locking in." You might need to keep people inside (i.e., quarantine). Is the hospital ready to authorize use of force ... and how much force?

Security forces need to have an effective lock down plan in place, to include all entrances and exits from the building and potentially between the Emergency Department and other departments (besides the obvious entry points like the ambulance bays and the main lobby). Thought also needs to be given to less obvious entrances such as the loading dock, exterior stairwells, cafeteria entrances and bridges or underground tunnels between buildings. Failure to secure access can become costly both in financial and in human life. Caring for patients is a noble cause; unnecessarily getting contaminated and dying from it, is not.

During the planning phase, should security need to lock down the hospital or Emergency Department, two questions need to be asked. How committed should they be; is security prepared to use force to prevent unauthorized entry or exit. Is the hospital prepared to allow force to be used? The second question How to obtain manpower to adequately cover the entrances and exits? Is relying on the local police department a practical consideration? If the event has occurred in your city or town, they may be deployed elsewhere. Many times emergency plans are written from an independent position (i.e., the hospital's or the city's). Each plan may require the use of the same resources, in different places, at the same time. For example, the hospital plan calls for the use of local police to back fill it's own security staff while the city plan calls for the police to be used to close city streets, direct traffic or close highways. (or if the hospital plans on having the fire department set up a decontamination site at the hospital, while they are tied up at an incident scene). Pre-planning as a community can help alleviate these types of problems before they happen. Establishing personal relationships with local leaders (elected, appointed, civic, and religious) can make this process easier and allow for better flow during an actual emergency.

Other options to gaining manpower include the calling in of additional off duty security officers, or pulling in officers from outlying buildings to the area of the incident within the hospital.

The important question to ask yourself are: Can we lockdown, what type of force will be authorized to enforce it, where will I get the manpower from? Does my hospital have enough manpower to lock down or lock in? An important point to consider when working with outside agencies is what happens when city is in "lockdown" and traffic flow is stopped. How can we as a hospital get our staff into facility. Think about immediately after the September 11, 2001 attacks when New York City was "closed." PD and Security should be aware to let certain individuals (hospital staff) in. (An awareness of hospital staff identification cards is helpful here.)

While securing the building that the Emergency Department is in, other logistical operations will still need to be staffed. Many patients will present to the Emergency Department by ambulance, it is likely that many more will present by private vehicle. There is a good chance that there will end be more vehicles than space to park them. Off site parking with shuttles may be needed. Vehicle traffic moving through the hospital campus will be needed in order to receive ambulances (and allow them to leave as well). Especially in urban areas, where parking can be a premium, gridlock can quickly result; no one will be able to move. It is possible that closing down city streets to civilian traffic, especially those within the hospital campus, may become a hospital security staff responsibility. This will be particularly true if the local police are deployed at the incident site.

Other emergency department responsibilities for the security team may include setting up the decontamination area. Also associated with the physical set up of decontamination is the ability to coral patients and send them through the decontamination process if it is needed. For hospitals that do not have helipads on the roof of the building, the securing of the landing zone will become the job of the security department, as well.

All of these roles will require manpower, teamwork and above all practice of a well thought out plan. Once a security plan is in place, it needs to be practiced and improved upon. All disaster planning should be works in progress and constantly evolving from lessons learned during drills.

9.6 Notification of an Incident and Preparation to Receive Patients

Once the ED is contacted regarding the likelihood of receiving patients from a terrorist event, the hospital's emergency plan should be immediately put into effect. Time will not be on the side of the emergency department. Your notification of the event may occur after patients have already entered the department.

Two important questions that will guide the department's response will be; How many patients are expected or involved in the incident? (Remembering that just because 100 patients were involved in the incident, many more "worried well" may be heading your way) What type of event will you be dealing with: biological, chemical, radiological or incendiary?

Establishing a command post within the hospital and sending a representative from the emergency department are important first steps. It is critical to open communications both internally (within the hospital) and externally (with other hospitals, EMS, CMEDs, and officials at the incident). The person in charge of emergency department operations should appoint a communications officer with assistants. These could be nursing, paramedic, PCA, or secretarial staff.

Staffing may become an issue quickly. The process of calling back/calling in staff needs to be started and delegated to the administrative staff at once. Many hospital plans allow for the holding over of staff as well. Incoming personnel will need directions on where to park and how to enter the building. Local security and police will need to know to allow these people into the hospital.

Other options to increase staffing include utilization of EMS and Nursing Education personnel, medical reserve corps and students involved in training programs.

Most hospitals have both an EMS department and a Nursing Education Department. These staff members can be used to fill either clinical roles or incident command positions. One Pittsburgh hospital's plan allowed for the use of the EMS department to be available to either the Emergency Department as additional staff or to the local incident commander for use in Incident Command System (ICS) or in treatment positions. Most Nursing Education Departments consist of 2–10 staff members who can also be put into service quickly.

Medical Reserve Corps have been set up by some states. These are either retired healthcare workers, or those who now work outside of the healthcare field. They have volunteered to assist in the event of a disaster or mass-casualty incident (MCI). The concept is similar to that of the military reserves.

The drawback to this system is that some or all of these healthcare providers may be unfamiliar with local operations, protocols and may have been out of practice for years. If this system is used by a hospital, a mustering of the medical staff reserves should take place as part of the normal disaster drill. Taking some time to give an orientation to the hospital, the computer system and some MCI training can help decrease the amount of time needed for "on the job training" during the incident itself.

Always remember to keep the plan simple. Do not want to run the risk of writing something no one will be able to follow when the disaster is occurring. Realize that this is the time when most staff will be seeing it for the first time.

Medical reserve preparedness can be increased by having licensing bodies allow for healthcare professionals licensed in one jurisdiction to practice in another during an emergency. Preparing "temporary admitting privileges" for physicians is also another item that can be pre-planned in advance to assist in the use of the medical reserves.

Another option to increase staff is to use senior students to supplement the licensed staff. Arranging for the short term emergency licensure or certification of senior students can also be pre-planned with the state department of public health. As an example, on September 11, 2001 the Hartford Hospital Emergency Department used paramedic students who had graduated the week before (who had not received their licenses yet) as additional ED staff at the paramedic level. The same could be done with nursing, respiratory therapy, or other allied health students.

This type of emergency licensing is something that needs to be planned by with the state department of health and senior hospital staff before the need arises.

A final method of gaining staff is to utilize the National Disaster Medical System (NDMS). NDMS is part of FEMA and they can deploy Disaster Medical Assistance Teams (DMAT) to an area to supplement hospital staff. Many times during a natural disaster such as a hurricane these teams are pre-deployed to an area. During a terrorist event it may take them some time, from hours to days to be able to respond to an area. In New York City after attacks on September 11, 2001, the Rhode Island 1 DMAT was at the federal rendevous point in Newburgh, NY at 4:30am on September 12, 2001 and was on the ground in the city later that day.[1]

9.7 Additional Preparation

Retrieving and organizing the hospital's disaster cache is another activity that needs to be performed at this time. Equipment technicians, nurse's aides or PCAs can do this and distribute it as needed. The contents of the cache should be established according to local need and as part of the hospital disaster plan. Additional beds may need to be retrieved at this time as well.

If staffing allows, a physician, senior resident or nurse may quickly gather information regarding the type of incident and the appropriate treatment. Likely symptoms can also be researched. If time allows, a quick briefing of this information can be relayed to senior medical leaders for further dissemination. Special needs for equipment can be identified at this time. Examples include the need for decontamination, the process for decontamination, antidotes, and effective treatments. Other needs may also be identified, such as for large amounts of medications, antibiotics or radiological measuring devices.

Communication with state and local health departments may prove valuable at this time. They may have a lot of important intelligence regarding epidemiology of incident and can provide technical expertise and support.

9.8 Decontamination

Once the need for decontamination is identified, the facility will need to prepare to administer it. This can be down in either a specially prepared room before entry into the emergency department or outside the hospital in tents with showers and hoses. Some hospitals have agreements with local fire departments to provide decontamination. However reliance solely on the local fire department may not be advisable; just like the police department, they may be deployed at the incident site and not be available.

Many patients arriving by ambulance will have had a decontamination done in the field by public safety officers (Fire, EMS, Hazmat). Patients who come by private vehicle will not; they and whoever drove them to the hospital may need to be decontaminated.

The hospital will need to make predetermined decision that anyone coming in from the field is either OK to enter or needs to be completely decontaminated.

Some basic concepts for all patients who need decontamination:

1. Removal of patient clothing will remove > 80% of contaminants.

2. Warm soapy water with some vigorous scrubbing will remove most contaminants.

3. Detection devices should be set up outside of the decontamination area, and before the patient enters the emergency department. Knowledge of what you looking for here is important. This is again a place in which your Health Department or possibly the military (CST) or Fire Department could help.

4. Set up your decontamination area so that patients who are cleaned are not re-contaminated. Setting up a decontamination trailer backwards will cause this to happen.

5. Consider using a surrogate marker (food coloring, fluorescein) to validate full decontamination.

6. Decontamination depends on contaminant. Poison Control, Department of Environmental Protection (DEP), Department of Public Health (DPH), etc., staff may be able to aid in identifying decontamination needs.

Once patients start arriving, determining if they have been decontaminated or not will be important. A likely clue will be what they are wearing. Patients without their own clothes *will* have most likely been decontaminated.

9.8.1 Who Needs to be Decontaminated

Of the likely patients to be seen from a terror event, only those exposed to chemical or radiological attacks will need to be decontaminated. Victims of biological attacks will be infectious and may need to isolated or quarantined. Although, with a biological attack, it is likely that some casualties will present to the emergency department before a pattern is recognized. A plan to mitigate this possibility is strongly advised.

Patients exposed to explosive or incendiary devices need not be decontaminated, other than routine cleaning and irrigation of wounds. The exception to this would be those who were exposed to a dirty bomb or toxic substance from the explosion.

Once patients have been decontaminated, they can be treated according to their injuries.

9.9 Staff Needs

For prolonged ED operations, certain needs must be taken into account. With additional staff called in, supplemental food will need to be provided.

To decrease the likelihood of contaminating other parts of the hospital, it is probably better to bring food to the department rather than send the staff to the cafeteria.

There will also be a need for staff rest and sleeping quarters as the event progresses. The longer a staff member goes without sleep, the greater the possibility for errors and poor judgement. Many hospitals have dormitories and call rooms that can be used for this purpose. Staff shower and lavatory facilities will also be required, separate from the general public (to decrease the possibility of contamination).

Terrorism does not only affect the hospital, it has an impact on the entire community. As such it should be planned as a community event with leaders from outside of the hospital. Staff will work more diligently if they do not have to worry about their children and families. Childcare can help alleviate some of this worry for the staff. Some hospitals have childcare facilities in house, others do not. A relationship with the local school system and churches may be helpful.

As an example, the CT-1 DMAT team actually has a formal arrangement where members who are not deployed on missions will look out for the family members of those who are deployed. This may be as simple as a phone call or two, to as complex as making childcare or eldercare arrangements. It has had a reassuring effect on the team members who are out on deployments, unable to fulfill obligations at home and on their family members as well. This could be a role for a social worker or mental health professional, hospital volunteers or the Red Cross.

9.10 Post Incident Return to Normal Operations

Once a terrorist event is contained and the response phase for ED staff has been completed, the process of taking the system out of emergency response mode and putting it back into day to day operations starts.

The CISD should be required of all personnel prior to their being allowed to return to normal operations / shift work. Early integration of mental health teams can head off feelings of guilt, helplessness, frustration, and anxiety by emergency providers after a terrorist event.

The CISD defusings can be career and lifesaving for the providers involved. Providers needing professional follow-up care can be identified at an early stage and be assisted with putting their lives back into perspective and order after these events.

During CISDs, emergency providers are given the opportunity to discuss the events that they were involved in, including areas that did not go as planned or that did not end with good results. The environment is one of support and no assignation of blame is placed on any provider. A responsible director will arrange for shift coverage while he stands his crew down for debriefing (both for CISD and normal debriefing) and rest and relaxation. For many small departments this may be accomplished in as little as a single day or two. For larger departments a more thought out and organized approach may be needed. This process can be planned, just like the rest of the disaster plan.

Long term psychological evaluation need to be made available; many times the effects of a terrorist attack do not manifest until days or weeks after the event. Some of these manifestations may need long term psychological care and this should be provided to any EMS provider who needs it.

Lastly, a final event debriefing should occur, separate from the CISD debriefing. This should include reviewing lessons learned from the event and the plan for applying those lessons to future ED responses and into the overall emergency response plan. By reflecting on all the information gathered at an incident, from patients, providers, department heads and municipal leaders, we can learn about areas of the response that went well and areas that did not. From that knowledge, changes can be made to address the shortcomings of the original plan. This is not done to assign blame, but to prevent loss of life and decrease suffering in the future and ultimately to learn from the experience.

Planners need to emphasize inclusive preparedness. A Hospital does not operate in isolation and must break down barriers such as thinking that it is alone in preparing. A hospital should work with multiple agencies and partner with them to plan. Knowing one's resources is paramount.

References

1. Dan Avstreih. The Rescue, 9.11.01: Two weeks at ground zero. *Brown Alumni Magazine Online*, November December 2001. http://www.brownalumnimagazine.com/storydetail.cfm?ID=373 (Accessed January 29, 2006)
2. Lab Safety Supply, *Disaster Preparedness & Response.* Janesville, WI, Lab Safety Supply, p. 54, Fall 2001

10 Pediatrics: Special Considerations for Children

JAMES F. WILEY, II

10.1 Introduction

As terrorist activities have increased and civilian targets for terrorism have become more common, the critical need to develop comprehensive systems of care for pediatric victims of weapons of mass destruction has emerged as a national priority in the United States of America. In recognition of the importance of this priority, a national consensus conference on pediatric preparedness for disasters and terrorism convened in New York City during February 2003 and was reconvened in Washington, D.C. in November 2005 (Table 10.1). Over 70 pediatric specialists, representatives from key government agencies and liaisons for national pediatric organizations attended this conference. Their work has served as a touch point for a new emphasis on the special needs of children in emergency preparedness planning.

The major outcome of this conference was the development of recommendations and guidelines for pediatric care following a biological, chemical or nuclear attack. These recommendations were structured within eight key areas: (1) pre-hospital and emergency care, (2) hospital care, (3) emergency preparedness, (4) terrorism preparedness and response, (5) mental health needs, (6) school preparedness and response, (7) training and drills, and (8) future research and funding. The conference also made priority recommendations that cut across these major areas [1].

The priority recommendations for hospital preparedness focus on ensuring ALL hospitals are prepared to take care of pediatric victims. Children's hospitals must provide the lead role in preparing prior to an event and directing the care of children in general hospitals during an event. For general hospitals, pediatric training and the availability of 48 hours of pediatric specific medicine and equipment to care for their average daily number of pediatric patients plus a surge of 100 additional children is crucial to this preparedness goal. Additional recommendations focus on assessing specific community pediatric vulnerabilities. This risk assessment then guides proper pediatric training, medicines, and equipment for the region. Pediatric care and treatment guidelines within all hospital emergency operations and preparedness policies are vital to a successful response to a terrorist attack. General hospitals should partner with their regional pediatric centers to ensure that the children in their community will receive the highest level of pediatric care during a terrorist event [1]. In the wake of the atrocity at Beslan, Russia, where children suffered specifically to further terrorist goals, the need to build emergency preparedness infrastructure for children has taken on a new urgency [2].

10.2 Children: Special Vulnerabilities

Children possess unique characteristics that place them at a disproportionate risk of injury from terrorist activities relative to adults. As such, emergency planning that does not account for children's physiology, cognitive capability and developmental needs will fail to protect them during an event. This section outlines key pediatric differences and proposes important considerations in hospital planning to account for children's physical weaknesses relative to adults.

Table 10.1 Priority Recommendations from Pediatric Preparedness for Disasters and Terrorism: A National Consensus Conference, February 2003*

All hazards preparation and planning
    Pediatric-specific triage system used by all pre-hospital and hospital personnel in mass-casualty incidents involving children.
    Pediatric equipment and medicines on all EMS vehicles, including those needed to respond to weapons of mass destruction.
    Prepare all hospitals to care for children with children's hospitals taking a leading role in training pre-event and direct care during an event.
    Maintain a 48-hour supply of pediatric equipment and medicines in all hospitals to manage current average number of pediatric patients and a 100 additional patients.
    Designate a pediatric resource center in every regional and state disaster plan to include, at a minimum, pediatric critical care, pediatric trauma care, and pediatric burn care.
    Include a detailed pediatric component in Web-based hospital resource availability networks.
    Ensure pediatric specialty experts are involved with regional and statewide emergency preparedness planning.
    Require pediatric medical guidance for all Disaster Medical Assistance Teams (DMATS) including specific pediatric members during deployments.
    Ensure adequate pediatric supplies to all DMAT basic loads.
    Primary care providers (PCPs) and urgent care centers (UCCs) should prepare, practice and update an office disaster plan.
    PCPs and UCCs should encourage home disaster preparedness including distribution of the Family Readiness Kit.
    All government plans should provide for communication, health care delivery, contacting and reuniting families with their children.
    All government plans should provide for placement, medical and mental health care, shelter and guardianship for children with injured or deceased family members.
    All biological, chemical and radiological terrorism medication provision plans should keep all necessary medications in appropriate dosages and forms available for administration to children including the National Pharmaceutical Stockpile, Push packs and any State and Local Health Department deployment.
    Design decontamination systems for children of all ages including infants, parentless children, non-ambulatory children and children with special needs.
    Enhance pediatric mental health infrastructure as a necessary part of emergency preparedness.
    Conduct pediatric emergency preparedness drills in every school every year.

Agent specific treatment recommendations
    Any new vaccines developed should undergo appropriate testing in children.
    Mark 1 Auto injector kits should be used as initial treatment in children with severe, life-threatening nerve agent toxicity when IV or precise IM dosing is not available or is logistically impractical.
    Expedite approval of the pediatric auto injector kit.
    Develop plans and distributions systems that ensure potassium iodide (KI) administration with 2 hours of exposure to radioactive iodine to all children who need it.
    Adhere to graded dosing of KI whenever possible but allow for standard 130 mg KI dosing if graded dosing is impractical and administer KI to children at the lowest possible threshold (≥ 5 cGY projected internal thyroid exposure).

---

* Updated recommendations from the November 2005 conference are due out late Summer, 2006.

Analysis of respiratory patterns in children indicates that they have higher respiratory rates than adults. Minute ventilation (tidal volume or size of the breath multiplied by the number of breaths per minute) is also increased. As a result, children may receive higher doses of aerosolized agents including infectious, chemical, and radiological substances [3,4]. Higher dose would correlate with greater degree of illness among children vs. adults with the same exposure. Agents that are heavier than air, such as nerve agents and vesicants, accumulate near the ground. Because of their smaller size, children may be exposed to a higher concentration of these agents than adults in the same area [5,6]. Finally, children have less respiratory reserve and higher oxygen utilization than adults [4,7]. Therefore, pulmonary agents that produce airway and bronchial disturbances, such as chlorine, phosgene, and riot control agents ("tear gas") might cause more life threatening respiratory distress in children.

Children are at greater risk of morbidity and mortality due to traumatic injury. In trauma situations, the force of the trauma, such as an explosion, is transmitted over a smaller surface area, thus magnifying the amount of traumatic injury in the child [8]. Relative to the adult, a child has a larger head size that translates into a higher frequency of head injuries in children with its attendant sequelae. Pediatric circulation allows maintenance of a normal blood pressure despite the loss of up to 50% of blood volume. However, this is at the expense of underperfusing important organs such as the liver, gastrointestinal tract, and kidney. This ability to compensate is due to the generation of high concentrations of catecholamines in response to injury [9]. As a result, children managed by inexperienced personnel may receive care after adults who have similar or even lesser injuries in a mass-casualty situation. Because traumatic force is transmitted to underlying organs through the relatively plastic pediatric skeleton, children are more apt to develop pulmonary contusion, an injury that can be difficult to detect in its early stages.

Children have a higher body surface area to mass and a more permeable skin than adults. As a result, they are more prone to serious consequences of dermal exposures from chemical agents such as nerve gas and vesicants. The large surface area exacerbates insensible heat loss and fluid loss in children with burns. Convective heat loss with hypothermia can be a serious problem in children undergoing wet decontamination. Children also have lower glycogen and fluid reserves and are more prone to ketosis and dehydration in the setting of vomiting and diarrhea, a common consequence of biological, chemical and radiological weapons [6].

The pediatric immune system is less robust, especially those under 2 years of age. This makes children more prone to infectious agents and to agents that compromise immunity such as vesicant agents and nuclear agents. In addition, children's bone marrow is more susceptible to malignant transformation induced by radiation exposure and chemical mutagens. This susceptibility makes cancer risk higher in children than in adults with the same exposures [5,10].

Cognitively, children have limited reasoning ability. They are dependent on adults to recognize danger and avoid hazards. Their psychological immaturity places them at great risk because they have limited coping skills. Serious mental illness can result not only to direct victims of a terrorist attack but also to witnesses of the attack, even in the absence of physical injury [11,12].

Ideally, children should be cared for by personnel with specific training in pediatrics and pediatric emergency care. However, in a disaster situation, these resources may be quickly overwhelmed. Nationwide there are 56 freestanding children's hospitals and over 5000 general hospitals [13]. Most children's hospitals run at or near capacity year round. In Connecticut, there are two children's hospitals with a combined total of 174 inpatient pediatric medical/surgical beds, 36 pediatric intensive care beds, and 24 emergency department beds. These hospitals serve an estimated population of 612,816 children less than 19 years of age [14]. There are 30 remaining general hospitals and one Veteran's Administration hospital that currently have limited pediatric services. Clearly, a major disaster of the magnitude of Beslan, Russia (150 children killed, 500 injured, over 50% critically) would quickly overwhelm existing pediatric resources in Connecticut. Therefore, in Connecticut and elsewhere, it is imperative that general hospitals, including those with limited existing pediatric resources, develop additional pediatric capacity.

Several key interventions are necessary to mitigate negative outcomes for children during disaster care. Training in pediatric assessment and triage with pediatric specific protocols, such as the Jump-START system helps prevent undertriaging of seriously ill or injured children when they are evaluated with adults (Figure 10.1) [15]. Personnel designated for hospital triage should familiarize themselves with these protocols and practice them regularly on simulated pediatric victims during mass casualty drills. Appropriate treatment of children begins with correct assessment that identifies critical resuscitation needs. Pediatric assessment and care is taught in several standardized courses. Table 10.2 summarizes these courses and the intended audience.

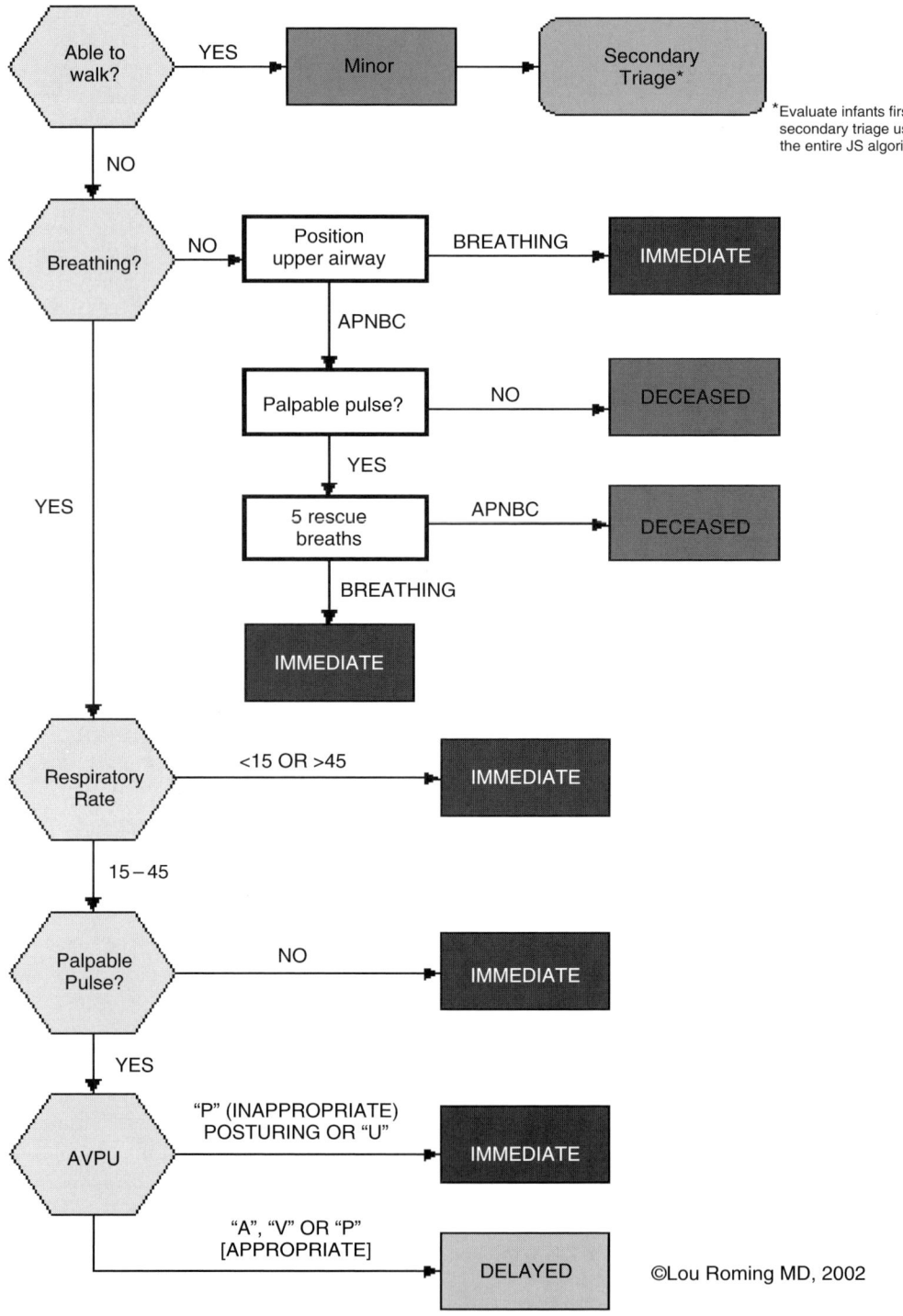

Figure 10.1 JumpSTART Pediatric MCI TrigaeProtocol© developed by Lou Romig. (Reprinted with permission.)

Table 10.2 Standardized courses that teach pediatric assessment, triage, and care

Course title	Intended audience	Organization/contact information
Pediatric advanced life support (PALS)	Paramedics, physician's assistants, nurse practitioner, nurses, and physicians	American Heart Association, at 800/242-8721, or at www.americanheart.org.
Pediatric education for the prehospital provider (PEPP). PALS renewal may be offered with some courses.	EMT and paramedics	American Academy of Pediatrics, American College of Emergency Physicians at www.peppsite.com,
Emergency nurses pediatric course (ENPC). PALS renewal may be offered with some courses.	Nurses	Emergency Nurses Association, email at jmika@ens.org or call Course Operations Department of the ENA National Office, phone (800) 900-9659.
Advanced pediatric life support (APLS, may be combined with PALS certification in some courses)	Physicians, physician's assistants, and nurse practitioner	American Academy of Pediatrics (AAP) at 800/433-9016, ext 4795 or the American College of Emergency Physicians (ACEP) at 800/798-1822, ext 3292
Pediatric disaster life support (PDLS)	Physicians, Nurses, Nurse Practitioners, and Physician Assistants	American Medical Association, Phone: (508) 856-4101 E-mail: carol.shustak@umassmed.edu

Proper equipment size and correct pharmaceutical dosing present significant obstacles to quality pediatric care in a general hospital. Systems for pediatric equipment use and drug dosing such as the Broselow–Luten system provide a standard approach for general hospitals to ensure proper medication therapy with minimal error. The color-coded Broselow–Luten organizes equipment and provides specific drug dosing information based on a weight reference. When weight is known, then the proper equipment and drug doses can be read directly off the reference. When the weight is not known, a tape can be used to determine the weight range based on the patient's height. The corresponding color on the tape provides equipment sizes and drug doses based on this weight. Expansions of this system allow for organization of equipment by these color designations. A new adaptation of this system, the Pediatric Disaster Assistance Tool (PDAT), developed by Drs. Wiley and Baum, supplies a readily available resource for the provision of timely and accurate treatment of children exposed to weapons of mass destruction (Figures 10.2 and 10.3). Additional pediatric information in pdf or html format for download is available at the following websites www.bt.cdc.gov/children (Centers for Disease Control) [16], www.aap.org/terrorism/index.html (American Academy of Pediatrics) [5], and www.ems-c.org/disasters/framedisasters.htm (Emergency Medicine Services for Children). Care priorities for children based on specific agents are discussed below.

From the behavioral standpoint, children require much greater supervision than adults. Children under 4 years of age may not be able to understand instructions and are likely to be uncooperative with medical personnel when frightened. Keeping families together as much as possible while delegating control of children to their parents will minimize disruption of important procedures such as wet decontamination. In the setting where a parent or older sibling is not available or is too sick to provide supervision, personnel with the ability to rapidly establish rapport with children must provide the needed supervision. Child life specialists, social workers, schoolteachers, and day care workers represent personnel who can assist with this important task. This response capability

PURPLE

BIOLOGICAL AGENTS

Anthrax   Rx: Ciprofloxacin 150 mg IV q 12 h
 Alt: Doxycycline 22 mg IV q 12 h
 Prophy: Ciprofloxacin 150 mg po q 12 h
Botulinum toxin   Rx: Trivalent antitoxin (Type A-B-E)
 Alt: Heptavalent antitoxin, investigational
 Prophy: Pentavalent toxoid vaccine (Type A-B-C-D-E)
Plague   Rx: Streptomycin 100 mg IM q 12 h
 Alt: Gentamicin 15 mg IV q 8 h, or
 Prophy: Ciprofloxacin 150 mg po q 12 h
Ricin   Rx: None
 Alt: None
 Prophy: Protective mask to avoid inhalation
Smallpox   Rx: None
 (Vaccinia immune globulin only for certain complications)
 Alt: Vaccination / revaccination of exposed persons
 Prophy: Vaccination
Tularemia   Rx: Streptomycin 100 mg IM q 12 h
 Alt: Gentamicin 15 mg IV q 8 h
 Prophy: Ciprofloxacin 150 mg po q 12 h
Viral Hemorrhagic Fevers
 Rx: Ribavirin 300 mg IV load
 then 160 mg IV q 6 h x 4 d
 then 80 mg IV q 8 h x 6 d

10 KG

CHEMICAL AGENTS

Blister Agents
 Rx: BAL 25 mg IM q 6 h, 1st 2 d
 (if Lewisite or Phosgene)
Cyanide
 Rx: Na-nitrite 100 mg IV,
 then Na-thiosulfate 500 mg IV
Nerve Agents
 Rx: Atropine 0.2 mg IV
 (IM if hypoxic), await atrop. effect,
 then 2-PAM 500 mg IV / IM
Pulmonary Agents
 Rx: None
Riot Control Agents
 Rx: None

RADIATION AGENTS

"Dirty" Bomb
 Rx: Blast / Burn protocol

Nuclear Reactor
 Rx: Potassium iodide 32 mg
 (if I-131 suspected & > 5 cGy)

11 KG

Figure 10.2 Pediatric disaster assistance tool. Sample section for treatment of a 10–11 kg. Child, Side A, treatment for specific agents. Adapted by Carl Baum and Jim Wiley for the Broselow–Luten Coloring Kids System, Vitalsigns® (all rights reserved).

is a key element to successful general hospital care of children.

10.3 Children and Agent-specific Vulnerabilities

Limited information specific to children for weapons of mass destruction currently exists. This section addresses specific issues relative to recognition of pediatric exposure to weapons of mass destruction and treatment modifications. Recommendations typically reflect individual cases reported in the literature or consensus expert opinion.

10.3.1 Biological Agents

Category A agents define potential biologic weapons that are available, easily disseminated and carry a high mortality rate with expectation of major public health disruption. Currently, the designated category A agents include anthrax, smallpox, plague, tularemia, the viral hemorrhagic fevers, and botulinum toxin. Details regarding pathogenesis, clinical findings, identification and treatment for these agents are covered in Chapter 4.

10.3.2 Anthrax

Dissemination of 2 g of weapons grade anthrax spores, amounting to 20–200 million infectious doses, occurred through the United States of America mail system in the months of September and October, 2001. Potential exposures and cases were identified in New York City, Connecticut, Washington, D.C. and Florida. Despite the large dose, only 11 cases of inhalational anthrax and

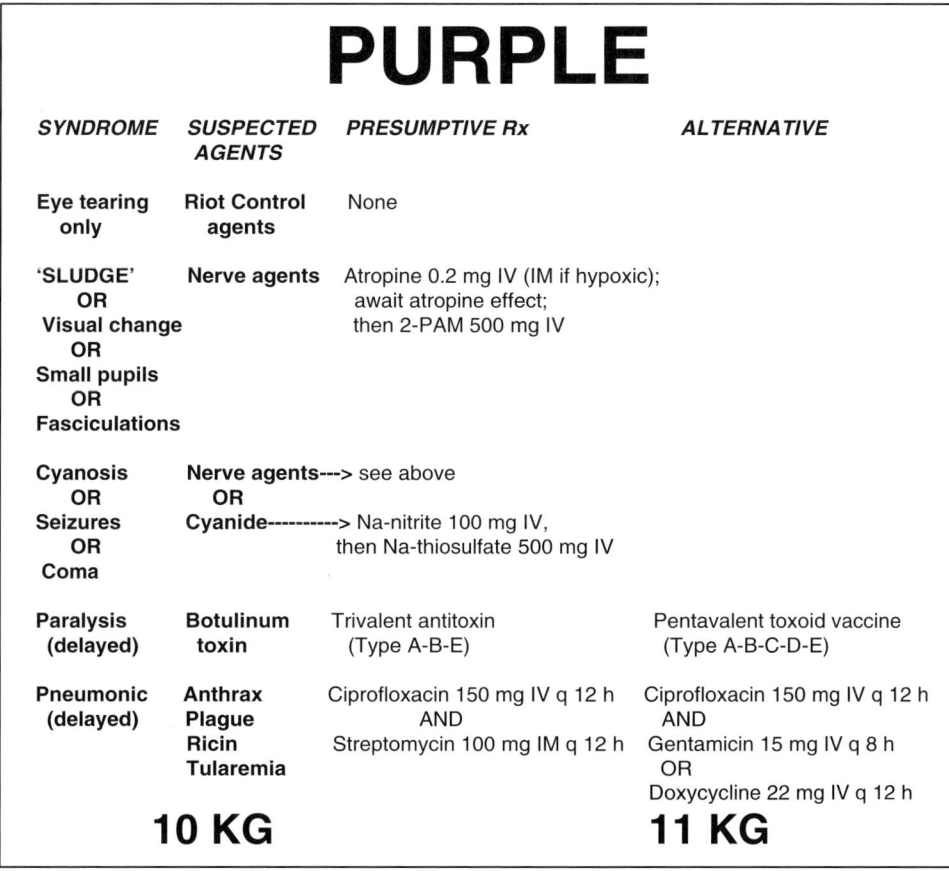

Figure 10.3 Pediatric disaster assistance tool. Sample section for treatment of a 10–11 kg. Child, Side B, Treatment based on presenting syndrome. Adapted by Carl Baum and Jim Wiley from the Broselow–Luten Coloring Kids System, Vitalsigns® (all rights reserved).

11 cases of cutaneous anthrax resulted [17]. One case of cutaneous anthrax infection was found in a 7-month-old male infant who had crawled around on the floor in an office space at the New York City Headquarters of a major news organization. The child developed a large area of infection on the arm that was initially misdiagnosed as cellulites and treated as an outpatient after surgical debridement and a single does of intravenous antibiotics. Subsequently, the child returned with worsening symptoms. Because of the lack of response, he was admitted to the hospital with a diagnosis of Brown Recluse Spider Bite. Ultimately, a diagnosis of anthrax was made based on the history of possible exposure and PCR confirmation of anthrax DNA in a skin biopsy of the lesion and in serum. The infant's course was complicated by hyponatremia, hemolysis, DIC, and renal insufficiency. He made a complete recovery [18]. This case represents the only documented case of biological terrorism in a child. The previously undescribed systemic effects in this child raise the question of differential susceptibility to complications of cutaneous anthrax in children. No pulmonary cases occurred and also did not occur in this child despite obvious exposure. Whether children are less susceptible to this form of disease after deliberate exposure remains an important question for further investigation.

Because of possible engineered resistance, ciprofloxacin is the drug of choice for infection with suspected weapons-grade anthrax. Typically, this drug is not recommended in children under 12 years of age due to reports of adverse effects on cartilage growth in young animals. However, in the setting of anthrax disease or exposure, the risk of contracting or not treating resistant anthrax infection outweighs the potential for an adverse effect of ciprofloxacin. For acute infection, ciprofloxacin is given intravenously in a dose of 10–15 mg per kg every 12 hours up to the adult maximum of 400 mg for 60 days. For prophylaxis the same dose of ciprofloxacin is given orally for up to 60 days after exposure. Both treatment and prophylaxis regimens should be changed if the anthrax isolates are susceptible to penicillin. Appropriate alternatives in this instance include intravenous penicillin G and oral amoxicillin [17].

When ciprofloxacin is in short supply, doxycycline becomes the drug of choice despite its adverse effects in children; weakening of bones in infants and dental staining in children under 8 years of age. Children over 8 years of age should receive doxycycline 100 mg IV every 12 hours for 60 days to treat acute infection and the same dose orally for prophylaxis. Children under 8 years of age should receive 2.2 mg/kg up to 100 mg intravenously as above for acute infection and orally for prophylaxis [17].

An inactivated anthrax vaccine, anthrax vaccine adsorbed, was given experimentally to adults potentially exposed to anthrax spores in 2001. Limited data are available to determine the efficacy of postexposure vaccination. However, the extended time for potential infection would possibly give vaccinated persons a chance to mount some immunity prior to infection. There is no data regarding safety or efficacy of anthrax vaccine in children [19].

10.3.3 Smallpox

Smallpox has an estimated 30% mortality rate among unvaccinated children and adults. Clinical findings among children and adults do not differ significantly. Varicella (chickenpox) infection in children can mimic certain features of smallpox infection. Several resources exist to help differentiate these infections [16]. Also, routine vaccination against varicella has markedly reduced the number of cases in the pediatric population.

Although eradicated as a natural source of infection in the 1970s, smallpox samples were kept by the USA and the former Soviet Union. In response to the terrorist attacks of September 2001, the United States of America began several steps to mitigate against the threat of smallpox dissemination, including resumption of a national smallpox vaccination program. The initial focus of the program was to vaccinate up to 500,000 public health professionals and hospital personnel to serve on vaccination response teams. Subsequently, attention has turned to developing plans through the public health infrastructure for mass vaccination of the entire US population in the event of a smallpox outbreak. Current recommendations for mass smallpox vaccination are the same for children and adults.

Despite this plan, institutions and government agencies have withheld approval for new pediatric studies of safety and efficacy for the Wyeth Dryvax Variola Major vaccine [20]. A systemic review of major complications and mortality following smallpox vaccination based on US experience from 1963 to 1968 did find that infants less than 1 year of age had greater risk for post-vaccinial encephalitis and generalized vaccinia than other age groups [21]. Limited data from adult volunteers suggest that current vaccination risks are equal to or less than these historical risks [22,23].

10.3.4 Plague

When aerosolized, *Yersinia pestis*, organism responsible for plague, causes pneumonic plague, a disease with a 25% mortality rate. Intramuscular streptomycin (15 mg/kg twice daily up to 1 g) or intravenous gentamicin (2.5 mg/kg three times daily) are the therapies of choice in children. However, in the setting of a mass casualty, it is unlikely that adequate supplies of these drugs would be available and intravenous therapy with ciprofloxacin (see anthrax treatment above), doxycycline (see anthrax treatment above) or chloramphenicol (25 mg/kg four times daily) are recommended [24].

10.3.5 Tularemia

Tularemia is naturally occurring and has several different manifestations including ulceroglandular, glandular, oculoglandular, oropharyngeal, pneumonic, typhoidal, and septic forms. A pneumonic infection is most likely following an aerosolized release. Treatment recommendations for children are the same as for plague [25].

10.3.6 Viral Hemorrhagic Fevers

The virus families Filoviridae, Arenaviridae, Bunyaviridae, and Flaviviridae comprise the viral hemorrhagic fevers. Specific agents, such as Ebola virus, Lassa and Yellow fever cause a clinical syndrome of fever, rash, DIC and hemorrhage 2–21 days after exposure with mortality ranging from <1% to 90% depending on the infecting organism. Intravenous ribavirin is recommended for clinically evident viral hemorrhagic fever of unknown origin or identified arenavirus or bunyavirus infection. Dosing is weight-based and the same for children and adults. Oral dosing is recommended in mass casualty settings. The pediatric dose is 30 mg/kg once followed by 15 mg/kg twice a day for 10 days [26].

10.3.7 Botulinum Toxin

Aerosolized botulinum toxin produces a descending paralysis by preventing acetylcholine release at the motor end plate. Children and adults would be expected to have the same clinical presentation. However, children, especially infants, would be expected to be more vulnerable to paralysis and respiratory failure following exposure. Equine botulinum antitoxin is the primary therapy. Indications and dosing are the same for adults and children [27].

10.3.8 Chemical Agents

The main classes of weaponized chemicals include nerve agents, vesicants, pulmonary agents, cyanide and riot control agents. Detailed discussion of pathophysiology, clinical manifestations and treatment are found in Chapter(s) 6. Similar to biological agents, little pediatric data exist concerning effects of chemical warfare agents. Some data regarding vesicant exposure comes from reports of pediatric victims exposed during the Iran–Iraq War [28]. Evidence also suggests that many children died from chemical exposures, possibly a combination of vesicants and nerve agents in the village of Halabja during Saddam Hussein's Anfal campaign.

Wet decontamination is recommended following liquid exposures to nerve agents, vesicants and pulmonary agents [5]. Decontamination should be performed by personnel wearing appropriate personal protective equipment (PPE, see Chapter 7). Wet decontamination ideally should be provided in the field prior to hospital transport or outside of the hospital structure if required for patients arriving for care. Life-saving resuscitation measures such as airway support with endotracheal intubation and emergent antidotal therapy should be given concomitantly with decontamination. All clothing and jewelry must be removed and double-bagged in plastic. This measure alone typically removes between 80–90% of contamination. Victims should have skin and hair washed and irrigated with tepid water and mild soap. Any eye exposure should receive copious normal saline irrigation [29]. Warm clean clothing and blankets for children who undergo wet decontamination will help prevent hypothermia from convective heat loss during the procedure.

10.3.9 Nerve Agents

Chemical nerve agents produce marked inhibition of the enzyme, acetylcholinesterase, and thereby prevent the breakdown of acetylcholine at muscarinic, nicotinic and central nerve synapses. The clinical effects of bronchorrhea, miosis, diaphoresis, vomiting, diarrhea, salivation, lacrimation and urination derive from enhanced cholinergic transmission at pre- and post-synaptic muscarinic nerve terminals. Fasciculations and then paralysis follow initial depolarization and then depolarizing blockade of nicotinic receptors at motor end plates. Nicotinic receptors are also found at the presynaptic symapthomimetic synapses in the spinal cord. Stimulation at these sites leads to dilated pupils, tachycardia and hypertension. Nerve agent effects at central nervous system synapses cause coma and seizures. One series described a preponderance of central and sympathomimetic effects in children under 2 years of age after organophosphate poisoning [30]. Although the spectrum of physical findings after nerve agent exposure in children will be similar to adults, pediatric patients are likely to be sicker due to increased dose and greater vulnerability to the toxic effects of nerve agents (see above).

Atropine, pralidoxime, and benzodiazepines counteract the effects of nerve agents. Atropine provides drying of secretions with reversal of bronchorrhea serving as the endpoint for treatment. Atropine may also provide protection against seizures. Pralidoxime, when given in a timely manner, prevents irreversible binding of the nerve agent to acetylcholinesterase and prevents paralysis. Benzodiazepines also treat seizures and provide improved outcomes in animal exposure studies. In the USA, atropine is the only antidote packaged as an autoinjector specifically for children (Atropen™). This autoinjector kit does not contain pralidoxime. Table 10.3 provides weight-based dosing recommendations for hospital treatment of nerve agent exposure [31].

Children represent a major challenge in delivering effective field treatment in the USA due to no availability of a comprehensive pediatric nerve agent kit. Currently, expert opinion recommends the Mark I kit as the preferred treatment for children down to the age of 3 years as follows [32]:

1. 3–7 years or 13–25 kg : 1 Mark I autoinjector (2 mg Atropine/ 600 mg Pralidoxime)
2. 8–14 years or 26–50 kg : 2 Mark I autoinjectors (4 mg Atropine/1200 mg Pralidoxime)
3. Over 14 years or >51 kg : 3 Mark I autoinjectors (6 mg Atropine/1800 mg Pralidoxime)

Children under 3 years require weight-based dosing as per Table 10.3. The AtroPen™ may be used based on weight in situations where Mark I administration to children is specifically prohibited by regulations or legislation: Under 7 kg, 0.25 mg autoinjector; 7–18 kg, 0.5 mg autoinjector; 18–40 kg, 1 mg. autoinjector [31].

10.3.10 Vesicants

This category consists of the alkylating mustard agents, especially sulfur mustard and the chemical arsenical agent, lewisite. These agents cause irritation and chemical burns of the eyes, skin, and respiratory tract. Higher exposures lead to bone marrow inhibition and gastrointestinal tract injury. Developed during World War I, lewisite was never used extensively and has not been stockpiled to a very large degree. In contrast, sulfur mustard exists in large amounts and was recently used by Saddam Hussein against Iranian troops and Kurds in the past two decades. Pediatric exposure data from these events indicate that children may develop clinical effects rapidly after mustard exposure and have more extensive skin lesions [28]. Mustards have no antidote. The most important treatment is rapid decontamination within minutes of exposure. Severe exposures to lewisite may benefit by therapy with British antilewisite (BAL, Table 10.3).

10.3.11 Pulmonary Agents

Chlorine and phosgene comprise the commonly weaponized pulmonary agents. They also are prime chemical weapons of opportunity given their ubiquitous use in industrial chemical production. Irritation of the eyes, nose, and throat are common, especially with chlorine. Bronchospasm and pulmonary edema follow serious exposure. Pulmonary edema may occur 2–4 hours after chlorine exposure and anywhere from 6 to 24 hours after phosgene exposure. Treatment is supportive and does not differ from adults. Children are more vulnerable to the effects of these agents as previously discussed in section 10.2 [29].

10.3.12 Cyanide

Cyanide, the notorious poison used in the Nazi gas chambers, causes cellular anoxia and death

Table 10.3 Antidotes for children exposed to chemical warfare agents

Agent	Indication	Treatment
Nerve agents[a]	Cholinergic effects: Bronchorrhea, bradycardia, miosis, tearing, drooling, vomiting, and diarrhea	Atropine 0.05–0.1 mg/kg IM or IV (minimum 0.1 mg, maximum 5 mg) every 2–5 minutes as needed for marked secretions or bronchospasm.
	Nicotinic (motor end plate): Fasiculations, muscle weakness, and paralysis	Pralidoxime 25–50 mg/kg IV (maximum 1 gm), IM (maximum 2 gm) repeat in 30–60 minutes as needed and then every hour for up to 2 doses as needed. Pralidoxime may be given continuously as infusion of 10–15 mg/kg/hour (maximum 600 mg/hr)
	CNS: Seizures or prophylactically in severe exposure	Lorazepam 0.1 mg/kg IV, IM (maximum 4 mg) OR Midazolam 0.2 mg/kg IM (maximum 10 mg) OR Diazepam 0.3 mg/kg IV (maximum 10 mg)
Lewisite	Bone marrow suppression and GI tract symptoms	British anti-lewisite (BAL) 3 mg/kg every 4–6 hours for severe symptoms
Cyanide	Dyspnea, coma, seizures, and apnea	Sodium nitrite (3%): Hgb (estimated, g/dL) Dose (ml/kg) 10 0.27 12 0.33 14 0.39 Maximum 10 ml. Sodium thiosulfate (25%) 1.65 ml/kg (Maximum 50 ml)

[a] see text for discussion of autoinjectors and Atropen™.

by its direct inhibition of electron transport in the mitochondria. From the standpoint of a chemical weapon, it is only effective in closed spaces. Rapid treatment with sodium nitrite and sodium thiosulfate is necessary to salvage exposed victims. Weight-based dosing in children is based on estimated hemoglobin and is essential to avoid untoward effects of excess methemoglobinemia from sodium nitrite (Table 10.3) [29].

10.3.13 Riot Control Agents

Modern riot control agents include the commonly available pepper spray (*Oleoresin capsicum*), CN (1-chloroacetophenone, Mace™) and CS (2-chlorobenzylidene). These agents are chemical irritants of the skin, eyes, upper airways, and gastrointestinal tract. Typically, they are incapacitating but not lethal. However, close exposure in enclosed areas has caused serious upper and lower airway disease in children. Pulmonary deaths have occurred in previously healthy people.

Treatment requires removal from exposure, decontamination and supportive care and does not differ significantly from adults [33].

10.3.14 Radiation

Extensive information exists regarding the health effects of radiation exposure in children. Experience from survivors of Hiroshima, Nagasaki, and Chernobyl indicate that, when controlled for exposure level, radiation-induced cancers occur more frequently in children than in adults. Protection from radiation exposure consists of evacuation and shelter. Potassium iodide provides protection from thyroid uptake of radioactive iodine, an isotope commonly found in nuclear power plants and likely released after an incident [34]. Table 10.4 lists age and weight-based dosing recommendations, including how to prepare potassium iodide solution. The solution is stable for 7 days in the refrigerator and should be given daily until authorities indicate that it is no longer needed [35].

Table 10.4 Potassium Iodide Administration in Children Exposed to 0.05 Gray (5 rad) or More of Radioactive Iodine (FDA, 36)

Age	KI Dose (mg)	Volume of solution prepared from a 130 mg Tablet[a], ml (tsp)
12–17 yrs. (≥70 kg)	130	40 (8)
4–17 yrs (<70 kg)	65	20 (4)
1 mo–3 yrs	32	10 (2)
Birth–1 mo.	16	5 (1)

[a]Home preparation: Crush one 130 mg KI tablet in a small bowl into a fine powder. Add four teaspoons (20 ml) of water and mix. Add four teaspoons (20 ml) of raspberry syrup, low-fat chocolate milk, orange juice, or flat soda. Resulting mixture is 16.25 mg KI per teaspoon (5 ml). Dose as above. If using 65 mg KI tablet then use same instructions as for 130 mg KI tablet, but double the volume administered.

10.4 Mental Health Considerations in Pediatric Victims of Terrorism

Several studies have documented a high incidence of anxiety, depression and post-traumatic stress disorder in children exposed to disaster [36–38]. Risk factors for these adverse psychiatric outcomes include prior history of mental illness in the child, lack of coping by parent or caregiver, specific externally obvious signs of post-traumatic stress disorder in the father, repeated media exposure to scenes from the disaster and proximity to the disaster [39–41]. With respect to proximity to the disaster, researchers have demonstrated that the subjective perception of threat to life (either self or close family member) is more important than preordained objective features [42]. Finally, children who experience greater pain during hospital recovery are at higher risk of serious psychiatric sequelae later on [43].

Effective mental health interventions for pediatric disaster victims arise from a developmental understanding of children's psychological capabilities and needs [44]. The aforementioned risk factors for mental health pathology can be used to set up appropriate surveillance systems in the wake of a disaster [45]. Promotion of family cohesiveness, limitation of repeated exposures of children to trauma during and after the disaster event and reestablishment of routines (school, play, etc.) all bolster innate resilience in children. Health care workers must be careful not to engage too aggressively in therapeutic behavioral interventions shortly after a disaster. Certain aspects of cognitive behavioral therapy, such as having the victim describe their experience; can actually be detrimental if the victim feels coerced into doing so, such as in a group therapy setting. Rather, experienced disaster workers recommend ongoing monitoring of children at risk with timely intervention for symptoms of anxiety, depression and posttraumatic stress disorder [46].

References

1. National Center for Disaster Preparedness. Pediatric preparedness for disasters and terrorism: a national consensus conference, Columbia University Mailman School of Public Health, Executive summary 2003 at http://www.childrenshealthfund.org/CHF2286VFinal_adj.2.pdf(accessed12/3/2004).
2. Glasser, P. Baker. Hostage takers in Russia argued before explosion: Chechen gave orders by phone, investigators say. *Washington Post*, page A01, Tuesday, September 7, 2004.
3. E. K. Motoyama. Respiratory physiology in infants and children. In: (E. K. Motoyama and P. J. Davis eds) *Smiths' anesthesia for infants and children*, 11–67. St. Louis: Mosby, 1996.
4. K. J. Sullivan and N. Kissoon. Securing the child's airway in the emergency department. *Pediatr Emerg Care*. 18:108–118, 2002.
5. American Academy of Pediatrics, Committee on Environmental Health and Committee on Infectious Diseases. Chemical-biological terrorism and its impact on children: a subject review (RE9959). *Pediatrics* 105:662–670, 2000.
6. E. L. Lynch and T. L. Thomas. Pediatric considerations in chemical exposures: are we prepared? *Pediatr Emerg Care* 20:198–208, 2004.
7. J. R. Hill and K. A. Rahimtulla. Heat balance and the metabolic rate of newborn babies in relation to environmental temperature; and the effect of age and of weight on basal metabolic rate. *J Physiol* 180:239–265, 1965.
8. P. R. Holbrook. Pediatric disaster medicine. *Crit Care Clin*. 7:463–470, 1991.
9. R. M. Perkin and D. L. Levin. Shock in the pediatric patient: Part 1. *J Pediatr*. 101:163–169, 1982.

10. American Academy of Pediatrics Committee on Environmental Health. *Radiation disasters and children*, 111(6, part 1):1455–1466, 2003.
11. R. H. Gurwitch, M. Kees, S. M. Becker, M. Schreiber, B. Pfefferbaum, and D. Diamond. When disaster strikes: responding to the needs of children. *Prehospital & Disaster Medicine.* 19(1):21–28, Jan–Mar 2004.
12. C. W. Hoven, C. S. Duarte, and D. J. Mandell. Children's mental health after disasters: the impact of the world trade center attack. *Curr Psych Reports*, 5(2):101–107, 2002.
13. National Association of Children's Hospitals and Related Institutions and National Association of Children's Hospitals: Fact sheets at www.childrenshospitals.net (accessed 12/8/04).
14. A. S. Adomako, I. Melese-d'Hospital. State-by-State Profiles: The Integration of pediatric care components into the EMS system at ww.emsc.org/State/framestate.htm (accessed 12/8/04).
15. L. Romig. Pediatric triage. A system to JumpSTART your triage of young patients at MCIs. *Journal of Emergency Medical Services.* 27(7):52–58, 60–63, 2002.
16. http://www.bt.cdc.gov/agent/smallpox/diagnosis/index.asp (accessed 2/11/05)
17. T. V. Inglesby, T. O'Toole, D. A. Henderson, J. G. Bartlett, M. S. Ascher, E. Eitzen, A. M. Friedlander, J. Gerberding, J. Hauer, J. Hughes, J. McDade, M. T. Osterholm, G. Parker, T. M. Perl, P. K. Russell, K. Tonat, and Working Group on Civilian Biodefense. Anthrax as a biological weapon: updated recommendations for management. *JAMA*, 287(17):2236–2252, 2002.
18. A. Freedman, O. Afonja, M. Chang, et al. Cutaneous anthrax associated with microangiopathic hemolytic anemia and coagulopathy in a 7-month-old infant. *JAMA*, 287:869–874, 2002.
19. T. Jefferson, V. Demicheli, J. Deeks, P. Graves, M. Pratt, and D. Rivetti. Vaccines for preventing anthrax. *Cochrane Database of Systematic Reviews*, (2):CD000975, 2000.
20. R. S. Baltimore and H. B. Jenson. Should smallpox vaccine be tested in children? *Current Opinion in Infectious Diseases.* 16(3):237–9, 2003.
21. T. J. Aragon, S. Ulrich, S. Fernyak, and G. W. Rutherford. Risks of serious complications and death from smallpox vaccination: a systematic review of the United States experience, 1963–1968, *BMC Public Health* 3:26, 2003.
22. L. M. Jacobs, K. Emanuelsen, C. McKay, and K. Burns. Bioterrorism preparedness—Part II. Smallpox vaccination in a hospital setting. *Connecticut Medicine*, 68(1):27–35, Jan. 2004.
23. M. Haim, M. Gdalevich, D. Mimouni, I. Ashkenazi and J. Shemer. Adverse reactions to smallpox vaccine: the Israel Defense Force experience, 1991 to 1996. A comparison with previous surveys. *Military Medicine.* 165(4):287–289, 2000.
24. T. V. Inglesby, D. T. Dennis, D. A. Henderson, J. G. Bartlett, M. S. Ascher, E. Eitzen, A. D. Fine, A. M. Friedlander, J. Hauer, J. F. Koerner, M. Layton, J. McDade, M. T. Osterholm, T. O'Toole, G. Parker, T. M. Perl, P. K. Russell, M. Schoch-Spana, K. Tonat, and Working Group on Civilian Biodefense. Plague as a biological weapon: medical and public health management. *JAMA*, 283(17):2281–2290, 2000.
25. D. T. Dennis, T. V. Inglesby, D. A. Henderson, J. G. Bartlett, M. S. Ascher, E. Eitzen, A. D. Fine, A. M. Friedlander, J. Hauer, M. Layton, S. R. Lillibridge, J. E. McDade, M. T. Osterholm, T. O'Toole, G. Parker, T. M. Perl, P. K. Russell, K. Tonat, and Working Group on Civilian Biodefense. Tularemia as a biological weapon: medical and public health management. *JAMA.* 285(21):2763–2773, 2001.
26. L. Borio, T. Inglesby, C. J. Peters, A. L. Schmaljohn, J. M. Hughes, P. B. Jahrling, T. Ksiazek, K. M. Johnson, A. Meyerhoff, T. O'Toole, M. S. Ascher, J. Bartlett, J. G. Breman, E. M. Eitzen Jr. M. Hamburg, J. Hauer, D. A. Henderson, R. T. Johnson, G. Kwik, M. Layton, S. Lillibridge, G. J. Nabel, M. T. Osterholm, T. M. Perl, P. Russell, K. Tonat, and Working Group on Civilian Biodefense. Hemorrhagic fever viruses as biological weapons: medical and public health management. *JAMA*, 287(18):2391–405, 2002.
27. S. S. Arnon, R. Schechter, T. V. Inglesby, D. A. Henderson, J. G. Bartlett, M. S. Ascher, E. Eitzen, A. D. Fine, J. Hauer, M. Layton, S. Lillibridge, M. T. Osterholm, T. O'Toole, G. Parker, T. M. Perl, P. K. Russell, D. L. Swerdlow, and K. Tonat Working Group on Civilian Biodefense. Botulinum toxin as a biological weapon: medical and public health management. *JAMA.* 285(8):1059–1070, 2001.
28. A. Z. Momeni, M. Aminjavheri. Skin manifestations of mustard gas in a group of 14 children and teenagers: A clinical study. *Int J Dermatol* 33:184–187, 1994.
29. F. M. Henretig, T. J. Cieslak, and E. M. Eitzen. Biological and chemical terrorism. *J Pediatr* 141:311–326, 2002.

30. Pediatric expert advisory panel. Atropine use in children after nerve gas exposure. Info Brief. 1:1–7, Spring 2004 available at http://ncdp.mailman.columbia.edu/AtropineAutoInjectorV1N1.pdf accessed March 9, 2005.
31. F. M. Henretig, T. J. Cieslak, J. M. Madsen, E. M. Eitzen Jr., and G. F. Fleisher. The emergency department response to incidents of biological and chemical terrorism. In *Textbook of Pediatric Emergency Medicine*, 4th ed (G. F. Fleisher and S. Ludwig ed.) pp. 1763–1784. Philadelphia (PA): Lippincott Williams and Wilkins, 2000.
32. J. F. Wiley II. Riot Control Agents. In *Pediatric Terrorism and Disaster Preparedness Resource*. (G. Foltin, D. Schonfeld, and M. Shannon, eds). American Academy of Pediatrics, August 2005 (*Online resource available*).
33. Committee on environmental health. Radiation disasters and children. *Pediatrics* 111: 1455–1466, 2003.
34. US Food and Drug Administration, Center for Drug Evaluation and Research. Home preparation of procedure for emergency administration of potassium iodide tablets to infants and children. Using 130 milligram (mg) tablets. Rockville, MD, Center for Drug Evaluation and Research; 2002. available at: http://www.fda.gov/cder/drugprepare/kiprep130mg.htm accessed March 9, 2005.
35. C. V. Russoniello, T. K. Skalko, K. O'Brien, S. A. McGhee, D. Bingham-Alexander, and J. Beatley. Childhood posttraumatic stress disorder and efforts to cope after Hurricane Floyd. *Behavioral Medicine*. 28(2):61–71, 2002.
36. N. Laor, L. Wolmer, M. Kora, D. Yucel, S. Spirman, and Y. Yazgan. Post-traumatic, dissociative and grief symptoms in Turkish children exposed to the 1999 earthquakes. *Journal of Nervous & Mental Disease*. 190(12):824–832, Dec. 2002.
37. W. Yule, D. Bolton, O. Udwin, S. Boyle, D. O'Ryan, and J. Nurrish. The long-term psychological effects of a disaster experienced in adolescence: I: The incidence and course of PTSD. *Journal of Child Psychology & Psychiatry & Allied Disciplines*, 41(4):503–511, May, 2000.
38. J. Asarnow, S. Glynn, R. S. Pynoos, J. Nahum, D. Guthrie, D. P. Cantwell, and B. Franklin. When the earth stops shaking: Earthquake sequelae among children diagnosed for pre-earthquake psychopathology [see comment]. Comment in: *J Am Acad Child Adolesc Psychiatry*. 39(2):141–142, 2000.
39. M. Korol, B. L. Green, and G. C. Gleser. Children's responses to a nuclear waste disaster: PTSD symptoms and outcome prediction. *Journal of the American Academy of Child & Adolescent Psychiatry*. 38(4):368–375, Apr. 1999.
40. B. Pfefferbaum, S. J. Nixon, P. M. Tucker, R. D. Tivis, V. L. Moore, R. H. Gurwitch, R. S. Pynoos, and H. K. Geis. Posttraumatic stress responses in bereaved children after the Oklahoma City bombing. *Journal of the American Academy of Child & Adolescent Psychiatry*. 38(11):1372–1379, Nov. 1999.
41. B. Pfefferbaum, D. E. Doughty, C. Reddy, N. Patel, R. H. Gurwitch, S. J. Nixon, and R. D. Tivis. Exposure and peritraumatic response as predictors of posttraumatic stress in children following the 1995 Oklahoma City bombing. *Journal of Urban Health*. 79(3):354–363, Sep. 2002.
42. E. Caffo and C. Belaise. Psychological aspects of traumatic injury in children and adolescents. *Child & Adolescent Psychiatric Clinics of North America*. 12(3):493–535, 2003.
43. R. H. Gurwitch, M. A. Sullivan, and P. J. Long. The impact of trauma and disaster on young children. *Child & Adolescent Psychiatric Clinics of North America*. 7(1):19–32, vii–viii, Jan, 1998.
44. A. M. La Greca, W. K. Silverman, and S. B. Wasserstein. Children's predisaster functioning as a predictor of post-traumatic stress following hurricane Andrew. *Journal of Consulting & Clinical Psychology*. 66(6):883–892, Dec. 1998.
45. R. S. Pynoos, A. K. Goenjian, and A. M. Steinberg. A public mental health approach to the postdisaster treatment of children and adolescents. *Child & Adolescent Psychiatric Clinics of North America*. 7(1):195–210, Jan. 1998.

11 The Role of Psychiatry and Social Services in the Hospital Response to Bioterrorism

JULIAN D. FORD

11.1 Introduction The Psychological Dimension of "Terror" in Bioterrorism

Psychiatry and social services play a critical role in addressing the public health impact of terrorism and disasters (Norris, Young, Ford, Ruzek & Gusman, 1997). Terrorism and disasters expose people not only to physical danger and pathogens, but also to psychological trauma [1,2] (Norris, Friedman, Watson, Byrnes, Diaz, & Kaniasty, 2002). Terrorism is by definition intended to cause psychological fear and a sense of dread and helplessness due to life-threatening danger [3], and which precisely fulfills the criteria for "traumatic stress" in the American Psychiatric Association's Diagnostic and Statistical Manual (1994). Post-traumatic stress in the wake of disasters has been implicated as a contributor to physical illness and medically unexplained health problems [4,5], as well as mental health problems, and therefore represents a major public health concern. This chapter will provide an overview of the psychological sequelae and interventions that hospitals can provide to prevent or ameliorate persistent post-traumatic stress psychosocial impairment in the wake of terrorism.

11.1.1 The Challenge: Managing the Psychological Impact of Real or Potential Biological Contamination

Biological contamination, or the threat thereof, can lead to a contagion of fear that travels by vector similarly to the spread of actual physical harm [6].

Clear evidence of this psychological contagion was provided by the response to the 1995 sarin attack in the Tokyo subway. More than 500 persons came to the Emergency Department at a nearby hospital within the first few hours following this attack and more than 5500 sought medical evaluations subsequently. Although some persons had severe physical symptoms related to nerve gas exposure (of whom 12 died), more than 90% were "acute psychological casualties—worried well—who feared they might have been exposed to sarin gas" [7]. The hospital, like most, was unprepared for the flood of psychological casualties, and did not at first identify the need for psychiatry personnel because of the focus on addressing the medical sequelae of chemical contamination. Psychiatry and social service professionals were called upon, but only after the medical staff and clinicians were overwhelmed by the demand for not only diagnosis and treatment but also information and guidance. Psychiatry and social service staff and clinicians also found themselves largely unprepared to address the sheer volume and intensity of stress reactions, having primarily had experience in the assessment, care, and placement of patients whose acute crises occurred in the context of chronic psychiatric disorders.

The medical and psychiatric/social service response to patients and family members who are experiencing an acute sense of psychological terror must be grounded in an understanding of the nature of psychological terror. Fear of a specific threat or anxiety in anticipation of exaggerated potential threats are far more readily managed than terror, because terror combines anxiety and fear as well as a sense of horror, disbelief, helplessness, and profound and permanent loss [8]. The challenge to healthcare practitioners and organizations posed by terrorism is how to help victims, families, and providers themselves to understand and recover from the shock of psychological terror. Meeting this challenge does not require psychotherapy and cannot be done solely by pharmacological treatment (although strategic use of targeted pharmacologic agents may play a role, see below). The key is to replace terror with a sense of control and the real possibility of a future that is not poisoned by prolonged suffering and almost certain death. The "cognitive appraisals" (beliefs, interpretations) that people exposed to terrorism have about their *culpability* in and *ability to manage* the "damage" they are actually or dread experiencing, and to *regain a life worth living*, can make the difference between experiencing a psychological breakdown or coping effectively in the face even of catastrophic harm and loss [9]. Not only psychiatry and social services providers but all healthcare providers can contribute to the restoration of hope in the face of terror. However, this cannot be done by simply exhorting people to be positive or to believe that somehow things will get better, because terror overrides such superficial encouragement. Instead, it is essential to tangibly increase the person's ability to predict and control immediate aspects of their lives by making threats visible, intrusions preventable, and losses grieved.

11.1.1.1 Unpredictability

The ability to exert meaningful control in any situation depends upon being able to predict both what is likely to happen next and what can be done in the form of "course corrections" that increase the likelihood of positive outcomes and reduce the chance of negative outcomes. When certain aspects of a crisis are unpredictable or not known (e.g., the extent of exposure to toxic chemicals or gas, and the degree of toxicity conferred by exposure), it is essential to provide information that re-focuses victims, family members, and first responders on the aspects of the situation that are predictable. Information about the mechanisms of action and likely physical effects and signs associated with a variety of toxic agents is widely available. However, this information may inadvertently increase the sense of terror for some persons, unless they also are given information relevant to other concerns which are more basic and yet tend to be lost in the panic when terror strikes. For example, knowing when and how it will be possible to make contact with loved ones from whom one has been separated, or that food and shelter can be depended upon while the crisis is being dealt with, can restore the sense that there are some ways in which important aspects of life still are predictable despite other as yet unresolved threats.

11.1.1.2 Uncontrollability

Being able to anticipate a near- and long-term future that is manageable involves knowing how to take practical steps that restore not only predictability but also the sense of being able to exert meaningful control. Terror forces people to live with uncontrollability, and the ability to exert control often cannot be quickly or completely restored. Toxic exposure can lead to physical reactions that often cannot easily or immediately be reversed, but the steps that not only the healthcare provider but also the patient or other persons concerned can take to manage and mitigate the harmful sequelae can be described and formed into a plan that restores some sense of control. Here too, it is important to focus not only on dealing with the direct source of threat, managing the effects of toxic exposure, but also to regaining a sense of control over other background concerns that reconnect the individual with "normal" life. Without denying or minimizing the severity of the threat and the importance of immediately addressing basic health concerns, getting help in gaining control of concerns such as basic bodily nourishment, privacy, communication with family and key support persons, and being able to make a difference by helping and protecting others, can help people to begin to regain the ability to think calmly and clearly.

11.1.1.3 Reversing the invisibility and violation of terrorism

When a sense of being able to anticipate and have some meaningful control over at least some important upcoming events has been re-established, there is a further challenge involved in sustaining this newly restored (and still fragile, after the shock of having been blindsided by terrorism) sense of control and hope. Terrorism is particularly traumatic because the agent or its mechanism of action is invisible (e.g., toxic gas, but also instruments of destruction that are hidden in plain sight by terrorists who cannot be distinguished from ordinary people, such as in the use of improvised explosive devices). Further, the harm that terrorism causes is not just frightening but moreover a pernicious and pervasive violation of the integrity of people's bodies (e.g., poisoning, disfiguration, and amputation) and of the trust that people place in one another [8]. These effects cannot be fully reversed, and should not be minimized, but they can be mitigated by communicating information that helps the patient understand what is happening to their body in a manner that is open and transparent (rather than rendered invisible by the cloak of silence or technical terminology), and that explicitly demonstrates the provider's trustworthiness by involving the patient in a collaborative relationships as a fully informed consumer and an equal and respected partner in decision making. Although this may seem like nothing more than the basic foundation for establishing a positive "working alliance" with any patient [10], this collaborative stance is particularly crucial in treating persons affected by terrorism in order to reduce rather than inadvertently exacerbate a sense of helplessness in the face threats that are invisible and profound violations.

11.1.2 Recognizing Acute and Repeated Exposure to Traumatic Stress: Direct, Threatened, and Witnessed

Terrorism unfortunately very clearly illustrates why psychological trauma is not limited to direct exposure to physical harm. As is evident from the Tokyo sarin incident—but also equally in other terrorist incidents with higher magnitudes of lethality (e.g., September 11th, 2001)—most victims of terrorism are not severely physically injured or harmed. Physical injury does increase the risk of subsequent psychological impairment (e.g., post-traumatic stress disorder, PTSD, or depression), but others also are at risk for PTSD if they: (a) could have been severely harmed but were not, or (b) witnessed devastating incidents in which others were harmed, or witnessed others experiencing pain and suffering in the aftermath of disaster [1,2]. Credible threats that do not occur, and close calls and near misses, can be as psychologically traumatic as direct exposure to severe physical harm—and may potentially have an even greater shock value, due to the ability of people to imagine even greater catastrophes than those that actually happen. Witnessing pain and suffering, or the horrors of dismemberment or massive property destruction, also can be traumatic—indeed even when witnessing terrorism occurs primarily through media, the effects can be traumatizing for children [11] or adults [12]. In the medical arena, a major unrecognized source of psychological trauma in the wake of terrorism is witnessing the suffering of others while awaiting emergency medical care.

Individuals who have experienced other psychological traumas or socioeconomic adversities or life stressors (e.g., poverty, immigration, racial discrimination [12]) prior to terrorism exposure are at elevated risk for developing PTSD [13] and other forms of persistent psychological impairment [12]. Prior traumatization does not appear to have an inoculation effect, but rather a sensitization effect which is consistent with the alterations in critical areas of brain functioning related to stress reactivity and stress management that have been found in PTSD [14]. However, living with the persistent and immediate threat of terrorism on a daily basis does not necessarily lead to PTSD: a survey of a large community sample of Israeli adults found that few (9%) had PTSD and most were optimistic about their own future (82%), their ability to cope with terrorist incidents (75%), and their country's future (67%), and did not wish to receive professional treatment for stress (72%), despite generally feeling unsafe (60–68%) and sub-clinically depressed (59%) [15]. Thus, remaining healthy and functional in the face of repeated exposure to or persistent threats of terrorism, and past experiences of other forms of psychological trauma, may require strong social support systems and active positive coping [12].

11.1.3 Traumatic Grief: Shock, Loss and Complicated Bereavement

Survivors and witnesses, as well as the family and close friends or associates of persons killed or severely harmed in terrorist incidents, often experience profound losses that compound the shock of the psychological trauma caused by terrorism [11]. Traumatic grief (also referred to as complicated bereavement) involves a combination of traumatic stress reactions (which lead the person to attempt to avoid reminders of terrifying or emotionally devastating experiences, including losses) and grief reactions (which lead the person to be preoccupied with thoughts of lost loved ones or other losses). Thus, traumatic grief involves a tension between avoidance of unwanted memories a need to mourn through painful remembrance, which can become a debilitating vicious cycle.

Terrorism causes not only the loss of important relationships due to death but also due to losses that involve a failure to conserve or replace crucial resources (e.g., housing, social services, employment, and neighborhood contacts). A study in rural China showed that a community distant from the epicenter of an earthquake was less adversely affected in terms of residents' quality of life and stress reactions than a more proximate community—but the more geographically distant community received less support and thus showed poorer outcomes and less positive change in quality of life at a 9-month follow-up than the more directly affected community [16]. While a return to the *status quo ante* is impossible, earthquake survivors who believe that their personal and social resources were still largely intact fared better psychologically than those who rated resources as either increased or decreased.

Culture provides a lens through which people interpret losses and seek help during and in the aftermath of disaster or terrorism. Culture includes secular and religious belief systems, support networks and resources, ritual practices and traditions, language and dialects, and national and group/tribal loyalties. Despite culture's pervasiveness and potency, little is known about how culture affects the impact of and recovery from disasters [1,2]. Most studies of the post-traumatic sequelae of disaster or terrorism have not systematically examined ethnic or cultural differences. Of those that include ethnicity as variable, several report that ethnicity is a predictor of post-traumatic psychosocial impairment, with increased short-term (but not long-term [17]) risk for Hispanics living in New York City in the wake of September 11th and greater risk for African American children and Hispanic and African American adolescents and adults after hurricanes [1,2]. Communities representing different cultures also may metabolize disasters differently. A study of disaster survivors found that younger age was a risk factor in Mexico, older age in Poland, and mid-adulthood in the United States [1,2]. Another study found that the gender difference in PTSD intrusion and avoidance symptoms and bereavement reactions were greater in a sample of hurricane survivors in Mexico than in the United States, and in the latter cohort African–American women and men showed less difference on these symptoms than Caucasian women and men [1,2]. These findings indicate that it is not culture alone but a complex combination of historical and current sociocultural factors that influence post-disaster adjustment. In ethnoculturally diverse communities, the types and sources of help that affected individuals and families seek and benefit from are likely to vary depending upon the extent to which they are embedded in pre-existing social networks and connected to indigenous resources (e.g., secular and faith-based organizations) that are familiar to each ethnocultural group. Across cultures disaster survivors are more likely to seek help from health care professionals or lay healers than from mental health providers (Adams, Ford, & Dailey, 2004). Thus, public health providers, traditional healers, opinion leaders, and "trusted advocates" within communities affected by disaster or terrorism may be the best sources of both programmatic guidance and front line assistance for ethnoculturally diverse individuals, families, and societies. Careful and respectful ethnographic observation of norms, traditions, and resources within different cultural sub-groups is an essential prerequisite to providing post-disaster or terrorism assistance. The community that existed before a disaster or terrorist incident is never the same as what exists in the aftermath, and these changes are a source of psychological loss that requires culturally sensitive social and medical healthcare. For example, displacement was found to be a risk factor for cardiovascular morbidity among survivors of the Lebanese Civil War [18].

11.1.4 Unique Effects on First Responders and Their Families

Emergency responders (e.g., fire, police, EMS, search and rescue, emergency management, military, and construction and transportation personnel) and recovery workers (e.g., Red Cross, Salvation Army, FEMA, or other disaster or emergency relief volunteers and personnel) enter the disaster setting with preparation and relatively well-defined roles and responsibilities—"with a job to do," rather than as "a victim." However, the line between responder and victim often blurs in the midst or aftermath of disaster (e.g., emergency responders often are killed or injured, lose team members to death or injury, and witness death, suffering, and destruction). First responders and recovery workers receive and provide a great deal of emotional/social and practical support—but only for a relatively limited time. First responders surveyed soon after rescue and relief operations often acknowledge experiencing traumatic stress reactions (both during deployment and afterward), but typically describe them as manageable and transient unless exacerbated by co-worker deaths or recurrent or particularly horrific traumatic incidents or by subsequent work or life stressors (Orner, 1995). For example, interviews with 51 Oklahoma City body handlers (many of whom were inexperienced and knew someone killed) revealed low levels of self-reported peri-traumatic stress or depression symptoms that decreased significantly after 1 year [19]. A small proportion (<10%) reported acute and chronic PTSD symptoms (and also physical health and alcohol use problems) initially and a year later. Four years later, firefighter rescue workers and 27 of their partners [20] reported little evidence of psychiatric disorders including PTSD.

However over half of the partners described firefighters as having continuing symptomatic difficulties, suggesting that under-reporting may obscure actual symptom prevalence. Although most first responders do not report difficulty with PTSD or psychosocial symptoms, the lasting impact of traumatic stress on first responders is not limited to anxiety, but also may involve depression or suicidality and substance abuse [19]. The interview study of first responders' primary partners provided no evidence of heightened risk of family problems or divorce—although one third of the partners reported that their relationship with their spouse had changed permanently since he had been deployed to respond to the Oklahoma City bomb site [20]. A number of factors have been empirically identified that place first responders at risk for serious and persistent post-traumatic stress problems (Table 11.1). None of these indicators should be considered definitive in identifying first responders who need psychiatric or social services [13], but they provide a basis for careful observation that can prevent failures by healthcare providers to proactively detect responders who are in need of specialized post-traumatic interventions over time.

11.2 Management of Acute Traumatic Stress and Grief Reactions in Patients and Staff

The first job for hospital-based psychiatry and social services providers in the wake of terrorist incidents is to identify and manage the acute traumatic stress and grief reactions of patients first and also of staff. Healthcare providers and hospital staff are first

Table 11.1 Risk factors for persistent psychosocial and vocational impairment among first responders

Pre-traumatic vulnerability
   Lower levels of prior education
   Younger age
   Single/unmarried
Traumatic exposure
   Witnessing severe physical harm and suffering (e.g., burns and dismemberment)
Peri-traumatic reactions
   Acute stress disorder
Post-traumatic life experiences
   Stressful life events following a traumatic rescue or recovery deployment
Post-traumatic coping and social support
   Use of alcohol or drugs to cope with stress
   Avoidant coping and emotional numbness
   Problems with anger and irritability
Social isolation and reduced involvement in social support networks

to reduce the burden on medical and nursing providers and staff). PFA provides a guide for mental health-informed and trauma-informed assistance to affected victims, families, and first responders in the immediate wake of critical incidents. In the form of "second aid" and "third aid" PFA involves the delivery of brief mental health interventions in the first weeks and months after critical incidents and into the longer term recovery phase (see below).

PFA involves four essential functions which flow in a sequence (Table 11.2) but in actual fact often occur simultaneously: In abbreviated form, the functions are to "direct" the person to resources that can assist with basic immediate needs, "protect" the person from further harm or unnecessary additional stress, "select" coping responders, albeit typically not right at the disaster epicenter. Even highly experienced and seasoned providers and staff (e.g., Emergency Department clinicians and staff) can experience post-traumatic reactions when their unit is flooded for hours and days with horrifically injured and extremely psychologically distressed patients and family members. These reactions often are described as "vicarious trauma" or "secondary trauma," but in fact they are no different than the "direct" trauma experienced by witnesses and responders.

11.2.1 Psychological First Aid: Protect, Direct, Connect, and Select

The first step in addressing the psychological needs of people seeking healthcare in the wake of terrorist incidents is to provide "psychological first aid" (PFA). The PFA is not in the purview primarily of psychiatry or social service providers, but they can provide essential training and consultation to medical, nursing, and other health professionals and hospital staff in providing PFA. The goal of PFA is to help distressed persons to regain the capacity to modulate their emotions and think clearly so that they can benefit from needed medical care and not use medical services as a means of getting psychological help (i.e.,

Table 11.2 Psychological first aid functions

(I) Direct: Engagement
Goal: To provide helpful direction to affected persons based on observing the context and persons (including responders) with whom contact may be made, respond to contacts initiated by affected persons, initiate contact in a non-intrusive and helpful manner, listen and respond effectively to immediate needs and concerns expressed or demonstrated by affected persons, and enhance motivation for adaptive coping by affected persons.

(II) Protect: Safety and Orientation
Goal: To ensure immediate safety, comfort, orientation, and access to resources by affected persons, and to protect them from unnecessary exposure to traumatic or other stressors.

(III) Select: Stabilization and Self-Regulation
Goal: To help affected persons to recognize (in tolerable amounts and ways), understand (in practical terms that do are easily remembered and utilized at times of stress in which cognitive capacity may be reduced), and modulate expectable changes in emotional reactivity (i.e., to keep reactions within a manageable range of intensity or to recover and resume manageable levels if extremely intense or dissociated reactions occur).

(IV) Connect: Connectedness
Goal: To promote a feeling of connectedness (i.e., that other people care about and can help you, and that you can care about and help others), by providing respectful, non-intrusive, and supportive ongoing relationship to people directly or by being involved in systems that can provide ongoing support and help affected people get back on their feet and regain their lives.

strategies that can enable the person to feel more in control and hopeful, and "connect" the person with other people who can together form (or reconstitute) a viable mutual support system. This is not psychiatric evaluation or treatment, but is a means to re-establish affected persons' essential personal and social resources [21] and provides an opportunity to begin the process of psychiatric triage by identifying persons who show signs of persistent clinically significant psychological distress.

The focus in PFA is on determining the person's primary concern, from the person's own point of view, and how you can help them make progress in achieving that goal within your role. PFA involves paying attention to one's own emotional and physical reactions, and using PFA skills to manage these reactions effectively so that as a provider you can think clearly and be helpful. PFA follows the basic code of "primum non nocere" (first do no harm), by orienting all healthcare provider to not do anything that creates further stress, confusion, or pressure for affected persons unless this is absolutely necessary to ensure safety or resolve crises. The process in PFA is to observe first, then ask simple respectful questions, and then say what you will do to help (preferably describing a plan that involves affected persons as full partners, rather than simply doing things for or to them). PFA establishes a vital human connection and provides accurate simple information that addresses affected persons' immediate concerns, thus helping to contain and control terrifying and still potentially highly dangerous situations and to build an alliance with affected person that will make them willing to work with responders and providers.

11.2.2 Mitigating the "Second Disaster:" Providing Psychological Surge Capacity

After the initial catastrophic impact of a terrorist incident (which may last only minutes or for many days), the two major risks for affected persons and communities are that the response efforts may inadvertently worsen conditions (iatrogenesis) or may be insufficient to meet their needs [22]. The former case has been described as the "second disaster," where well-intended response and recovery efforts backfire and create additional problems or even traumas for affected persons and their families and communities. For example, the media and helpers descended upon bereaved families in the immediate aftermath of the Oklahoma City bombing, until the Red Cross Disaster Mental Health Services helped the community establish a Family Center that had very carefully controlled access and provided families with evidence-based grief counseling.

The latter case of insufficient system capacity to meet rapidly spreading mental health needs is virtually inevitable both in the immediate aftermath and in the mid- to long-term recovery phase when the initial heroic efforts and the honeymoon period of initial recovery are followed by exhaustion on the part of not only affected persons but also responders and the overall response system [22]. The best scenario is one where a multistage psychiatry and social service response is planned well in advance, with provisions for rapid deployment of experienced disaster mental health responders during the first days and weeks after an incident, followed by continued gradual deployment of fresh mental health providers both from within and outside the affected communities over the next several months in order to prevent the existing mental health system from becoming overwhelmed by subsequent "surges" in psychiatry and social service cases. A model for strategic psychiatry preparedness and staged deployment can be found at www.ctrp.org.

11.2.3 Identification and Brief Preventive Interventions with High Risk Individuals and Families

Despite the benefits of psychiatric and social services, most people in disaster-affected communities do not seek help for stress or psychological problems (Adams et al., 2004), although persons with prior mental health problems are the most likely to seek specialized help (Adams et al., 2004) [20]. Both physical health care and mental health services tend to show small but significant increases in utilization in the wake of disaster or terrorism, and some (5%) patients show decreases in utilization. Help-seekers more often turn to medical than psychiatric or social (mental health) providers, as is the case generally in healthcare. For example, adults surveyed in the United States and Canada reported contacting their physician for antidepressant, sleep, or anxiolytic medications shortly after September 11th, but there appeared to be no increase in the use of specialty mental health services (see Adams et al., 2004 for a summary of these studies).

Addressing the needs of people suffering from pre-existing mental and physical health problems or bereavement, particularly if they have increased their substance use, is a first priority in order to engage survivors and emergency workers on their own terms and with a focus on supporting natural recovery processes and preventing long-term risks. Disaster survivors tend to both receive and provide a great deal of emotional/social and practical support—but only for a relatively limited time (i.e., most relief efforts end within 3 months) and unevenly, so that many with the greatest needs (e.g., stigmatized racial or ethnic groups; people with less education) suffer the greatest relative loss in resources and receive the least assistance [1,2].

Symptoms of unwanted memories ("intrusive re-experiencing"), extreme attempts to avoid unwanted memories (e.g., increased substance use, unwillingness or inability to travel to places or engage in activities that are reminders of trauma), "marked" arousal (e.g., jumpiness, tension, anxiety, irritability, inability to sleep, excessive vigilance due to fear of re-traumatization), and at least three symptoms of dissociation (i.e., numbing, feeling in a daze, depersonalization, derealization, and amnesia) (which may occur only during the traumatic exposure) constitute an *Acute Stress Disorder* (ASD) if they persist between 2 days and one month, and impair the individual's functioning (American Psychiatric Association, 1994). *Post-Traumatic Stress Disorder* (PTSD) involves similar symptoms which must persist for at least one month and significantly interfere with sociovocational functioning, specifically: (a) unwanted trauma memories, (b) purposeful attempts to avoid trauma memories and reminders or an involuntary numbing of emotions and detachment from relationships, and (c)"marked" arousal (American Psychiatric Association, 1994).

Incidence data from several studies including motor vehicle accidents, assaults, burns, and industrial accidents suggest that as many as 20% of adults who experience a traumatic accident or assault develop ASD [13]. Several prospective studies reviewed by Bryant [9] indicate that ASD is a risk for *but not an automatic predictor* of PTSD. As many as eight in ten persons who develop ASD go on to develop PTSD between 6 months and two years following trauma exposure. Yet, the proportion of individuals with ASD who develop PTSD differs substantially, from as high as 78% to as low as 30% (O'Donnell et al., 2001; Schnyder et al., 2001). Ehlers and Clark [23] and Brewin [13] conclude that ASD should be considered a sign of potential long-term psychiatric risk and treated immediately if it causes clinically significant impairment, but in most cases providing brief education about the effects of stress on the body [14] and the importance of healthy self-care (e.g., nutrition, sleep) and social support, is the best immediate plan of action.

Based on evidence that extreme immediate mental and physical stress reactions is an indicator a survival-based (as opposed to ordinary) biological adaptation [14], and that survival adaptations may be functional in crises but can interfere with normal memory [14] and self-regulation [24] processes, Brewin [13] developed a Trauma Screening Questionnaire that asks affected persons to simply say "yes" or "no" to PTSD's five symptoms of intrusive re-experiencing and five symptoms of hyperarousal. In studies with train crash survivors and victims of violent assaults, Brewin [13] found that endorsing six or more of these 10 items within the first few days following trauma accurately (>90% overall efficiency) identified persons who developed PTSD.

11.2.4 Triage and Acute Psychosocial and Psychopharmacological Treatment

The first systematic approaches to early psychosocial intervention in the wake of trauma were developed to address the effects of war trauma (e.g., shell shock, combat fatigue) on military personnel, and later to assist emergency medical service workers in the wake of deployment [e.g., "Critical Incident Stress Management"(CISM)]. A review of the outcomes of randomized controlled trials of single-session interventions in the aftermath of traumatic exposures concluded that single-session psychological interventions had no discernable benefit for individuals who had experienced motor vehicle accidents, assault, burns, or other potentially traumatic injuries or medical conditions (e.g., miscarriage, childbirth), with two possible exceptions among 11 studies [23]. Studies involving acute life-threatening accidents or violent assaults and longer follow-up periods (i.e., 3 months to 3 years) showed no benefit, and in two cases adverse outcomes, following a single session of psychosocial intervention. Although CISM most often is provided in a group format, no randomized studies have been conducted with group debriefing.

The best documented approach to brief multi-session psychosocial intervention in the acute period following exposure to psychological trauma is cognitive behavioral therapy (CBT). CBT involves several component interventions, including: (a) education about traumatic stress and PTSD, (b) "imaginal exposure" (i.e., a detailed repeated oral review of the traumatic event(s)), (c) "in vivo exposure" (i.e., activities placing the individual in proximity to reminders of the traumatic event(s)), (d) cognitive restructuring (i.e., identification and reformulation of thoughts or beliefs that sustain a sense of fear, helplessness, or horror), and (e) stress management skills (e.g., relaxation or breathing techniques). Three studies by Bryant [9] provided 5–6 weekly counseling sessions beginning about two weeks after a motor vehicle accident or assault to adults with ASD. CBT was superior to supportive counseling in reducing the severity of PTSD, depression, and anxiety symptoms at post-treatment and follow-up assessments between 4 months and 4 years later.

Despite these encouraging findings, many (25–40%) of CBT-treated patients still develop or fail to remit from PTSD. Ehlers and Clark [23] describe an alternative approach to the delivery and testing of CBT designed for acute trauma survivors who were at highest risk for developing PTSD. Motor vehicle accident survivors "had to meet PTSD criteria and report at least moderately severe symptom severity" after a "3-week self-monitoring phase" (p. 821). At that point, 3 months had elapsed since the accident, and participants were randomized to up to 12 weekly sessions of CBT, a single session with a clinician and self-help materials, or "repeated... infrequent, assessments of PTSD symptoms" (p. 821). The CBT model was 2–3 times longer than that provided previously, delivered at a later time after the traumatic incident (i.e., 3–6 months vs. 1–3 months), and also relied more upon cognitive restructuring than on imaginal or in vivo exposure. Ehlers and Clark [23] suggest these changes may account for the substantially lower rate of drop-outs from their CBT intervention—in fact, there were no dropouts. At a 6-month post-treatment follow-up assessment, approximately 1 year after the accident, participants receiving CBT were substantially more likely to be free of PTSD (86–89%) than the single session or self-assessment participants (approximately 40%) or than a cohort in a naturalistic longitudinal sample from the same population (approximately 30%).

Pharmacological interventions are not as well developed for persons acutely recovering from exposure to traumatic stressors, but recent evidence from a case study and a small randomized clinical trial suggests that prescribing the noradrenergic beta-blocker propanolol within the first few hours of a traumatic accident or assault may prevent the development of PTSD's persistent arousal symptoms or the re-emergence of PTSD in persons who had PTSD in the past [25]. Studies are underway testing other pharmacological agents, such as neuropeptide Y, corticotrophin releasing factor antagonists, opioids, benzodiazepines, and selective serotonin reuptake inhibitors, but no firm evidence as yet firmly supports any early pharmacotherapy strategy for acute trauma survivors. Morgan et al. [25] also warn that pharmacological treatment should be carefully prescribed and monitored in order not to inadvertently create an iatrogenic trade off between immediate relief from distress and subsequent risk of either dependence (e.g., ongoing use of benzodiazepines) or disruption of healthy biological recovery processes necessary for trauma survivors to learn that the threat or harm actually has ended. The latter outcome could increase the risk of PTSD by blocking crucial learning and memory processes [14].

Although replication with survivors of terrorism and disaster are required, the scientific results suggest several features of an acute intervention model. Intervention as early as the first day and in the next 1–2 weeks should focus on bolstering natural support systems and coping resources, and on education about post-traumatic symptoms that teaches practical approaches to managing expectable stress reactions. Post-traumatic coping skills should include simple but effective cognitive techniques for processing intrusive memories—conceptualized as expectable stress reactions that reflect the person's active attempts to make sense of shocking events and the ongoing aftermath—neither encouraging nor discouraging the recall or disclosure of such memories so that this is viewed as a choice rather than a therapeutic requirement. Guidance should be provided to victims, families, and informal and formal role models and caregivers about what types and degree of symptomatic impairment is sufficient to warrant mental health or medical professional evaluation, and how they can use available resources to help themselves and each other to restore reasonable functioning.

Screening for *persistent* post-traumatic impairment should not be conducted for 2–3 months, although healthcare and social service providers, educators, and clergy should be prepared to help people recognize and make practical changes to address potentially maladaptive coping strategies (e.g., increased alcohol use), and to identify and treat or refer individuals with severe impairment during this period as they would ordinarily: Persons experiencing persistent post-traumatic health or mental health problems 3 months or more following a terrorist incident or disaster should be given treatment designed to enable them to: (a) shift from fragmented or ruminative recalling of isolated moments or aspects of traumatic events to a coherent narrative, (b) identify and manage dysphoric thoughts or beliefs concerning symptoms that, if unchecked, can lead to problematic attributions (e.g., mental defeat, hopelessness) and affects (e.g., despondency, guilt, shame, rage), and, (c) pace the recall of trauma events in order to prevent flooding, extreme avoidance, or dissociation (Table 11.3).

11.2.5 Critical Incident Stress Management with Hospital Staff and First Responders

Although CISM has not been evaluated in controlled research trials, it is widely used as an approach to helping hospital staff and first responders to recognize and effectively manage the emotional toll that working with traumatized patients, victims, or family and community members has on them as helpers. Often, staff and responders are directly traumatized themselves, if they or their families are exposed to life threatening danger, or if they witness extreme suffering or death. When done optimally (Dyregrov, 1997), CISM provides an inclusive and non-pathologizing (i.e., everyone is included, not just those who are particularly severely distressed) forum in which staff and responders can construct a shared memory of the positive as well as traumatic and stressful aspects of their work in a crisis or disaster, and provide mutual support that reduces the sense of being "alone" that often occurs in the aftermath of terrible or terrifying experiences. CISM for staff and responders is *not* intended to be (and should never be done as) a confrontational or emotionally provocative process; indeed the focus is on helping each person feel a greater sense of closure and social support, rather than to "fall apart" or "vent" emotions (which can do more harm than good).

CISM for hospital staff or first responders requires two types of role models, first that of trained "peers" (i.e., staff or responders who did not work in this incident but are experienced in this type of work and circumstances), and second that

Table 11.3 Risk factors for persistent psychosocial and vocational impairment in individuals directly or indirectly exposed to disaster or terrorism

Pre-traumatic vulnerability
   Female gender
   Low educational or socioeconomic status
   Unattached marital status (single, divorced, separated, or unmarried but co-habiting—but not widowed, unless acutely bereaved)
   History of anxiety or mood disorders or anxiety proneness, PTSD, and family history
   History of life stressors and disruptions

Traumatic exposure
   Exposure to life threat or extreme violence
   Physical injury
   Witnessing death, extreme violence, or destruction
   Working in the rescue operations
   Exposure to graphic media coverage (e.g., repeated television viewing of disaster)

Traumatic Loss
   Death of a family member or close friend
   Job or financial loss
   Loss of home or possessions

Peri-traumatic reactions
   A panic attack
   Extreme initial distress or dissociation

Post-traumatic coping
   Coping via increased substance use
   Avoidant approaches to coping
   Post-traumatic alienation and bitterness
   Over-identification with victims

Post-traumatic Symptoms, life functioning, and experiences
   Persistent or new intrusive re-experiencing or hyperarousal symptoms one month later
   Persistently impaired psychosocial functioning and mental health treatment seeking
   Additional life stressors (e.g., financial, housing, employment, and family separations)
   Complicated bereavement

Protective factors
   Social support (e.g., spousal, family, peers, neighbors, school, and co-workers)
   Conservation of socio-environmental resources (e.g., home, employment, and relationships)
   For children, parental post-traumatic adjustment
   Psychological preparedness, active coping, and coping self-efficacy
   Optimism and trust in relation to other people and social institutions

of a mental health or social service professional who also was not a direct responder in this incident but is experienced in conducting CISM. As co-leaders, the peer and mental health/social service professionals can consult with facility or team administrators and supervisors to determine the best timing, group composition, place, manner of invitation, and precautions for CISM discussion sessions (see Young et al. [22] for detailed guidelines). There is no predetermined "formula" for when, where, with whom, or how to provide CISM, but there is a universal goal: to enable staff and responders to come away from traumatic deployments with a sense of being a valued, effective member of a team that made a difference in the wake of terrorism for victims, patients, family members, and their communities.

11.2.6 Coordinating the Acute Crisis Response Effort with Ongoing Care for Psychiatric Patients

Several studies found that poor mental health was associated with reporting post-disaster psychological problems (Jehel et al., 2003; North et al., 1999; Shariat et al., 1999; Silver et al., 2002; Rosenheck, & Fontana; 2003a, 2003b) and receiving formal services for those problems (Boscarino et al; 2002; Moyers, 1999; Rosenheck et al., 2003a, 2003b; Weissman, Kushner, Marcus, & Davis; 2003). However, Help-seeking by psychiatric patients did not increase greatly after 9/11 (Rosenheck et al., 2003a, 2003b; Weissman et al., 2003), but prior mental health problems were associated with mental health service utilization in New York City (Boscarino et al., 2002) and with requests for psychotropic medications (Boscarino, Galea, Ahern, Resnick, & Vlahov, 2003; Kettl, & Bixler, 2002; McCarter, & Goldman, 2002). Psychiatric services thus must not only assist victims, responders, and affected families but also ensure that resources are allocated in the wake of disaster so that persons with pre-existing psychiatric disorders are able to continue to receive services in timely and measured manner.

11.2.7 Connecticut's Response; The Center for Trauma Response, Recovery, and Preparedness

Within hours after the tragic events of September 11th, training and supervisory support were requested by hundreds of behavioral health professionals and personnel in Connecticut who recognized that they needed immediate guidance to adapt their skill sets and responsibly provide acute and long term services to individuals, families, organizations, and communities while "first doing no harm." Many already had been asked by media, schools, and civic, business, and religious organizations to provide guidance for directly or indirectly affected adults and children.

In the midst of setting up a mental health command center in the state Department of Mental Health and Addiction Services (DMHAS) Commissioner's office as an adjunct to the overall state incident command center established by the Governor and the Office of Emergency Management, administrators from DMHAS and the state Department of Children and Families (DCF) reached out to the academic centers at the University of Connecticut and Yale University to for disaster mental health consultation. The state-academic partnership began to organize the spontaneously mobilizing behavioral health professionals within the first week following September 11th.

11.2.7.1 Initial training

Connecticut's initial full-day behavioral health disaster response training on September 16th drew upon curricula previously developed for a national network of disaster mental health teams in the Department of Veteran's Affairs [22] and of crisis response teams working in schools and with police agencies by the Yale Child Study Center. Attendees were deployed as a *de facto* virtual behavioral health crisis response and recovery team (CRRT) under the coordination of DMHAS and DCF to serve as contacts for evacuees and bereaved families, to staff Connecticut's outreach services to survivors and family members in New York City, to assist Connecticut emergency responders following deployment to New York City, and to coordinate local agency responses in the most affected towns and cities. The CRRT also served as the repository for the collection and dissemination of resources and protocols for safe and effective post-traumatic crisis management and recovery counseling interventions well in advance of the next disaster.

Over the next month, the state-academic partnership team developed an organizational plan and operational policies and procedures for the establishment of an ongoing administrative, services, and research infrastructure that subsequently became the Center for Trauma Response, Recovery, and Preparedness (CTRP; see www.CTRP.org for a description of the CTRP organizational structure, sample public and professional education services and curricula, and a resource repository for behavioral health, social service, medical, and educational professionals, victims of all ages and families, first responders, administrators, and researchers). Grant funds from the SAMHSA Centers for Substance Abuse Treatment (CSAT), Substance Abuse Prevention (CSAP), and Mental Health Services (CMHS) to DMHAS provided the basis for CTRP initiatives over the next three years.

11.2.7.2 Public education and outreach

Immediately following September 11, CTRP faculty consulted with DMHAS, DCF, and a public relations firm in order to develop public service materials, media presentations, and fact sheets that informed the entire State population (Fan, 2002) about expectable behavioral health sequelae of this complex disaster and its aftermath, and about ways to seek help and resources available to provide help. This coordinated public information campaign reached every area of Connecticut within the first three months following September 11, 2001 through statewide and local media, in Spanish as well as English language. Collaboration with public health, public safety, emergency management, and behavioral heath providers or agencies in designing and implementing media campaigns reduced the amount of inaccurate and conflicting information that could have led to unwarranted fears or other adverse reactions in directly and indirectly affected communities (e.g., a sense of helplessness and vulnerability, xenophobia, unfounded fear and panic).

11.2.7.3 Community outreach

Outreach for bioterrorism preparedness served as a vehicle for enhancing existing behavioral health services and supports by invigorating the collaboration between providers and diverse communities and consumers within a context that utilizes and empowers indigenous community support structures (e.g., faith-communities). The CTRP provided ongoing assertive outreach to diverse racial, ethnic and cultural communities, given the prominent role that culturally specific needs, customs, norms, values, strengths, and vulnerabilities of individuals, families, and communities play in both preparedness for and recovery from disaster. Culturally informed outreach provided an opportunity to engage providers and consumers in recognizing and anticipating the several key risk factors (e.g., prior trauma history; social isolation) and the potentially clinically significant peritraumatic stress reactions that require attention in the wake of disaster.

11.2.7.4 Statewide network of behavioral health response teams and prevention consortia

Consultation and technical assistance provided by CTRP to local and state agencies and providers (including the FEMA funded crisis counseling program) led to the development of five regional CRRTs with more than 450 active members who have a training curriculum and participate in semi-annual live disaster response simulations co-facilitated and critiqued by disaster mental health experts and organizations such as the American Red Cross. A parallel network of community prevention consortia (CPC) also was established with multi-constituency working groups that represented (a) highly affected towns and cities near New York City in Southwestern Connecticut and (b) high risk special populations throughout Connecticut (e.g., families of color, immigrant communities with pervasive trauma histories). This network of 250 prevention specialists was involved in the development of a web-accessible Prevention Toolkit that was adapted by CTRP faculty and staff from evidence-based protocols from the disaster response fields. CPCs assist community mental health and substance abuse agencies in expanding their "target" groups of patients to include people whose behavioral health problems are situationally based (e.g., bereaved families, first responders) or who are at risk (e.g., frail elderly, military families), in effect expanding the provider's or agency's penetration into new markets. This led to a broadening of the range of services provided statewide to existing and new clients and to affected communities, including: (1) evidence-based screening for early identification of non/under-served affected people, through trauma exposure-risk screening, and (2) preventive education materials preparing people to proactively address the expectable reactions and prevent persistent problems through the use of natural support systems and existing services.

11.2.7.5 Professional education

Training and supervision, both acute and long term, provided a vehicle for communicating accurate information (to which behavioral health providers ordinarily are not privy) about a disaster's public health and safety impact and about the nature and steps being taken to mitigate future threats to public health and safety. CTRP faculty elaborated the initial training curriculum to create a multi-component behavioral health disaster response program delivered in stages over the next 10 months to more than two thousand behavioral health professionals and other providers of advocacy, spiritual guidance, health care, education, child care, elder care, and social services via the Internet and in more than 50 face-to-face trainings across the state.

Over time, training and supervision shifted developmentally to parallel the recovery process. Training and supervision increasingly focused on areas (i.e., persistent PTSD or substance abuse) and high risk (e.g., persons with severe mental illness or medical disabilities; refugees), underserved (e.g., monolingual non-English speaking, older adults) or resilient but cumulative affected (e.g., first responders) populations (see literature review above). Training and supervision for CRRT personnel included not only technical skills for assessment and intervention, but also information about the operational procedures for actual emergencies—with an emphasis on the need for operational flexibility as critical to making *in-situ* adaptations to unanticipated events.

11.2.7.6 Information technology system
CTRP developed a sustainable information technology infrastructure (Chandrasekhar & Ghosh, 2001), the Behavioral Health Regional Crisis Response Information System (BHRCRIS). The BHRCRIS supports a web-based database holding all pertinent information necessary to ensure an organized system for mobilization and deployment of CRRTs and CPCs on the CTRP website. The BHRCRIS enables the dissemination and tracking of information regarding team activities, related activities of DMHAS/DCF, selected training opportunities, and resources related to trauma and behavioral health crisis response.

11.3 Longterm Psychiatric Services in the Wake of Bioterrorism: After the Heroic/Honeymoon Phases

11.3.1 Post Traumatic Stress Disorder (PTSD): Course and Comorbidity
More than half of all American adults report having experienced at least one traumatic stressor, and approximately one in 20 men and one in 10 women develop PTSD at some time in their lives (Kessler, Sonnega, Bromet, Hughes & Nelson, 1995). Witnessing a severe injury or death (35.6% of men, 14.5% of women) and being in a life-threatening accident (25% of men, 14% of women) were the most prevalent types of trauma exposure reported. Although somewhat less prevalent, being the victim of a physical assault or rape (11–12% of men; 9–16% of women) also was prevalent.

Physical assaults occur in the context of community violence (2 million women, 3+ million men; Kilpatrick & Acierno, 2003) and domestic violence (3+ million annually; Frank & Rodowski, 1999), the latter affecting more than two million children as witnesses annually (Mitchell & Finkelhor, 2001). More than 2.5 million people are hospitalized as a result of injuries each year in the United States (Zatzick et al., 2002).

Post-traumatic stress symptoms are virtually universal in the first hours and days after exposure to traumatic stressors, but fortunately most such symptoms remit within the first 2–4 weeks [9]. PTSD often co-occurs with other mental health problems following disaster or potentially traumatic accidents or assaults, and there is preliminary evidence that PTSD precedes the other mental health sequelae (McMillen et al., 2002). Most immediately in the wake of a potentially traumatic disaster, accident, or assault, acute stress reactions occur universally although in variable and individualized forms [1,2,9]. Risk factors associated with the individual (e.g., gender, ethnicity, age, biological stress-reactivity, preparation and training, access to socioeconomic resources and social support) and the community (e.g., pre- and post-trauma socioeconomic resources, religious and cultural institutions).

A study of survivors of sexual assault (Rothbaum, Foa, Riggs, Murdock, & Walsh, 1992) found that 94% met all but the duration criteria for PTSD at an average of 14 days post-trauma. A study with nonsexual assault survivors (Riggs, Rothbaum & Foa, 1995) reported that 50% of the men and 70% of the women met all but the duration criteria for PTSD at an average of 19 days post-trauma. However, after another 3–4 months only 21% of the female assault survivors, 0% of the male assault survivors, and 47% of the female sexual assault survivors met criteria for PTSD. Bryant [9] also identified a 5% incidence rate of delayed PTSD (i.e., meeting diagnostic criteria at 2-year follow-up but not at 6-month follow-up) in a sample of motor vehicle accident survivors, and found that these individuals had elevated (although diagnostically sub-threshold) levels of PTSD symptoms at earlier assessment time points [an incidence level similar to that found at a three-year follow-up of motor vehicle accident survivors by Koren et al. (2001)].

PTSD often is comorbid with affective disorders, particularly depression, and substance abuse (Kessler et al., 1995). PTSD and unipolar depression share symptoms of anhedonia, emotional numbing, and social detachment, and have similar although not identical symptomatic features involving problems with sleep, anger, and avoidance. Comorbid PTSD and depression are associated with particularly severe risk (e.g., suicidality), functional impairment, and health care utilization (Kramer et al., 2003) compared to either disorder alone. Comorbid PTSD and substance abuse similarly is associated with medical and psychosocial morbidity.

11.3.2 Psychotherapeutic and Psychopharmacologic Treatments for Post-Traumatic Disorders

The three phases of psychotherapeutic and psychopharmacologic treatment for PTSD involve: (1) developing a working alliance, enhancing safety by stabilizing suicidality, impulsivity, and pathological dissociation, and acquiring or accessing core self-regulatory skills and sustaining beliefs and relationships that were lost or never attained in earlier development; (2) recalling trauma memories with a goal of achieving "mastery over memory" (Harvey, 1995)—a more inclusive, emotionally modulated, and organized autobiographical memory and a more mindful and self-determined orientation to present living and future planning; and, (3) enhancing meaningful ongoing involvement in viable interpersonal, vocational, recreational, and spiritual relationships and pursuits [26]. In practice, phase-oriented treatment often takes the form of a recursive spiral: the issues addressed and biopsychosocial processes involved in each phase frequently are returned to in subsequent phases. For example, the shame, guilt, and disgust associated with a sense of being damaged or a terror of rejection, betrayal, and abandonment tend to emerge anew in each treatment phase even after apparently having been dealt with in earlier phases of treatment. Across all theoretical models of psychotherapy, phase-oriented trauma treatment involves enhancing the recognition (rather than avoidance) of post-traumatic self-dysregulation in tolerable ways and amounts, in order to promote proactive self-regulation.

11.4 Conclusion

Hospital-based psychiatry and social service professionals have a crucial role to play in societal preparedness for and responses to the psychological trauma of disaster and terrorism. Most survivors are unaware of available services even after intensive public education campaigns (e.g., Project Liberty in New York City after September 11th). Unfortunately, not only medical, nursing but also psychiatry and social service professionals generally are not prepared to inform patients or address psychological trauma in routine practice, let alone as disaster responders. For example, only 3% of immigrant primary care patients who had prevalent PTSD due to exposure to political violence had ever been asked about violence exposure by their providers [27]. General practitioners documented only 6% of patient-reported symptoms of fatigue, anxiety, dyspnoea, skin problems, and backache as related to an airline crash disaster that these patients had survived, and diagnosed depression (7%) more often than PTSD (5%) (144).

A proactive approach is needed to prevent the delays and gaps in knowledge (by providers, as well as laypersons), access, coordination, and continuity of acute and follow-up mental health care that occurred despite often heroic efforts in the wake of past disasters and terrorist incidents [28]. An approach also is needed that helps survivors and affected individuals to recognize and enhance the positive beliefs and emotions (e.g., increased hope and trust as a result of experiencing compassion and being inspired by the courage of survivors and responders) that may emerge in disasters [29,30]. Given the propensity of disaster-affected persons to seek informal help through natural caregivers, attention must be paid to helping the helpers as well as caring for patients. The challenge to hospitals of dealing with the "terror" in terrorism are substantial, but the evidence base for effective psychiatric and social services interventions is growing rapidly and provides a solid foundation for the design of services that can address these vital needs [31,32].

Acknowledgments

Funding for the Center for Trauma Response, Recovery, and Preparedness was provided by a contract from the Connecticut State Department of Mental Health and Addictions Services to the University of Connecticut Health Center Department of Psychiatry (J. Ford, Principal Investigator) from grants awarded to the Connecticut State Department of Mental Health and Addictions Services from the Substance Abuse and Mental Health Services Administration, Center for Substance Abuse Treatment, Center for Substance Abuse Prevention, and Center for Mental Health Services (A. Evans, Principal Investigator).

References

1. F. Norris, M. J. Friedman, and P. Watson. 60,000 disaster victims speak: II, summary and implications of the disaster mental health research. *Psychiatry*, 65:240–260, 2002.
2. F. Norris, M. J. Friedman, and P. Watson. 60,000 disaster victims speak: I, an empirical review of the empirical literature, 1981–2001. *Psychiatry*, 65:207–239, 2002.
3. S. Clarke. Bioterrorism. *British Journal of Biomedical Science*, 59: 232–234, 2002.
4. J. Fagan, S. Galea, and J. Ahern. Relationship of self-reported asthma severity and urgent health care utilization to psychological sequelae of the September 11, 2001 terrorist attacks on the World Trade Center among New York City area residents. *Psychosomatic Medicine*, 65:993–996, 2003.
5. C. Engel, Jr. Outbreak of medically unexplained physical symptoms after military action, terrorist threat, or technological disaster. *Military Medicine*, 166 (12 Suppl):47–48, 2001.
6. M. J. Friedman. Toward a public mental health approach for survivors of terrorism. *Journal of Aggression, Maltreatment and Trauma*, 10(1/2):537–549, 2005.
7. K. Taneda. The sarin nerve gas attack on the Tokyo subway system: Hospital response to mass casualties and psychological issues in hospital planning. *Traumatology*, 11(2):75–85, 2005.
8. R. Malkinson, S. Rubin, and E. Witztum. Terror, trauma, and bereavement: Implications for theory and therapy. *Journal of Aggression, Maltreatment and Trauma*, 10(1/2):467–477, 2005.
9. R. A. Bryant. Predicting posttraumatic stress disorder from acute reactions. *Journal of Trauma and Dissociation*, 6(2):5–15, 2005.
10. M. Cruz and H. A. Pincus. Research on the influence that communication in psychiatric encounters has on treatment. *Psychiatric Services*, 53:1253–1265, 2002.
11. B. Pfefferbaum. Aspects of exposure in childhood trauma: The stressor criterion. *Journal of Trauma and Dissociation*, 6(2):17–26, 2005.
12. E. Cardena, J. M. Dennis, M. Winkel, and L. Skitka. A snapshot of terror: Acute posttraumatic responses to the September 11 attack. *Journal of Trauma and Dissociation*, 6(2):69–84, 2005.
13. C. R. Brewin. Risk factor effect sizes for PTSD: What this means for intervention. *Journal of Trauma and Dissociation*, 6(2):123–130, 2005.
14. J. D. Bremner. Effects of traumatic stress on brain structure and function: Relevance to early responses to trauma. *Journal of Trauma and Dissociation*, 6(2):51–68, 2005.
15. A. Bleich, M. Gelkopf, and Z. Solomon. Exposure to terrorism, stress-related mental health symptoms, and coping behaviors among a nationally representative sample in Israel. *Journal of the American Medical Association*, 290:612–620, 2003.
16. X. Wang, L. Gao, N. Shinfuku, et al. Longitudinal study of earthquake-related PTSD in a randomly selected community sample in North China. *American Journal of Psychiatry*, 157:1260–1266, 2000.
17. S. Galea, D. Vlahov, and H. Resnick, et al. Trends of probable post-traumatic stress disorder in New York City after the September 11 terrorist attacks. *American Journal of Epidemiology*, 158: 514–524, 2003.
18. A. Sibai, A. Fletcher, and H. Armenian. Variations in the impact of long-term wartime stressors on mortality among the middle-aged and older population in Beirut, Lebanon, 1983–1993. *American Journal of Epidemiology* 154:128–137, 2001.
19. B. Pfefferbaum, C. North, K. Bunch, et al. The impact of the 1995 Oklahoma City Bombing on the partners of firefighters. *Journal of Urban Health*, 79:364–372, 2002.

20. P. Tucker, B. Pfefferbaum, D. Doughty, et al. Body handlers after terrorism in Oklahoma City: Predictors of posttraumatic stress and other symptoms. *The American Journal of Orthopsychiatry*, 72:469–475, 2002.
21. J. Cwikel, J. Havenaar, and E. Bromet. Understanding the psychological and societal response of individuals, groups, authorities, and media to toxic hazards. In *Toxic Turmoil: Psychological and Societal Consequences of Ecological Disasters* (J. Havenaar, E. Bromet, and J. Cwikel eds) pp. 39–65. New York, Kluwer Academic/Plenum Publishers, 2002.
22. B. H. Young, J. D. Ford, J. Ruzek, M. J. Friedman, and F. Gusman. *Disaster Mental Health Services: A Guidebook For Clinicians and Administrators*. Menlo Park, CA, National Center for Post-Traumatic Stress Disorder, 1998.
23. A. Ehlers and D. Clarke. Early psychological interventions for adults survivors of trauma: A review. *Biological Psychiatry*, 53:817–826, 2003.
24. J. D. Ford. Treatment implications of altered neurobiology, affect regulation and information processing following child maltreatment. *Psychiatric Annals*, 35:410–419, 2005.
25. C. A. Morgan III, J. Krystal, and S. Southwick. Toward early pharmacological posttraumatic stress intervention. *Biological Psychiatry*, 53:834–843, 2004.
26. J. D. Ford, C. Courtois, O. van der Hart, E. Nijenhuis, and K. Steele. Treatment of complex post-traumatic self-dysregulation. *Journal of Traumatic Stress*, 18:467–477, 2005.
27. D. P. Eisenman, L. Gelberg, H. Liu, et al. Mental health and health-related quality of life among adult Latino primary care patients living in the United States with previous exposure to political violence. *Journal of the American Medical Association* 290:627–634, 2003.
28. J. D. Ford, W. F. Dailey, and K. Dean. Development of a behavioral health disaster preparedness system in the wake of September 11: Center for Trauma Response, Recovery, and Preparedness. In *On the Ground after September 11: Mental Health Responses and Practical Knowledge Gained* (Y. Danieli and R. Dingman, eds), pp. 158–166. Binghamton, NY, Haworth, 2005.
29. G. Bechtel, A. Hansberry, and D. Gray-Brown. Disaster planning and resource allocation in health services. *Hospital & Material Management Quarterly*, 22(2):9–17, 2000.
30. B. Flynn. Mental health response to terrorism in the United States: An adolescent field in an adolescent nation. *Journal of Aggression, Maltreatment and Trauma*, 10(3/4):755–768, 2005.
31. M. Heldring and H. Kudler. The primary care health system as a core resource in response to terrorism. *Journal of Aggression, Maltreatment and Trauma*, 10(1/2):541–552, 2005.
32. I. Kutz and A. Bleich. Mental health interventions in a general hospital following terrorist attacks: The Israeli experience. *Journal of Aggression, Maltreatment and Trauma*, 10(1/2):425–437, 2005.

Appendix 11.1

For the Healthcare Professional: When Disaster Strikes

Understanding and Managing Normal Reactions of Traumatic Shock and Grief

Thousands of healthcare professionals face the possibility that their patients may suffer severe physical disability and pain, as well as that their patients may die. Although unavoidable, exposure to human suffering and death (and to the emotional suffering that this causes for the patient's loved ones) is very stressful for the healthcare provider.

In many cases, providers cope very well by simply going on with their work, by turning to trusted colleagues to informally seek and give emotional support, and by finding a balance of rejuvenating activities outside the workplace. However, facing suffering, disability, and death day after day at work causes a cumulative drain on even the most resilient provider's physical, emotional, and social resources. Normal stress reactions can become nagging psychological problems, for example:

- *Emotional reactions: Feelings of shock, fear, grief, irritability, resentment, guilt, shame, helplessness, hopelessness, and emotional numbness (difficulty feeling love and intimacy or in taking interest and pleasure in day-to-day activities).*
- *Cognitive reactions: Confusion, disorientation, indecisiveness, worry, shortened attention span, concentration problems, memory*

loss, unwanted memories, self-blame, easily frustrated with others, and repeated annoying thoughts.

- *Physical reactions: Tension, fatigue, edginess, difficulty sleeping, bodily aches or pain, startled easily, racing heartbeat, nausea, change in appetite, change in sex drive, high blood pressure, headaches, inability to relax, problems with sleep.*
- *Interpersonal reactions: In relationships at school, work, in friendships, in marriage, or as a parent, such as: distrust, irritability, conflict, withdrawal, isolation, feeling rejected or abandoned, being distant, judgmental, or overcontrolling.*

These normal reactions are a signal that your body, emotions, and relationships are being strained by repeated exposure to trauma. More severe stress problems may develop if these early warnings are not dealt with, such as PTSD, anxiety disorders, depression, or problems with eating, sleep, or substance use:

- *Dissociation (feeling completely unreal or like you do not know yourself; having "blank" periods of time)*
- *Intrusive reexperiencing (terrifying memories, nightmares, or flashbacks)*
- *Extreme attempts to avoid disturbing memories (such as through substance use)*
- *Extreme emotional numbing (completely unable to feel emotion, as if utterly empty)*
- *Hyperarousal (panic attacks; rage; extreme irritability; intense agitation)*
- *Severe anxiety (paralyzing worry, extreme helplessness, compulsions or obsessions)*
- *Severe depression (complete loss of hope, self-worth, motivation, or purpose in life)*

The suffering, disability, or untimely death of a child, especially a very young infant, places a special physical and emotional strain on healthcare providers. We all instinctively want to protect vulnerable little ones, but necessary medical procedures often unavoidably cause pain. We all want to see children have a full and long life, but illness and physical abnormalities can take the life of a child before the child has ever really had a chance to experience life. Providers and parents must live with the feeling of deep regret, helplessness, dread, and confusion about why this has to happen to an innocent child they care for.

However, it is important to not become so used to children's suffering and death that you begin to feel indifferent or numb. *The challenge is to find a balance of not caring too little or too much—to not lose track of your feelings while also not letting your feelings dominate your life and impair your ability to work effectively and derive satisfaction from your life.* If you have experienced, or are experiencing, other draining stressors, worries, losses, or even life-threatening traumas, the suffering or death of a child for whom you are caring is particularly likely to intensify the stress and grief you are dealing with. This is only normal—everyone has a limit to how much they can cope with. It may be important to privately seek help from psychological or spiritual counselors, friends, or family members, to get support and assistance in coping with these other life concerns. It may also be helpful to reach out help your co-workers.

Here are some ways that healthcare providers reach out to get and give support for dealing with trauma and grief:

- *Develop a "buddy" system with a co-worker and informally stay in touch with your buddy every day.*
- *Encourage and support your co-workers in small ways that show that you respect, care for, and value them.*
- *Take care of yourself physically, with a regular regimen of good exercise, rest, and nutrition.*
- *Take a break when you feel your stamina, coordination, or tolerance for irritation diminishing.*
- *Talk informally to trusted colleagues about the personal impact of troubling incidents during or after each work shift.*

- *Talk about feelings as they arise, and be a good listener to your co-workers.*
- *Do not take anger too personally—it is often an expression of frustration, guilt, or worry.*
- *Give your co-workers recognition and appreciation for a job well done.*
- *Maintain as normal a routine and a pace of life as possible, but take several days to "decompress" gradually.*

Attend a debriefing with co-workers, to share your personal reactions and to get and give emotional support:

- *Understand that it is perfectly normal to want to talk about the tragedy, and equally normal not to want to talk about it, so you and everyone else can say only as much as you want or need to say.*
- *Remember that everyone has a different perspective on the incident, and yours may be helpful to someone else just as listening to others may help you to better understand what happened and how you feel about it.*
- *Expect disappointment, frustration, and conflict, and respect your own and others' rights to express these feelings—but do not get stuck in blaming: a tragedy provokes anger ("why did this have to happen?") that can lead to blaming co-workers or at parents or at "the system," and blame tends to be a source of more problems rather than of solutions.*
- *To get beyond blame, while acknowledging real problems, talk about how you and your colleagues can take steps to constructively make your work environment safer, more humane, more respectful, and more compassionate.*
- *Do not be surprised if you experience mood swings; instead of trying to vent every feeling all at once, focus on one feeling at a time so your emotions can begin to sort themselves out (and you can feel in control but not numb).*
- *Do not overwhelm yourself or others with your experiences; focus on understanding how the incident unfolded and how your thoughts and feelings developed—like re-playing a film that was going on fast-forward, slowly enough to see what really happened (which we all tend to miss because trauma seems to speed events up and we are just trying to survive).*

Taking every day one-at-a-time is essential in tragedy's wake. Each day is a new opportunity to FILL-UP:

Focus Inwardly on what is most important to you and your family today (see attached Focusing handout);

Look and Listen to learn what you and your significant others are experiencing, so you will remember what is important and let go of what is not;

Understand Personally what these experiences mean to you as a part of your life, so that you will feel able to go on with your life and even grow personally.

[Developed by Julian D. Ford, Ph.D. There is more information on the following websites to aid responders and communities affected by disaster (www.ctrp.org) and trauma (www.ptsdfreedom.org)]

Appendix 11.2

Coping Effectively with Extreme Stress: Focusing

Here's a practical way for you to deal effectively with feeling emotionally overwhelmed, confused, or shut-down.

Focusing involves three steps—**SOS**—to gain control of your emotions without hurting yourself or shutting-down.

Step 1: Slow down (Take a time out; calm your body; One thought at a time)

Start by telling yourself: "Slow down"—I can deal with this if I just do one thing a time."

Step 2: Orient yourself (Bring your mind and body back to present time/place)

Talk to yourself calmly: "I can look around and see that I am in a safe and familiar place. I can feel my body sitting in this chair and feel the floor under my feet. I can see the people I am with, and I know who they are and that I can trust them."

Step 3: Self check (How much distress? How much control? The worst ever?)

Ask yourself calmly and supportively, "Is this the worst I've ever felt? Are there still some ways in which I still feel in control and can deal with this situation effectively?"

Tell yourself, calmy and supportively, If I've gotten through other times feeling as bad or worse than this, I can get through this! I am still in control in some important ways, so I can handle this! There are people in my life who are helping me to get through this okay!"

Each of us can find a way to *slow down, get oriented,* and *check-in* with ourselves when we feel in crisis or very stressed—we just need to take the time to find, *and use,* our own ways of focusing.

Each time you use the *focusing* skill you are helping your body, your brain, and your spirit recover from trauma!

Each time you *focus* you are strengthening your personal resources and your commitment to recovery!

[Developed by Julian D. Ford, Ph.D. There is more information on the following websites to aid responders and communities affected by disaster (www.ctrp.org) *and trauma* (www.ptsdfreedom.org)*]*

12   Bioterrorism and Obstetrics
The Exposed Pregnant Patient

RENEE A. BOBROWSKI, JOHN F. GREENE, JR., AND JOEL SOROSKY

12.1   Introduction

This chapter focuses on the management of pregnant women in the setting of a bioterrorist attack. Pregnancy poses unique challenges for both maternal and fetal concerns. The mother is at increased risk for infection while the infectious agent and medications required for treatment can having a variety of effects on the fetus. This chapter will be limited to specifics of pregnancy as more detailed information is regarding the various biologic agents is contained elsewhere within this text.

12.2   Obstetrics Staff Training

Information regarding training for obstetrics staff in the area of bioterrorism is limited. The obstetrics team of care providers will function best in concert with their colleagues who are bioterrorism experts. Nevertheless, given the recent threats of bioterrorism, continuing education seminars would appear to be the optimal method of maintaining proficiency on the part of the OB team. Virtually all obstetrical units at tertiary care centers have standardized procedures and protocols for ensuring adequate staffing in the labor and delivery unit. This includes nursing, clerical, and ancillary personnel. Commonly, these protocols involve increasing the length of work shifts and calling staff in from home. The institutional "call rooms" facilities can be used to accommodate staff that need to remain in the hospital for several days.

Women go into labor and delivery regardless of a potential or on-going crisis. Access to labor and delivery must be maintained. Thus, the police and security personnel must be able to grant hospital access and triage healthy and unexposed women for routine obstetrical care. With a national cesarean section rate of greater than 30%, attention must be directed to scheduled cesarean sections and induction of labor. For elective and non-emergent planned or scheduled deliveries, a short delay of several days may be appropriate to optimally utilize the available resources for the immediate crisis.

A formal triage team should be formed that include leadership representation from anesthesiology, NICU, maternal fetal medicine, and general obstetrics. This triage team will prioritize care based upon the available resources and the medical need. Decisions from this triage must be successfully communicated to in hospital personnel as well as patients who may not be in the hospital but are scheduled for obstetrical intervention within the next several days. This leadership team must also reassure the community that adequate access to labor and delivery is available. A dedicated obstetrical phone triage person should be available to communicate information from the leadership team to the community. This phone triage person should also be available to handle scheduling and confirmation of information from both inside and outside of the institution. The phone triage person will also provide information regarding the obstetrical protocols that are in effect. This will also include the available to NICU beds.

12.3 Management of the Exposed Pregnant Woman

A pregnant woman is more susceptible to infection throughout pregnancy due to changes in the immune system. Thus the gravida is not only more likely to contract an infection but also to suffer a more complicated clinical course. In addition, treatment considerations should take into account the potential effects on the fetus. Diagnostic studies and treatment, however, should never be withheld on the basis of the pregnancy. If a study will assist in or change clinical management of the mother, it should be performed. Medications should be chosen to minimize the fetal risk but in some cases an ideal alternative is not available; the mother should be treated based upon her clinical situation.

The remainder of this chapter addresses various biologic agents, their maternal and fetal effects and management of the exposed gravida. Category A agents include smallpox, anthrax, plague, botulism, tularemia, and viral hemorrhagic fevers while Q fever, brucellosis, typhus and food and water safety threats are Category B agents reviewed.

12.3.1 Category A Biologic Agents
12.3.1.1 *Variola virus* (Smallpox)

Pregnant women are more susceptible to smallpox and maternal mortality is increased above that of the non-pregnant patient. Unfortunately vaccination did not appear to completely protect gravidas from smallpox mortality. The frequency of hemorrhagic smallpox is seven-fold higher during pregnancy with a case-fatality rate of 100% reported.

Varioloa virus is known to cross the placenta and cause fetal infection. First trimester fetal infection with variola major is associated with an increased rate of fetal loss and prematurity although the virulence of the strain may play some role. Transmission appears to be unpredictable. The reported incidence of congenital variola during epidemics varies widely from 9% to 60%. It is characterized by diffuse necrotic lesions of the placenta and giant dermal pox. However, the virus is not teratogenic.

Management of the pregnant woman infected with smallpox is primarily supportive as there are no approved therapies. Thus preventative and post-exposure vaccination and quarantine have been critical in the management of smallpox epidemics in the general population. The smallpox vaccine is a live-virus preparation that is contraindicated during pregnancy in non-emergent circumstances. Pregnant women should be cautioned against close contact with a recently vaccinated individual. If, however, a woman is at risk for smallpox due to direct exposure or close contact with a victim, the risks of smallpox far outweigh the risks of vaccination. If a woman requires vaccination while breastfeeding, she should not breastfeed until the scab has separated from the vaccination site.

The prophylactic administration of vaccinia immune globulin (VIG) to a woman who becomes pregnant shortly after vaccination or a pregnant women in attempt to reduce the maternal viral load and hence the risk for fetal infection has advantages and disadvantages. Documented cases of fetal vaccinia are extremely rare given the numbers of pregnant women who have been vaccinated during past smallpox outbreaks, clinical evidence for efficacy is insufficient to recommend routine administration and VIG is not without its risks.

The intravenous form (VIG-IV) is preferred for use in pregnancy although the FDA has approved it only for treatment of vaccine related side effects. If prophylactic VIG-IV is considered for a pregnant woman, timing of administration is critical as immunoglobulin use more than 10 days after vaccination may be less effective in preventing fetal infection. The intramuscular preparation (VIG-IM) should not be used in pregnancy since the preservative contains potentially teratogenic levels of mercury.

Suggestions for managing vaccinia exposed pregnancies are as follows. Women attempting pregnancy should not be vaccinated within 4 weeks of planning to conceive. If the vaccine is inadvertently administered during early pregnancy, termination is not recommended; the vaccine is not teratogenic. Women who have been inadvertently vaccinated should be counseled regarding the small risk and offered the option of VIG-IV administration providing it is within 10 days of the vaccine. If more than 10 days has passed since vaccination, VIG should not be offered. If a pregnant woman experiences a vaccine complication for which VIG is recommended, the intravenous preparation should be administered without hesitation. The Centers for Disease Control and Department of Defense maintain a registry for women in whom pregnancy is identified after vaccination.

12.3.1.2 Bacillus anthracis (Anthrax)

Information regarding anthrax during pregnancy is not available. The CDC, Infectious Disease Society of American and American College of Obstetricians and Gynecologists have formulated the following recommendations.

Pre-exposure vaccination is recommended for a small subset of individuals. The vaccine alone is not recommended for post-exposure use but can be used in combination with antibiotics. Although the vaccine contains no live or killed bacteria, vaccination of pregnant women is not recommended until further data are available. Antimicrobials are not indicated for asymptomatic individuals with low risk exposure. Prophylaxis is recommended for gravidas with anthrax exposure as determined by the local Department of Health. Prophylaxis consists of ciprofloxacin 500 mg orally every 12 hours for 60 days. If the bacteria are proven sensitive to penicillin, ciprofloxacin may be changed to amoxicillin 500 mg orally three times daily to complete a 60 day course. Cutaneous anthrax is treated with ciprofloxacin 500 mg p.o. twice daily for 60 days. In the event of inhalational, gastrointestinal or oropharyngeal anthrax, initial therapy is via the intravenous route with ciprofloxacin 400 mg q12 hours or doxycycline 100 mg q12 hours plus one or two additional antimicrobials (rifampin, vancomycin, penicillin, ampicillin, imipenem, clindamycin, and clarithromycin). The above regimens are also appropriate for women who are breastfeeding.

12.3.1.3 Yersinia pestis (Plague)

Similar to other potential bioterror agents, information regarding plague during pregnancy is limited. The most important factor in the management of plague is prompt institution of antibiotic therapy and pregnancy is no exception. The Working Group on Civilian Biodefense has developed guidelines for management of plague including antibiotic administration to all patients, either parenteral or oral depending upon the magnitude of the infection, supportive care and treatment of septic complications. The preferred antibiotic choices in adults include streptomycin or gentamycin although streptomycin is contraindicated during pregnancy. Therefore gentamycin 5 mg/kg intramuscular or intravenous once daily (or 2 mg/kg load followed by 1.7 mg/kg IM or IV 3 times daily) for 10 days is first-line therapy for pregnant women. Treatment alternatives include doxycycline (100 mg IV twice daily or 200 mg IV once daily), ciprofloxacin (400 mg IV twice daily) or chloramphenicol (25 mg/kg IV 4 times daily) 10 days. Prophylaxis for the pregnant woman is doxycycline 100 mg orally twice daily for 7 days. Since doxycycline can be hepatotoxic in pregnancy, liver function tests should be considered during therapy. Currently a plague vaccine is not available and while there has been interest in its development, no information regarding its use in pregnancy is available.

12.3.1.4 Clostridium botulinum (Botulism)

The botulinum toxin is a large molecule that theoretically should not cross the placenta, but data are lacking. Anti-toxin and supportive care of the mother are the mainstays of treatment just as with the non-pregnant patient. The FDA labels the anti-toxin as Pregnancy Category C.

12.3.1.5 Francisella tularensis (Tularemia)

Tularemia in pregnancy was last described in the literature 70 years ago. Post-exposure prophylaxis for pregnant women includes doxycycline 100 mg orally twice daily or ciprofloxacin 500 mg orally twice daily for 14 days. Treatment of tularemia in pregnancy consists of gentamycin 5 mg/kg IM or IV once daily for 10 days.

12.3.1.6 Viral hemorrhagic fever

Viral Hemorrhagic Fever (VHF) may be caused by any one of the four agents: Ebola, Marburg,

Lassa, and Congo-Crimean. Ebola infection is generally more serious during pregnancy with higher hemorrhagic and neurologic complications. It is also associated with a higher mortality (95% vs. 77% in non-pregnant victims). Mortality does not, however, differ between trimesters. The risk for spontaneous abortion appears to be higher in infected women. Treatment of Ebola in pregnancy is supportive care and correction of the hematologic abnormalities. Lassa Fever also has an increased mortality during pregnancy and this risk is highest during the third trimester. Ribavirin may decrease the fatality rate although it is a Category X medication. It has been suggested that delivery may improve maternal outcome in the setting of Lassa Fever.

If an obstetric or surgical procedure is indicated in a patient infected with VHF, the state health department and CDC should be consulted with regard to appropriate precautions during the performance of these procedures.

12.3.2 Category B Biologic Agents

12.3.2.1 Q fever

Q fever is caused by *Coxiella burnetii*. Chronic infection develops only in patients with a compromised immune system; pregnant women are among those at particular risk for chronic infection. Bacteria colonize and replicate in the placenta, uterus, and mammary glands when a woman is infected during pregnancy. The data suggest women with primary infection during pregnancy are at increased risk for abortion, premature delivery and in utero fetal demise, depending upon the timing of infection. The pathogenesis of fetal disease may be related to placental vasculitis and/or direct fetal infection. *Coxiella* has been detected in both the placenta and fetal viscera of infected pregnancies. Infection in animals may be spread at the time of delivery via aerosol from an infected placenta and infection of an obstetrician following an infected woman has been reported.

Concurrent use of doxycycline and chloroquine is the only effective in vitro bacteriocidal regimen although concerns have been expressed with regard to long term use of doxycycline during pregnancy. Treatment with trimethoprim–sulfamethoxazole (TMP–SMX; 160 mg trimethoprim and 800 mg sulfamethoxazole p.o. bid) has been shown to be effective in reducing the complications associated with Q fever during pregnancy. The development of chronic infection is not, however, prevented by TMP–SMX. A one year course of doxycycline and chloroquine following delivery is therefore recommended. *Coxiella* has been isolated from human breast milk and thus breastfeeding is contraindicated for woman with Q fever. Women with acute infection prior to pregnancy do not appear to be at increased risk for adverse obstetric outcomes.

12.3.2.2 Brucellosis

Brucellosis infection in pregnancy poses a substantial risk for spontaneous abortion with the highest risk in the first and second trimesters. Congenital brucellosis has been reported although transplacental transmission has not been well-documented. Rifampin 900 mg p.o. qd for 6 weeks has been recommended as the primary treatment for pregnant women with brucellosis. Alternatively, TMP–SMX or TMP–SMX plus rifampin have been used with evidence of a decreased rate of spontaneous abortion.

	Prophylaxis	Treatment	Vaccination	Special Considerations
Smallpox		Supportive	Contraindicated in non-emergent circumstances. Administer if direct exposure	Avoid contact with recently vaccinated individual. If vaccinated, do not breastfeed until scab falls off
Anthrax	Ciprofloxacin 500 mg p.o. q12 hours for 60 days. If sensitive: Amoxicillin 500 mg p.o. tid to complete 60 day course	Ciprofloxacin 400 mg IV q12 or doxycycline 100 mg IV q12. Plus one or two additional atimicrobials: See text	Not recommended during pregnancy	
Plague	Doxycycline 100 mg po bid for 7 days	Gentamycin 5 mg/kg IV or IM once daily for 10 days. Alternatives detailed in text		Streptomycin contraindicated in pregnancy. Monitor LFTs in pregnant women on doxycycline
Botulism		Anti-toxin and supportive care		
Tularemia	Doxycycline 100 mg po bid or ciprofloxacin 500 mg po bid for 14 days	Gentamycin 5 mg/kg IM or IV once daily for 10 days		
Viral Hemorrhagic Fever		Supportive care. Correction of hematologic abnormalities		Ribavirin: Category X. Consult health department for precautions if obstetric procedure planned
Q Fever		TMP–SMX during pregnancy; doxycycline plus chloroquine for 1 year following delivery		
Brucellosis		Rifampin 900 mg p.o. qd for 6 weeks; TMP–SMX or TMP–SMX plus Rifampin		

13 Operating Room Preparation for Mass Casualties

JOSEPH H. McISAAC, III

13.1 Introduction

Little, if anything, has been published on planning and training for mass casualties at the level of the operating room (OR). There is also a paucity of literature about the surgical and anesthetic treatment of patients exposed to weapons of mass destruction (WMDs). References that do exist are derived largely from military experience [1–5].

The preparation of the OR involves exactly the same thought process as that required to prepare the hospital as a whole. The functioning is broken down to fundamental tasks and workflow. Vulnerabilities under various stress scenarios are examined and mitigation strategies are devised. Once a plan is written, it is tested, practiced, and revised. Each iteration should escalate the difficulty in order to realistically simulate an event. Planning for a worst-case scenario is preferable to hoping for the best. Introduction of unexpected problems into training encourages flexibility and promotes creative problem solving for both the staff and the leadership. Analysis should be performed on several dimensions: Scale, critical systems, workflow, and inter-departmental communications/cooperation.

13.2 Individual Preparation

The first and most fundamental level of training occurs at the individual level. There exists a very large body of knowledge about nuclear, chemical, and biological threats which must be distilled to a level that is both useful and accessible to the end user (Guzzi, 2002). A physician needs to understand the pathogenesis and treatment of individual diseases, toxins, and syndromes. The nurse needs similar but less detailed knowledge. Technicians and ancillary staff need to understand the basics of self-protection and decontamination, especially as applied to their role on the unit. For example, the patient transport aid will need to know how to avoid personal contamination, how to protect the patient, how to clean the equipment, properly dispose of contaminated linen, and appropriate routes for transporting infectious and non-infectious patients between units. Good training, and confidence in that training through practice, is the best way to alleviate the fear of the unknown. The least medically sophisticated staff are the most vulnerable. Without them, a modern unit cannot function as they provide the support logistics necessary for physicians and nurses to deliver healthcare. Unfortunately, the support staff often are the last to receive training, if they receive any at all. Their inclusion in training should be considered a priority for unit leaders.

For the professional staff, a combination of self-education, consisting of selected readings and on-line courses, can be supplemented with periodic lectures and attendance at conferences. Ready access to technical documentation is highly recommended. Besides keeping departmental copies of key texts and treatment summaries, personal digital assistant (PDA) versions are highly advised. They can be downloaded from a number of sources as well as purchased from well known medical software retailers [6,7].

13.3 Departmental Plan

The departmental plan serves as a top-down, strategic approach to organization. It should be a simple, living, practical document developed jointly by the surgical service leadership. A unified plan, encompassing nursing, anesthesiology, and surgery is the best way to ensure synchronization of all three specialties. The plan should address key issues: who, what, where, when, and how. In other words: the mission, chain of command, communications, and logistics (Figure 13.1).

Hospital operative services normally are an amalgamation of several different groups who interact to receive, treat, and transfer patients along the "surgical axis" of the hospital. Patients usually originate from the Emergency Department and are transported to a holding area before being operated on in the surgical suite. They are then transported to a post anesthesia care unit (PACU) or to an intensive care unit (ICU), ultimately returning to a surgical ward. At least four diverse groups of personnel are involved in patient care: surgical nurses and technologists, ancillary staff (clerks, secretaries, and transport aids), surgeons, and anesthesia providers (anesthesiologists, anesthesia assistants (AAs) and certified registered nurse anesthetists (CRNAs)). During normal operations, each of these groups functions semi-independently to accomplish patient care. During a mass-casualty event, they need to be much more closely coordinated if they are to be successful. Although the HEICS model does not continue below the level of OR chief, it is logical that the same principles should apply. A single individual should have total authority over the functioning of the OR. This author's bias is that the individual should be a physician, probably a senior anesthesiologist, but other individuals could also assume that role. Directly under this OR chief would be representatives of nursing, surgery, and anesthesiology; each with authority to direct personnel of their respective specialty. Additional positions covering logistics and PACU should also be designated (Figure 13.2). In larger surgical suites, specialty departments (e.g.: orthopedics, neurosurgery, cardiothoracic) already exist. Often, they have entire wings dedicated to a single surgical specialty. It makes sense to maintain this same organization to the extent it facilitates patient care.

The key elements to any plan for mass-casualty care involve transition to a contingency mode, assessment of personnel and capacity, and maintaining logistical support. Sustainment and transition back to routine operations must also be considered. Upon alert that a mass-casualty incident is occurring, several actions must occur in rapid succession (Figure 13.3). First, the Mass-Casualty Plan should be reviewed by all leadership. There should be a brief meeting between nursing, anesthesiology, and surgery leaders to establish that all services are in synchrony. Contact should be made with the hospital EOC to determine the exact nature of the situation, types and numbers of casualties expected, and of course, the nature of suspected agents. A message should be broadcast to all active operating rooms, passing along what is known of the situation. Surgeons should be informed that they should finish in the most expeditious manner consistent with patient safety and stand ready to receive acute surgical trauma.

> The operating room is a major bottleneck in [mass casualty scenarios]. Therefore, its immediate use should be reserved for a few "absolute" indications such as compromised airway or the control of active bleeding endangering life or limb. Other surgeries are delayed to the second phase. Once in surgery, the fundamental approach is "damage control". Holcomb et al. . . . concluded their review on "damage control philosophy" as follows: "This situation demand that surgeons, accustomed to expending enormous resources and time on single patients,

---

Chain of Command
Priority Tasks
Patient Flow
Isolation
Logistics
Communications

Figure 13.1 Elements of operating room planning.

OR Preparation for Mass Casualties 185

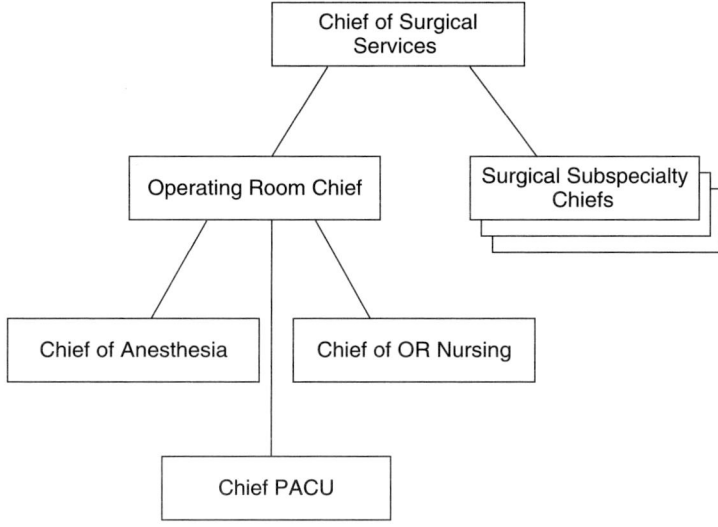

Figure 13.2 Operating room hierarchy.

Upon notification by HEOC:

- Briefly coordinate with Chief of OR Nursing to assess status (number of ORs available: immediately, in 30 minutes, and in 60 minutes)
- Notify all surgical teams of disaster (including pertinent information such as WMDs), instruct them to finish in the most expeditious manner, and prepare to receive trauma patients
- Activate disaster call-in tree to expand personnel
- Notify PACU and ICU to reduce patient load and/or expand capacity
- Instruct supply personnel to restock/overstock all locations
- Coordinate with Blood Bank, Pharmacy, and CMS to expect increased demands
- Coordinate with Surgical Chief to assess availability of surgeons
- Send liaison to ED to assess situation and report back (number and types of cases)
- Consider assembling contingency teams for "off-floor" response (airway emergency management, ED and ICU assistance)
- If airborne infectious disease is suspected, coordinate with Security and Facilities Management to institute isolation procedures

Figure 13.3 Operating room chief priority tasks for mass-casualty.

---

occasionally reset their priorities and rapidly provide only the minimal acceptable care. Providing care in this manner and moving those patients quickly through treatment will maximize care to as many patients as possible". [8,9]

Further elective surgery should be cancelled and patients sent back to their units or discharged, as appropriate. It is expected that surgical patients will not arrive for a period of time (transport, decontamination, triage) allowing some preparation to ensue. As ORs empty, they should be restocked with equipment and supplies. The military uses a form of "push" logistics, whereby supplies are sent automatically to the zone of anticipated fighting without needing to be specifically requested. A similar approach is warranted here. Fluids, drugs, sterile supplies and instruments should automatically be overstocked. Coordination should occur with Pharmacy, Blood Bank, and Central Sterile Supply to, likewise, push matériel towards "the front."

While the PACU and ORs are cleared of patients, augmentation of staff should occur. Telephone callback lists (disaster lists) should be activated. Telephone "trees" are much more effective when large numbers of personnel must be called. At three minutes per call, a 60-person list takes

180 minutes to complete! A branching structure can be completed much faster. Thought needs to be given to distribution of personnel between multiple institutions. Many physicians, especially, have privileges at several hospitals. In a widespread disaster, there must be an equitable distribution of providers. Core and supplementary lists are one possible solution.

In contrast to nursing and anesthesia staff, surgeons are usually much more dispersed between their offices, clinics, wards, and various ORs and ambulatory surgery centers. The Surgical Chief will need to have a means of tracking down these physicians. Establishment of protocols that include surgical office staff who usually know where their surgeons are working is a prudent step to rapidly increasing operative capacity. Likewise, maintaining address lists that can be passed to law enforcement or military personnel will allow communication with surgeons event when the telephone system is down.

Critical to good decision-making is accurate and timely information. Sending a liaison to the Emergency Department to act as the "eyes and ears" of the Chief of the OR is highly recommended and has proven effective during mass-casualty simulation drills at Hartford Hospital. This individual should be an experienced anesthesiologist. A critical care trained anesthesiologist would be ideal. This physician's role is to provide timely information on the situation, numbers of patients, and types of surgical cases pending. Although he or she can render assistance when needed, care should be taken not to get tied-up, unable to perform the primary role. This individual can also provide valuable feedback to the Chief of the ED on OR availability, as well. A dedicated means of communications between the OR liaison and the Chief of the OR must be available for this system to work.

Coordination with intensive care units should occur early to assess bed availability and begin preparations for ICU expansion. Surgeons and anesthesiologists trained in critical care are idea to manage ICU overflow areas, but all anesthesiologists and many surgeons, while not subspecialty trained, possess the ability to provide and supervise critical care patients in an emergency. CRNAs, most of whom are former critical care nurses, are also qualified to serve in this role, if necessary.

Consideration should be given to the establishment of rapid response teams. Most hospitals have a "code team" which responds to respiratory and cardiac arrests as needed. These teams usually consist of an anesthesia provider, a medical physician (MD or PA), a surgeon (MD or PA), a respiratory therapist, and several nurses. During mass casualties, it can be expected that there will be a significantly higher need for these services than normal. Extra contingency teams, either prepositioned in the triage area and ICUs, or kept in reserve in the OR, will ease the stress to find needed personnel quickly.

Perhaps the most problematic aspect of surgical mass casualty management is the distribution and management of surgical subspecialists during a crisis. In normal times, they function as autonomous providers, either individually or as parts of small groups. They usually manage their own patients and cross-cover for their specialist colleagues. A means of distribution of appropriate specialists between functional areas of the hospital (OR, Triage team, hospital wards) must be developed and tested beforehand by the department of surgery. Furthermore, a means of assigning cases must also be established. All surgeons possess common skills which potentially allow them to care for injured patients outside of their usual surgical specialty. For example, a gynecological surgeon could treat abdominal trauma; a plastic surgeon could stabilize an open fracture with a vascular injury in the absence of anyone with more specific skills. Large numbers of less urgent injuries can also be anticipated. Surgical teaching clinics, private medical offices, and nearby ambulatory surgery centers can also be recruited to handle the patient surge. Obviously, prior planning is essential to success of this model.

It should not be forgotten that even during mass-casualty events, routine surgical emergencies continue to occur and will need to be addressed (acute appendicitis, wound dehiscence and infection, emergency caesarian section, etc.). As a crisis prolongs, there will be an increasing backlog of emergency and urgent cases. A triage system is necessary to accommodate this patient stream while continuing to provide care for trauma victims. Many busy operating rooms already run at or near-capacity during normal operations. They manage contingency patients by keeping one or more operating rooms reserved for unscheduled cases. Often, these rooms run continuously throughout the day. After the first 8–12 hours of patient surge, staff fatigue will begin to take its toll. A transition to shift work will need to occur. Rotating 8–12 hour shifts with periodic breaks should be planned. Planning should include a means to accommodate large numbers of personnel to sleep in-house. Offices and lounges can be temporarily converted.

13.4 Expansion of Capacity

In most scenarios, all surgical suites can be opened up in a matter of a few hours. Outpatient ORs can be utilized rapidly since most scheduled procedures in these facilities tend to be short. Many hospitals have excess surgical space which is used for storage or other purposes. These rooms normally continue to have piped medical gasses and suction. They can be utilized as minor procedure rooms even if not equipped with anesthesia machines. Alternatively, ICU ventilators or even bag-valve-mask (BVM) devices with transport monitors can be substituted and intravenously-only anesthesia can be administered. Even office space can be transformed in this manner if needed. Endoscopy suites and regional anesthesia procedure rooms, likewise, may be pressed into service as surgical treatment rooms. Obstetrical caesarean section rooms, also can be used for non-obstetrical procedures, however, emergency c-sections will continue to occur and it is unwise to commit 100% of capacity.

The greatest problem occurs as traditional postoperative areas (PACU and ICU) rapidly fill up with the initial wave of post-operative patients. Increased throughput can be achieved by temporarily relaxing standards for discharge during the contingency and by expansion to adjacent spaces normally used for other purposes (i.e., ambulatory waiting areas). Nurse/patient ratios, similarly, can be temporarily altered to provide coverage to an expanded case-load. Under extreme circumstances, awake, stable, spontaneously ventilating patients should be transported directly to patient floors if necessary.

13.5 Patient Flow and Infectious Considerations

During mass-casualty contingencies involving WMDs, consideration should be given to patient flow and isolation; especially if virulent, airborne transmissible infectious agents may be present (pneumonic plague, smallpox, and SARS) (Figure 13.4). Early in an event, patients may make it to the OR before being identified as being contaminated or infectious. Under stressful, chaotic conditions, some patients may not receive full decontamination and continue to pose a risk to surgical personnel. A method for secondary decontamination should be available and practiced. Double gloves, waterproof surgical gowns and HEPA filtered respirators (PAPRs) will provide adequate protection, assuming all staff have been trained in advance. Hypochlorite continues to provide the best and most accessible universal decontamination.

Operating rooms are normally ventilated with filtered, positive pressure systems to keep out infectious contamination. When airborne transmissible infectious agents are present a reverse situation occurs. Negative pressure is desired to prevent dispersion of airborne agents to adjacent areas. Facilities management should be contacted to reverse the direction of airflow. This can best be achieved with prior planning and should be part of the facilities management contingency plan. It may, unfortunately, result in contaminated ductwork and HVAC equipment which will require decontamination before restoration to normal use. Portable, HEPA filtered forced air systems have been used to convert large rooms (gymnasiums) into negative pressure wards and should be considered a viable option, especially for expansion areas [10]. An alternative to air flow reversal is to

Patient selection

- Elective procedures will not be performed on patients with smallpox.
- Emergent procedures that entail life, limb, or eyesight will be the only surgeries performed on patients with smallpox.

Patient transport

- Patients will be transported to the OR via the most direct route in the hospital.
- The route should bypass the preoperative holding area.
- Patients will wear a surgical mask and he covered with a linen sheet during transport because this is emergency surgery, and the patient will not have been properly fit tested for an N95 particulate respirator mask.

Staff procedures

- The charge nurse will notify perioperative staff members and the surgical services chief of anesthesia about the patient with smallpox.
- The central material supplies (CMS) department will be notified by the charge nurse.
- Facilities managers will be contacted by the charge nurse.
- The facilities department will ensure the proper number of air exchanges per hour (i.e., a minimum of 15 air exchanges per hour, at least three of which must be fresh air) (1).
- Anesthesia personnel will coordinate recovery of the patient in the OR or intensive care unit with negative-pressure isolation.
- All staff members involved in the patient's care and transportation or cleaning of the OR involved will be vaccinated and wear an N95 mask, gloves, gown, and shoe covers.
- All staff members and patients who come in contact with smallpox should be vaccinated within seven days if they are not already vaccinated (2).
- Non-essential personnel will not be allowed in the OR at any time.
- In addition to the circulating nurse in the OR, an outside circulating nurse will be assigned strictly for the procedure.
- The outside circulating nurse will assist in bringing equipment and needed supplies to the room.
- If the facility does not have computers in the OR for documentation, the outside circulating nurse will be responsible for documentation. A paper chart is not to enter the OR because it may become a vector if contaminated. The inside circulating nurse will document all information on a dry erase board and either display the board to the outside circulating nurse through a core window or relay the information via telephone.
- The outside circulating nurse will not enter the OR and will bring supplies and equipment only to a designated door.
- The outside circulating nurse also will wear appropriate personal protective equipment (PPE) and an N95 respirator mask because the positive pressure of the OR could potentially blow organisms out to him or her.
- After perioperative staff members enter the OR, they will not be allowed to leave until the procedure is concluded.
- At the conclusion of the procedure, all PPE will be placed in a biohazard bag as staff members exit the room.

OR setup

- Each OR door will be labeled with airborne and contact precaution signs.
- Nonessential equipment will he removed from the rooms.
- To prevent contaminating supplies in cabinets and drawers that cannot be removed from the OR, personnel should not open cabinets or drawers after the patient has entered the room. Cover and seal all cabinets and drawers with plastic and tape.
- Personal protective equipment will he placed outside the entrance to the room.
- The outside circulating nurse will have a designated door for transport of supplies and equipment. This door will not be taped, so the outside circulating nurse will have access. A high-efficiency particulate arresting (HEPA) tilter machine will be placed in front of designated door access.
- All other doors will be taped shut.
- Place tape around the frame of the door and inside of the OR to prevent or decrease air flowing to the OR hallway.
- Tape a "do not enter" sign on the outside of the patient transport door.
- A HEPA filter machine will be placed in the OR in front of the nontaped door.
- These machines may expedite air filtration and are an added precaution to prevent outflow of organisms (3).
- At a minimum, all personnel will wear an N95 respirator mask, impermeable disposable gown, gloves, and shoe covers.
- If PPE gets wet or soiled during the procedure, personnel should change to clean, dry PPE.

Figure 13.4 Guidelines for Handling Patients With High Risk Airborne Diseases (Smallpox) in the OR [2].

> **Specimens**
>
> - Label specimens in accordance with hospital policy.
> - Notify the pathology department about any smallpox specimen before it is transported.
> - The specimen cannot be labeled "smallpox" because of patient confidentially.
> - Deliver the specimen to the pathology department immediately.
> - Document the specimen appropriately according to OR protocol.
>
> **Waste material**
>
> - All waste material, including tape from doors; all packaging, regardless of contamination; and all unopened disposable supplies will be placed in a red biohazard bag.
> - No clear bags will be used for waste in a smallpox-related procedure.
>
> **Linen**
>
> - Current linen standards are sufficient for decontamination of smallpox-contaminated linen (4).
> - Linens will be bagged and labeled "smallpox." This labeling is acceptable because linen cannot be traced to a specific patient.
> - The linen department will be notified before smallpox-soiled linen is sent to the laundry.
> - Linen should be handled with minimal agitation to prevent aerosolization (4).
> - The linen cart will be covered with a clear plastic bag for transport.
> - Linen bags will be transported immediately to the laundry service.
> - Linen should not be separated or sorted before laundering (4).
> - Use water soluble laundry bags to avoid separating.
>
> **Instruments**
>
> - Current instrument sterilization is sufficient for decontaminating and sterilizing instruments (4).
> - The CMS department will provide the OR with a red soak pan half-filled with approved hospital cleaning solution to soak contaminated reusable instruments.
> - Instruments should be kept moist until they are cleaned and decontaminated in accordance with hospital guidelines.
> - The instrument container should be labeled "smallpox" before it is transported from the OR to the CMS department. This labeling is acceptable because the container cannot be traced to the patient.
> - The CMS department should be notified before instruments are transported to the decontamination area.
>
> **Completion of case**
>
> - The HEPA filter machine will run for one hour after the procedure is completed or until a minimum of 15 air exchanges have taken place (3).
> - The OR then should be terminally cleaned according to facility standards.
> - After terminal cleaning, contact the facilities management department to make any adjustments or filter changes in the ventilation system.

Figure 13.4 Continued.

temporarily shut off the air-handling system in the affected area. Airflow modification is easiest to accomplish in a single wing or building and is specific to the particular HVAC configuration.

Anesthesia machines and ventilators will need to be decontaminated before use on non-contaminated patients. Infected fluids from irrigation, suction canisters, and sponges will need to be discarded with a higher degree of care than is the usual practice. Hospital vacuum lines are to be considered contaminated as will the pumps that they lead to. During transport to and from isolation, infectious patients need masks; outflow from BVM devices must be HEPA filtered. All personnel attending these patients should be in Level C protective equipment.

Linens and stretchers require high-level decontamination before reuse on non-contaminated patients.

13.6 Training Drills

The most difficult aspect of training is finding the time to practice the departmental plan in simulation drills. Many ORs run close to capacity during the day. Administrators are hesitant to cancel blocks of well paying surgery to accommodate un-reimbursed training. Paying staff overtime for weekend training is also financially unappealing. Even harder than funding training is getting busy surgeons to participate in large numbers. However, this is imperative if meaningful results are to be achieved. Hospital leadership must be committed from the very top if mass-casualty training is to be effective.

Periodic drills should be conducted on a small scale at the departmental level as part of routine "in-service" training. Setting aside one OR for simulation can allow large numbers to rotate through during the day. Multi-departmental scale exercises should occur at the bi-annual JCAHO mandated hospital disaster drill. This is the ideal time to test communications and coordination between hospital departments. Most critical is the identification and resolution of issues impeding the smooth flow of patients along the surgical axis: from the ED to the OR and on to the ICU, PACU, and surgical ward.

As with any infrequently performed skill, knowledge rapidly decreases with time. One innovative way to keep mass-casualty plans and WMD treatment protocols fresh is to post a laminated summary on the inside of every restroom stall. This virtually guarantees that every staff member will have to look at the plan at least once a day. Job Action Sheets, describing necessary tasks can be stored with the disaster plan and distributed when the initial alert is called. Each specialty in the surgical services should have a designated training officer assigned to ensure that periodic training is effective.

13.7 Communications

Small operative suites function well with face-to-face verbal communications. Larger facilities rely on telephones. Interdepartmental communications are usually by telephone or intranet (email). Prudent planning requires alternative communications in anticipation of disruption of these services. Cellphones and Internet/Intranet communications represent the two most vulnerable systems today. They can be expected to fail early in any large-scale disaster. Most hospitals maintain numbers of two-way radios for use during a communications crisis. These radios may be configured as discrete point-to-point lines or as parts of a network. In any case, proper radio and net procedure must be taught and practiced during every exercise if radios are to be effective in an actual crisis. Most professional communicators require all messages to be written first before being passed to a central point for transmission. In many locations, Amateur Radio Emergency Services (ARES) volunteers are available to assist hospitals with both internal and external communications during an emergency. Ultimately, a runner with a written message is the final fall-back option.

13.8 Security/Crowd Control

Most hospital operating suites are considered restricted areas and already have means to control access. During a crisis, there is a greater potential for unauthorized access to occur. Coordination with the Hospital Security Department should occur to maintain an appropriate balance between physical security and access for authorized individuals. At lease on security officer should be stationed in the OR. This officer can also serve as an alternate communicator if necessary.

13.9 Conclusion

A mass-casualty situation is simply an intensified version of what many ORs experience on a daily basis. Appropriate planning and frequent training will allow the staff to adapt and successfully treat the casualty surge. Fully decontaminated radiation and chemical exposed trauma patients can be treated in the usual manner. Partially decontaminated patients can be safely managed with proper precautions. Casualties exposed to airborne infectious agents may require extraordinary measures during transport and surgery to prevent dissemination of infectious agents throughout the facility.

References

1. A. Beasley, S. Kenenally, et al. Treating patients with smallpox in the operating room, *AORN Journal*, Oct., 2004.
2. D. J. Baker and J. M. Rustick. Anesthesia for Casualties of Chemical Warfare Agents, Textbook of Military Medicine, Part IV, Anesthesia and Perioperative Care of the Combat Casualty, Office of the Surgeon General, 1995.

3. www.facs.org/civiliandisasters/trauma.html, Unconventional Civilian Disasters: What the Surgeon Should Know, American College of Surgeons.
4. www.brooksidepress.org/Products/emergency_war_surgery_entrance.htm, Emergency War Surgery, Third Edition, The Borden Institute and Army Medical Department, Department of the Army, United States of America, 2004.
5. www.itaccs.com/traumacare/archive/04_04_Winter_2004/preparedness_for_bioterror.pdf, TraumaCare International, *Trauma Care*, 14(1), 2004.
6. www.nbc-med.org, Medical NBC, Office of the Surgeon General, Army Medical Department Center and School, US Army.
7. www.bt.cdc.gov, Center for Disease Control Bioterrorism Page.
8. B. -J. Gada, M. Michaelson, et al. *Current Opinion in Anaesthesiology*, 16(2): 193–199, 2003.
   L. M. Guzzi, The Anesthesiologist's Role in Nuclear, Biological and Chemical Warfare: A Response, *ASA Newsletter*, 66(3), 2002.
9. J. B. Holcomb, T. S. Helling, and A. Hirshberg. Military, civilian, and rural application of the damage control philosophy. *Mil Med* 166: 490–493, 2001.
10. R. A. Rosenbaum, et al. Use of a Portable Forced Air System to Convert Existing Hospital Space Into a Mass Casualty Isolation Area, *Annals of Emergency Medicine*, 44:6, December 2004.

14 Bioterrorism and Implications for Nurses and Nursing

JACQUELYN McQUAY

The world is a changed place since the events of September 11, 2001. Nurses, especially those who do triage in emergency departments are on the forefront of community disease surveillance. They must be aware of signs and symptoms that are non-specific and flu-like in nature, but may actually be indicative of exposure to biological or chemical agents used as weapons of mass destruction (WMD). Diagnosis and treatment may be delayed if the triage nurse does not have the knowledge to recognize features of a biological or chemical attack and initiate a response. The threat of WMD is a reality and nurses must have the knowledge, skills, and resources that are integrated into a community-wide plan and that offer victims the best hope for survival [1].

Historically, biological and chemical agents have been used throughout the years as WMD. They are relatively inexpensive and accessible and their use is likely to continue into the future. Acts of terrorism are intended to make a public statement. The mere thought of an exposure to a bioterrorist weapon provokes fear in many people. The psychological impact may far outweigh any physical effects and even a hoax can achieve the desired reaction.

The triage process begins with an assessment of a patient's airway, breathing, circulation and disability (ABCDs) along with a brief history. An acuity level is determined based on presenting signs and symptoms. There is a high likelihood that the discovery of a bioterrorist incident may occur in an emergency department so the triage nurse must be aware that exposure to a biological or chemical agent may mimic a naturally occurring disease process.

The use of a biological or chemical agent should be suspected when clusters of similar presentations are seen. Triage nurses should be suspicious of a potential bioterror agent exposure in any of the following syndromes [2]:

- infectious gastroenteritis
- pneumonia and sudden death of a previously healthy adult
- an unexplained widened mediastinum in a febrile patient
- specific rashes
- acute neurologic illness and fever
- generalized weakness with advancing cranial nerve impairment
- severe disease manifestations in previously healthy people
- large numbers of patients with fever, respiratory, and gastrointestinal complaints
- multiple patients from the same location with common complaints
- an endemic disease occurring during an odd time of the year
- large number of rapidly fatal cases
- large number of ill or dead animals
- large number of patients with sepsis, sepsis with coagulapathy, fever with rashes, and diploplia with progressive weakness

Biological agents are used as bioterrorist weapons because they are easy to manufacture, do not require sophisticated delivery systems and can kill or injure many people. Unlike chemical agents where symptoms are immediate, biological agents have a delay between exposure and clinical manifestations. The Centers for Disease Control (CDC) [3] has classified biological agents into three categories based on ease of transmission, severity of morbidity and mortality, and likelihood of use.

Category A agents are easily transmitted, may be transmitted person-to-person, have the potential for mass casualties and require a well-defined public health structure to manage it. Category B agents are generally transmitted through food and water sources, and have moderate morbidity and low mortality, and require assistance for management from the public health structure. Category C agents would have high morbidity and mortality but have not yet been used as WMD.

The following are all Category A agents and are believed to be the most commonly used agents being developed as weapons:

- anthrax
- smallpox
- tularemia
- plague
- botulism
- viral hemorrhagic fever (Ebola and Marburg)

14.1 Vulnerable Groups

Most medical planning for bioterrorism focuses primarily on the needs of the military or the population as a whole. Vulnerable groups such as children, pregnant women, the elderly, immunocompromised patients, and health care clinicians must be considered as a subset of the exposed population and special consideration must be given to them.

Children are more vulnerable to bioterrorism agents because their overall exposure and absorption is greater due to their body surface area to mass ratio. Smaller fluid reserves increase the risk of dehydration from vomiting and diarrhea. Since many biological agents cause vomiting and diarrhea, the hydration status of a child needs to be carefully monitored. Increased permeability in the skin of newborns and infants puts them at risk for higher absorption rates. Children also have increased respiratory rates with shorter tracheas, which may increase their vulnerability to inhaled agents. Finally, many high threat agents of bioterrorism are treated with antibiotics not approved for use in children.

Pregnant women may be move susceptible to infections, making them a vulnerable group to consider. Hormonal, biochemical, cellular and humoral changes suppress the maternal immune response. Stasis of secretions and increased local bacterial growth may be due to smooth muscle relaxation of the respiratory tract due to changes in progesterone levels. Numbers of circulating white blood cells are increased by neutrophil chemotaxis and natural killer cell activity are decreased. Humoral responses are also inhibited by large levels of circulating steroids. All these processes depress protective defense mechanisms of the pregnant woman, making her a susceptible host to biological or chemical agent exposure [4:p. 366].

The elderly represent the fastest growing segment of our population today. Inability to overcome disease and co-morbidities associated with physiological changes that occur put the elderly population at increased risk from a biological attack. The potential for drug reactions and adverse effects from antibiotics may also be increased. Decreased metabolism, perfusion, and other changes may alter the effects of any drug. People with renal insufficiency, e.g., may need appropriate adjustment for their medications. In addition, elderly patients may present atypically after a biological exposure and treatment regimes will need to be altered for them.

Immunocompromised patients are another vulnerable part of the population. Advances in medical therapies and the use of potent immunosuppressive or cytotoxic agents have resulted in a more compromised host than previously. Complications and death rates could be higher than expected in this group compared to the general population. In persons with HIV infection, there is a depression of cell-mediated immunity. This may place them at an increased risk for infection and post-infection complications following a terrorist attack. In addition, there is little information available on the most appropriate treatment of immunocompromised patients following a bioterrorist attack [4:p. 384].

Finally, health care clinicians are a vulnerable population at risk for exposure to a bioterrorist agent. In case of an exposure, strict isolation techniques should be employed until no longer necessary. Clinicians should be knowledgeable about disaster management guidelines and protocols and should have access to personal protective equipment. If indicated, clinicians should have prophylactic therapy to a suspected agent. Adequate food, water, exercise, sleep, and time for relaxation will enable the clinician to provide continued medical care during such an event.

14.2 Triage

An important component of preparations for illnesses and syndromes related to a bioterrorist attack includes some type of surveillance system to detect and monitor an outbreak. Triage nurses are in a unique position to collect clues to a deliberate exposure to a biological or chemical agent. Surveillance systems can detect and monitor the course of an outbreak and decrease morbidity and mortality.

There are several systems for surveillance of bioterrorism-related diseases or syndromes: those that monitor the incidence of bioterrorism-related syndromes and those that disseminate bioterrorism detection data from environmental or clinical samples to appropriate decision-makers [5:p. 912].

Effective surveillance for bioterrorist-related illness depends on prompt collection and reporting of data. Intervention is linked to rapid detection of a related exposure to an agent. Substantial delays in detection may result in increased morbidity and mortality. Bioterrorism attacks are unpredictable, so health care professionals must always be alert for the possibility of an outbreak and be prepared to address them in a coordinated manner. Triage nurses can play a vital role in early recognition and detection of exposure to bioterrorist agents.

Triage nurses who suspect an exposure to a bioterrorist agent should notify local health authorities. For example, a brisk increase in disease incidence, large number of patients presenting with similar but unexplained symptoms, diseases occurring outside a normally endemic area, those occurring at an unusual time, increased symptom severity or increased deaths should raise the level of alertness of the triage nurse. Local health authorities will notify the FBI and state health departments. The CDC and other government agencies may assist in investigating bioterrorist attacks but, generally, they fall under the jurisdiction of the FBI [3].

In the case of a large-scale bioterrorist exposure, health care professionals will need to treat as many victims as possible who have a chance of survival. Triage will be based on the greatest good for the most number of people in the shortest period. Triage is a dynamic process that changes constantly based on victim status and available resources. Presumptions of the type of bioterrorist exposure will guide triage decisions and management of patients including need for quarantine or specific isolation techniques.

Emergency medical management and triage decisions may be based on the following questions [2]:

- What are the goals and objectives of triage for the hospital?
- What are the goals and objectives of triage for the community?
- What are the causes of morbidity and mortality of the agent?
- What are the subsequent associated public health issues?
- What are the current resources?
- How long can the infrastructure support the current resources?
- What other resources can become available?
- Does triage address water, sanitation, food, shelter, and quality of life issues?
- Is there a facility to treat the "worried well"?

Triage categorization is essential during a large-scale bioterrorism exposure. This enables individual victim disposition as well as being a marker in a potential evolving epidemic. An epidemiological approach such as SEIRV uses five categories for triage categorization [2:p. 422]:

(S) Susceptible individuals (including those with incomplete or unsuccessful vaccinations)

(E) Exposed individuals (who are symptomatic and contagious)

(I) Infectious individuals (who are symptomatic and contagious)

(R) Removed individuals who are no longer sources of infection

(V) Vaccinated (who are successfully vaccinated)

Difficulty in triage comes form distinguishing those individuals actually exposed, those potentially exposed, those "psychologically" exposed, and those with multiple unexplained symptoms. Overtriage may also occur and accuracy will improve as more data are obtained.

Triage tags will be helpful in identifying victims and in determining priorities for treatment. They may also include basic medical information that follows the victim through the treatment. To be effective, triage tags must be simple, easy to understand, and should allow for a brief documentation. If a victim improves or deteriorates necessitating a new category, a new tag should be added on top with a brief description of the management decision recorded along with the date and time.

Triage management provides the "best opportunity" to survive but does not necessarily guarantee treatment or survival. Triage and resource allocation can be measured as "life saved" (L) per unit "effort" (E) or resources required [2:p. 425]. Critically ill or injured patients would have a low L/E value due to the high amount of resources needed. Victims who can be saved with a moderate amount of resources needed but would die without it them have a high L/E value. Triage categories should be disaster-specific and should help set thresholds for initiating care.

14.3 Hospital Expansion

A large-scale disaster requiring triage for a prolonged period would result in an effective medical response that would save the maximum number of lives. This might include a system that refuses medical assistance to those unlikely to recover. In 1998, under the direction of the Department of Defense (DOD) Preparedness Program (DPP), the Biological Weapons Improved Resource Program conducted a series of workshops designed to identify improved strategies to managing a large-scale biological terrorism attack [6]. From this project, a template was obtained for an interagency response that included the efficient utilization of a community's combined medical resources.

The modular emergency medical system (MEMS) is one component of the response and is designed to assess the need to rapidly enhance the community's medical capacity. In a large-scale biological weapon incident, it focuses on managing the large number of casualties, which overwhelms the existing medical capabilities and involves an outbreak of a disaster. MEMS provides systematic, coordinated and effective medical care to casualties. The response is based on the incident command system (ICS), which is a nationally recognized emergency response system. The MEMS plan also establishes a framework for which outside medical resources can assist local response efforts.

The MEMS response divides into two types of expandable patient care modules: The acute care center (ACC) and the neighborhood emergency help centers (NEHCs). These modules enable non-hospital facilities to become mass care centers. The ACC and NEHC are linked to a local hospital that oversees patient care, medical resources, and communication. The modules and hospitals can provide a vast array of care and services to victims of biological incidents as well as to the local normal patient population. The casualties and "worried well" would be triaged through the MEMS.

If hospitals reach full capacity, an ACC can be established in a nearby building to transfer and redirect patients who need non-critical, agent-specific supportive care. Transportation units would coordinate the transfer of all patients between the ACCs the NEHC and the hospitals. In addition, they would also transfer patients not exposed to the biological weapon to remote facilities to provide area hospital space.

The ACC provides inpatient medical services to those exposed to a biological weapon but do not require mechanical ventilation and/or those who are likely to die. Patients requiring higher standard of care will be admitted to a hospital until capacity is reached. In that event, patients will receive as much care as the ACC can provide. Restricting care at an ACC ensures that an efficient approach to patient care is delivered. Most patients will require similar treatment following pre-established clinical practice guidelines. This system also allows for grouping patients with similar symptoms following exposure thereby eliminating potential exposure to non-infected persons. Again, as with the triage process, healthcare practices will have to be reassessed regularly to effectively apply available resources to provide care for the greatest number of casualties. Patient care would be prioritorized to provide the best care available under existing conditions.

Responding medical personnel must be cognizant and understand that to deliver the necessary patient care for each patient is not optimal and may be hazardous. The rationale for limiting the care provided at the ACC is based on the following [6]:

- Hospitals are better equipped to treat critically ill patients and have more resources.
- Hospitals have better access to trained staff and it is more efficient to treat patients in one location.
- The ACC is designed for situations where the demand for healthcare exceeds existing resources. The ACC must be set up quickly and streamline its level of care to provide maximum good to the most people.
- Providing a designated level of care minimizes ethical decisions healthcare providers will need to make when limited resources are available.
- A designated level of treatment eliminates the healthcare professional's dependence on technology to provide mass care.
- An ACC may face logistical issues that affect the level of care that can be provided (e.g., an ACC set up in a school gymnasium could not provide oxygen. They would however offer space to provide needed agent-specific therapy and basic supportive care).

Pre-designated practice guidelines will allow healthcare clinicians of various backgrounds to provide care in a streamlined manner. The organization of the command of the ACC will de designed to compliment the existing local emergency command structure. The medical command center (MCC) will determine whether patients need to be admitted to a hospital or should be triaged to an ACC.

The ACC is physically designed into five 50-bed nursing subunits (or a 250 bed "pod"). The pod can admit patients when it is ready and fully staffed. When the current pod is at 70–80% capacity the next pod should be nearing completion and preparing to accepts patients. Upon arrival, patients are registered and evaluated for placement. The ACC is not designed to provide assessments in the registration area, but to log patients into an internal tracking system and assign a bed.

Suggested staffing requirements per 12-hour shift for a 50-bed nursing unit is a follows [6]:

- one physician
- one physician's assistant or nurse practitioner
- six RNs (or a mix of RNs and LPNs)
- four nursing assistants
- two clerical personnel
- one respiratory therapist
- one case manager
- one social worker
- two housekeepers
- two patient transporters

Creative planning may be necessary and mutual aid resources may be necessary to augment available staff. The local office of emergency medical services (OEMS) and metropolitan medical response system (MMRS) could fulfill personnel needs while awaiting outside assistance. Division of responsibility for different aspect of patient care will be based on the knowledge and skills of available staff members.

The overall effectiveness of the operations of the ACC depend on the ability of staff members to function within the organizational guidelines. Staff members should receive some sort of training that addresses the following [6]:

- mission of the ACC
- site orientation
- standard operating procedures
- responsibilities of each member of the ACC
- ICS and reporting structure
- personal protective measures including infection control, handling and disposal of infectious waste, agent-specific transmission prevention measures, etc.
- information on the agent and treatment modalities
- response to outside requests for information
- patient confidentiality
- patient records and documentation

Medical equipment and supplies should be predetermined and cached for emergency use. If prior stockpiling is not possible, emergency planners must determine mechanisms for rapid acquisition of needed supplies. Necessary pharmacological and therapeutic drugs must be readily available to the ACC as well as a mechanism for distribution to hospitals and NEHCs. Communities are expected to be self-sufficient for up to 72 hours, so law enforcement officials may be an available resource for pick-up and delivery following a biological attack.

Adequate procedures for environmental health and sanitation must be adhered to and include approved germicidial cleaning agents. Patient linen should be handled in accordance with standard universal precautions if not disposable and contaminated waste should be sorted and discarded in accordance with regulations. Universal precautions must be maintained for blood and body fluid exposure. Certain diseases or syndromes may require additional precautions to prevent further transmission.

Special attention must be paid to vulnerable populations such as children, the elderly and the immunocompromised. Healthcare providers will also have unique needs during these times. An isolated area away from the patient treatment area should be available so the staff can rest and debrief away from patients and visitors. Staff should also have access to separate toilet and shower facilities. It is also recommended that staff have the ability to address fears related to potential health risks, provisions for protection from exposure and daily incident updates.

In large-scale situations with high mortalities, an ACC may be utilized as a temporary morgue in accordance with established federal guidelines. The temporary morgue would provide initial processing of the remains until they can be transferred to an appropriate facility. Death notification would be done through official channels.

Hospice care with emphasis on symptom management and pain control may become a reality in a bioterrorist incident. Adequate supplies of pain medicine and protocols for its use must be an available component of emergency medical services provided at the ACC. Chaplains and social workers would be an essential part of an ACC and should be available around the clock to provide emotional, spiritual and supportive care.

An incident involving exposure to a biological or chemical agent would have a profound effect psychologically as well as physically on everyone involved. Clinicians as well as patients will respond to such an event and experience reactions of an acute stress disorder. Initially, the survivor will respond to the disaster and protect their own life as well as those around them. This immediate response is a stunned reaction with anxiety or confusion. This may subside into numbness, grief, despair, nightmares, or change in eating or sleeping habits. Left untreated, they may progress to post-traumatic stress disorder (PTSD). Failure to identify those at risk for acute stress disorder may result in a complicated and prolonged recovery. Being aware of potential symptoms and early referral for follow-up services may make a difference in prevention of PTSD [7].

14.4 Summary

Bioterrorism attacks and threats are a reality in today's world. Nurses, especially those who do triage in emergency departments are in a unique position to detect a possible or chemical attack. They must be knowledgeable of signs and symptoms of exposure and initiate an immediate response to prevent delay in intervention.

Education is the key to defense against bioterrorism and nurses need to be educated in biological and chemical emergency management. Appropriate content for education includes the following [8]:

- awareness of major biological and chemical agents
- technical skills related to clinical patient care, triage, decontamination and treatment
- incident command system
- understanding bioterrorism surveillance and response systems
- collaboration with other agencies
- flexibility to work under chaotic and changing conditions
- teamwork and the ability to work effectively under stress
- current therapeutic modalities and the national pharmaceutical stockpile
- management of psychosocial issues during a mass disaster
- HAZMAT incidents
- personnel protective equipment

Disaster awareness and preparation is an essential component and hospitals must take an active role in development of formal plans. Nurses must examine their own preparedness with regard to a disaster response and potential problems that might affect the ability to respond. They should be able to answer the following questions [9]:

- What are the natural disaster risks in your area?
- Are there seasonal challenges?
- Is there a plan for disruption of utilities at your facility?
- Is there a backup communication system?
- If the hospital was disable is there a plan to deal with the situation?
- Are there enough supplies on had in case of a disaster or what is the mechanism for delivery if needed?
- Are there agreements with nearby facilities to support your institution in case of a disaster?
- Are you prepared to deal with WMD?
- Do you know how to activate your hospital's emergency management plan?

Special populations who are vulnerable to bioterrorist attacks include children, the elderly, pregnant women, those who are immunocompromised as well as health care professionals who care for the patients. Surveillance systems can detect and monitor the course of an outbreak and decrease morbidity and mortality.

In the case of a large-scale bioterrorist exposure, health care professionals will have to treat as many victims as possible and care will be based on the greatest good for the most number of people in the shortest period. This will be done within a dynamic triage process that is constantly changing based on victim status and available resources.

A large-scale disaster may require the assistance of outside resources and non-hospital facilities to become mass care center based on an incident command system. Part of this expanded response will include hospice care with an emphasis on symptom management and pain control. An incident involving exposure to a biological or chemical agent will have psychological as well as physical effects on everyone and failure to identify those at risk for an acute stress disorder may result in a complicated and prolonged recovery. Being aware of potential symptoms and early referral for follow-up services may make a difference in prevention of PTSD.

References

1. Emergency Nurses Association Position Statement on Weapons of Mass Destruction, 2002.
2. Frederick Burkle. Mass casualty management of a large scale bioterrorist event: an epidemiological approach that shapes triage decisions. *Emergency Medicine Clinics of North America*, 20:409–436, 2002.

3. Centers for Disease Control and Prevention. Interim recommended notification procedures for local and state public health department leaders in the event of a bioterrorist incident, 11 October 2001, http://www.bt.cdc.gov.
4. S. White, et al. Medical management of vulnerable populations and co-morbid conditions of victims of bioterrorism. *Emergency Medicine Clinics of North America*, (20):365–392, 2002.
5. D. Bravata, et al. Systemic review: surveillance systems for early detection of bioterrorism-related diseases. *Annals of Internal Medicine*, 140(1):910–924, 2004.
6. Nunn-Lagar-Domenici. Domestic Preparedness Program by the Department of Defense. 1–32, December 1, 2001.
7. D. Persell, et al. Preparing for Bioterrorism: Category A Agents. *The Nurse Practitioner*, 26:(12) 12–27, 2001.
8. T. Veenema. Chemical and biological terrorism preparedness for staff development specialists. *Journal for Nurses in Staff Development*, 19(5):215–222, 2003.
9. D. Kim, et al. Disaster management and the emergency department. *Nursing Clinics of North America*, 37(1):171–188, 2002.

15 The Role of Pharmacy in Emergency Preparedness

ROBERT S. GUYNN

The United States currently faces an environment rife with challenges to our interests and security. Unlike the nuclear threat of the cold war, the threat of foreign and domestic terrorism has visited upon us repeated insults resulting in well-documented death and destruction [1]. While terrorism perpetrated against the US in foreign lands is largely the province of the State Department, Pentagon and Federal law enforcement and intelligence agencies, preparing for terrorism on US turf requires the additional and concerted efforts of other Federal, State, local government, private health care, and emergency response agencies. It is at the regional, state, and local levels where the pharmacy practitioner community can and must step up and make significant contributions to the public welfare. When one considers the impact of a chemical or biological attack on this nation, it is clear that the most definitive response involves, fundamentally, a mass dispensing or vaccination problem. Pharmacy practitioners are key players in both activities.

Among the challenges facing hospital pharmacy directors engaged in the continued provision of pharmacy services during a public health emergency are the continued operation of systems, supply channels, and personnel. Planning and preparation hold the best promise for successful crisis management [2]. Directors can consult guidance documents provided by such organizations as the American Society of Heath System Pharmacists (ASHP) [3] and the CDC as a starting point [4] and then proceed to:

- Consult with the institution's public safety coordinator and local health authorities to determine the local history of, and planning for, natural and manmade disasters as well as their plans for potential terrorist attacks with weapons of mass destruction (WMD),
- Conduct a review of the hospital's disaster planning documents to reveal the administration's currently defined pharmacy responsibilities and suggest modifications as necessary,
- Assess vulnerabilities to critical operational systems including communications, suppliers, distribution channels, drug information, and automated systems (dispensing, compounding and health care information systems), and develop backups (and backups for the backups) when appropriate,
- Review, update and test contact lists for staff members and establish lists of household members,
- Look outside the four walls of the hospital to suppliers, state/national professional associations (hospital and pharmacy), and public health planning authorities (state and local), to determine resource availability and extra-institutional roles and obligations.

Among the topics to be explored at this point, include: stockpile requirements, staff support, emergency personnel augmentation, mutual aide, and re-supply. All of these systems and their backups need to be updated and reviewed with applicable staff periodically. Additionally, system backups need to be posted in the department's disaster plan manual and be accessible to charge pharmacists on every shift.

Development and maintenance of hospital pharmaceutical stockpiles must be accomplished in coordination with state and local public health planners, state hospital and pharmacy associations, the institution's Pharmacy and Therapeutics Committee, and contract suppliers. Care must be taken to develop and maintain stockpiles that are relevant, manageable, reasonable, and sufficient to meet projected needs of the community for at least the first 72 hours of an emergency. The CDC has identified and published a list [5] of biological agents with application as WMDs. Anthrax, Plague, Small pox, Botulism, and Tularemia are some of the disease states possible in this context. Typical antibiotics include tetracyclines, fluoroquinolones, and penicillin analogues [6]. Quantities sufficient to provide prophylaxis for hospital staff, public officials, public health personnel, and emergency responders and their families (staff support), will need to accommodated. The Federal Government has made funds available to hospitals to establish these stockpiles through the Health Resource Services Administration (HRSA) and the CDC. Additionally, some state and city governments have allocated funding for this purpose. Funding issues and sources evolve rapidly. Hospital administrators and pharmacy managers need to stay close to their state/national hospital and pharmacy associations for updates and application information.

With regard to public health emergencies precipitated by chemical agents, again, the CDC list is exhaustive [5]. Based utility and efficacy, the nerve agents have been characterized as being among the most attractive chemical WMDs to terrorist groups. Indeed, in recent years nerve agents have been inflicted upon civilian populations in Japan and Iraq [7,8]. An attack by a nerve agent will be relatively overt in nature, resulting in casualties rapidly. Typical nerve agents include Sarin, Tabun, and Vx. Depending upon the specific nerve agent and dose, immediate nervous system failure and death can result. Antidotes include:

- Atropine sulfate: an anti-cholinergic,
- Pralidoxime chloride (2PAM): an acetyl cholinesterase reactivator,
- Diazepam: a benzodiazepine used in this context as an anti-convulsant employed to reduce the severity of acetylcholine-induced convulsions.

To be successful, exposure to nerve agents must be rendered promptly. To this end, the CDC has developed and forward deployed their CHEMPACK (Figure 15.1), containerized antidote kits at the community level as part of the Strategic National Stockpile (SNS) [9,10]. These CHEMPACK containers are available in two configurations each designed to treat about 1000 patients:

- Emergency Medical Service (EMS) Container
  Most items packaged as auto-injectors, most useful for first responders.
- Hospital Container
  some auto-injectors included but the majority of doses in multi-dose vials to facilitate Emergency Room and patient unit use.

It is to be noted that, at present, the CHEMPAK containers do not contain ophthalmics needed to deal with the visual disturbances and painful eye symptoms associated with the miosis (constricted pupils) seen with exposure nerve agents. These ophthalmic symptoms are best treated with commercially available ophthalmic dosage forms

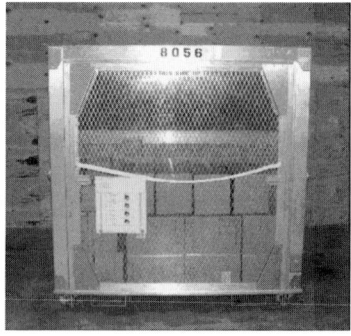

Figure 15.1 Typical CHEMPACK container.

of 0.5% tropicamide/0.5% phenylephrine HCl or 1% cyclopentolate HCl.

While the CDC states: "CHEMPACK participation is voluntary for public health agencies," [9] it is clear that most jurisdictions have (or will) take advantage of the CHEMPACK program. Hospital pharmacies have been identified as logical locations for the storage and maintenance of prepositioned CHEMPAK containers. The justification for this includes:

- Statewide distribution of hospitals.
- Well-known locations within a community.
- Pharmacist/custodians are well-qualified licensed personnel in facilities with existing DEA registrations.
- Facility characteristics:
  - Secure
  - Already meet state and federal requirements for the storage of controlled drugs (C-IV, diazepam)
  - Climate controlled (lighting, temperature, ventilation, and humidity)
  - Constantly staffed (and monitored).
- Quality assurance personnel and practices already in place:
  - Management of expiration dates
  - Organic staff capable of upgrade/retrofit/remediation actions as needed

The challenge to most pharmacy directors will be the allocation and preparation of dedicated space to accommodate the container(s) [9]. Each container requires about 50 square feet of floor space plus a isles and maneuvering space. Containers must also be sequestered or caged to limit access to unauthorized persons and be covered by intrusion detection devices (Figure 15.2). A dedicated analog phone line and 115 VAC with UPS backup must be available to support the remote monitoring equipment. All CHEMPACK assets remain the property of the CDC SNS. As is the case with the establishment of local pharmaceutical stockpiles, hospital pharmacies can secure grants to fund accommodations for their

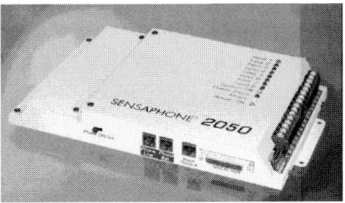

Figure 15.2 Sensaphone® remote monitoring device.

hospital and community CHEMPACK containers from the HRSA, CDC and some state agencies.

15.1 Strategic National Stockpile

The Department of Homeland Security (DHS) and the Centers for Disease Control (CDC) have created and maintain the Strategic National Stockpile (SNS) [1], in an effort to support US states and possessions in their mounting of a credible response to public health emergencies. CDC's Strategic National Stockpile (SNS) has large quantities of medicine and medical supplies to protect the American public if there is a public health emergency (terrorist attack, flu outbreak, earthquake) severe enough to cause local supplies to run out. Once Federal and local authorities agree that the SNS is needed, medicines will be delivered to any state in the U.S. within 12 hours. Each state has plans to receive and distribute SNS medicine and medical supplies to local communities as quickly as possible. As mentioned previously, hospitals and communities must plan to rely on their own assets for 72 hours. In addition to the above described CHEMPACK, the SNS consists of:

- 12 Hour Push Pack [2]: 12 strategically pre-positioned push packs distributed in such a way as to be available to any U.S. jurisdiction within 12 hours of a declared public health emergency. These push packs consist of 50+ tons of medical supplies, equipment and pharmaceuticals, designed to deal with the broad spectrum of potential bioterror agents. Due to the nature of its contents, the majority of SNS tonnage will likely be distributed to a state's hospitals (Figure 15.3). Such items as cases of IV solutions, ventilators,

204 Preparing Hospitals for Bioterror

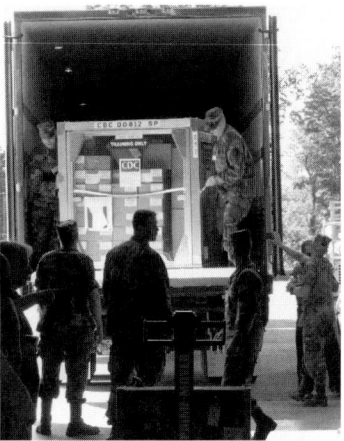

Figure 15.3 Portion of the SNS being delivered.

antibiotics and controlled drugs are primarily used in the institutional setting.

- VMI (Vendor Managed Inventory) [3]: Ongoing shipments of pharmaceuticals and medical supplies that are focused to the threat which is designed to begin arrival 36 hours after the public health emergency declaration.
- Chempak [4]: Chemical agent antidotes pre-positioned at the local level and a component of the 12 hour push pack.
- Additional automated drug packaging equipment in two containers shipped only when determined necessary (Figure 15.4).

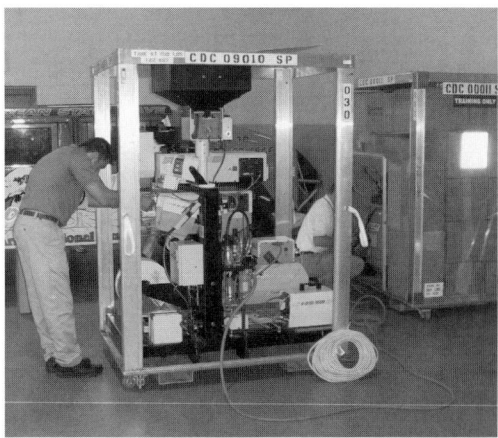

Figure 15.4 Automated drug packaging machine.

Hospital pharmacy directors and managers need to be mindful of the broader role of pharmacy beyond the walls of their institution, since the bulk of prophylaxis and/or vaccination will occur in distributed "points of dispensing" (POD's). The "textbook" POD [5] has been defined by the CDC as serving up to 50,000 citizens and is located away from hospitals in distributed community venues, typically schools, health clinics, civic centers, fire stations, etc.

15.2 Staffing Concerns in a Crisis

The greatest challenge to health care workers and public safety personnel in the face of a public health emergency will be one of balance. Such events have the potential to be "up close and personal," profoundly affecting our families, friends, neighbors, and community. Hospitals and emergency response resources will be stretched, requiring the full commitment of their staffs. Personnel will be torn between their jobs, families, and community responsibilities. Community leaders, public health planners, and hospital administrators (and pharmacy directors) need to engage in some serious planning [1] to ensure the presence and effectiveness of first responders, hospital staff members, public health personnel, and other community emergency response personnel in the face of such emergencies. Expectations, training and family care are necessary elements of such planning and preparation. As previously discussed, local stockpile provisions need to be established with household/family considerations included. The workforce needs to be informed of such provisions.

The need for emergency staff augmentation will vary significantly with the scenario. Most state legislatures have already taken steps to suspend state licensure requirements in the face of a declared public health emergency. Connecticut's act is representative and has a provision for volunteers who are: "appropriately licensed, certified or registered in another state or territory of the United States or the District of Columbia, to render temporary assistance within the scope of the profession for which a person is licensed, certified or registered, in managing a public health emergency in this state" [3]. Hospital pharmacy and human resource managers must participate in discussions and planning sessions with state pharmacy and hospital associations, health departments, and other health professional licensing authorities, to establish procedures for the credentialing and incorporation of health professionals from other settings and states into the workforce in the event your personnel resources become overwhelmed, fatigued, or otherwise depleted.

15.3 Training and Participation of the Pharmacy Staff in Community Preparedness Efforts

The ASHP Statement on the Role of Health-System Pharmacists in Emergency Preparedness, suggests that hospital administrators, "Encourage and enable pharmacy personnel employed by the institution to participate in local, state, regional, and federal emergency preparedness planning and to volunteer for community service in the event of a disaster." [3] Hospital pharmacy directors, likewise need to promote the involvement of staff members at all levels (clerks, technicians, students, pharmacists and managers) in their communities' public health emergency response planning, disaster drills, and, when needed, actual events. Although it is acknowledged that staff members owe their primary allegiance to their employer whenever the institution's disaster plan is activated, there is considerable room and numerous scenarios whereby staff members can effectively participate in their community response without neglecting the needs of their employer institutions.

When dealing with a crisis, we often do not have the luxury of certainty of cause, effect, or resolution [2]. Despite this characteristic lack of definition, pharmacy management can enhance the department's response to such events through encouraging staff participation in the growing number of public health emergency simulation exercises being conducted across the country. Institutional pharmacy practitioners need to be "plugged-in" to the overall city, state, and regional public health emergency response planning activities. Involvement vehicles include, but are not limited to, city and state health departments, state hospital associations, pharmacy professional organizations, and pharmacy colleges.

With regard to the Strategic National Stockpile, the CDC is engaged an aggressive training effort including a week long in-residence "Stockpile School" in Atlanta, regional abbreviated "SNS road shows," and on-line tutorials which are open to interested parties. These programs are fully funded by the CDC. Additionally, the CDC supports a series of conferences, drills, and exercises at the state level, which include planning conferences, desktop (paper) exercises, and full-blown multiday SNS exercises, which provide vehicles for familiarization, competencies, and process improvement. Pharmacists should participate in local efforts as well as get out to observe such exercises in other cities, regions, or states when the opportunity arises. Of particular value are the lessons learned in the wake of an event or exercise.

15.4 Conclusion

Considerable coordination of effort is required to support effective preparation for, and response to, a public health disaster. Critical factors to a credible response of a public health emergency include availability and distribution of pharmaceuticals, as well as the availability and placement of qualified personnel to facilitate such distribution. The pharmacy community (institutional, retail, academic and regulatory) are instrumental assets to successful preparation and response.

References

1. Significant Terrorist Attacks Against the United States and its Citizens 146-2001, *Center for Arms Control and Non-Proliferation.* http://www.armscontrolcenter.org/terrorism/101/ timeline.html
2. W. P. Johnston, and P. L. Stepanovich. Managing in a crisis: Planning, acting, and learning. *Am J Health-Syst Pharm.* 58:1245–1249, 2001.
3. ASHP Statement on the Role of Health-System Pharmacists in Emergency Preparedness, *Am Soc Health-Syst Pharm.* 2003. http://www.ashp.org/emergency/counter terrorism.cfm

4. A. S. Khan, A. M. Alexander, et al. Biological and Chemical Terrorism: Strategic Plan for Preparedness and Response—Recommendations of the CDC Strategic Planning Workgroup. *CDC MMWR*, 49(RR04);1–14, 2000. http://www.cdc.gov/mmwr/preview/mmwrhtml/rr4904a1.htm
5. Emergency Preparedness & Response: Agents, Diseases and Other Threats, *CDC*. http://www.bt.cdc.gov/agent/
6. Prevention and Treatment of Injury From Chemical Warfare Agents, *The Medical Letter*, 44:1, 2002. http://www.medicalletter.org/freedocs/reprints.pdf
7. Terrorism Questions and Answers, Council on Foreign Relations, 2004. http://cfrterrorism.org/groups/aumshinrikyo.html
8. Research and Investigations: Nerve Gas used in Northern Iraq on Kurds, Physicians for Human Rights, 1993. http://www.phrusa.org/research/chemical_weapons/chemiraqgas2.html
9. Continuation Guidance – Budget Year Five, Attachment J–CHEMPACK Public Health Preparedness and Response for Bioterrorism, *CDC*, 2004. http://www.bt.cdc.gov/planning/continuationguidance/ docs/chempack-attachj.doc
10. Strategic National Stockpile, *CDC*, 2005. http://www.bt.cdc.gov/stockpile/
11. Conn. Public Act No. 03-236, AN ACT CONCERNING PUBLIC HEALTH EMERGENCY RESPONSE AUTHORITY, http://www.cga.ct.gov/2003/act/Pa/2003PA-00236-R00HB-06676-PA.htm

16   The Clinical Engineering Department Role in Emergency Preparedness

DUANE MARIOTTI

For decades the Joint Commission on Accreditation of Healthcare Organizations (JCAHO) has required hospitals (and other accredited agencies) to have a "disaster plan" and show functionality of this plan via semi-annual drills. Clinical Engineering or Biomedical Engineering Departments may or may not participate in these drills. However, experience has shown that in an actual crisis all staff have a role in the emergency response.

What is a disaster?

The ideal definition of a disaster is a short term event which overloads the ability of normal agencies to respond in a timely and expected manner. Basically a disaster is when you have more going on than you have people or solutions to correct. This may sound familiar to hospital (and field service) technical staff. Frequently, there is a "crisis" in the Operating Room or Intensive Care Unit that requires immediate intervention.

As an example, at midnight a telemetry transmitter in the step-down unit fails. The nurse has some free time, changes the lead wires, and changes the battery and still nothing on the central monitor. She goes to the drawer where the spare telemetry transmitters are and swaps out the defective unit, places a defective sticker on it and leaves a message so it can be picked up and repaired in the morning.

Same scenario, but when the nurse goes to the drawer, there is no spare transmitter. She has the Clinical Engineering technician on call paged and connects up the transport defibrillator/monitor to the patient so the ECG may be monitored. The technician comes in, pulls a spare transmitter off the on-call shelf and assists the nurse with connecting it to the patient. He assures the ECG is present at the central station, sees that all other waveforms look acceptable and goes home and back to bed.

A little different scenario: The nurses all realize that only one patient's ECG is available on the central station. No other ECG's are displayed. There are suppose to be sixteen patients displayed on that central station. The second central station is only displaying half the ECG's.

All three of these scenarios are crises. In healthcare, crises are dealt with routinely. The word "triage" (to sort), is routinely used in medicine to determine who gets what resources when, based on their medical condition. But, the last scenario is a disaster. There are not spare transmitters for twenty-three patients, there is not enough staff to check every transmitter, and while the Clinical Engineering department has a loner central station monitor, that does not appear to be the cause of the failure. These patients arc in a step-down unit for advanced ECG monitoring, and it is not available.

This is an example of an internal disaster in a hospital. Other internal disasters may include sewer pipe breakage and sewage knee deep in the basement of the hospital, water main breakage (or any flooding), significant network failures, a hazardous materials spill, a hostage situation or a fire.

External disasters also have impacts on hospitals. Typically these disasters impact the community and result in additional patient loads. Patient loads may not only be due to injuries, but inability to refill prescriptions, inability to get follow up care (such as dialysis or oxygen), and lack of normal medical (family physician) avenues. Hospitals, due to their planning, may be the only place in a community with lights, heat and food when all else may appear dark and hopeless; thus, a beacon to the community. Typical external disasters which affect hospitals are well known and include wild land fires, floods, tornados, earthquakes, hurricanes, and terrorist events.

If you work in a hospital there is a good chance at some time in your career you will have to respond not just to a crisis, but a disaster.

16.1 Lessons Learned

As response to disasters are infrequent events, learning from past disasters and what worked and did not work, is very valuable. In clinical engineering, this means contacting your peers who were affected by the disaster and determining what went well and what did not. All of the information gained should be added to your personal and departmental disaster plan.

Some events which have provided significant after action lessons learned include:

- The Kansas City Hotel Walkway Collapse—7/17/81—This is considered the advent of emergency medical and urban rescue response [1].
- The Oklahoma City Bombing—4/19/95 [2].
- The Columbine High School Shootings—4/20/99 [3].
- The Texas Floods due to Tropical Storm—Allison 6/9/01—The largest known evacuation of patients in the United States under less than ideal conditions (prior to Katrina) [4].
- And of course September 11, 2001.
- Hurricane season of 2004–5 in Florida and the Gulf Coast [5].

Many emergency preparedness planners look to where terrorist events are common and how hospitals respond to these events for "best practices." Israel is, unfortunately, where most of this information has been of great value.

While the above events were national in scope, many communities have experienced their own significant events, some planned, some not planned, that have resulted in changes to the way that hospitals in the community respond to crisis. In the Seattle metropolitan area we have had chemical plant mishaps resulting in hundreds of sick residents, snow and ice storms which crippled transportation in the region (Seattle does not do well with snow), evacuation of a two hundred bed hospital due to lack of power (during the day with on-going surgeries), and the World Trade Organization (WTO) event (content.lib.edu/wtoweb) which did not result in many patients, but in transportation, significant facility, security and safety concerns.

Every community most likely has its own example of events. While it is important to learn from national events, it is also critical to learn and communicate how to improve on the local level. Many Clinical Engineering groups, organizations and communities did this in preparation for Y2K. Meetings were held, information and ideas were exchanged and plans were developed. However, Y2K had a definitive end date. Emergency preparedness requires the same communications, but on a routine and ongoing basis.

Emergency planning does not have to be "over the top." Look at your hospital, your community and determine what may be situations that you need to respond. Are there railroad tracks in town? Do they carry hazardous materials? What if one (or more) derailed and started leaking? (South Carolina) Is the hospital located near a sports stadium? What if something occurred at the stadium and hundreds of people flooded the hospital? (Wisconsin) What is your threat of wildfires? What if you had to evacuate the hospital due to fires in the forests? (California) How do you prepare for a hurricane? Earthquake? Start small and plan as best you can, talk with your peers at other hospitals, maybe even create a community wide engineering disaster plan. Like in the Y2K planning efforts, it is best to share insights and capabilities prior to the event. This may even be formalized with mutual aid agreements signed among a group of hospitals at the engineering department or senior administrative level. Mutual aid agreements formalize the plan, but the plan should be routinely practiced.

Of all the lessons learned, the most critical one is that you will do what you practice, not what is in the manual. In other words, practice as close to real as possible. The military and civilian emergency planners have learned this. As required by the JCAHO, the hospital has two drills per year to test the emergency preparedness plan. Has the Clinical Engineering department participated in these drills? Do they know that the drill is ongoing? Is it just another routine day, or does staff practices what they would do in a disaster situation?

16.2 Priorities

There is one primary understanding of emergency preparedness planning for healthcare organizations: Protect Staff, Protect Patients, and Protect Facility.

Staff is the most important resource in a hospital. Physicians, nurses, technicians, engineers, and ancillary personnel all are part of the team. If anyone section of that team fails, the primary mission of the hospital—provide safe patient care—is in jeopardy. Therefore protection of staff in whatever manner possible from disease, building collapse, and hazardous materials is paramount.

Most patients are susceptible to any external crisis. Many are not ambulatory, frequently on medications that affect judgment, and are very vulnerable. Protection of patients is one reason hospitals exist and must be included in any emergency planning. The features put in place to protect staff, frequently are the same measures required to protect patients. There is a mutual benefit.

While a hospital is primarily the staff, specialized facilities are required for treatment of patients. CT Scanners, Operating Rooms, etc., are all part of the facility as are medical gas distribution, food preparation, etc. Without the facility there is no safe place for patient care and treatment. Hospitals in parts of the country with potential for hurricanes and earthquakes have learned these lessons. Building codes have been implemented to assist with assuring facilities are available. (National Building, Life Safety and National Electrical Code promulgated by the National Fire Protection Association and implemented in many communities is an example.)

16.3 Incident Command System

The Incident Command System (ICS) is part of the comprehensive National Incident Management System (NIMS). Participation in some form of ICS is critical to span of control and positive outcomes of a disaster event (ICS is discussed in detail in Chapter 20). The ICS is based on the principal that there is a single person in charge. At the top of the chart that is the "Incident Commander." There are four branches under the Incident Commander: Operations, Logistics, Planning, and Finance. Clinical Engineering as a support service is typically part of the Logistics Branch in ICS for hospitals. Operations are primarily associated with direct patient care as well as triage and specialty operations in the Emergency Department. FEMA has excellent on line classes in both ICS and NIMS that senior Clinical Engineering staff should participate.

It is important to understand in a disaster situation that one person is in charge: The Incident Commander. That person communicates with the Logistics Chief who provides Clinical Engineering with tasks and responsibilities. Clinical Engineering should not "freelance" projects, but communicate its actions (or planned actions) within the ICS.

16.4 Communications

When reviewing disaster situations failure of communications is typically one of the three most mentioned areas for improvement. Therefore any planning with Clinical Engineering departments should include communications. Communications has many aspects, internal communication among staff, communications with the hospital command center, communications with vendors and parts suppliers, communications with families and other loved ones.

Typically hospitals have some form on internal radio communications system. The larger and more complex the campus, the more complex the radio system. Is Clinical Engineering part of this radio system? Are radios provided to Clinical Engineering staff for immediate use in a disaster? Are they used on a routine (daily) basis for internal communications so staff is aware of use?

Does the radio system assigned to the Clinical Engineering department have ability to communicate with the system used by the Facilities Engineering Department for coordination? With the hospital command center?

Frequently telephone communications (including cellular phone) will fail in a crisis. If not immediately, then batteries will fail and there will be a host of other problems. It is important that communications planning is not based solely on cellular phones as means of back up communications. Planning should include what to do if the hospital telephones fail. Sometimes a roll of quarters and the pay phones in the lobby are the only telephone communications hospitals have available.

Most vendors use toll free 800 numbers. These numbers may fail in a crisis. What is the direct non-800 number to access vendors? What is the vendor's telephone outage plan? What is the vendor's disaster plan? How does vendor communicate with field service representatives in a disaster? Is there a standardized plan where field service representatives respond to specific high acuity hospitals to get dispatched to other locations by the hospitals? Or, is there no plan at all—unfortunately this has typically been the experience.

Ideally any service contract should include complete documentation on the vendors' disaster response, contingency, and business resumption plan. This plan must include actions for a disaster in the hospital location, as well as a disaster at the vendors corporate headquarters or telephone answering location. Informing the vendor that in the event of a major catastrophe, you want a service technician to immediately respond to the hospital and then practice contacting vendor and requesting emergency disaster response during your disaster drills will significantly improve the vendor's understanding. Further, home phone numbers of local service technicians, managers and directors—solely for emergency purposes—have significant value and create additional understanding and communication among the vendor and hospital community.

There are some questions for communications planning:

Who are you going to call?
How do you contact them 24 by 7?
How do you contact them if no telephones?
What do you do if you can not locate them?

Most of us use the answers to the top two questions routinely to contact field service representatives. We need to build on these plans to assure that the vendor's plans are as resilient as possible.

16.5 Departmental Staff Care

How does staff assure that family members are OK? Typically staff will function much more efficiently in a disaster situation once they are aware that their immediate loved ones are OK. How is this done? Does the hospital sponsor emergency planning events for families? Is information provided as part of orientation? Is the family disaster plan reviewed and taken into account during the hospital drills? How does one prepare her family for a hurricane, knowing she will be in the hospital during the event? Are plans made to include sheltering of families during disaster plans?

There are no easy answers, but a little family planning goes a long way. Seattle is separated by bridges. Failure of the bridges due to high winds, earthquake or terrorist event is possible. My wife works on one side of the bridge, I on the other. It is not much, but in event of a crisis, we were both responsible for the children on the side of the water we were on. As I worked at the hospital, I knew there would be lights, etc., and a safe haven for myself and the children I could pick up. My wife had our home or would try to get to the hospital once she had the children on her side of the bridge. We actually had a windstorm and earthquake and in both cases, while not ideal, this plan worked. Staff (and others) will use the hospital as a safe haven and family refuge—build it into your plans.

Additional family planning includes resources for staff and family to sleep and eat at the hospital. Consider gasoline availability for vehicles, carpooling and other resources for moving families around.

16.6 Individual Preparedness

Individual preparedness is the mindset that we must accept as part of the position. Hospitals are critical part of any community disaster planning and response. Disasters have an impact and while as many folks when faced with a disaster can just go home, patient care demands that hospital employees remain on the job. You will be expected to perform during a disaster and most of us will experience at least one disaster during our careers.

Individual preparedness includes basic family planning, home emergency kits, and family communications plans. The American Red Cross [6] and others have excellent examples of this. The information is readily available on the Internet.

Individual preparedness is a mindset. If you live in the Midwest, there will be a tornado at sometime. On the Gulf Coast, there will be hurricanes, in the west, there will be earthquakes. Hopefully, they will be minor or miss you, your family, and your hospital. But if not, you do not have the choice of not being prepared. A little preparation for an event will pay significant dividends should it occur.

16.7 Departmental Preparedness

Departmental preparedness starts with some basic orientation. Are all staff familiar with the hospital's emergency preparedness plan, is the review of plan included in employee (volunteer, student, and contractor) orientation? Is there a Clinical Engineering departmental disaster plan? Ideally this should be about one page in length. Is the review of departmental plan included in the departmental orientation? Is the plan practiced during hospital drills and improved based on experience? Is Clinical Engineering part of the Hospitals Emergency Preparedness Committee?

Is emergency powered lighting available in the clinical engineering shop? Emergency power receptacles? It is difficult to repair something if you cannot power it or see it.

Most Clinical Engineering departments should create a small "Disaster Kit" that can be used in a crisis should the shop area have to be evacuated or worse (Figure 16.1). This kit contains basic items such as a small tool kit, VOM, basic safety supplies, flashlights, paper copy of the medical equipment database, pens, papers and pencils.

Some Clinical Engineering departments have created actual disaster carts (Figure 16.2). These carts contain spare equipment (typically monitors, pulse oximeters, oxygen regulators, etc.), heavy duty (12 G) extension cords of various lengths (10–100 feet), spare ECG cables, NIBP components, and other "consumable" items for ICU monitors (Table 16.1). Flashlights, bull horns, basic tools, suction regulators, and many other items. Typically these carts are made up from equipment that would be surplussed or traded in.

16.7.1 Medical Technology

Clinical Engineers might not consider it emergency preparedness, but they have routinely performed emergency preparedness activities. Equipment that malfunctions during emergency power tests due to lack of power, receive uninterruptible power supplies. Complete spares of critical equipment such as bedside ICU monitors are typically found in biomedical inventories. Spare parts to allow rapid repair and minimize downtime for routine devices such as defibrillators are stocked in biomedical shops. The very best means of technology preparedness is to manage all of the medical technology to maximum performance on a daily and routine basis.

212 Preparing Hospitals for Bioterror

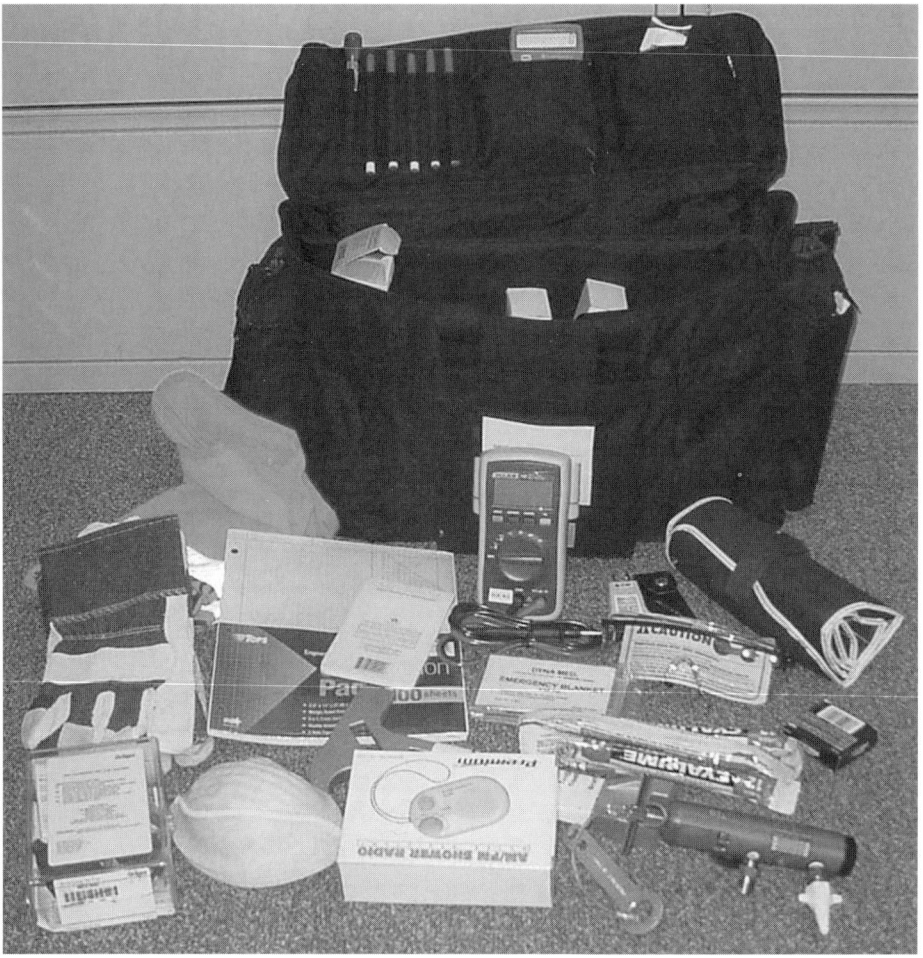

Figure 16.1 Clinical engineering jump kit.

There are many critical medical devices in a hospital. Some of these devices such as lasers may not be required during an emergency situation. Other devices such as ventilators may be in short supply. It is important for every hospital to determine what its critical (typically life support) technologies are and assure sufficient inventory to meet daily needs in a cost-effective manner. If a hospital is typically renting ventilators on a daily basis, ventilators will be in short supply in a crisis.

Hospitals consist of many clinical departments. Typically it is best to review the needs of each department to function in a crisis mode and continue to deliver patient care. Based on the hospital, the community and the department each will be unique in some manner. There are similarities.

Is there sufficient emergency power for all departments to provide a minimal level of emergency functionality? This is not just the critical care areas, but support areas such as pharmacy and laboratory. Are the proper devices connected to emergency power circuits? An excellent example are blood bank refrigerators and bone freezers. Are

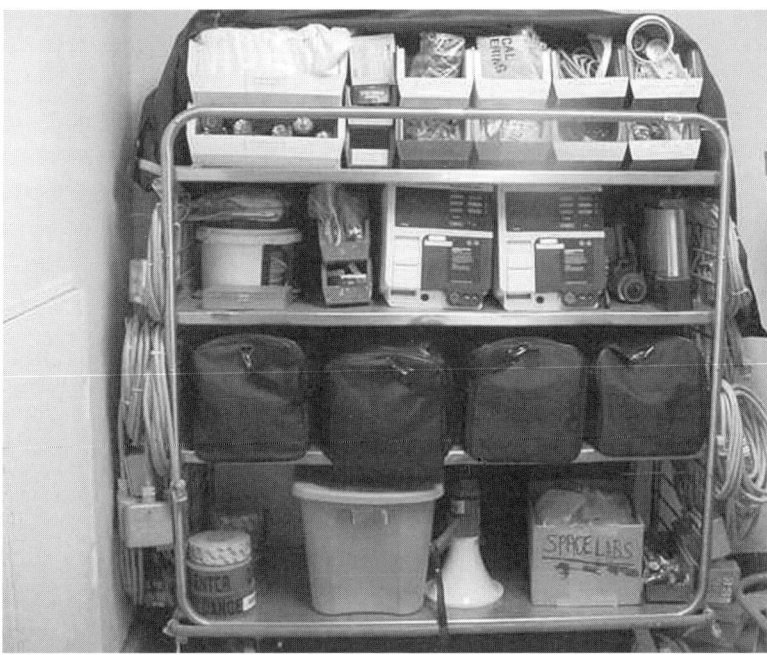

Figure 16.2 Clinical engineering disaster cart.

these critical devices alarmed, with remote indication of alarms and are the alarms on emergency power? For certain critical items what is the back up plan. Are there additional blood refrigerators in other areas of the hospital?

Many devices in the laboratory are interfaced or driven by computers. Are these devices connected to emergency power and also an uninterruptible power supply to assure continuous operation? Are redundant devices maintained for critical lab studies such as basic chemistry and blood gas studies? Are some of these devices configured to be mobile to be relocated to patient care areas?

Have special consideration been made on how to support ventilator dependent patients? There are disposable ventilators available which may provide clinical staff time to determine a clinical course. These disposable ventilators are only of value if respiratory therapy staff have worked with them and they are available for immediate patient use. This is especially true with some of the potential bioterrorism concerns.

It is not nice to think about, but has the hospital and the community developed a mortuary plan? Is the hospital morgue deceased holding area on emergency power? What options are available? How many deceased patients can the hospital manage easily? These are all questions that require consideration.

In the surgical suite, how are spare medical gasses provided? How are instruments sterilized? In some hospitals, there are flash steam sterilizers connected to a self-contained steam boiler on emergency power to assure some minimal level of steam sterilization. Are the central sterile processing area lights and support equipment on emergency power?

Radiology is a key component of most patients diagnostic testing. With the advent of PACS and other digital systems, it is critical to assure that patients can be treated independent of the IT infrastructure and network functionality. In some

Table 16.1 Clinical engineering disaster cart inventory

Physio control	Defibrillator	LIFEPAK 9	Nelcor	Pulse oximeter
Physio control	Defibrillator	LIFEPAK 9	Nelcor	Pulse oximeter
Physio control	Defibrillator	LIFEPAK 9	Nelcor	Pulse oximeter
Physio control	Defibrillator	LIFEPAK 9	Nelcor	Pulse oximeter
Physio control	Defibrillator	LIFEPAK 9	Nelcor	Pulse oximeter
Physio control	Defibrillator	LIFEPAK 9	Nelcor	Pulse oximeter
Physio control	3 Lead ECG cable	One dozen	Nelcor	Pulse oximeter cable (12)
Physio control	Paper	One box	Nelcor	Pulse oximeter sensors (12)
Miscellaneous items				
6 Mini mag flashlights	2 Butane soldering irons		**Monitor accessories**	
16 Mag flashlights (2 D-cells)	2 Bull horns		6 Adult NIBP hoses	
4 Standard flashlights (Hosp. white)	6 Rolls danger tape		6 Neonatal NIBP hoses	
12 Wall suction regulators	2 Rolls kapler chem suit tape		2 Adult CO_2 adapters	
1 100′ 4-Plex extension cord in bucket	24 #2 Pencils		3 Lab chart paper folded—boxes	
1 14′ Extension cord	24 Bic ballpoint pens		2 Lab chart paper rolls—boxes	
1 12′ Extension cord	3 Small adult adult/child manometer		24 Disposable O_2 sensors	
1 7′ Extension cord	4 Sets kapler chemical suits		12 $SPCO_2$ cables	
1 40′ 4-Plex extension cord	2 Roll tool kit misc. hand tools		12 Pressure cables	
1 30′ 4-Plex extension cord	2 Cases bottled H_2O		6 Temp probe	
2 20′ 4-Plex extension cord	50 EA green & red chemlites		12 Telemetry lead sets	
1 12′ 4-Plex extension cord	14 Isolation suits		12 5-Lead ECG cable	
1 10′ 4-Plex extension cord	20 Particle masks		12 3-Lead ECG cable	
13 15′ 4-Plex extension cord	7 Clinical engineer vests		NIBP cuffs disposable—2 boxes each	
1 15′ 3-Plex extension cord	2 Suction manifolds outlets		Adult small 17–25 cm	
18 Electronic thermometers	6 Cutting blades		Adult med 23–33 cm	
3 Fluorescent lights (6 D-cells)	4 Four in one tool		Adult large 31–40 cm	
	12 PR Cotton gloves		Child reg. 12–19 cm	
	24 O_2 Regulator w/wrench		Neonatal size 1	
	24 O_2 Cylinder wrenches		Neonatal size 2	

hospitals CT scanners and angiography suites are on emergency power to assure patient access. This may not be required in all facilities, but some significant level of planning needs to be considered for all imaging modalities. It is critical that the physician has quick access to films and other test results to diagnose the patient. Radiology systems should be "stress tested" on a routine basis to assure that independent of normal power, network, IT infrastructure, etc., that films or displays are available for physician diagnosis and treatment.

16.8 Vendor Preparedness

Most hospitals have relationships with medical equipment vendors. These relationships range from formal full-service contracts to ad hoc parts purchasing and many intermediary forms. Most hospitals depend on medical equipment vendors for some level of service and failure of vendor to provide that service, during a disaster may be detrimental to patient care.

Clinical Engineering departments should strive to have spare technology and work arounds for all patient care related systems. While this is not always possible, the more work arounds, spare equipment, and planning to prepare for outage contingencies the better prepared the Clinical Engineering department will be to manage a disaster.

Vendors, especially those on contract, should be included in the disaster planning. Specifically what is the vendor's disaster plan? What is the local versus the national disaster plan? What do you expect as a contractual agreement to be the vendor's response to a hospital disaster?

In rural communities, just having the vendor agree to do all that is possible to show up within 24 hours of a disaster may be the best that is expected. In urban areas specific high risk hospitals such as University hospitals and/or designated trauma centers should receive immediate (self dispatch) priority to a disaster situation. Other hospitals in the community should agree that the vendor will respond to the trauma center and not be relieved until all hospitals have been called and validated that the vendor is not required at any other hospital. Of course, many vendors have multiple service representatives, so they may be dispatched to those critical hospitals as determined by the community.

Parts availability is and continues to be a concern in our global economy. Rapid air transport, worldwide requirements, minimization of inventory all work together to form a recipe for parts shortages in a disaster. The best tool hospitals have is to assure local parts inventories and assure that uptime commitments are met, including after action discussions of any significant down time due to failure to receive parts. If parts are not available during non-disaster situations, parts availability may be severely compromised during a disaster. Work with the vendor community to minimize parts issues at every opportunity, including offering hospital space for critical parts.

It is clearly the hospital's responsibility to work with those vendors critical for continued patient care and assure that the vendor understands its role in the hospital's overall emergency preparedness plan and response.

16.9 Business Resumption Planning

While this is a new buzz word in today's Information Technology (IT) planning, it has really been occurring for years in the Clinical Engineering field. Basically, do you have what you need to recreate your "business" to allow relatively seamless operations independent of the affects of a disaster?

Is there a list of all FDA devices with software in your facility? Is spare software or mirrors available for this technology in-house or from the vendor? What is the vendor's current response for replacing software of the generation of technology installed in your hospital?

Is the Clinical Engineering business able to function after the disaster? Most importantly is the medical equipment database backed up routinely, secured offsite and in paper form?

Are critical paper records stored in a secure location or in electronic format in a redundant manner?

Do all FDA regulated servers have routine backups of entire database and operating systems? Are these backups stored in a secure off site location?

Business resumption planning may be as simple as installing UPS's on critical components so that the systems have one less mechanism to fail.

16.10 Departmental Response

Despite your best wishes your hospital has been affected by a disaster. As most Clinical Engineering departments do not function 24×7, the time of day when the disaster occurred has significant impact on how the response is implemented.

Could the section below be done in a more formal—less conversational—manner?

What mechanism is in place to assure that all Clinical Engineering staff (including students, interns and vendors that may be on campus) are accounted for? How do you know who is out of the building? Where are they? Who called in sick? Who has the day off? Are there satellite shops? Are all shops and staff accounted for? It is the responsibility of everyone in the department to assure all staff is accounted for. Priority should be placed upon assuring all staff are accounted for initially in a crisis situation. An attempt to locate missing staff shoud be made. Staff not accounted for should be reported to the Command Center.

Departmental EICS

Who is in charge of the Clinical Engineering Department? Is the Director in the hospital or out of state at a convention? Who is in charge in the Directors absence? What needs to be done? All departments as part of good management have an organizational plan as to who has authority at what levels. The larger the department the more important these lines of authority are. These lines of authority are maintained in a disaster situation. The person in charge of the department assures all staff is accounted for and then responds reports to the hospital command center.

A simple checklist (Table 16.1), can be used by the senior person to initiate the Clinical Engineering Department Incident Response Plan. This checklist is just an example. Every department should have a list that is tailored to its staffing levels, facility, and responsibility. This checklist should be reviewed and modified after every drill and actual disaster.

In the ideal situation, all staff are accounted for and collects in one location. The person in charge designates someone responsible for the collection point. This person remains at the collection point (main shop) for the immediate duration of the incident. Someone is assigned the responsibilities to answer the telephone and record all issues. If the telephone is not functioning, then that person becomes a runner from the hospital command center to the collection point. The department specific response plans also provide suggestions for other activities, such as support to the Emergency Department. Teams to critical care and other areas to assure operation of equipment and to assist, in general, with disaster needs.

During the normal work day most critical patients are located in areas undergoing treatment (endoscopy, operating rooms, labor, and delivery, etc.) and critical care areas (intensive care units, post anesthesia care units, etc). Clinical Engineering staff should be sent from the collection point to these areas of patient intensity. Most Clinical Engineering staff have areas of specialization, anesthesia, operating room, ventilators, etc. The technical staff responsible for these areas should check in, be recorded as to where they are going, and then assume a sweep of these critical areas to assure that patient technology is functioning appropriately. Significant issues (medical gas failure, power outages affecting patient care, etc.) should be immediately reported to the hospital command center. Upon completion of their initial "sweeps" technical staff should report back to the collection point to provide information on what was observed and receive a new assignment.

If the event is one that will result in injuries to the public then staff should be assigned specifically to support the Emergency Department.

For every predetermined protocol, vendors critical for patient operations should be contacted to immediately respond to the hospital to support any potential failures of medical technology.

Depending on the magnitude of the disaster staff will be worried about their families. Staff may also be assigned to a clinical area for an extended amount of time (specifically, operating room and emergency department). It is important that staff are rotated and receive frequent breaks, food and ability to activate their family disaster plan and contact loved ones.

Disasters create a significant amount of activities in a short period of time. With some planning and a couple of drills, it is very easy to accomplish. Planning is an ongoing activity. It includes assuring that everyone knows who is off and called in sick on any given day. Whenever staff leaves the main hospital campus for an off-site meeting, off-site clinic, etc. that information is known. Staff are familiar with the ICS, with family emergency planning and with the Clinical Engineering Departmental Disaster Plan.

Many hospitals have responded to significant events and done very well. Staff know who is in charge, and everyone has radios and alpha-numeric pagers. In a crisis, everyone checks in on the radio and is assigned (almost by default) to their areas of responsibility. Satellite shops closest to ICUs have responsibility for those units. The person in charge reports to the hospital command center, states everyone in Clinical Engineering is accounted for and provides information on what has been observed.

If all disasters occurred during normal work hours, or if they were known in advance, like hurricanes it would be great. Unfortunately, that is not realistic. Departments need to have plans for after hours disasters. Some such as tornados and earthquakes may be self evident and staff can self report to the collection point. Others may not be well advertised and a call out plan is required to assure enough staff to assist with the disaster. Since Security is in house at all times, they can dispatch via alpha numeric pagers that a disaster has occurred. The on-call technician is now the person in charge and initiates response to the hospital as well as activating the telephone tree.

Resumption of normal business operations is an important part of disaster management. It is critical to go back and assure that everything truly is functioning properly. Depending on the disaster this may be simple or very complex. As an example: After a significant earthquake, everything that is attached to the walls must be tested to be assured it is still attached properly. Clinical Engineering technicians know most of the hospital and may join Facilities Engineering or other teams that are doing secondary and tertiary surveys of individual clinical units and facilities in general. Some areas of concern, network closets, dedicated air conditioning units for MRI and CT and other high-tech medical equipment, medical gas manifolds, compressors and piping, steam and sterilization capacity, dialysis water systems.

16.11 Putting it all Together

Some keys to successful implementation of Disaster Response include:

Clinical Engineering participates in the hospitals disaster committee.

Clinical Engineering has a departmental disaster plan and immediate action check list. Clinical Engineering Department orientation includes review of the departmental disaster plan.

Clinical Engineering maintains a departmental "disaster kit" (Figures 16.1 and 16.2) that is readily available and is checked semi-annually.

Clinical Engineering Technicians are made aware of their importance to the operation, and requested to review data and implement a family emergency plan.

Key vendors have field service representatives assigned specifically to your hospital in event of a disaster.

Clinical Engineering has access to the hospitals various communications systems and implemented a system for after hours access to all technical staff.

A roll of quarters is in the departmental disaster kit so in case all else fails so you can use the pay phone.

The Clinical Engineering inventory and data restoration procedures for your FDA software based technology is up to date.

Critical information in the Clinical Engineering department is stored in a reliable and redundant manner.

The Disaster plan is practiced on a routine basis. Information gathered from the plans is used to improve existing plans.

Routinely the managers of Clinical Engineering programs in surrounding hospitals meet to discuss relevant topics, including Emergency Preparedness. A signed "Mutual Aid" agreement may be a work product of this peer group.

Hopefully, you will never need any of this, but it will have taken minimal effort to implement and you just never know in today's world.

Appendix   Disaster Action Sheet Normal Work Hours Hospital Clinical Engineering

1. All staff immediately report to clinical engineering (CLE) main shop area. Check in, accounted for and pick up radio on CLE channel.
2. Emergency group page all staff of event.
3. Locate any staff not accounted for.
4. Supervisor or designee is in charge of all staff and assigments.
5. One technician assigned to main shop to answer primary phone number.
6. All staff to monitor radios on CLE channel during entire event.
7. Director or senior supervisor reports to command center and checks in on behalf of CLE with staff status.

8. Technical radio person reports to hospital radio room and provides support as required.
9. Disaster cart and two technicians to emergency department for support.
10. Allocate one staff member to radiology emergency calls.
11. Allocate one staff member to biomedical emergency calls.
12. If decon is required—decon support team responds to emergency department to support decon activities.
13. If internal disaster—two members of CLE to area affected by internal disaster to support medical equipment issues—may request other resources from senior person.
14. If significant event (earthquake, etc.) roving checks of ORs and ICUs are initiated to assist with equipment issues—one technician team to OR and PACU, one team to upper ICUS and work down, third team to lower ICUS and work up. Imaging team to radiology.
15. Assure internal infrastructure in clinical areas is functional—emergency power, medical gasses, network, telephone, etc.
16. Initiate activation of key service vendors to respond to hospital.
17. Assist at command center with phones, radios, medical equipment needs, etc.
18. All staff to maintain communication of activities and issues to senior person at command center.
19. Consider length of incident—determine overtime needs or stop time and break staff into two teams for continued 24 hour coverage.
20. Consider overnight coverage—send staff home for rest prior to need—relief staff early in am.
21. Debrief after incident.
22. Document the good, the bad and ideas for improvement.

References

1. http://www.engineering.com/content/ContentDisplay?contentld=41009033
2. (www.oklahomacitynationalmemorial.org)
3. www.cnn.com/SPECIALS/2000/columbine.cd/frameset.exclude.html
4. (www.chron.com/allison)
5. http://en.wikipedia.org/wiki/2005_Atlantic_hurricane_season
6. http://www.redcross.org/services/prepare/0,1082,0_ 77_,00.html

17 Amateur Radio Support for Hospitals

MARINA ZUETELL

Executive Summary

Hospitals and the healthcare system are dependent upon reliable and redundant communication systems. When these systems fail, as they often do during a disaster or other event that puts an overload on normal ways of conducting business, there needs to be an ultimate, reliable fall-back solution. Volunteer communications experts, known as Amateur Radio operators can provide communications and hold things together until the commercial phones and radio systems can recover.

17.1 What is Amateur Radio?

Amateur Radio is a technical hobby that teaches people how to use a two-way radio to communicate. Many people use the hobby to acquire new friends, contest, talk to the space shuttle, bounce signals off the moon, and experiment with radio and other technical aspects of the hobby. The Federal Communications Commission (FCC) has granted the Amateur Radio Service access to a wide variety of the radio spectrum, with the stipulation that it be used to develop new radio technologies and provide emergency communications [1]. The term "Amateur" denotes that the operators are unpaid volunteers, not that they are unprofessional or unskilled. They are also called "hams," although the derivation of that term is lost to history.

There is one aspect of the hobby that serves a more serious mission—that of Emergency Communications. Amateur radio operators use their hobby to provide backup and emergency communications during disaster situations, and when normal communications fail. They like to communicate, and they volunteer their skills and interest by helping the agencies and organizations who rely on communications to fill the gap when things go wrong. Hurricanes, floods, earthquakes, tsunamis, and other geological events can cause complete or partial failure of the normal phone, cell phone, and commercial radio systems. So do man-made events such as the collapse of the World Trade Center towers or a large terrorism or bioterrorism event, where regular communication systems are overloaded or compromised.

There are two commonly known groups who provide these emergency communications. One of these is sponsored by the ARRL (Amateur Radio Relay League) [2]—the national organization for amateur radio; and the other is sponsored by the federal and local governments, an offshoot of the old Civil Defense system. Different operating requirements and restrictions apply to each.

- *Amateur Radio Emergency Service* (*ARES*®)— Public service communications have been a traditional responsibility of the Amateur Radio Service since 1913. In those early days, such disaster work was spontaneous and without previous organization of any kind. In today's Amateur Radio, disaster work is a highly organized and worthwhile part of day-to-day operation, implemented principally by the ARES and the National Traffic System (NTS), both sponsored by ARRL [2].

- *Radio Amateur Civil Emergency Service* (***RACES***)—and other amateur public service groups are also a part of ARRL-recognized Amateur Radio public service efforts. Founded in 1952, the RACES is a public service provided by a reserve (volunteer) communications group within government agencies in times of extraordinary need. During periods of RACES activation, certified unpaid personnel are called upon to perform many tasks for the government agencies they serve. Although the exact nature of each activation will be different, the common thread is communications [3].

    The Federal Emergency Management Agency (FEMA) provides planning guidance and technical assistance for establishing a RACES organization at the state and local government level. A comprehensive RACES manual, *Guidance for Radio Amateur Civil Emergency Service*, is available on the FEMA Web site [4].

- Emergency service is one of the basics of the Amateur Radio Service and there is sometimes confusion about ARES, the ARRL arm of emergency services and RACES, the government arm of amateur emergency services. ARES is activated before, during, and after an emergency. Generally, ARES handles all emergency messages, including those between government emergency management officials. As an example, the ARRL recruited ARES team members from all over the country to provide communications in response to the Katrina and Rita Hurricanes. They supported field kitchens, mobile meal delivery, shelters, and wherever else they were needed, around the clock, for about six weeks. RACES, on the other hand, almost never starts before an emergency and is active only during the emergency and during the immediate aftermath, if government emergency management offices need communications support. RACES is normally shut down shortly after the emergency has cleared. Radio operations are limited to one hour of training per month, and team members can only be called upon by a government agency when there is a formal emergency declaration.

17.2 What Motivates "hams" to Volunteer their Time, Skills, and Equipment?

It is significant that Part 97 of the Federal Communications Commission's (FCC) Rules and Regulations states, as the first principle under "Basis and Purpose," the following: *"Recognition and enhancement of the value of the amateur service to the public as a voluntary non-commercial communication service, particularly with respect to providing emergency communications."* [5]. Amateur radio operators are encouraged to provide community and public service response to various agencies and organizations, as a return for the use of the radio spectrum they utilize.

There are only about 15–20% of the licensed amateur radio operators who take this to heart and really volunteer their time—and they have a ball doing it! Parades, marathons, rallies, races, etc. all enjoy the support of amateur radio providing communications. Of a more serious nature are those who belong to and participate in the activities of the ARES and RACES teams in their communities. Those who do, usually spend a lot of time training and preparing for that big event when their services are REALLY needed. The recent hurricanes in the Gulf Coast are a perfect example of this. Amateur Radio operators came from all over the country, at their own personal expense, to provide communications for the beleaguered government and non-government organizations.

17.3 External Hospital Communications

Hospitals need to be able to communicate with a variety of organizations and agencies "7 × 24 × 365." (Seven days per week, 24 hours per day, and 365 days per year). When these communication systems fail or are overloaded, it places a huge stress on the facility's ability to serve its patients and provide safe and effective healthcare. During a routine business day, hospitals have a variety of means for communicating internally and with other hospitals, emergency medical systems (EMS), vendors, suppliers, health departments, as well as patients and their families. If this is disrupted, because of a large mass-casualty incident, a natural or man-made disaster, or even just a technological failure, communications becomes a huge problem. Building communication redundancy and flexibility into the hospital response system is a vital necessity. There are a variety of ways to do this:

(a) Most hospitals already have a variety of radio communication systems, in addition to the normal land-line and cellular telephone systems. Sometimes these radio systems can take up the slack, but often they become overloaded as well. The Hospital Emergency Administrative Radio (HEAR) system is relatively common across the United States in hospitals and EMS units. It is often used for EMS units to notify hospitals that there are incoming casualties or patients. This system was developed in the 1970s and not much has been done to modify it, although there is some newer equipment available. The technology is old enough that it is unlikely that it can ever be brought up to current interoperability standards (APCO-25) [6]. Other radio systems, in addition to, or replacement of, the HEAR system include UHF, VHF, 800 MHz, and others commonly used by public safety agencies (Fire, EMS, police). These are used for day-to-day to communicate with the hospitals, but often become overloaded when some unanticipated large-scale event occurs.

The Amateur Radio Service has multiple segments of all of these bands, which allows it to be more versatile and responsive to various communication needs than many of the public safety radio systems.

> UHF/VHF/HF—These terms indicate various bands of the radio spectrum, each with its own characteristics for distance, penetration, and inter-agency communication. Ultra-high frequency (UHF: 300–3000 MHz) has shorter wave-length, but greater penetration within a building; Very-high Frequency (VHF: 30–300 MHz), has somewhat longer wave-length and distance, but works less well within the facility compound. High-frequency (HF: 1.8–30.0 MHz) is used for long-distance communications—across state or national boundaries, depending on the frequency band and antenna used [7].

(b) HF issues—there are a number of technological challenges to be aware of when using HF frequencies in the healthcare environment. Radios which transmit on these frequencies are often higher-powered than those on the UHF and VHF bands, and the antennas often have a stronger radiation pattern, which have the potential to interfere with medical telemetry and other biomedical equipment. Careful location and polarization of the antenna in or above patient-care areas needs to be taken into consideration when installing HF radios in a hospital setting.

Communication systems for hospitals, and other health-care entities, depend on reliability, constancy, and redundancy. Systems need to be reliable; they need to be there all the time and they need to be redundant. There are multiple examples of how systems can fail; what other systems can replace or supplement them, and, when all else fails, who comes to the rescue.

Examples: Why not put in actual hospital names and references to news articles? Hurricaine Katrina? ***Mostly they are anecdotal from local experiences, and were not ever publicized.***

- King County, WA—December 1998—A large metropolitan hospital suffered a failure of a co-generation electrical system. A routine test of the cutover from commercial power to a new $5.9 million hospital co-generation system, with the failure of a $10.00 part, caused the evacuation of an entire hospital, potentially life-threatening patient care events and huge loss of revenue. Most of the patients transferred out were not returned to the hospital after power was restored. This power failure lasted over 8 hours.

- King County, WA—2001—a lightning strike to a metropolitan hospital took out hospital switchboard for several hours. Another hospital in Pierce County, WA took a lightning strike to a radio antenna, which completely melted the fiberglass mast and the metal parts of it. This was not discovered until they noticed that the coaxial cable was charred, and the radio was not working.
- Whatcom Co., WA—2002—There have been two separate instances of communication disruption to an entire community, including 9-1-1 systems, when someone dug up the fiber-optic lines feeding the county communications system. Both disruptions lasted several hours. During these periods, there was no way for patients to contact emergency services, or for hospital to contact staff, patients, vendors, or ambulances. Both instances took several hours to restore service.
- Clallam County, WA—February 2004—A Port Angeles hospital reported that the entire community had lost Internet, 800, long distance, Metro call paging as well as cell phone coverage. The call came via wireless cell phone from a cell tower on Vancouver Island, B.C. This single Verizon cell phone was apparently the only means of communications outside of Port Angeles that the hospital was aware of. Their contingency plan, should they need aero-medical evacuation or other assistance would be to use this phone or someone would go to the nearby Coast Guard Station which had communication with Seattle Coast Guard. Due to topography (Olympic Mountains) there is no line of sight communications from Seattle to Port Angeles. Apparently a second cable failed at about 1500 which caused a more significant loss of communication. Reason for the failure of fiber-optic cables is still unknown.
- Lewis County, WA—February 2004—Approximately 8:40 AM, the hospital's internal phone system went dead. Investigation identified that the UPS (Uninterruptible Power Supply) failed, which shorted out the ability to turn on the back-up battery function. The hospital's emergency fail-safe phones were turned on manually and were affected also. Some did not have dial tones. Some could make calls out of the facility, but could not get calls in. Additionally, staff members reported that they could not call out on their cell phones. Power was returned to the telephone system about 9:55 AM by re-wiring around the UPS. Hospital communications were limited for 2–3 hours [8].

17.4 Redundant Systems and Pathways

Every hospital communication system should have multiple routes for incoming and outgoing messages. Phone and electrical systems should have multiple access points to the facility, and multiple Central Office connections. Single-point access paths are bound to fail eventually. In addition to multiple access points, there should be a variety of systems to perform similar functions. Reliance on any single communication system could result in serious adverse events for the hospital. The capacity to do this depends on the telecommunications and information technology departments within the facility. Technology is expensive and complex, but lack of communications can be even more expensive in the long run.

Amateur Radio can contribute significantly to recovery from a communications failure by providing backup emergency communications until normal systems are restored. In each of the above mentioned events, amateur radio operators were called in to provide communications to support the hospital mission. Depending on the facility, these resources were used to greater or lesser degree. But each facility learned that the amateur radio operators really could provide the necessary links to keep life-safety and basic, essential communication functioning. Amateur radio has the advantage of being frequency-agile (meaning the ability to change frequencies and bands readily, which most public-safety and commercial radios cannot do), communications-savvy, and knowledgeable as to what services operate on which frequency bands. They can usually contact the necessary agencies, or route information to them, using the assigned amateur radio frequencies, or by linking the radio to a telephone-patch.

Amateur radio operators commonly support many different communication activities. These include hospital–hospital, hospital–emergency operation center (EOC), hospital–field sites (usually mass-casualty incidents), and hospital–medical suppliers. Wherever portable communications are needed, amateur radio operators can usually go.

Another support mission that they sometimes fulfill is to provide communications for National Disaster Medical System (NDMS) exercises; and occasionally support the Disaster Medical Assistance teams in exercises and deployments [9].

17.5 Where can a Hospital or Healthcare System Find Amateur Radio Resources?

Often the best recruiting source is within the staff of the facility, or within the ranks of hospital volunteers, or even patient populations. Recruitment ads in hospital newsletters, employee and patient bulletin boards, etc. often produce immediate results. However, often times staff members will be required to perform their professional assignments during a disaster, and will not be available for "radio" duty. They can be useful for making that initial call, or serving until outside volunteers can arrive.

If internal recruiting does not work, then contacting the local ARES Emergency Coordinator and requesting their assistance is the next step. Usually, the local emergency management agency will know who that is; or you can access the ARRL Web page to find out [10]. This will give you a list of the Section Managers by region, and contacting them for assistance should produce results.

Once you have identified some radio operators, then the task is to form them into a hospital-focused team. This is the job of the Emergency Coordinator, but he or she will need help from the healthcare providers, for they need some orientation to hospital culture, operations, and hierarchy. In many locations, there may not be enough operators to dedicate to a specific mission, and they will be shared with emergency management, search and rescue, and other mission-oriented tasks. There are some hams who choose not to support these other government-focused groups, but would be really enthusiastic about supporting "their" hospital, so it is definitely worth asking the question, or sending out a special invitation.

The operators will need some training to familiarize them with how the hospital works, and special needs and concerns when working in this environment. Some suggested topics include:

- Orientation to Hospital environment and culture
- Health Insurance Portability and Accountability Act (HIPAA) Awareness
- Hospital Emergency Incident Command System (HEICS)
- Medical radio systems
- First Aid, CPR, and Blood-borne pathogens
- Working in a professional/business environment
- National Incident Management System (NIMS) Awareness
- Weapons of Mass Destruction (WMD) Awareness

(The last two of these classes are ones that are required of hospital personnel if they are recipients of Homeland Security grants.)

Most ham radio operators have their own radios, and are well prepared to bring their kits with them, however, an appropriate antenna installed on the hospital roof will vastly improve the signal strength and distance that the operator can reach, when talking to facilities or agencies outside the hospital. This will also lessen the effect of any radio signals within the hospital environment. To go one step further, installing amateur radios in a secure location within the building will speed up the process of getting communications up and running when they are needed. It takes time to bring in equipment, set it up, test it, and then start operations.

It is important that radio operators be given regular access to the installed radio equipment. They need to be familiar with the operation of it, and also to verify that it is operational when needed. There have been frequent instances where roofers have taken down antennas, or someone has cut the coaxial feed-line, or the radios become inoperable for some other reason. Without regular testing, they might not be available when really needed. Additionally, it is beneficial for the radio operators to train and interact with the hospital staff, so that they become comfortable with the hospital environment. Incorporating radio operators into the twice-yearly required disaster exercises familiarizes both sides with how each functions in an event.

In the event of a switchboard or power failure situation, internal communications can be carried out within the hospital campus, using portable radios between departments or floors. The UHF band usually works best because of the wavelength and penetration characteristics. This usage can be combined with external-to-the-hospital communications, using the amateur radio antenna installed on the roof. If this were a localized emergency, the outside antenna could be used to stay in contact with public safety or other hospitals, and the portables could be used to communicate and coordinate between hospital departments. There are a few areas of the buildings where radio waves do not penetrate well, such as shielded radiology suites, basement areas, etc., but for a limited time this support should be adequate.

Amateur radio is not limited to purely voice transmission. There are a number of digital forms of communications that allow the conversion of computer digital information to radio analog signals which can be sent over the airwaves, and then converted back to computer format at the receiving end. This facilitates the sending of large amounts of data, such as lists of supplies, damage assessment reports, or even E-mail. In the near future, higher transmission speeds and bandwidth will allow pictures, maps, and the like.

Additionally, there is another protocol that incorporates the use of Amateur television to send live video feeds from the field, such as a mass-casualty incident, back to the hospital or emergency operations center. While not used widely as yet, this format has tremendous potential for keeping the emergency managers or Emergency Department personnel apprised of what the scene looks like. It also has the capability of providing damage assessment information via either portable cameras in so-called windshield surveys, or through fixed camera sites in key areas.

17.6 Hospital Disaster Plan

Make sure that the hospital's Disaster Plan incorporates using Amateur Radio for back-up communications; and that there is a slot on the Organization chart for Communications (which is different than the Liaison-Public Information Officer position.) Often, the technical communications position falls under Logistics, but not always. Also make sure that you invite the volunteers to practice and train with the hospital when it conducts drills and exercises. The ham radio person should have a vest, and a Job Action Sheet, like every other member in the HEICS plan of action.

For further information, an excellent handbook called "Amateur Radio: A Communications Resource for Hospital Emergencies," written by April Moell, WA6OPS, published in 1996, is available from the author [11].

17.7 Summary and Conclusions

Hospitals depend on reliable and redundant communications to provide safe and effective healthcare to patients. Most of the time, wired and wireless telephone systems provide the majority of the communication "transactions"; and some use of public safety or commercial radio systems are used to augment this. Treatment orders, tests,

Ø = Zero; "I." = Island; "Is." = Islands

COMMON PREFIXES OF COUNTRIES (2004)

UPDATED 4/04

PREFIX	COUNTRY	PREFIX	COUNTRY	PREFIX	COUNTRY	PREFIX	COUNTRY	PREFIX	COUNTRY
1AØ	Sov. Mil. Order of Malta	C8-C9	Mozambique	H4	Solomon Is.	OJØ	Market Reef	VK9L	Lord Howe I.
1S, 9MØ	Spratly Is.	CA-CE	Chile	H4Ø	Temotu Province	OK-OL	Czech Republic	VK9M	Mellish Reef
3A	Monaco	CEØX	San Felix & San Ambrosio Is.	HA	Hungary	OM	Slovak Republic	VK9N	Norfolk I.
3B6, 3B7	Agalega & St. Brandon Is.	CEØY	Easter I.	HB	Switzerland	ON-OT	Belgium	VK9W	Willis I.
3B8	Mauritius	CEØZ	Juan Fernandez Is.	HBØ	Liechtenstein	OX	Greenland	VK9X	Christmas I.
3B9	Rodriguez I.	CE9	Antarctica	HC-HD	Ecuador	OY	Faroe Is.	VO	Canada
3C	Equatorial Guinea	CM	Cuba	HC8-HD8	Galapagos Is.	OZ	Denmark	VP2E	Anguilla
3CØ	Annobon I.	CN	Morocco	HFØ	South Shetland Is.	P2	Papua New Guinea	VP2M	Montserrat
3D2	Fiji Is.	CO	Cuba	HG	Hungary	P4	Aruba	VP2V	British Virgin Is.
3D2	Rotuma I.	CP	Bolivia	HH	Haiti	P5	North Korea	VP5	Turks & Caicos Is.
3D2	Conway Reef	CT	Portugal	HI	Dominican Republic	PA-PI	Netherlands	VP6	Pitcairn I.
3DA	Swaziland	CT3	Madeira Is.	HJ-HK	Colombia	PJ2, PJ4	Bonaire, Curacao	VP8	Antarctica
3V	Tunisia	CU	Azores	HKØ	San Andres & Providencia	PJ5-PJ8	St. Maarten, Saba, St. Eustatius	VP8	Falkland Is.
3W	Vietnam	CV-CX	Uruguay	HKØ	Malpelo I.	PJ9	Netherlands Antilles	VP8	South Georgia I.
3X	Guinea	CYØ	Sable I.	HL	South Korea	PP-PY	Brazil	VP8	South Shetland Is.
3Y	Bouvet I.	CY9	St. Paul I.	HO-HP	Panama	PPØ-PYØF	Fernando de Noronha	VP8	South Orkney Is.
3Y	Peter I I.	D2, D3	Angola	HQ-HR	Honduras	PPØ, PYØS	St. Peter & St. Paul Rocks	VP8	South Sandwich Is.
4J-4K	Azerbaijan	D4	Cape Verde	HS, E2	Thailand	PPØ, PYØT	Trindade I. & Martim Vaz Is.	VP9	Bermuda
4L	Georgia	D6	Comoros	HV	Vatican	PZ	Surinam	VQ9	Chagos Is.
4P-4S	Sri Lanka	DA-DL	Germany	HZ	Saudi Arabia	RA-RZ	European Russia	VS6	Hong Kong
4U_UN	United Nations HQ	DU-DZ	Philippines	I	Italy	RA-RZ	Asiatic Russia	VU	Andaman & Nicobar Is.
4U_ITU	ITU Headquarters	E2	Thailand	ISØ, IMØ	Sardinia	R1FJ	Franz Josef Land	VU	Laccadive Is.
4W	Timor-Leste	E3	Eritrea	J2	Djibouti	R1MV	Malyj Vysotskij I.	VU	India
4X, 4Z	Israel	E4	Palestine	J3	Grenada	SØ	Western Sahara	VY	Canada
5A	Libya	EA-EH	Spain	J5	Guinea-Bissau	S2	Bangledesh	W	USA
5B	Cyprus	EA6-EH6	Balearic Is.	J6	St. Lucia	S5	Slovenia	XA-XI	Mexico
5H-5I	Tanzania	EA8-EH8	Canary Is.	J7	Dominica	S7	Seychelles	XA4-XI4	Revilla Gigedo
5N-5O	Nigeria	EA9-EH9	Ceuta & Melilla	J8	St. Vincent	S9	Sao Tome & Principe	XT	Burkina Faso
5R-5S	Madagascar	EI-EJ	Ireland	JA-JS	Japan	SA-SM	Sweden	XU	Cambodia
5T	Mauritania	EK	Armenia	JD1	Minami-Torishima	SN-SR	Poland	XV	Vietnam
5U	Niger	EL	Liberia	JD1	Ogasawara	ST	Sudan	XW	Laos
5V	Togo	EM-EO	Ukraine	JT-JV	Mongolia	SU	Egypt	XX9	Macao
5W	Western Samoa	EP-EQ	Iran	JW	Svalbard	SV/A	Mount Athos	XY-XZ	Myanmar
5X	Uganda	ER	Moldova	JX	Jan Mayen	SV-SZ	Greece	YA	Afghanistan
5Y-5Z	Kenya	ES	Estonia	JY	Jordan	SV5	Dodecanese	YB-YH	Indonesia
6V-6W	Senegal	ET	Ethiopia	K	U.S.A.	SV9	Crete	YI	Iraq
6Y	Jamaica	EU-EW	Belarus	KC4	Antarctica	T2	Tuvalu	YJ	Vanuatu
7O	Yemen	EX	Kyrgzstan	KC6	Palau	T3Ø	West Kiribati Is.	YK	Syria
7P	Lesotho	EY	Tajikistan	KG4	Guantanamo Bay	T31	Central Kiribati Is.	YL	Latvia
7Q	Malawi	EZ	Turkmenistan	KHØ	Marianas Is.	T32	East Kiribati Is.	YN	Nicaragua
7T-7Y	Algeria	F	France	KH1	Baker & Howland Is.	T33	Banaba I.	YO-YR	Romania
8P	Barbados	FG	Guadeloupe	KH2	Guam	T5	Somalia	YS	El Salvador
8Q	Maldive Is.	FH	Mayotte	KH3	Johnston I.	T7	San Marino	YT-YU	Serbia & Montenegro
8R	Guyana	FJ	Saint Martin	KH4	Midway I.	T8	Palau	YU3	Slovenia
9A	Croatia	FK	New Caledonia	KH5	Palymra & Jarvis Is.	T9	Bosnia-Herzegovina	YV-YY	Venezuela
9G	Ghana	FK/C	Chesterfield Is.	KH5K	Kingman Reef	TA-TC	Turkey	YVØ	Aves I.
9H	Malta	FM	Martinique	KH6-KH7	Hawaii	TD	Guatemala	YZ	Serbia & Montenegro
9I, 9J	Zambia	FO	Austral I.	KH7K	Kure I.	TE	Costa Rica	Z2	Zimbabwe
9K	Kuwait	FO	Clipperton I.	KH8	American Samoa	TF	Iceland	Z3	Macedonia
9L	Sierra Leone	FO	French Polynesia	KH9	Wake I.	TG	Guatemala	ZA	Albania
9MØ	Spratly Is.	FO	Marquesas I.	KL7	Alaska	TI	Costa Rica	ZB2	Gibraltar
9M2, 9M4	West Malaysia	FP	St. Pierre & Miquelon	KP1	Navassa I.	TI9	Cocos I.	ZC4	UK Sov. Base on Cyprus
9M6, 9M8	East Malaysia	FR	Reunion I.	KP2	Virgin Is.	TJ	Cameroon	ZD7	St. Helena I.
9N	Nepal	FR/E	Europa Is.	KP3-KP4	Puerto Rico	TK	Corsica	ZD8	Ascension I.
9Q-9T	Democratic Rep. of Congo	FR/G	Glorioso Is.	KP5	Desecheo I.	TL	Central African Republic	ZD9	Tristan da Cunha & Gough Is.
9U	Burundi	FR/J	Juan de Nova Is.	LA-LN	Norway	TN	Congo	ZF	Cayman Is.
9V	Singapore	FR/T	Tromelin I.	LO-LW	Argentina	TR	Gabon	ZK1	South Cook Is.
9X	Rwanda	FS	Saint Martin	LU	South Georgia I.	TT	Chad	ZK1	North Cook Is.
9Y-9Z	Trinidad & Tobago	FT5W	Crozet Is.	LU	South Shetland Is.	TU	Ivory Coast	ZK2	Niue
A2	Botswana	FT5X	Kerguelen Is.	LU	South Orkney Is.	TY	Benin	ZK3	Tokelau Is.
A3	Tonga	FT5Z	Amsterdam & St. Paul Is.	LU	South Sandwich Is.	TZ	Mali	ZL-ZM	New Zealand
A4	Oman	FW	Wallis & Futuna Is.	LX	Luxembourg	UA2	Kaliningrad	ZL7	Chatham Is.
A5	Bhutan	FY	French Guiana	LY	Lithuania	UJ-UM	Uzbekistan	ZL8	Kermadec Is.
A6	United Arab Emirates	G	England	LZ	Bulgaria	UN-UQ	Kazakhstan	ZL9	Auckland & Campbell Is.
A7	Qatar	GC	Wales	M	England	UR-UZ	Ukraine	ZP	Paraguay
A9	Bahrain	GD	Isle of Man	MD	Isle of Man	V2	Antigua & Barbuda	ZR-ZU	South Africa
AA-AK	USA	GH	Jersey	MI	Northern Ireland	V3	Belize	ZS8	Prince Edward & Marion Is.
AP-AS	Pakistan	GI	Northern Ireland	MJ	Jersey	V4	St. Kitts & Nevis		
BS7	Scarborough Reef	GJ	Jersey	MM	Scotland	V5	Namibia		
BT	China	GM	Scotland	MU	Guernsey	V6	Micronesia		
BV	Taiwan	GN	Northern Ireland	MW	Wales	V7	Marshall Is.		
BV9P	Pratas I.	GP	Guernsey	N	USA	V8	Brunei, Darussalam		
BY	China	GS	Scotland	OA-OC	Peru	VE	Canada		
C2	Nauru	GT	Isle of Man	OD	Lebanon	VK	Australia		
C3	Andorra	GU	Guernsey	OE	Austria	VKØ	Heard I.		
C5	The Gambia	GW	Wales	OF-OI	Finland	VKØ	Macquarie I.		
C6	Bahamas	GX	England	OHØ	Aland Is.	VK9C	Cocos (Keeling) Is.		

BAND PLAN FREQUENCY ASSIGNMENTS

23-cm, 1240-1300 MHz ARRL Band Plan

MHz	Use
1240-1246	ATV #1
1246-1248	Narrow-bandwidth FM point-to-point links and digital, duplex with 1258-1260 MHz
1248-1252	Digital communications
1252-1258	ATV #2
1258-1260	Narrow-bandwidth FM point-to-point links and digital, duplexed with 1246-1252 MHz
1260-1270	Satellite uplinks
1260-1270	Wide-bandwidth experimental, simplex ATV
1270-1276	Repeater inputs, FM and linear, paired with 1282-1288 MHz, 239 pairs every 25 kHz, e.g., 1270.025, 1270.050, 1270.075, etc., 1271.0-1238.0 MHz uncoordinated test pair
1276-1282	ATV #3
1282-1288	Repeater outputs, paired with 1270-1276 MHz
1288-1294	Wide-bandwidth experimental, simplex ATV
1294-1295	Narrow-bandwidth FM simplex services, 25 kHz channels
1294.5	National FM simplex calling frequency
1295-1297	Narrow bandwidth weak-signal communications (no FM)
1295.0-1295.8	SSTV, FAX, ACSB, experimental
1295.8-1296.0	Reserved for EME, CW expansion
1296.0-1296.05	EME exclusive
1296.07-1296.08	CW beacons
1296.1	CW, SSB calling frequency
1296.4-1296.6	Crossband linear translator input
1296.6-1296.8	Crossband linear translator output
1296.8-1297.0	Experimental beacons (exclusive)
1297-1300	Digital communications

ARRL 70-cm Wavelength Band Plan, 420-450 MHz

MHz	Use
420.00-426.00	ATV repeater or simplex with 421.25 MHz video carrier control links and experimental
426.00-432.00	ATV simplex with 427.250 MHz video carrier frequency
432.00-432.08	EME (Earth-Moon-Earth)
432.08-432.10	Weak-signal CW
432.100	70 cm CW/SSB calling frequency
432.10-433.00	Mixed-mode and weak-signal work
432.30-432.40	New beacon band
433.00-435.00	Auxiliary/repeater links
435.00-438.00	Satellite only uplink/downlink
438.00-444.00	ATV repeater input with 439.250 MHz video carrier frequency and repeater links
442.00-445.00	Repeater inputs and outputs (local option)
445.00-447.00	Shared by auxiliary and control links, repeaters and simplex (local option); 446.00 MHz national simplex frequency
447.00-450.00	Repeater inputs and outputs

ARRL 33-cm Wavelength Band Plan, 902-928 MHz

MHz	Use
902-904	Narrow-bandwidth, weak-signal communications
902.0-902.8	SSTV, FAX, ACSB, experimental
902.8-903.0	Reserved for EME, CW expansion
903.0-903.05	EME exclusive
903.07-903.08	CW beacons
903.1	CW, SSB calling frequency
903.4-903.6	Crossband linear translator inputs
903.6-903.8	Crossband linear translator outputs
903.8-904.0	Experimental beacons exclusive

ARRL 33-cm Wavelength Band Plan, 902-928 MHz (cont.)

MHz	Use
904-906	Digital communications
906-907	Narrow bandwidth FM-simplex services, 25 kHz channels
906.50	National simplex frequency
907-910	FM repeater inputs paired with 919-922 MHz; 119 pairs every 25 kHz; e.g., 907.025, 907.050, 907.075, etc., 908-920 MHz uncoordinated pair
910-916	ATV
916-918	Digital communications
918-919	Narrow-bandwidth, FM control links and remote bases
919-922	FM repeater outputs, paired with 907-910 MHz
922-928	Wide-bandwidth experimental, simplex ATV, Spread Spectrum

ARRL 2 Meter Wavelength Band Plan, 144-148 MHz

MHz	Use
144.00 144.05	EME (CW)
144.275-144.300	Propagation beacons
144.06-144.10	General CW and weak signals
144.10-144.20	EME and weak-signal SSB
144.200	National SSB calling frequency
144.200-144.275	General SSB operation, upper sideband
144.275-144.300	Beacon band
144.30-144.50	OSCAR subband plus simplex
144.50-144.60	Linear translator outputs
144.60-144.90	FM repeater inputs
144.90-145.10	Weak signal and FM simplex
145.10-145.20	Linear translator outputs plus packet
145.20-145.50	FM repeater outputs
145.50-145.80	Miscellaneous and experimental modes
145.80-146.00	OSCAR subband – satellite use only!
146.01-146.37	Repeater inputs
146.40-146.58	Simplex
146.61-146.97	Repeater outputs

ARRL 2 Meter Wavelength Band Plan, 144-148 MHz (cont.)

MHz	Use
147.00-147.39	Repeater outputs
147.42-147.57	Simplex
147.60-147.99	Repeater inputs

ARRL 6 Meter Wavelength Band Plan, 50.0-54.0 MHz

MHz	Use
50.000-50.100	CW and beacons
50.060-50.080	U.S. beacons
50.100-50.600	SSB
50.125	SSB DX calling frequency
50.200	SSB domestic calling frequency (Note: Suggest QSY up for local & down for long-distance QSOs)
50.400	AM calling frequency
50.600-51.000	Experimental and special modes
50.700	RTTY calling frequency
50.800-50.980	Radio Control (R/C) channels, 10 channels spaced 20 kHz apart (new)
51.000-51.100	Pacific DX window
51.000-52.000	Newly authorized FM repeater allocation
51.100-52.000	FM simplex
52.000-52.050	Pacific DX window
52.000-53.000	FM repeater and simplex
53.000-54.000	Present radio control (R/C) channels, 10 channels spaced 100 kHz apart

ICOM®

SOUTHERN CALIFORNIA REGIONAL NOTE: Southern California, plus other major metropolitan cities throughout the country, may adopt local 2 Meter band plans slightly different than what appears here. See your local Icom dealer for more local details. 6836

Figure 17.1 Amateur Radio Spectrum Chart showing band allocations [12].

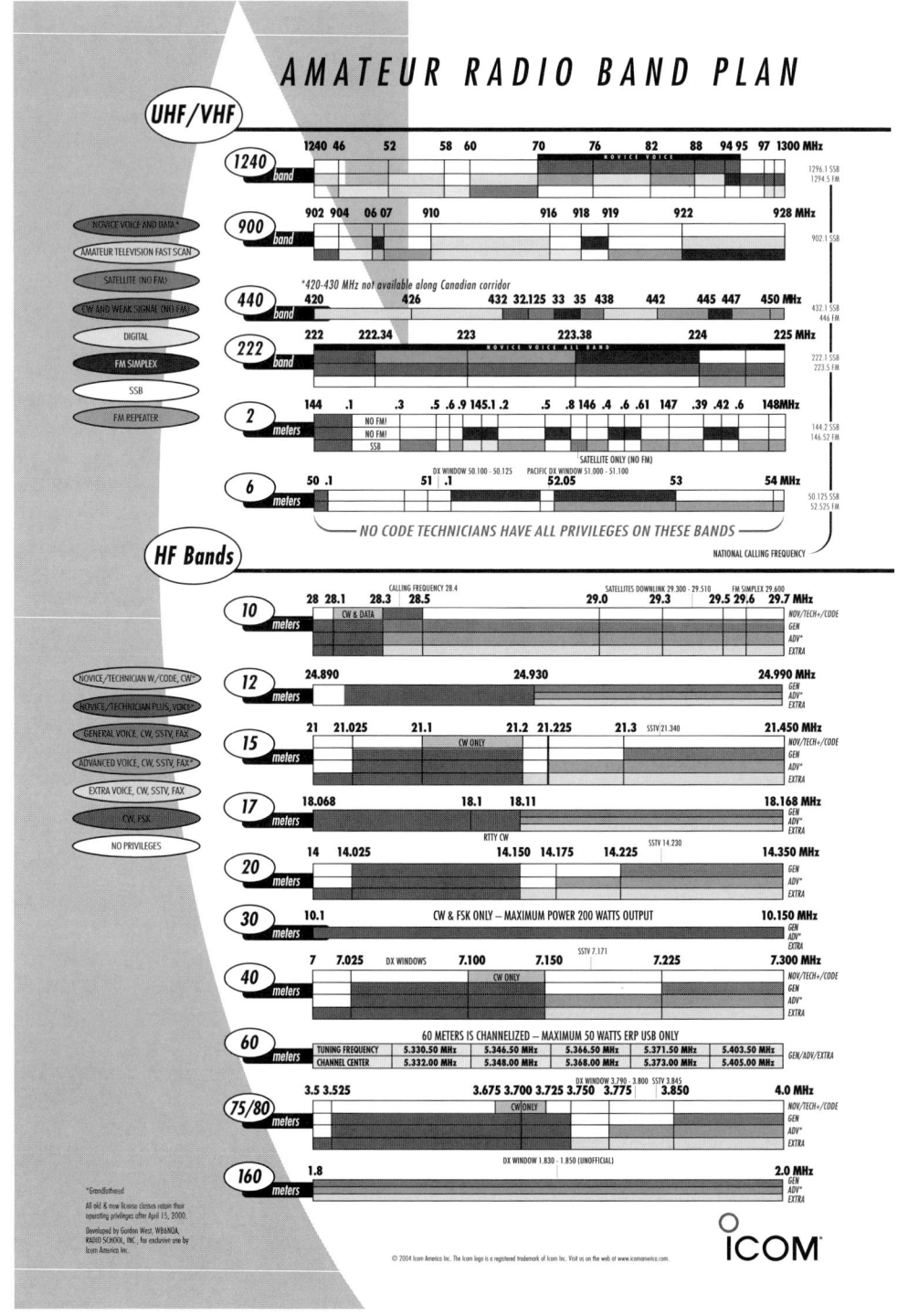

Figure 17.1 Continued.

information requests, supplies, and pharmaceutical orders are all relayed by some form of telephone, radio, or computer system. Patients are delivered or discharged using phones, radios, etc. What would happen if, suddenly, all these communication systems failed?

Hospital disaster plans should include alternative communication methods, and they should be practiced right along with other elements of an exercise or drill.

Amateur radio operators, also known as hams, are experienced, trained emergency communicators who are volunteers. Their services are free; they really enjoy performing their special service and using their skills. They usually bring their own equipment, although having equipment in the hospital ready to go will speed up the response time. They can provide both internal and external communications; and they have use of a wide variety of radio frequencies and modes. They can free up hospital personnel to perform patient care, and leave the monitoring of radios, and sending and receiving messages to those who really like to do it.

Amateur Radio is an excellent resource that should be included in every hospital's planning for response and recovery.

References

1. http://www.access.gpo.gov/nara/cfr/waisidx_04/47cfr97_04.html
2. http://www.arrl.org
3. http://www.races.net/
4. <http://www.fema.gov/library/civilpg.shtm>
5. http://www.access.gpo.gov/nara/cfr/waisidx_04/47cfr97_04.html
6. ftp://www.fcc.gov/pub/Reports/rpts5001.txt
7. http://www.ntia.doc.gov/osmhome/allochrt.html
8. Marina, Zuetell. Providing efficient healthcare when the phones fail. *Washington Family Physician*, 31(2): 30–32, 2004.
9. http//:www.fema.gov/news/newsrelease.fema?id=11927
10. http//:www.arrl.org/FandES/field/org/smlist
11. http//:www.hdscs.org
12. http//:www.icomamerica.com/amateur/

Additional Resources

http://www.emcomm.org/
http://www.ww7mst.org

18 Hospital Power: Critical Care

JAMES F. NEWTON, P. E.

A severe thunderstorm, a construction crew digging in the wrong place, an earthquake, hurricane, ice storm, or even a squirrel that finds its way into a substation can leave a medical facility without normal power for a few minutes, a few days, or even longer. The situation is further complicated by the expectations of hospital administrators, doctors, patients, and the general public that their hospital will be fully functional under any circumstance, regardless of the unpredictability or severity of the situation. Understanding code requirements, performing a hazard vulnerability analysis, and understanding what role the medical facility has in the community during an emergency are all essential to designing a safe and reliable hvac system for a hospital (Figure 18.1).

The loss of normal power at a medical facility, whether the result of a natural disaster or system failure, is a situation that every health care engineer must anticipate. Certain hvac equipment is required by the National Electric Code or mandated by the authority having jurisdiction (AHJ) to be connected to the emergency power system of a hospital. Hvac systems that are not code required or mandated for connection to the emergency power system may still need to operate to meet the facility's needs during a number of critical situations.

Performing a hazard vulnerability analysis as outlined by the Joint Commission on Accreditation of Healthcare Organizations (JCAHO) is the best way to begin to establish the extent of the hvac emergency power requirements that are above the minimum required by code or otherwise mandated. The first step, however, is to understand the code requirements.

18.1 Code Required Systems

The National Electric Code (NEC) and National Fire Protection Association Standard for Healthcare Facilities (NFPA 99) require certain hvac systems to be connected to the emergency power system in a hospital. The following is a summary of those hvac systems:

Generator-related equipment

- Fuel pumps;
- Damper operators and controls;
- Ventilation and combustion air fans; and
- Remote radiator fans.

Fire safety systems

- Smoke control systems including exhaust fans, air-handling equipment, and controls;
- Stair pressurization equipment and controls; and
- Kitchen hoods.

Heating equipment to maintain inside design temperature where the outside design temperature is lower than +20 °F

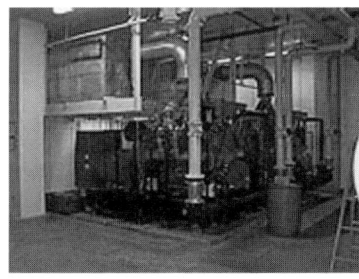

Figure 18.1 The 1.2 MW generators shown here are the heart of the emergency power system at this hospital.

- Operating rooms and associated support spaces;
- Labor and delivery rooms and associated support spaces;
- Recovery areas;
- Intensive care and coronary care units;
- Nurseries;
- Protective and infectious isolation rooms;
- Emergency treatment spaces; and
- General patient rooms.

Supply, return, and exhaust air systems serving the following areas

- Surgical and obstetrical delivery suites and associated support spaces;
- Intensive care and coronary care units;
- Protective and infectious isolation rooms;
- Emergency treatment spaces;
- Exhaust fans for fume hoods and radio-isotope hoods; and
- Ethylene oxide evacuation and anesthesia evacuation systems.

The hvac systems and equipment listed above are considered to be the minimum requirements in an acute care hospital. Additional state and local requirements will add to the minimum requirements. These requirements should be understood prior to the start of any design.

18.2 Recommended Systems

With respect to the operation of a hospital, it is important to understand the need for those hvac systems that may not be mandated for connection to the emergency power system to remain in service during a loss of normal power. Often, it is only after the hospital experiences a loss of power for an extended duration that deficiencies are uncovered.

Outlined below are the systems and equipment frequently overlooked due to a lack of understanding of the equipment and procedures needed during a loss of power.

The following should be placed on emergency power under most circumstances.

- Building automation system:
  Head-end computer;
  Control panels;
  Control air compressors and dryers; and
  Any electric controls serving systems on emergency power.
- Refrigeration system and controls for food storage and clinical laboratory refrigerators and freezers.
- Hvac systems serving telecommunication rooms and computer rooms.
- Water chillers, pumps, and controls for MRIs, CT scanners, and linear accelerators—city water cooling as a redundant source of cooling may be allowed in some jurisdictions.
- Autopsy room exhaust air systems and refrigeration systems for body cold boxes.
- Supply, return, and exhaust air systems serving bone marrow treatment areas.
- Supply and general exhaust air serving the clinical laboratory to maintain pressure relationships.
- Electric heat tape for exposed piping, absorption chillers to prevent crystallization, oil sump heaters on electric centrifugal chillers.

It is critical that the criteria for the systems required to be connected to emergency power be established as early in the design phase as is possible. Major system decisions are dependent on an early understanding of these issues. As an example, the number of air-handling units (AHU) and what departments they will serve can have an impact on the size of the mechanical rooms, as well as the size of the emergency generator.

18.3 HVAC System Impact on Generator Size

Hvac systems have a significant impact on the emergency power system of a hospital. The connected load of the hvac equipment can range from 3 to 6 W/sq ft in an acute care facility. This is generally 50–60% of the entire load on the emergency generator plant. With the typical cost of an emergency generator plant ranging from $800 to $1200/kW of generator capacity, the cost of adding 100 hp of motor load could be as high as $90,000.

It goes without saying that care must be taken when determining what hvac equipment is required to be connected to the emergency power system. Establishing an appropriate balance between the cost of adding equipment to the emergency generator and the risk of not having hvac service during a loss of power is a difficult task.

Mechanical cooling is one of the most difficult issues to resolve in establishing the criteria. There are certain departments of a hospital that should have provisions for providing air conditioning even when normal power is not available. The operating suite, post-anesthesia care units, and the intensive care units are areas of the hospital where patient safety may be compromised if the rooms are outside certain temperature and humidity requirements. In certain warm and humid climates, consideration should be given to providing mechanical cooling in all patient rooms and diagnostic and treatment areas.

18.4 What can Happen during the Loss of Normal Power

At a recent planning meeting to discuss a major expansion to the operating suite of a 350-bed hospital, the director of facilities described what happened during the loss of normal power at his facility. It was 3 p.m. and the temperature was 95° with extreme humidity. A line of severe thunderstorms had resulted in a loss of normal power at the hospital. The emergency generators were running hot and concern was growing that they may shut down due to the high temperature.

As the outage continued into the second hour, the situation was becoming much more severe inside the hospital. The AHUs that are required to be connected to the emergency power system for ventilation of the critical areas were running. The problem was that the minimum outside air dampers were open and the system was pumping hot and humid air into the critical areas. Fortunately, the scheduled surgeries for the day were complete, but doctors and nurses were calling from all areas of the hospital with urgent requests for cooling as concern for patient safety grew. The power was back by 6 p.m. and the conditions slowly improved.

After the event, the director of facilities was under pressure from the hospital administrators and doctors to explain how this could have happened. They were amazed to find out that cooling was not available after a power outage caused by something as common as a thunderstorm. The answer could be traced back to a value engineering decision made during the last hospital expansion. The chiller plant needed additional capacity to serve the proposed expansion and a new emergency generator and electric centrifugal chiller were proposed for the chiller plant.

One cooling tower, one condenser water pump, one primary chilled-water pump, and one secondary pump were to be added to the new emergency generator in addition to the new chiller. Unfortunately, the cost for this solution was value engineered and the emergency generator was deleted after the bids for the expansion project were over budget.

Providing air conditioning to critical areas during a loss of normal power can require a significant amount of electricity. A typical 300-bed hospital will require approximately 300 tons of cooling to offset the cooling load in the critical areas of the facility. Even the most efficient, water-cooled, electric centrifugal chiller would require approximately 300 kW of emergency power when all ancillary pumps and cooling towers are included.

The cost of connecting this mechanical cooling system to an emergency generator could be as high as $360,000. The range of these costs will obviously vary on each project, however, the magnitude of the costs justify an analysis of alternate strategies for providing mechanical cooling upon a loss of normal power.

18.5 Alternate Cooling Strategies

There are many strategies that will allow a facility to achieve partial mechanical cooling during a loss of normal power. A central chiller plant where at least one chiller is driven by something other than an electric motor—a natural gas-fired absorption chiller, natural gas engine-driven chiller, or steam absorption chillers—are the most common choices. Other less common strategies are coupling a generator directly to the electric chiller or some form of thermal storage. Any of these strategies should be part of a larger energy strategy.

Trying to guess what energy prices will do over the course of the next five years or even five months is nearly impossible. The best recommendation for managing the volatility of energy prices over the life of an hvac system is the same advice given for good fiscal planning—diversify. A carefully thought-out energy strategy that does not rely on any single energy source for all heating or cooling needs can have many benefits.

The ability to switch to the least expensive fuel to produce chilled water during times of peak demand will lead to lower utility costs than the competing hospital who has decided to take the lowest first cost approach to chilled water and steam production. A secondary benefit to the diversification of energy usage is the ability to produce chilled water for the critical areas of the hospital with minimal investment when compared to the cost of electrically driven chillers or direct-expansion equipment connected to the emergency power system.

18.6 Emergency Generator Coordination

Another issue that must be considered in the design of a safe and reliable hvac system is the effect of the major hvac systems on the generator. It is clear that if the emergency generator is running and all of the hvac motors were transferred onto the emergency generator simultaneously, the generator would probably shut down due to the inrush current.

To avoid this situation, it is advisable to integrate a staggered restart into the sequence of operation of the major hvac equipment after a loss of normal power. A similar situation may occur if the variable-frequency drives (VFDs) have across-the-line bypass as an option. Larger motors should have some form of reduced voltage starters included as the bypass.

The design criteria for systems that have motors controlled by VFDs and are connected to the emergency generator may be different than systems connected to the normal power system. AHUs, fans, and pumps controlled by VFDs will contribute harmonic distortion into the emergency power system that will lead to a degradation of the generator. The emergency power system is much less forgiving than the larger normal power system and the harmonic distortion will reduce the service life of the generator if the distortion is not properly mitigated.

A separate harmonic analysis should be conducted on the emergency power system to ensure the system is in compliance with IEEE 519 "Recommended Practices and Requirements for Harmonic Control in Electric Power Systems."

18.7 Commissioning

A hospital is a complex building with many systems that must interact for the facility to operate under a number of different conditions. The continuity of hvac services during a power outage is dependent on the interdisciplinary coordination of design professionals, owners, and subcontractors. This is a reality that sometimes yields unintended results. Building systems commissioning can be part of the solution to ensure that the hvac and building systems perform according to the design intent. These services can be a small price to pay when you reflect on the potential consequences.

18.8 Conclusion

Understanding the role of a hospital in the community during an emergency situation where normal power is not available and determining what functions within the hospital must remain operational in that emergency are the basis for many of the hvac design decisions on a project. The right decisions will ultimately provide the hospital with a safe and reliable hvac system during a loss of normal power. Commissioning the building after the construction is complete is the best insurance the owner, engineer, and contractor have that the system will operate as intended when the inevitable loss of power occurs.

19 Electromagnetic Interference

JOSEPH H. McISAAC, III

19.1 Overview of EMI

The modern world is increasingly dependant upon electronics. It is difficult today to find a useful device that is not dependent on the transistor or integrated circuit. From the computer to the cellular telephone to the automobile, the common theme is the extensive use of low-powered digital electronics. Hospitals make even greater use of these devices than average. Even the ubiquitous paper chart is giving way to the electronic medical record. Along with this convenience comes the risk of electromagnetic interference (EMI). EMI is not new, European agencies established standards as early as 1936. In the United States, EMI requirements were instituted via MIL-STD-461 for government work and in 1979 by the Federal Communications Commission under Part 15 regulations [1,2]. Presently, medical devices are covered under the Food and Drug Administration (US) [3] and International Electrotechnical Commission (Europe) [4,5] (see Figure 19.1).

The EMI can be natural (static electricity, lightning) or man-made. It can be intentional, such as the effect from a high altitude detonation of a nuclear weapon (HEMP) or unintentional, as a byproduct of a digital circuit (see Figure 19.2). It can be radiated or conducted [1].

All electronic devices function according to Maxwell's Laws [1]. The movement of electric charges generates an electromagnetic field which propagates through space as a wave. The wave contains both an electric field vector and a magnetic field vector which are coupled together (see Figure 19.3). Either field can couple to an electronic device through capacitive (E-field) or inductive (B-field) coupling; the device functioning as an antenna.

Narrow-band (<1% center frequency) RF from 0.2 to 5 GHz tends to be very high energy and produce permanent failures. Wideband RF consists of short, often repetitive pulses over much broader spectrum. Energy is less concentrated but more likely to find system resonance and thus disrupt function. Frequencies below 10 MHz propagate

---

Association for the Advancement of Medical Instrumentation, http://www.aami.org

- American Medical Association Council on Scientific Affairs, "Report 4: Use of wireless radio-frequency devices in hospitals," http://www.ama-assn.org/ama/pub/article/2036-2918.html
- ANSI Accredited Committee C63, http://c63.ieee.org/
- ECRI, http://www.ecri.org
- FDA/CDRH EMC web page, http://www.fda.gov/cdrh/emc/index.html
- FDA/CDRH recommendations for wireless medical telemetry, http://www.fda.gov/cdrh/emc/wmt2.html
- FDA/CDRH Safety Alerts, Public Health Advisories, and Notices, http://www.fda.gov/cdrh/safety.html
- FDA MedWatch safety information and adverse event reporting program, http://www.fda.gov/medwatch/
- University of Oklahoma Center for the Study of Wireless EMC, http://www.ou.edu/engineering/emc/
- UK Medical Devices Agency, "Mobile Communications - Summary"

Figure 19.1 FDA Recommended Sites for Resources and Standards.

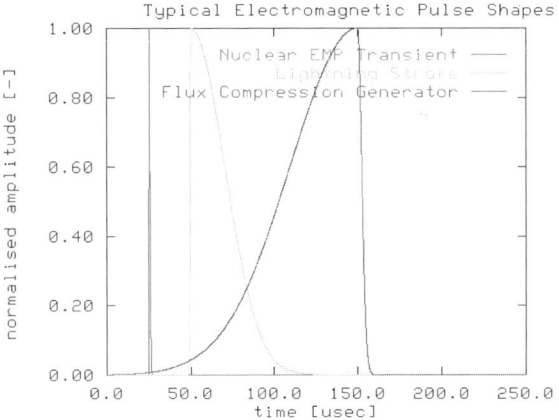

Figure 19.2 Typical Electromagnetic pulse shapes [15].

This author has measured electric fields as high as 10 kV/m induced by an 8 W, 800 MHz hand-held radio at the surface of a medical device [9]. This is 1000 times greater than the IEC standards and results from the electric near-field generated in the vicinity of an antenna. Conway and Jones [10] demonstrated that, "[i]n a clinical setting, high-power-output devices such as a two-way radio may cause significant interference in ventilator function. Medium-power output devices such as mobile phones may cause minor alarm triggers. Low-power output devices, such as Bluetooth appear to cause no interference to ventilator function."

Conducted EMI enters most commonly along power connections to a device. Transients induced locally from other devices (switching power supplies and electric motors) or over the power grid (lightning, HEMP) can gain direct entry without proper safeguards. Common mode voltages can develop on patient lead wires and device interconnects. When these lines are greater than 0.1 wavelength, they become efficient antennas [1].

Most modern equipment is well-protected against local static discharge. Lightning, on the other hand, can induce conducted transients as high as 40 kA with rise time of 20 ns resulting in a 40 kV to 250 kV voltage spike, depending on the proximity of the strike [11].

well via conduction. Frequencies above 100 MHz are efficient for radiation coupling [6,7].

Once the energy has propagated into a circuit, there is the potential for interference. Low energy EMI can occur in digital circuits as a propagation delay or by exceeding the triggering threshold of a logic device. Analog devices tend to show increasing effects as power increases and will usually recover after the EMI subsides. Digital systems usually require resetting or re-locking after an event [8]. At higher energy levels, permanent damage to low-power integrated circuits can occur.

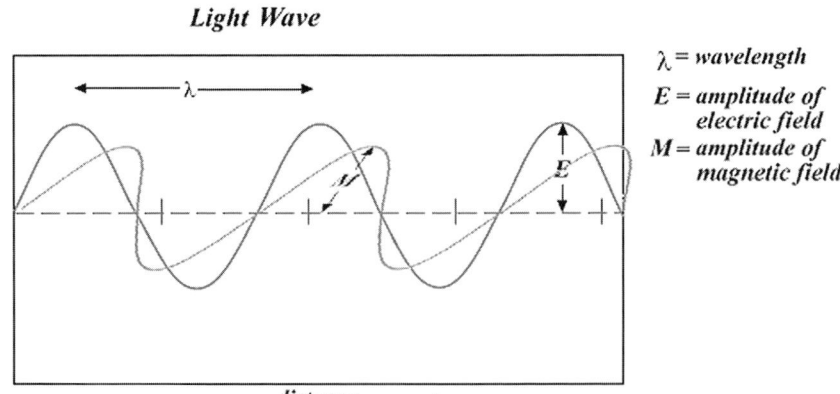

Figure 19.3 Electromagnetic field vectors [25]. (Permission is granted to copy, distribute and/or modify this document under the terms of the *GNU Free Documentation License*, Version 1.2 or any later version published by the Free Software Foundation; with no Invariant Sections, no Front-Cover Texts, and no Back-Cover Texts Subject to *disclaimers*.)

19.2 Intentional EMI

As terrorist threats are increasing world-wide, society's dependence on information and automated mission-critical and safety-critical electronic systems create an attractive target for covert operations outside physical barriers. This can manifest both as a "force multiplier" or as an isolated technique to disrupt infrastructure. "EM susceptibility of new high-density Information Technology (IT) systems working at higher frequencies and lower voltages is increasing." Intentional EMI (IEMI) is further facilitated by the proliferation of technological advances that have produced high-energy radiofrequency (RF) sources and more efficient antennas [6,7,12].

The classic IEMI paradigm is the result of the high altitude detonation of a nuclear weapon. Nine countries, the US, UK, France, Russia, China, Israel, Pakistan, India, Iran, and North Korea are thought to have this technology [13]. A high-altitude detonation of 1 megatons at 50–500 km (high enough to prevent blast effects at the surface) produces a burst of X-rays, neutrons, and gamma rays which strip electrons from the air molecules resulting in 1–3 MeV-energy Compton electrons. This transient electrical current induces a radiating RF field of 1000 V/m in the 15–250 MHz band. This is enough to cripple sensitive equipment in a 600–5000 km circle below the blast, as anything with electrical wiring becomes a receiver [14]. Enough to cover the entire United States. The affected area can actually extend much farther. A 90 percent of the Low Earth Orbit Satellites (LEOS) would be lost within a month as ionized debris interacts with the earth's magnetic field. As these fields spread out, they induce low-frequency fields which couple with long-distance power lines to induce high voltages which trigger widespread disruption of electric power circuits (see Figure 19.4) [13].

19.2.1 E-Bombs

On a smaller scale, much work has been done to develop small scale EMP devices which can act at the local battle field level. In fact, a well-written US government paper is available on the Internet which describes the theory and development of non-nuclear ultrawideband EMP bomb, complete with schematics [15].

> "The best-known type consists of an explosive packed copper cylinder surrounded by a helical, current carrying coil. Upon detonation, the explosion flares out the cylinder, short-circuiting the coil, and progressively reducing the number of turns in the coil, thus compressing the magnetic flux. Large flux compression generators have produced tens of gigawatts, and they can be cascaded—connected end to end—so that the output from one stage feeds the next. [16]"

Clearly any country with advanced technology could construct a crude device. Any well-financed terrorist with an advanced degree in electrical engineering should be able to grasp its design (see Figure 19.5).

Narrowband microwave devices can also be constructed. They range from the high-power, high-tech Shiva Star (1 TW) at Kirtland Air Force Base in New Mexico, to commercial microwave radar sets (20 kW; $20k–50k), to a simple waveguide attached to a microwave oven (1500 W, $250) [16]. Indeed, a most effective medium-sized directed energy weapon can be constructed from an ionizing laser coupled to a high power microwave source [17]. The cylinder of ionized air (a plasma) around the beam will efficiently transmit radiofrequency energy below its plasma cutoff frequency. This can be conveniently directed into buildings to disrupt digital equipment at significant standoff distances (see Figure 19.6).

19.3 Mitigation

Despite its potential for creating electronic mayhem, EMI, whether intentional or not, can be reduced or eliminated in all but the most severe cases through proper design and mitigation techniques [1,2,14]. A thorough vulnerability analysis of existing equipment, especially high value items, will result in a number of effective strategies (see Figure 19.7).

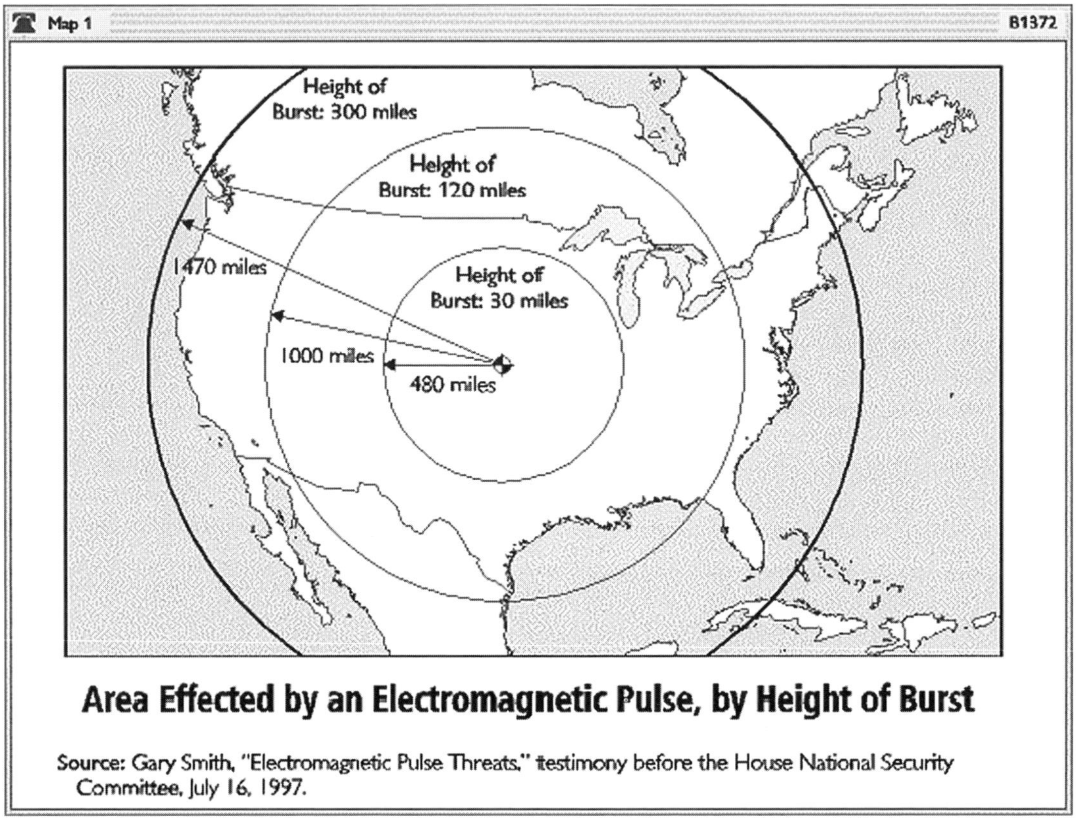

Figure 19.4 HEMP Footprint [26].

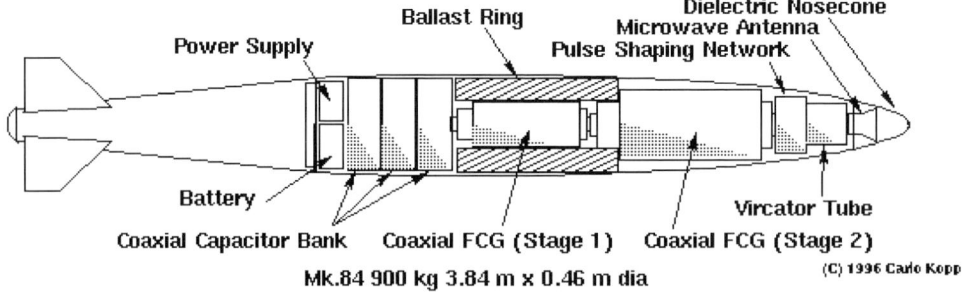

Figure 19.5 E-bomb [15].

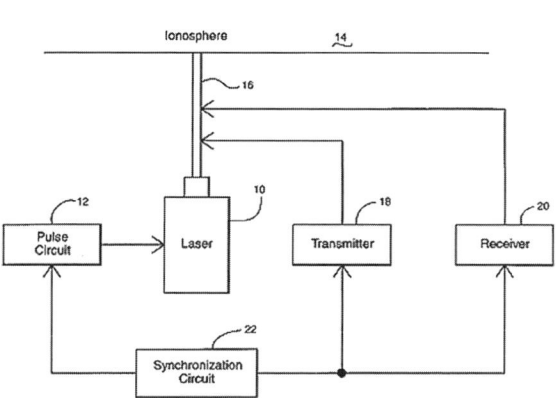

Figure 19.6 Ionizing laser antenna for IEMI device.

Grounding	Testing
Shielding	Monitoring
Filtering	Physical security
Optical coupling	

Figure 19.7 Effective strategies for EMI mitigation.

19.3.1 Grounding

Grounding is the most overlooked factor when hardening against EMI. The avoidance of ground-loops is critical to reducing interfering signals. A ground is simply a current return path. The best grounds are obtained using low impedance, single point grounds, or a ground plane. At audio frequencies, low resistance is the most important factor in reducing impedance. At higher frequencies, capacitive and inductive reactance must also be considered. Wide, short (<1/20 wavelength) flat ribbons are the preferred means of grounding at RF frequencies. Ground-loop currents can also occur without any direct contact, due to capacitive and inductive coupling. Optical coupling of digital signals is another way to prevent ground-loop currents from flowing between devices. Even micro-amps across micro-ohm ground impedances will result in enough signal to interfere with sensitive analog devices. Consideration should be given to long-term bonding of components. Corrosion of contacts can increase impedance as well as lead to non-linear effects such as rectification [2,18,19].

19.3.2 Filters and Shielding

Conducted emissions along power and signal transmission lines are best dealt with by shielding and filtering. Modern electronics produce high levels of fast transients which are readily conducted through the power mains. Standard EMI power filters do an excellent job of attenuating these unwanted signals and will work equally well against most modest IEMI. High quality shielded cable (preferably balanced line) with terminal ferrite EMI filters will prevent common mode transients from entering the equipment. Unused connectors should be covered with conductive caps. Power and signal cables should be unplugged when not in use. This prevents high energy EMI such as that from a HEMP event from conducting into critical equipment. This measure is especially critical during times of heightened vigilance. Small, hand-held equipment sealed in conductive foil or polymer ESD bags will likewise have substantial shielding from high intensity IEMI. External antennas, in addition to good lightning grounds, should be coupled to the inside transmission line through a gas discharge tube. This will rapidly shunt both lightning and HEMP impulses to ground, rather than into sensitive radio equipment. Cabinets should always be closed with their EMI gaskets properly seated. Ventilation holes are second only to cables in their ability to allow breach. All perforations of the Faraday cage act as slot antennas. They can be retrofitted with copper screen, bonded to the case to reduce this phenomenon. Care must be taken to avoid reducing air flow excessively.

19.3.3 Backup Systems

While an expensive option, thought should be given to having backup systems for mission critical devices. Often, several members of a class of device may be idle. Placing these in a physically secure, EMI-hardened state will ensure their survival after an event. Uninterruptible power supplies, which can filter both transients and power sags will allow orderly shutdown during power failures. This is important if hard drives are to avoid a crash during momentary voltage drops.

19.3.4 Security Approach

Monitoring for IEMI of high value, high risk targets such as government installations has been advocated by several authors [6,7,14]. This probably exceeds the capabilities of most medical facilities. Physical security, on the other hand, should be routine at all facilities. Access to power and wired communications should be prevented. Much has been written regarding radiated threats, but it is much easier to inject EMI into a building when there is easy access to its infrastructure. Parfenov et al. have shown that signals as low as 0.4 V injected into the power or earthing circuits of a commercial building can cause disruption of telephone equipment. A pulsed signal of several kV can cause catastrophic destruction of equipment [20]. Buffer zones around all buildings should be designed and monitored. Critical equipment should be located towards the interior of the building, away from outer walls and always have uninterruptible power supplies.

19.3.5 Testing

Nitsch [21] demonstrated that the more complex the system, the lower the power level necessary to cause equipment disruption. Hoad [22] examined the susceptibility of i486® and Pentium4® computers in a mode stirred reverberation chamber. They demonstrated, unexpectedly, that more modern systems with higher clock rates had more immunity. They speculate that the newer systems had better internal shielding to accommodate the faster speeds.

Flintoft [8] demonstrated that measuring the re-radiated spectrum can be used to predict the susceptibility of a device at field strengths below that which cause actual failure. "Specifically, non-linear behavior in the cross-modulation products... was observed as the incident field strength approached that required to cause equipment failure" [−5 dB and below]. This suggests

Make use of available resources such as EMC professionals and publications and Internet web pages on the subject of medical device EMC;

- **Assess** the electromagnetic environment of the facility (e.g., identify radio transmitters in around the facility) and identify areas where critical medical devices are used (e.g., ER, ICU, CCU, NICU);
- **Manage** the electromagnetic environment, RF transmitters and all electrical and electronic equipment, including medical devices, to reduce the risk of medical device EMI and achieve EMC;
- **Coordinate** the purchase, installation, service, and management of all electrical and electronic equipment used in the facility to achieve EMC;
- **Educate** healthcare facility staff, contractors, visitors, and patients about EMC and EMI and how they can recognize medical device EMI and help minimize EMI risks;
- **Establish and implement written policies and procedures** that document the intentions and methods of the healthcare institution for reducing the risk of medical device EMI and achieving EMC;
- **Report** EMI problems to the FDA MedWatch program and communicate EMI/EMC experiences to colleagues in open forums such as medical/technical publications and conferences.

Figure 19.8 FDA recommendations for health care facilities [27].

a useful, non-destructive, and non-disruptive test of radiated immunity for high value systems. ANSI C63.18 [23] can be used for most other systems to detect vulnerabilities. TIR 18 [24] from the Association for the Advancement of Medical Instrumentation is recommended by the FDA (see Figures 19.8 and 19.9). Strong consideration should be given to obtaining the services of a consultant who specializes in EMI/TEMPEST assessment and mitigation.

19.4 Summary

Intentional and unintentional EMI is a growing threat to the integrity of health care organizations. It has the ability to degrade or totally disrupt healthcare delivery. It is imperative that biomedical engineers understand the problem and institute robust mitigation programs to ensure the ability to survive in a crisis.

- Because of their responsibility for the safe functioning of patient care equipment, clinical/biomedical engineers should be the focal point for EMC, EMI mitigation, and EMC/EMI education/training within the health care organization.
- Purchase, installation, service, and management of all equipment (medical, communications, building systems, and information technology) used in the facility should be coordinated to assure EMC. Clinical/biomedical engineering, facility management, information systems, materials management, and risk management personnel should all be aware of the possibility for equipment interactions and the need for coordination.
- EMC/EMI should become a permanent responsibility of the health care organization's Safety Committee.
- Staff, visitors, and patients, including home-care patients, should be educated regarding the nature of EMI and how they can recognize and help prevent it.
- EMC should be considered in the site selection, design, construction, and layout of health care facilities.
- Clinical/biomedical engineers should work with facility management, telecommunications, information systems, materials management, and risk management personnel to manage the electromagnetic environment of the health care facility.
- The institution's administration or its designate, e.g., the Safety Committee, should promulgate policies and procedures that clearly set forth the intentions of the institution regarding management to achieve EMC including, among other things, the designation of areas of the facility where the use of common hand-held RF transmitters (e.g., cellular and PCS telephones, two-way radios) by staff, visitors, and/or patients is to be managed or restricted.
- Ad hoc radiated RF immunity testing should be considered when EMI is suspected, when RF transmitters are likely to operate in proximity to critical care medical devices, in prepurchase evaluation of new types of RF transmitters to determine their effect on existing medical devices, in prepurchase evaluation of new electronic medical devices, and when checking for age-related changes in medical device RF immunity. Ad hoc testing can be used to estimate the minimum distance that should be maintained between a specific RF transmitter and a specific medical device to mitigate EMI. Policies and procedures for EMI mitigation should be based on objective information, such as that obtainable by ad hoc RF immunity testing.
- RF transmitters purchased for use in the facility should have the lowest possible output power rating that can be used to accomplish the intended purpose.
- Electrically powered medical devices purchased for use in the facility should meet EMC standards.
- Electronic medical devices used in intense electromagnetic environments, such as near ambulance radios or in electrosurgery, should have EMC specifications suitable for these environments.
- Clinical/biomedical engineers should consider tracking "no problem found" service calls by the location, date, and time of the reported malfunction. This can help associate malfunctions with sources of electromagnetic disturbance (EMD).
- EMI problems should be reported to the manufacturer and to regulatory authorities.
- The health care organization may want to consider obtaining the services of an EMC professional for assistance in characterizing the electromagnetic environment, solving specific problems, and/or educating staff.

Figure 19.9 AAMI TIR 18 Summary Recommendations [24].

Refernces

1. C. Paul. *Introduction to Electromagnetic Compatibility*, pp. 42–77. Wiley, 1992.
2. H. Ott. *Noise Reduction Techniques in Electronic Systems*, 2nd Edition, p. 6. Wiley, 1988.
3. Modifications to the list of recognized standards. *Federal Register*, 69(191): 59240, 2005.
4. International Electrotechnical Commission, International Special Committee on Radio Interference, CISPR 22, Fifth edition, 2005–04.
5. International Electrotechnical Commission, International Special Committee on Radio Interference, International Standard 60601-1-2, Edition 2:2001 consolidated with amendment 1:2004.
6. W. A. Radasky, C. E. Baum, and W. W. Manuem. Introduction to the special issue on high-power electromagnetics (HPEM) and intentional electromagnetic interference (IEMI), *IEEE Transactions on Electromagnetic Compatibility*, 46(3): 314–321, 2004.
7. W. A. Radasky. An update on intentional electromagnetic interference (IEMI), Annual EMC Guide, Interference Technology, 2004.
8. I. D. Flintoft, et al. The re-emission spectrum of digital hardware subjected to EMI, *IEEE Transactions on Electromagnetic Compatibility*, 45(4): 576–583, 2003.
9. J. H. McIsaac. Interference to Anesthesia Devices by Radio Transmitters, unpublished paper, The Hartford Graduate Center, 1996.

10. R. P. Jones and D. H. Conway. The effect of electromagnetic interference from mobile communication on the performance of intensive care ventilators. *European Journal of Anaethesiology*, 22: 578–583, 2005.
11. I. M. Zhou and S. Boggs. Effect of high frequency cable attenuation on lightning-induced overvoltages at transformers. Rural Electric Power Conference, 2002. *IEEE*, pp. A3-A3_7. 5–7 May 2002.
12. W. D. Prather, et al. Survey of worldwide high-power wideband capabilities, *IEEE, Transactions on Electromagnetic Compatibility*, 46(3): 335–343, 2004.
13. D. Dupont. Nuclear explosions in orbit. *Scientific American*, June, 2004.
14. J. F. McNulty. Critical infrastructure protection: Using TEMPEST technology to forestall EMP damage, Interference Technology Annual EMC Guide, 2004.
15. C. Kopp. The Electromagnetic Bomb—A Weapon of Electrical Mass Destruction, Air Chronicals, *USAF CADRE Air Chronicals*, October, 1996.
16. M. Abrams. Dawn of the E-Bomb. *IEEE Spectrum*, 24–30, November 2003.
17. T. Anderson, et al. US 6,650,297, Laser driven plasma antenna utilizing laser modified maxwellian relaxation, November 18, 2003.
18. W. D. Kimmel and D. D. Gerke. *Electromagnetic Compatibility in Medical Equipment: A Guide for Designers and Installers*, pp. 103–126. IEEE Press and Interpharm Press, New York, 1995.
19. K. L. Kaiser. *Electromagnetic Compatibility Handbook*, CRC Press, Boca Raton, 1995.
20. Y. V. Parfenov, et al. Conducted IEMI threats for commercial buildings. *IEEE Transactions on Electromagnetic Compatibility*, 46(3): 404–411, 2004.
21. D. Nitsch. Susceptibility of some electronic equipment to HPEM Threats. *IEEE Transactions on Electromagnetic Compatibility*, 46(3): 380–389, 2004.
22. R. Hoad. Trends in EM Susceptibility of IT Equipment. *IEEE Transactions on Electromagnetic Compatibility*, 46(3): 390–395, 2004.
23. American National Standards Institute Accredited Standards Committee C63 (EMI).
24. Technical Information Report (TIR) 18, *Guidance on Electromagnetic Compatibility of Medical Devices for Clinical/Biomedical Engineers*. AAMI TIR 18-1997. Arlington, VIA, Association for the Advancement of Medical Instrumentation, 1997.
25. http://en.wikipedia.org/wiki/Image:Light-wave.png
26. G. Smith. Electromagnetic Pulse Threats, testimony before the House National Security Committee, July 16, 1997.
27. www.fda.gov/cdrh/emc/emc-in-hcf.html
28. IEEE EMC Society Committee TC-5, "High Power Electromagnetics" International Electrotechnical Commission (IEC) subcommittee 77C, "EMC: High Power Transient Phenomena."

20   Chapter for Simulation for Bioterrorism

THOMAS C MORT AND STEPHEN DONAHUE

20.1   Introduction to Simulation

High-fidelity mannequin simulation: Is it a new modality of education or is it simply a technology advancement of what is already embedded in each us from childhood? Learning to ride a bike, ice skate, hit a baseball, or a downhill ski takes practice over an extended period of time for most children coupled with plenty of time and instruction from a mentor. As a child, we engage in sporting events and play games to develop and mature our physical, emotional, social, and intellectual skills. This technique of learning by doing and experiencing mistakes, receiving correction and then starting all over again is steadfast in our growth as a child but is often neglected in adulthood.

Adults in the medical community are expected to perform with accuracy and efficiency in the delivery of patient care, even in emergency crises. However, our current methods of instruction and education may underestimate the complexity of today's technology and our ability to quickly absorb new information such that we can then perform a task, operate a piece of equipment or follow a protocol/algorithm even under normal working conditions. This perilous assumption is not only unsafe, but it is doubtful that can personnel educated in this manner can perform confidently, efficiently and correctly when faced with a clinical situation that can only be described as "on demand" during an acute crisis. Our current method of in-servicing personnel on newly written protocols and new equipment may benefit from an update to reflect the degree of time and effort that must be expended to truly master new skills. To illustrate this point, if the hospital introduces a new brand of defibrillator with biphasic technology and deploys them throughout the institution following a mandatory in-service, should we expect personnel to be well-versed in the use the new defibrillator? Will a brief 10 minutes in-service or lecture provide the basis for personnel to respond with ease, conviction, confidence, and efficiency, plus understand the new technology following a brief discussion? Envision the havoc and potential misapplication of the technology when the staff are being asked to incorporate the new equipment in a patient care crisis about 4 months later. It is quite obvious that the crucial steps of "drilling" personnel on the intricacies of proper and efficient equipment use is missing from this type of educational endeavor. Ill-prepared personnel may be likely to falter in their performance of acute care skills potentially leading to patient injury. While it may be difficult to find many in the medical field willing to pronounce that there are significant problems with the system and the way medical care is delivered, claims by the Institute of Medicine estimates nearly 100,000 lives lost each year due to medical errors [1]. Though not all "medical errors" are related to crisis management, simulation-based education may allow an inroad for improving competency, team work, and individual performance that may lead to a reduced number of medical errors.

20.2   History of Simulation

Though introduced to medicine as early as the late 1960s, mannequin-based simulation training accelerated in the late 1980s and early 1990s. High-fidelity mannequin-based simulation training remained, however, isolated to only a handful of medical centers. The technology is exploding of late and several simulator systems are now professionally manufactured and commercially available. The distribution of this technology, however, is still in its infancy as is the incorporation of this educational modality across the spectrum of medicine. If one steps back and analyzes what takes place around us, one would observe simulation training in nearly every aspect of our lives. The emergency personnel who provide police, fire, ambulance, and disaster intervention use simulation training to various degrees to recreate situations they are likely to face during the delivery of their services. The SWAT team trains week in and week out but may only rarely be called upon to deliver "on demand" services in an emergency [2]. However, their ability to respond, to react, and to defuse a crisis will be dependent, in most cases, on their prior training. They will respond spontaneously in an acute crisis but their reaction will be based on a foundation of training that is designed to improve the likelihood of responding correctly, thus saving innocent lives, as well as, possibly their own.

Simulation-based training and education is new only to the medical profession: it has been employed since ancient times when armies pursued training and testing during war games so to allow soldiers and their leaders the ability to gauge their response to conflict, danger, injury, overwhelming odds, and the confusion of a battle. As far back as China in 3000 BC, war games incorporated simulation in battlefield preparation of warriors by re-enacting gladiator and jousting competition incorporated rigorous training rituals, scenarios and repetitive practice rounds to better prepare the warrior for the execution of his craft during the extreme conditions they confronted. The modern era soldier encounters high-tech simulation in many aspects of his training. This allows the soldier to be exposed to common and uncommon or rare battle situations where a precise and deliberate response can be practiced, tested, corrected, and matured under extreme conditions. Likewise, the race car pit crew is criticized when the pit stop of 18 seconds should have taken only 13 seconds. The pit crew trains repeatedly to hone in their skills and roles to maximize efficiency in the least amount of time. Imagine such training for the cardiac arrest team or other associated medical crises internal or external to the hospital locale.

The airline industry has aggressively adapted flight simulation as a mainstay in individual and crew flight training for routine flight and crisis management in its efforts to safeguard the public. Though both industry and the public applaud the flight simulation training, the use of simulation has not been widely challenged as a valid education-training tool for airline pilots or other industries that incorporate such training and education technology (nuclear power, military, utility industry, and safety aspects of the manufacturing industry). The proof of success and efficacy of simulation training is considered self-evident in many arenas. However, medicine is extending considerable research efforts to validate simulation-based training and education in regards to learning, teaching, retention of skills, validation and certification for licensing [3].

A human mannequin simulator is similar in concept to a flight simulator but often pales in comparison in sophistication, complexity and hence, cost. Nonetheless, both offer the ability to provide a venue for routine training and re-enactment of acute and rare problems. Technological advances have brought the previously static "dummy" to a dynamic, complex mannequin that can provide physiological changes. Wheezing or a thready pulse, can be interpreted by the examining student. Output from monitoring devices reflect changes in the patient's vital signs in response to interventions by the student. Audio feedback from the mannequin replicates cries of anguish or pain, history taking, complaints, and even accolades to the student. The power of such a teaching tool is awesome but it must be applied in a constructive manner by individuals capable of developing a simulation curriculum that fosters learning and teaching [2]. The purchase of a high-fidelity human simulator is only the first step toward offering this educational adjunct to the curriculum of the student trainee. The mannequin, itself, does not teach without a dedicated and well-trained staff of educators who are willing to expend a considerable amount of time, effort, and money toward better preparedness of the student trainee, regardless of their current level of education.

20.3 Adaptation of Simulation to Medicine

The medical profession has recently seen a marked interest in simulation as an educational adjunct to the standard methods of teaching and training students, i.e., lectures, reading, journal club, mock interviews, case presentations, and bedside/operating suite/clinic apprenticeship. Work hour limitations, financial restrictions, paradigm shifts in the delivery of medical care to fewer highly trained individuals supervising many less highly trained medical care providers and generational alterations have and will continue to revamp our methods of teaching and learning [4–6]. Simulation is increasingly being utilized for training medical personnel. In addition to the ability to remediate, certify, validate or evaluate the student's clinical acumen, it can assess critical thinking and leadership skills, one's communication capabilities, the ability to prioritize in problem solving, the effective use of monitoring and laboratory/radiographic data, the efficient use of resources, organization of care, distribution of workload and stress management. Simulation is not the panacea nor a replacement for lecture-based learning, reading a journal, viewing a educational CD, attending a conference, or pursing bedside teaching rounds. It provides a powerful adjunct to the apprentice model of medical education [7–9]. As evidence accumulates in support of simulation methodologies and better defines its advantages, benefits and limitations, we will experience a paradigm shift from the "old" to the "new". However, the purchase of a "high-fidelity human simulator" will not, alone, guarantee success. The clear advantage of individual and team training using a simulation model cannot be realized without dedicated faculty, a well-developed curriculum, the provision of time and substantial financial resources to ensure that the future care providers are adequately prepared.

High-fidelity patient simulation, with a full-size computer-linked mannequin, offers an ideal venue for presentation of critical events that can be managed by medical personnel without risk or harm to a patient. These simulated events can be presented following a lecture series to reinforce and clinically apply the concepts or they may be presented without any background introduction so as to assess the student's response to other previously "old" review topics or brand new material. This may provide valuable feedback on the students' adaptation, response and stress management during exposure to unknown clinical problems. Clinical cases or scenarios can be based on pre-programmed clinical situations that serve as a foundation of a curriculum. The exact scenarios can be repeated in a variety of ways: to a variety of students to allow gauging the skills of the students amongst or against their peers or expose the student to a repeated scenario at various time periods (i.e., baseline, three months, six months, twelve months) to assess their skills and retention of clinical material, judgment and critical thinking [10–12]. Likewise, videotaping the scenarios in realistic re-creations of clinical settings will provide a hard copy for future reference and review by both the student and the instructor. This technology, as compared to the present pedagogic-apprentice methods of learning and teaching offers an advanced ability to provide feedback to the educators who then have the opportunity to assess students' performances using standardized cases and to determine whether the educational objectives set out in the curriculum are being matched by performance in a clinical setting. This methodology compares favorably to the current method in which the mentor must grade the student based on her observing the student on rounds or a brief interaction in the hospital hallway or at the patient's bedside [3]. The ability of the instructor to properly and accurately evaluate the effectiveness of non-simulator based education is currently limited to a grade on a written examination or performance during a clinical experience.

The students attend typically work and/or teaching rounds, attend lectures and conferences, and then acquire hands-on teaching at the bedside to varying degrees. The students are expected to acquire knowledge, judgment, leadership skills, autonomy and interactive group working and cooperation skill by these relatively archaic teaching encounters. The development and maturation of technical skills and a keen sense of problem-solving abilities based on the learning objectives of the rotation are lofty but rarely mastered during the rigors of the training period of a one-month rotation. The clinical experience offered to the student, especially in the initial stages of training has a number of limitations, including a restricted enthusiasm, eagerness and motivation of the faculty (or more senior residents) to allow students to provide hands-on patient management. It is common that the students are relegated to an observation role and the ability to acquire hands-on skills will vary broadly. Because of patient safety constraints, students may not be given the autonomy to manage a critically ill patient due to patient safety concerns. Moreover, the student may be limited to certain cases by choice of the supervising staff or residents, potentially missing the more challenging, interesting, rare or potentially catastrophic clinical conditions.

These are the types of cases, in particular, that would provide considerable educational benefit for the student under risk-free conditions. The experienced practitioner may reminisce that "trial by fire" is a great teaching tool and should play a major role in maturing and seasoning the less experienced. However, taking in to consideration teaching principles and concerns for patient safety, learning under such conditions is not optimal for either party. Confusion, embarrassment, loss of self-confidence, and bewilderment on the student's part while placing the patient in harm's way is always a possibility, regardless of one's preparedness and education. Imprinting a horrific experience in the mind of the student is one teaching method that is long lasting but the concern for patient safety in an emergency situation should be paramount. This situation can now be replicated by high-fidelity simulation and therefore can be confronted in our educational process for the adult student in a risk-free, less threatening and appropriate teaching environment [3,10–12]. The student's actions, behaviors and response to such an emergency can now be assessed, corrected, fortified and groomed by no-risk hands-on high-fidelity mannequin training. This methodology will fill in the gaps of the student's curriculum that have been long regarded by some as being unable to meet the goal of acquiring critical thinking skills, judgment, leadership, communication, prioritization, and distribution of workload despite the best efforts of educators in providing to the student what appears to be an adequate patient exposure [4].

The ability to practice and train without risk is an obvious quest of any practitioner who is immersed in today's brand of medical care. Some may argue that the current methods of education have served us well and the traditional pedagogic or apprenticeship style of teaching and learning is fine. However, one should consider that we are surrounded by "simulation training" in many aspects of our lives and it is accepted and embedded in many fields of industry, safety, sports, and recreation. Even within medicine, medical students experience mock interviews with actors posing as patients. We "drill" during ACLS training. A student may practice suturing material together in the confines of a call room to better her dexterity and speed. Unfortunately, we have imbedded into our education method an approach of learning new tasks with the mentality of "see one, do one, teach one". This may not always be acceptable practice.

20.4 Basic Elements of Simulation Education

Measuring performance by the individual or the team has been a focus of simulation-based medical education whereas it efficacy for learning and training has received less strenuous attention. Both facets should be attainable goals for fortifying the current methods of training personnel. Simulation in a controlled environment offers the advantages of experiential learning (learning via experiences) and reflective practice. Reflective practice refers to one's analysis of his own or others experiences in the attempt to gain a new perspective of the said events [13]. The goal being to incorporated these findings into one's practice for the betterment of patient care. The epic text by Schön in 1983, *Educating the Reflective Practitioner*, discussed how professionals think in action [14]. Learning is viewed as the integration of reflection and experience. Schön stressed that knowledge, skill and expertise are implicit in practice and often occur spontaneously by the practitioner. This has been coined "knowing-in-action" and basically refers to the practitioner's spontaneous response and thinking processes ("knowing") during the act of delivering, in this case medical care or attending to a medical emergency ("action"). This is further delineated by two forms of reflection on "knowing-in-action" which purports that we should think about what we are doing or have experienced [14]. First, "reflection-in-action" is typically prompted by unexpected events that prompt a "reflective conversation" either internally or externally to one's self, to discuss the event, its implications, its etiology, its treatment, the role participants are playing or should play and avoidance or preventive strategies in the midst of the event. This type of reflection "on demand" may be difficult due to its rapid pace but the experienced and seasoned practitioner may portend an improved ability to "reflect" during the actual event. Following this instantaneous, "real-time" reflection on the said event as it is happening, the practitioner can develop a response to what is occurring. Thus, the practitioner is performing "research" or "real-time experimenting at the bedside" during the actual event.

"Reflection-on-action" takes place following the event and allows for thinking about the prior situation, causations, implicating factors, its etiology, etc., in a similar fashion to "reflection-in-action." The follow-up analysis should lead to a better understanding of the event and the deployment of preventive, avoidance, or treatment strategies. The individual or members of the team who were involved in an "event" may debrief themselves to gain a better understanding of their thoughts and behaviors. This should prompt improvement in one's critical thinking, highlight areas of weakness and strengths, and encourage open discussion and analysis to improve one's preparation for the next event [14]. Highly motivated practitioners who link their professional position to life-long learning may be individuals who more actively "notice" or seek information that can be harnessed to potentiate their education, hence, they may be those who actively pursue their own analysis of the events and solicit feedback and criticism from their colleagues in a more rigorous manner than those less inclined [3,14,15]. Once the reflective process takes place, it is the level of commitment by the individual (or department, governing body, etc.) that plays a pivotal role in initiating change one's own practice. There lies great educational benefit to reflecting on one's own actions and responses to routine and emergency care, as we should in nearly all areas of our personal and professional existence. We practice "reflection-on-action" in a delayed fashion when we discuss patient care issues or cases at the monthly interesting case conference or morbidity and mortality conference but the built in delay may allow certain key components of the "event" to languish and possibly be "lost to follow-up" [14,15].

It has been recommended that the design of a curriculum for an educational encounter, in this case, a simulated medical or surgical crisis, consist of three phases: preparation of the students for the "event," execution of the "event," and a period of time to debrief and reflect on the event that took place. For example, a mock bioterrorism drill may be developed based on these three guiding suggestions as outlined in Figure 20.1 [3].

Students not only benefit from the training session itself, but the instructors should solicit feedback from the "students" on how to improve the learning experience as well as repair the problems and shortcomings that were found within the "system" during the event. For example, more time devoted during the preparation phase to review of equipment, protocols and guidelines or the limitations noted by personnel donning

> A. Preparation for the event
>   1. Lecture on nerve gas exposure (agents, effects, treatments, differential diagnosis) or mandatory review of information on web based curriculum
>   2. Provide handout/review article related to "event"
>   3. Review of relevant equipment, isolation issues, decontamination procedures transportation issues, communication, hierarchy of responsibility for patient care, systems' review of institutional response
>   4. Review of the mannequin (limitations, physiological signs, and symptoms)
> B. Execution of the event
>   1. Mock drill of patient (mannequin) exposed to presumed bioterrorism toxin in the community, transported to medical facility, transfer of care to hospital personnel, isolation, decontamination drill, patient assessment, personnel practicing with protective garments, delivery of required medical care, transport and transfer of care within hospital
> C. Debriefing and reflection (with or without video tape review of event)
>   1. Participants reflect on their actions, behaviors, and responses
>   2. Solicit feeling and emotions of experiencing the event as an individual and as a member of the team
>   3. Provide constructive criticism, corrective actions, review skills, pinpoint deficiencies and provide positive reinforcement of their accomplishments
>   4. Reevaluate the event and suggest improvements or alterations in both the preparation for and execution of the event

Figure 20.1 Event—mock bioterrorism drill focusing on nerve gas exposure.

20.5 Post-Simulation Period: Debriefing and Reflection

(de-brief (Webster's dictionary)—Pronunciation: (")dE-'brEf; Function: *transitive verb*: to interrogate (as a pilot) usually upon return (as from a mission) in order to obtain useful information. Synonyms: catechize, interrogate, examine, inquire, query, question, quiz).

Debriefing and reflection may be the most critical component of the simulation exercise and should encompass a review of the events, a display of the students' emotions toward their actions, responses and behaviors, the facilitator/instructor display of compassion and empathy and finally, providing explanations for bettering the students' actions and behavior in a constructive manner [3]. The debriefing session should be entertaining, practical and interactive for the participants to better describe the clinical events that they either personally took part in or observed during the scenario. Students may have difficulty with some emotional aspect of the training session coupled with difficulty discussing these feeling during the debriefing. Frustration, anger, immature comments, fear of failure or overconfidence, excessive stress or the inability to actively participate in patient (Mannequin) care may surface during the event. The debriefer should facilitate the discussion of these emotions in a supportive manner (Figure 20.2). Positive reinforcement for desired emotional traits as well as actions and response are encouraged. Discussion of differences of opinion and viewpoints between the participants should be encouraged but held in check to remain in a positive, non-confrontational and

protective garments in the difficulty encountered with assessment of pulse, skin temperature, airway management skills, auscultation of breath sounds. Better preparation may include incorporating computer screen-based simulator scenarios that allow real-time feedback to the student handling the "computer generated emergency". This method was found to be superior when the students were later tested in their handling of anesthetic emergencies in a mannequin based simulator, as compared to those who prepared by studying a handbook [3,16].

> Offer a safe, educational atmosphere not bounded by obvious time constraints.
> Offer verbal feedback and constructive criticism augmented by audio-visual technology (if feasible).
> Encourage metacognition or self-learning and self-assessment (reflective learning).
> Promote communication and debriefing among team members.
> Sponsor a culture change to improve the attitude toward "errors" in medicine.

Figure 20.2 Goals of debriefing [3].

empathetic atmosphere. A non-threatening atmosphere can be reinforced by the knowledge that the educational process is confidential (if it is) and this may encourage solicitation of the student's honest appraisal of the team and individual capabilities, strengths and weaknesses.

The ability to capture the interest, enthusiasm and participation of the students should occur in the first few moments following cessation of the clinical scenario. A brief summation of the clinical scenario with an expression of gratitude for the student's participation in an upbeat manner may be a good introduction to the debriefing session. Following this, the instructor should seek feedback from the students about their own performance, either individually or as a group, what were their strengths and weaknesses, would they change anything if confronted with the same scenario again. The debriefing discussion should be guided by the instructor to maintain focus on the subject matter and one should focus on the significant value in supporting the student's active participation in their own critique.

The instructor may have a pronounced impact on the absorption of course material by the student. The delivery of the material may be affected by one's tone of voice, clarity of voice, facial and body mannerisms, demeanor, and pleasantness (or the lack there of). Many other factors may influence the success or failure of student learning including the student's attention span, absorption pattern of course material, enthusiasm for simulation and his willingness to partake in the current or future simulations. Portrayal of confidence, compassion and leadership in a non-confrontational manner balanced with a constructive critiquing style creates a more favorable atmosphere for learning [17].

The commencement of debriefing/reflection may be at the conclusion of the scenario or the scenario may "freeze" (pause) to emphasize teaching points, defuse a deteriorating situation, redirect the students or limit student embarrassment or frustration. If the simulated clinical case is brief (5 minutes) then concluding with debriefing may be the best approach. Interruption with verbal redirection or explanation may be best to improve the simulation experience and to optimize the educational benefits if the scenario is attended by junior or less experienced students or the clinical case is of extended duration (>20 minutes) [3,17,18]. However, experienced, senior level trainees may be best left alone to complete their clinical scenario to be followed by an in depth debriefing and reflection on their actions, behavior, and responses.

Videotape analysis is a very useful component of debriefing for both the instructor and the student. A recording of the session for review of the entire scenario or only for the review of a particular action performed or decision made during the scenario can be invaluable. Student may deny or refute actions, behaviors or comments made during the scenario or may display disbelief with the instructors' assessment of their performance. Conversely, video recordings can be used to illustrate examples of communication, teamwork, leadership, critical thinking, and problem solving. A recorded video provides hard data that may be archived for review and comparison at a later time [19–21]. Below is listed a group of educational based terms often witnessed by the instructor during a simulation based teaching scenario (Figure 20.3). These are key elements that the educators must appreciate to better understand the art of teaching and learning when dealing with a wide range of students with varying abilities, understanding, defense mechanisms and understanding of the course material [22].

20.6 Crew Resource Management

The basis for coalescing a group of individuals to work together in a constructive, efficient and effective manner is the optimal objective of nearly any industry or business. Putting together a selection of intelligent, well-trained workers, staff members, specialists, professionals, experts or a group of diversely educated and skilled personnel may be painstaking and time consuming, sometimes with less than optimal output. Consider the time and effort professional sport teams put into fundamentals, teamwork and constant drilling and practice. They condition in the off-season,

Convergent search process Several specific cues leading to a similarity-matching process that leads to a likely response, i.e. tachycardia, shortness of breath, hypoxemia, wheezing, immobile-bedridden patient → pulmonary embolus

Divergent search process Broad category-cue leads to a multi-answer query based on frequency-gambling, i.e., a differential diagnosis of *Wheezing* → asthma, URI, pneumonia, ETT occlusion, main stem bronchus intubation, pulmonary edema, pulmonary embolus

Slips of the Tongue untoward, unsolicited comments about behavior, actions or responses

Slips of Action due to preoccupation or distraction

Maladaptive behaviors amongst poor performers

1. Thematic vagabonding (flitting from issue to issue in a superficial manner as an escape behavior to avoid facing their helplessness)
2. Encysting: opposite of vagabonding; topics are lingered over and small details attended to in excess. Both reveal a poor self-assessment and intellectual inadequacy

Skill based performance

Inattention
Over-attention

Rule-based performance

Misapplication of good rules
Application of bad rules

Knowledge based performance

Overconfidence
Out-of-sight, out-of-mind mentality
Problems with causality, complexity
Biased reviewing of subject

Figure 20.3 Elements for the educator to understand [23].

commence the season with practice and a preseason game schedule to prepare for the real games. The season is essentially 10–12 months in duration with the motivation of stardom, endorsements and monetary gain. Conversely, the fire, police, counter-terrorist, anti-riot professionals, military personnel, and SWAT team members drill and fine tune their skills on a frequent and regular basis. Despite the intensive training, some may only rarely or never employ these special skills in an act to preserve life and limb. Surprisingly, those in the medical field who are very likely to face an acute, life-threatening crisis, will only on occasion train or practice acute care skills despite the fact that life and limb are involved. This disparity may be addressed with an aggressive approach to improving and better maintaining one's acute care skills. This may be accomplished by incorporating high-fidelity simulation training into our educational practices.

Imagine stepping onto a plane with an inexperienced crew who has never worked together as a team. One would be foolish to accept this level of experience and training, but this very scenario plagues our system of medical care delivery. The aviation industry, as many others have, adapted simulation training as a means of training their crew for optimal human performance under normal and adverse, crisis conditions. They gel the team members by teaching them "crew resource management" principles (Figure 20.4).

Consider the issue of patient safety, and imagine a practitioner who makes a clinical mistake; immediately after realizing the error, he or she will experience an emotional reaction that is powerfully instructive—but this may only be instructive for the next patient. What if educators could replicate such an experience with a much greater impact than simply discussing it at a case conference. Representing the case in a simulated environment allows students to "live through" a compendium of important, rare and difficult cases in a fraction of real-time? The benefits from simulation-based education may, in part, be due to the focus that complex information may be better understood and

1. Leadership skills
2. Critical thinking
3. Communication
4. Prioritization of care (triage)
5. Effective use of monitoring
6. Effective and efficient use of resources/equipment
7. Organization of care
8. Distribution of workload amongst team members
9. Stress management

Figure 20.4 Key Elements of Crew Resource Management (CRM) [3].

retained more efficiently than would be the case with traditional teaching methods [3].

Incorporating crisis resource management (CRM) may enable the students to consolidate knowledge, behaviors, interactions with colleagues, attitudes and skills to achieve an improved understanding of the significance of their performance in general, and in particular, how their performance impacts on patient safety and the quality of healthcare they provide. A video-assisted reflective process powerfully reinforces learning. Crisis resource management courses demonstrate the value of simulation in bridging the gap between "knowing" and "doing" and keeping the focus on patient safety [24–26].

20.7 Moulage vs. Mannequin Training

Training students in a simulated environment without actual patients is a potential method of teaching new skills and improving patient safety [27]. In its current format, disaster and bioterrorism training (and testing) relies heavily on actors as patients (moulage). The realism of a moulage environment is limited by replication of acute physiological alterations in a patient actor (i.e., diminished breath sounds, wheezing, tachycardia, weak pulses [27]. Little literature is available to answer the effectiveness question of "moulage" vs mannequin simulator for training. Previous studies have suggested that simulators could potentially improve trauma training [28–30]. Lee et al. [27] found that the clinical effectiveness of the simulator was equal and in several areas, superior, to patient actors in a trauma assessment training testing format.

20.8 Medical Professionals: Little Things Mean a Lot

Simple tasks can be erroneously performed, forgotten, or neglected by the novice as well as the experienced care provider. Calling for help, performing a history/physical examination, confirming or even checking vital signs before instituting aggressive treatment, discontinuing medications that are obviously contributing to patient morbidity and simply preparing and using airway equipment when indicated [31]. The literature has supported the fact that students' clinical experiences correlate with their level of confidence in practical application of that experience. Hands-on clinical experience was found to be the most important variable in building confidence during patient encounters [31,32]. Fincher and Lewis [33] support the relationship between self-acknowledged competence and the frequency of performing a given task or exercise. Due to concerns of patient safety, students cannot be given the freedom to manage a critically ill patient. High-fidelity patient simulation offers an ideal venue for replication of critical events that can be managed without risk or harm to a patient by using scenarios that are pre-programmed, may be repeated, and videotaped in realistic re-creations of dynamic clinical settings such in the community setting, within a helicopter, ambulance, the operating room, critical care unit, or emergency department (Figures 20.5 and 20.6). Simulation technology therefore presents educators with the opportunity to assess students' performances using standardized cases and to determine whether the educational objectives set out in the curriculum are being matched by performance in a clinical setting. A more detailed analysis of the trainee's performance, beyond simply the proper execution and completion of the CRM principles can be beneficial for improving the student's understanding of patient care principles; fostering reflective learning through self-analysis of leadership style and skills including cooperation and interaction with peers, subordinates, and superiors; and making appropriate personnel adjustments necessary for optimum delivery of medical care within a chaotic environment.

Further, many of the recognized shortfalls (e.g., knowledge deficits or decision making failures) uncovered during simulation training may be a useful focus for research in this new modality of medical education [17,21,34]. This is particularly true as simulation based validation, certification, or privilege-based assessment increases in frequency and acceptance in the medical community.

```
Pre-hospital response

    City vs. small town
    Air and ground ambulance transport issues
    Training and equipment

Emergency department

    Triage
    Trauma mass casualty
    Training
    Equipment
    Physician, nursing and ancillary/support staff
```

Figure 20.5 First responders: potential areas of simulation drills.

```
Isolation, training, preparation, etc.

    Individual medical/surgical departments
    Critical care response
    OR management of infected or contaminated
        patients
    Coordination between departments
        i.e., PACU/ICU/ED
    Nursing
    Hospital administration
    Human resources
    Finance
    Pharmacy
    Support/ancillary staff
    Command and control
    Security
    Clinical engineering/biomedical engineering
    Facilities management
    Hospital power supply
    Communications
    Information services
       Data security
       Data communication reliability
       Sensors and detectors for bioterror agents
```

Figure 20.6 Second tier of responders: potential areas of simulation drills.

20.9 Simulation Drills for Bioterrorism

The individual institution must decide what its level of commitment to preparedness is desired and required by the local and regional populace it serves. The development of a relationship with local, regional and national agencies involved in preparedness is the first step in involving the hospital and its personnel. Incorporating plans and protocols should not be left to the addition of a written report that is placed in the notebook labeled, "Policies & Procedures" and then expecting hospital personnel to be aware and prepared to act on such proceedings in an acute crisis. This is a setup for potential disaster. The main objectives of drills are two-fold: evaluate both the "system" issues and the human performance. The essential components of the system must be intact for the personnel to perform optimally, and conversely, the personnel must be capable of using the system to deliver the desired medical care. For example, if the well-trained out-of-hospital emergency personnel cannot triage the patient properly to the main facility due to a faulty communication chain of command, this demonstrate a system failure. Conversely, if the ICU and operating room personnel are not aware of the hierarchy of chain of command and the steps required to decontaminate an "exposed" victim who has slipped past the confusion of the emergency department, both system and personnel deficiencies exist. People cannot be expected to perform adequately if they lack training, their experience is deficient or marginal and they are not confident and comfortable working within a well-planned system. There is little doubt that a well run disaster drill is dependent on a well conceived plan that has been tested so to allow the "kinks" to be worked out and coupled with personnel who have been briefed, educated and have trained with the protocols, equipment and system issues. A recent survey of UK clinicians regarding the presentation and management of victims of chemical and biological agents suggested there are significant gaps in the knowledge and training of these individuals in regards to understanding decontamination, presenting features, and recommended therapies. Only a minority had participated in relevant training exercises related to bioterrorism [35]. Moreover, though recently updated protocols and incident plans have been enacted, many physicians who provide "frontline" care of victims of bioterrorism remain poorly integrated into the institution care schema [36]. Furthermore, some of the more straightforward steps in resuscitation, i.e., airway management, may be hampered by clinicians donning anti-chemical protective gear during the rendering of acute resuscitative measures. The cumbersome gear and its altering of the clinicians' comfort, dexterity and their sensory and tactile input from the patient may impact the delivery of medical care in a crisis. Likewise, personnel must be accustom to locating the gear and dressing themselves in an expeditious manner hence, training and drills designed to meet this objective are warranted [37,38]. Some examples of drills that may be run in one's institution are noted below (Figures 20.7 and 20.8). The value of running such a drill is that weaknesses, deficiencies and points of system breakdown may be identified then corrected. This will benefit all levels of patient care delivery irregardless if bioterrorism or mass casualties are involved. Conversely, identification of strong points within the system may allow one to optimally adjust other similar systems throughout the institution.

20.10 Conclusion

High-fidelity simulation has enormous potential for training in this safety conscious environment. Incorporating this modality will encourage the students to be an active participant in their own learning in a risk free setting with the possibility

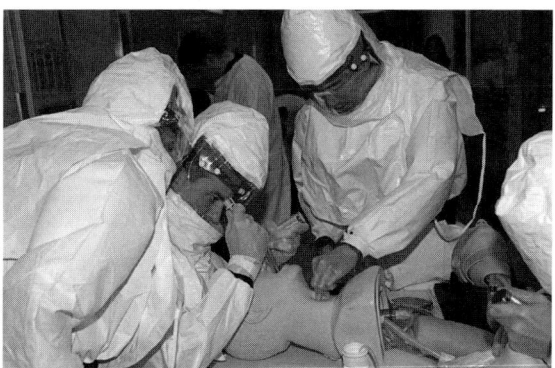

Figure 20.8 Anesthesiology residents practicing intubation skills during simulation training at Hartford hospital.

of immediate feedback and reflection. Simulation based curriculum can be standardized and focused to the level of the learner with the ability to assess skills, critical thinking and teamwork. This unique teaching environment provides an opportunity to identify discrepancies between what is expected of the student and what the student can actually deliver. This is indeed, 'a good idea whose time has come' [39,40].

References

1. L. T. Kohn, J. M. Corrigan, M. S. Donaldson, eds. For the Institute of Medicine Committee on Quality of Health Care in America. To Err Is Human: Building a Safer Health System. Washington, DC, National Academic Press, 2000.
2. J. A. Gordon, Wm. Wilkerson, D. W. Shaffer, and E. G. Armstrong. "Practicing" medicine without risk: students' and educators responses to high-fidelity patient simulation. *Acad Med*, 76;469–472, 2001.
3. W. Dunn (ed.) *Simulators in Critical Care and Beyond*, Simulation-A Revolution in Medical Education, 1st Edition, pp. 35–81. Society of Critical Care Medicine Press, Des Plaines, IL, 2004.
4. S. D. Issenberg, S. Pringle, R. M. Harden, S. Khogali, and M. S. Gordon. Adoption and integration of simulation-based learning technologies into the curriculum of a UK Undergraduate Education Programme. *Med Ed*, 371:42–49, 2003.

---

1. Communication based drills
   a. telephone, walkie-talkie, or wireless system
2. Single or multiple patients through system (moulage/actors or mannequins)
   a. transportation only (1st responder in community to ED, 1st responder to OR/ICU via ED)
   b. transportation & triage
   c. transportation, triage, patient care
3. Announced/planned vs impromptu/surprise drill
4. Decontamination system
5. Personnel protective equipment
6. Medical/surgical response to bioterror
   Airway issues
   Acute resuscitation
   Basic and advanced patient care
   ACLS

Figure 20.7 Single or multiple areas for testing/drilling for bioterrorism preparedness.

5. M. L. Good. Patient simulation for training basic and advanced clinical skills. *Med Ed*, 37(1):14–21, 2003.
6. G. B. Healy. The College should be instrumental in adapting simulators to education. *Bull ACS* 87:10–11, 2002.
7. D. M. Gaba and A. DeAnda. The response of anesthesia trainees to simulated critical incidents. *Anesth Analg*, 68: 444–451, 1989.
8. J. H. Devitt, M. M. Kurrek, M. M. Cohen, et al. The validity of performance assessments using simulation. Anesthesiology, 95: 36–42, 2001.
9. D. M. Gaba. Improving anesthesiologists' performance by simulating reality. *Anesthesiology*, 76: 491–494, 1992.
10. M. J. Freidrich. Practice makes perfect: risk-free medical training with patient simulators. *JAMA*, 288:2808–12, 2002.
11. D. Gaba, S. Howard, K. Fish, B. Smith, and Y. Soub. Simulation in anesthesia crisis management: a decade of experience. *Simul Gaming*, 32(2):175–93, 2001.
12. S. B. Issenberg, W. C. McGaghie, I. R. Hart, et al. Simulation technology for health care professional skills training and assessment. *JAMA*, 282(9):861–865, 1999.
13. J. M. Agutter, D. F. Arch, N. Syroid, D. Westneskow, R. Albert, D. Strayer, J. Bermudez, Weinger, and B. Matthew. Evaluation of Graphic Cardiovascular Display in a High-Fidelity Simulator, *Anest Analg*, 97(5):1403–1413, 2003.
14. D. Schön, *Educating the Reflective Practitioner*, pp. 23–34. Jossey-Bass, San Francisco, 1990.
15. P. M. Lyon, and A. Brew. Reflection on learning in the operating theatre. *Reflective Practitioner*. 4:5, 2003.
16. H. A. Schwid, G. A. Rooke, and P. Michalowshi. Screen-based anesthesia simulation with debriefing improves performance in a mannequin-based anesthesia simulator. *Teach Learn Med*, 12:92–95, 2001.
17. M. Shapiro. *Debriefing in Simulation Training*. New England SimMan User's Group, Foxwoods, CT, May 2003.
18. J. B. Sexton, E. J. Thomas, and R. L. Helmreich. Error, stress, and teamwork in medicine and aviation: cross sectional surveys. *BMJ*, 320:745–749, 2000.
19. P. Croskerry. The importance of cognitive errors in diagnosis and strategies to minimize them [Review]. *Acad Med*, 78:775–780, 2003.
20. C. Beach, P. Croskerry, and M. Shapiro. Center for Safety in Emergency Care. Profiles in patient safety: emergency care transitions. *Acad Emerg Med*, 10:364–367, 2003.
21. K. S. Cosby and P. Croskerry. Patient safety: a curriculum for teaching patient safety in emergency medicine. *Acad Emerg Med*, 10:69–78, 2003.
22. J. J. Schaefer and R. M. Gonzalez. Dynamic simulation: a new tool for difficult airway training of professional healthcare providers. *Am J Anesthesiol*, 4:232–241, 2000.
23. J. T. Reason. *Human Error*, pp. 67–75. Cambridge, England, Cambridge University Press, 1990.
24. W. B. Murray, and P. A. Foster. Crisis resource management among strangers: principles of organizing a multidisciplinary group for crisis resource management. *J Clin Anesth*, 12:633–638, 2000.
25. V. Chopra, B. J. Gesink, J. De Jong, et al. Does training on an anesthesia simulator lead to improvement in performance? *Br J Anaesth*, 1994; 73: 293–297.
26. R. H. Blum, D. B. Raemer, J. S. Carroll, N. Sunder, D. M. Felstein, and J. B. Cooper. Crisis resource management training for an anaesthesia faculty: a new approach to continuing education. *Med Ed*, 38(1):45–55, 2004.
27. S. K. Lee, M. Pardo, D. Gaba, Y. Sowb, R. Dicker, E. Straus, L. Khaw, D. Morabito, T. Krummel, and M. M. Knudson. Trauma Assessment Training with a Patient Simulator: A Prospective, Randomized Study. *J Trauma* 55(4):651–657, 2003.
28. R. L. Marshall, S. Smith, P. J. Gorman, et al. Use of a human patient simulator in the development of resident trauma management skills. *J Trauma*, 51:17–21, 2001.
29. D. Treolar, J. Hawayek, J. R. Montgomery, et al. On-site and distance education of emergency personnel with a human patient simulator. *Mil Med*, 166:1003–1006, 2001.
30. T. M. Krummel. Surgical simulation and virtual reality: the coming revolution. *Ann Surg*, 228:635–637, 1998.
31. P. Morgan and D. Cleave-Hogg. Comparison between medical students' experience, confidence and competence. *Med Educ*, 36:534–539, 2002.
32. P. L. Harrell, G. W. Kearl, E. L. Reed et al. Medical students' confidence and the characteristics of their clinical experiences in a primary care clerkship. *Acad Med* 68:577–579, 1993.
33. R.-M. Fincher and L. A. Lewis. Learning, experience, and self-assessment of competence of

third-year medical students in performing bedside procedures. *Acad Med* 69:291–295, 1994.
34. D. M. Gaba, K. J. Fish, and S. K. Howard. *Crisis Management in Anesthesiology*, pp. 88–93. Churchill Livingstone, Philadelphia, 1994.
35. S. Wimbush, G. Davies, and D. Lockey. The presentation and management of victims of chemical and biological agents: a survey of knowledge of UK clinicians. *Resuscitation* 58(3): 289–292, 2003.
36. D. Lockey and G. Davies. The challenges of deliberate chemical/biological attack. *Resuscitation* 58(3):293–296, 2003.
37. R. Flaishon, A. Sotman, A. Friedman, R. Ben-Abraham, V. Rudick, and A. Weinbroum. Laryngeal mask airway insertion by anesthetists and non-anesthetists wearing unconventional protective gear: a prospective, randomized crossover study in humans. *Anesthesiology*, 100(2):267–273, 2004.
38. R. Flaishon, A. Sotman, R. Ben-Abraham, V. Rudick, D. Varssano, and A. Weinbroum. Antichemical Protective Gear Prolongs Time to Successful Airway Management, *Anesthesiology*, 100(2):260–266, 2004.
39. H. R. Champion and A. G. Gallagher. Surgical simulation—a "good idea whose time has come", *BJ Surgery*, 90(7):767–768, 2003.
40. H. A. Schwid, G. A. Rooke, B. K. Ross, and M. Sivarajan. Use of a computerized advanced cardiac life support simulator improves retention of advanced cardiac life support guidelines better than a textbook review. *Crit Care Med*, 27:821–825, 1999.

21 Simulation II: Preparing for Biodisasters

RICHARD R. KYLE, JR.

Disclaimer

All specific commercial product references and contact information are offered for comparative use only; no endorsement is implied by and no financial interests are associated with the author. All statements and opinions are the author's, and are not official positions or policies of the Uniformed Services University, the Department of Defense, or the US federal government.

Objectives for the Reader

- Utilize criteria for evaluating biodisaster simulations;
- Apply principles of designing and producing simulation scenarios;
- Identify technical and personnel resources required for a successful biodisaster preparation program

Key Words

Patient simulation
Simulation personnel
Simulation scenarios
Team training
Weapons of mass destruction

21.1 Audience

This chapter is for all who are now or may become part of a clinical facility biodisaster plan and wish to work toward making themselves and their colleagues better prepared. Despite the vast differences in intent behind the two causes of biodisaster, competency in responding to intentional bioterror are equally valuable in responding to most "natural" biological generators of mass casualties.

21.2 Premise

The ideal way to become and remain proficient in a task is to practice it. Individual knowledge as well as teamwork skills required to successfully respond to biodisasters are learnable, but both fade in the absence of use. Simulation is an ideal way to learn and maintain the abilities required to minimize the consequences of rare but devastating events. Specific simulations can be constructed and delivered to meet the unique needs of the different kinds of biodisaster responders: first responders saving lives en mass, clinicians in the emergency department saving lives one at a time, crises managers allocating resources to save as many lives as possible. Simulation offers all learners the advantages of applying themselves to scheduled disasters at minimal added expense and disruption to existing activities. In exchange, the participants gain self-confidence in their own abilities as well as in those of their colleagues.

21.3 Unique Contribution of Simulation

The concept behind simulation is identical to the very essence of formal education: "Instructors" systematically abstract key concepts and actions from the distractions of the real world and create a presentation with these concepts highlighted for their emphasis and appreciation, while "students" attempt to ingest and incorporate their exposure to these concepts filtered through their individually experienced pasts. However, simulation is unique by providing students in traditional educational programs the opportunity to *apply* their learning to solve realistic problems in realistic settings with realistic resources and with realistic consequences of their actions. Specifically for biodisaster, simulation is an effective way for the students to reach their goal of competency in performing unusual tasks in unusual environments.

Beyond individual occupational expertise, success or failure in any biodisaster will depend greatly upon each participant's competence in communication, collaboration, cooperation, leadership, and followership. The seeds for many famous disasters sprouted in the gaps between non-cooperative "tribes" (e.g., Desert 1: covert military rescue, Challenger: manned space launch, Tenerife: commercial aviation, Chernobyl: nuclear power). In crafting and executing biodisaster simulations, improvements in resource allocation can be considered, performed and evaluated. For example, Dr. Dianne Rekow wants dentists to contribute to disaster relief and crisis management [1]. Simulation allows various practitioners to role-play their contributions to scenarios, evaluate their actions, and refine them.

There are no passive roles in simulation. Since the ultimate goal of clinical education is for students to become competent enough to assume total responsibility for their own actions, simulation is an excellent method for transforming theoretical understanding into competent action. Many of the student and instructor postures, positions, actions and inactions accepted in clinical education with live patients are antithetical to clinical education with simulated patients. In the former, the instructor often stands between the patient and the students while performing actions on or for the patient while speaking to the students. In the latter, instructors may say just enough to define the situation, turn over the patient to the student, and then leave the room. Students learn as they practice problem solving and skill mastering in a risk-free environment. The instructors' mission is to craft an event that tells a story in the guise of a treasure hunt using logical consequences to guide the students as they work toward success.

21.4 Scenario Resources

While simulation is an educational tool useful for augmenting existing learning programs, it does require dedicated people, equipment and spaces.

21.4.1 People and their Labels

Students are all those who participates in the simulation experience but are naive to its design and construction. In simulation, "students" are expected to be dynamic contributors, and if they are not, their instructors have failed them either by poorly designing their role within the scenario or by inadequately conveying what is expected of them. Students should be assigned roles and expected to progress in their learning. The only time students should ever doubt their responsibilities is when that uncertainty is an intentional teaching objective of the instructors.

Instructors contribute clinical and teamwork expertise to the scenario design and construction. Most participate during the simulation execution, usually observing student performance and often acting additionally as controllers to introduce realistic changes within scenarios as they proceed. Some instructors may be experienced simulation professionals.

Simulation professionals contribute simulation expertise and performance to the scenario design, construction, and execution. They translate the instructors' teaching objectives into realistic representations. Some are also clinical content and educational experts in their own right.

Clinical and *clinician* refer to any situation and person directly involving patient care. Likewise, non-clinical and non-clinician refer to any situation and person involving management and allocation of care resources not including direct patient care, even if such a manager were formally trained in a clinical discipline.

Actors are participants that are seen and or heard "on stage" by the students. They usually contribute gentle guides to the flow of the scenario, are fully aware of the plot, and fill a supporting cast role to the production. Their character is always subservient to those played by the students (otherwise, students surrender initiative). People playing the actors are either not known to the students, or if known, are not in the students' evaluative chain of command (otherwise, students surrender focus). However, the roles that the actors play should be well known, easily conveyed with a simple introduction, (e.g., "I'm just the EMT-trainee that brought in your patient") and they help move the story along when the students fail to pick up on an important clue (e.g., "Do you want me to answer that phone for you?").

Professional Human Patient actors [as in objective structured clinical examinations (OSCEs)] can provide their expertise in portraying specific illnesses and evaluating student performance. In addition, "walk-on" amateurs make for good nonclinical actors, especially as the voices of robotic patients, (e.g., the woman in the office down the hall with three children may realistically vocalize for the female robotic simulator's delivery). In all cases, live actors should be employed as patients when the patients' primary mode of communicating clinical information is through movement, touch, and verbal conversation. They may also be used when students are expected to perform noninvasive procedures.

21.4.2 Device Simulators

Patient simulation devices offering a wide range of features and presentation capabilities are now available for a wide range of acquisition and use/upkeep costs. They can be as simple as rubber fore-arms for intravenous (IV) placement (good for making the students carry out all the time and gear consuming tasks in gaining IV access without damaging real human arms) or as complex as the high-fidelity, full-body, real-clinical monitor-driving, drug- and ventilation-responsive, operator-intensive, fixed-site machines. The best device is the one that allows students to take clear, decisive actions that lead to success or failure in achieving the teaching objectives of their instructors. In all cases, these complex simulation devices should be employed as patients when the patients' primary mode of communicating clinical information is through clinical monitors and when the students are expected to perform invasive procedures.

21.4.3 Rooms and Environments

The *stage* is wherever the action is expected to take place. Most clinical simulations will take place in a recreation of a specific clinical environment and will be located far away from real patient care to minimize the possibility of contaminating real treatment objects with dysfunctional fake ones. Emergency-management simulations can take place in real emergency management centers, provided that the faked training signals and altered communication links used during the exercise are restored to their original "real" configuration (e.g. the ICBM missile attack training tape that was left in place and almost started WW III). Like the robotic patients, the fidelity of the stage environment needs to be no more elaborate than what is essential to convey the desired story, but realistic enough to introduce undesirable distractions.

Regardless of the stage and of the type of scenario, both audio and video *recordings* are made of students' words and actions. It is essential for students to review these recordings immediately after their session, so that they themselves can assess their performance and determine where *they* need to improve their competencies. Participating in a simulation is like eating a meal; assessing one's own performance is like digesting that meal. Likewise, this feedback is extremely valuable for simulation professionals and instructors in assessing how well their scenario design and execution fulfilled their goal of helping the students expand their competencies.

The *simulation control area* is usually adjacent to the stage, and houses all the remote control devices that the simulation professionals use to manipulate the sights and sounds experienced by the students. The control area should be sight- and sound-isolated from the stage to decrease distractions and increase realism. Students can participate successfully in simulation exercises without ever seeing the control area or meeting the simulation professionals, although a walk-through before or after the exercise may help them understand the degree of support entailed to produce their experience.

The pre-brief/de-brief room is usually near the stage, and is used to gather together all students before and after their simulation experience. Any conference room of appropriate size and typical teaching aids (white boards, video displays and projectors, etc) will suffice.

21.5 Scenario Creation

Use the following series of questions and answers as a framework to construct an effective scenario.

Start with answering the following questions:

Who are your students and how many are there?
What are their current competencies?
What are your teaching objectives?
How do you want your students changed by their simulation experiences?

The answers to the above questions will suggest answers to the following questions:

What is the setting of the scenario?
Where are the students' developing competencies to be employed?
Where is the simulation scenario to be staged?

Who are all the various players?
What roles do your students play?
What roles do your actors and, if needed, robotic characters play

What are the script elements that are *essential* to satisfy all the above?
What are the script elements that are *desirable* to augment all the above?
What are the script elements that are *non-essential* and that may confound all the above?

What resources are required to produce the scenario?

21.6 Scenario Examples

The three following examples illustrate the principles and tools of simulation applied as learning experiences tailored to the specific needs of the participants. These examples could be produced separately as three independent exercises but are even more effective when exercised together as part of the response to a single defined incident. Note that in each example the entire essence of the simulation is captured within a single sentence that defines who, where, and what:

1. A few clinical students in their emergency department perform hands-on treatment of bio-intoxicated patients;
2. Many non-clinical students in their Emergency Operations Command Center allocate resources during a bio-contaminant outbreak in their Treatment Facility;
3. Many clinical and non-clinical students just outside their treatment facility perform crowd control, decontamination, and triage of crowds demanding help.

In the first scenario, the world of the simulation is limited to just a few beds within the simulated emergency department (ED). For this kind of simulation to be an effective learning experience, the patients, both the humans on stage and the humans controlling the robots from off stage, must present themselves very realistically. The "audience members" that they are trying to convince are learning to be bio-agent experts through their responses to the realistic presentations of the patients, so the patients must be thoroughly competent in the content and the expression of the content.

The number of students is limited to how many clinicians usually contribute in treating one ED patient times the number of simultaneously simulated ED patients. Thus, the population of the entire ED along with all the ED augmenters will not all "fit" into this kind of simulation all at one time. However, given the nature of ED work, workloads, staffing and the relative short duration of the scenario, this simulation could be offered regularly, with small subsets of the student population assigned to "staff" the simulated ED. Given the numerous re-certification requirements of ED clinicians (ACLS, ATLS, etc.), perhaps a rotating scheduled "training day" could be crafted so that no one clinician's experience of a bio-mass-casualty event is more than six months old.

In the second scenario, the world of the simulation is the entire treatment facility that is contending with an outbreak of a bio-contaminant like SARS, but the exercise itself takes place in the facility's Emergency Operations Command Center (EOCC). If a real EOCC is unavailable this scenario can be produced in a typical conference room. For the simulation to be an effective learning experience at least one member of each "tribes" required during a real disaster in the EOCC must attend the simulated one; thus there will be administrators, network operators, nurses, physicians, public information and security personnel, support staff, technicians, etc. This kind of simulation uses an acute and overwhelming health problem of the kind that Alfred Hitchcock called "The McGuffin"—something around which the story is built and that drives the action but the specific nature of which is irrelevant. Those who function in the EOCC do not treat the infected patients; they are responsible for the command, control, communication, collaboration, and overall resource allocation that determines how effective those who do the hands-on treatment will be.

It is mostly through their interaction with other students that exercise participants will learn how to become crisis-management experts. It is the responsibility of the simulation "ringmaster" to gently emphasize that the students' learning should be focused upon behaviors that improve allocation of resources in a crisis and reduce frictions. Also, this kind of simulation is ideal for cross-training personnel between the different tribes that send representatives to manage a disaster response.

In the third scenario, the world of the simulation is the surroundings (e.g., parking lots) of the treatment facility that are flooded with mass casualties seeking help during a bioterror outbreak. For the simulation to be an effective learning experience, those playing the would-be patients must be very persistent in seeking their goal—access to the ED for treatment.

A primary objective for the students in this scenario is to learn the consequence of poor crowd control. Dry runs should be held in a typical conference room prior to execution outdoors with all the actual equipment and clothing. These dry runs will help the students familiarize themselves with not only their immediate area of responsibility, but also the value for communication across the different segments of the entire process of crowd control. The subsequent wet runs (and real water is a requirement) will clearly illuminate logjams and inadequacies in preparations by any treatment facility for the onslaught of large numbers of contaminated casualties.

21.6.1 Real World Mass Casualty Decontamination General Principles

Expect no less than a 5:1 ratio of unaffected to affected casualties;

Decontaminate casualties as soon as possible;

Decontamination is disrobing—more removal is better, total is best;

Copious water flushing is a good mass decontamination method, although soap may also be necessary to remove oily liquids (and washing with soap is a way casualties will expect to cleans themselves).

All responders in contact with casualties should observe standard precautions;

Collection and disposal of "Dirty" clothing and the dead is critical;

All treatment facilities down-wind of disaster sites become part of the problem.

21.7 Example 1: Clinical Students

Clinicians diagnose and treat patients with viral hemorrhagic fever (VHF) in an emergency department. See CDC Viral Hemorrhagic Fever Fact Sheet in Appendix.

21.7.1 Students

Clinical ED personnel and all other clinical personnel called to augment the ED.

21.7.2 Instructors' Teaching Objectives

Familiarization with diagnosis and treatments of the wide-ranging types and overwhelming numbers of patients generated by bioterror event.

Reminder that Standard Precautions in the ED are always essential.

21.7.3 Students' Goals

Correctly care for all types of patients expected in the ED during a bio-agent event.

Correctly identify unfamiliar agents.

Inform appropriate disaster managers of presence of unusual agents.

21.7.4 Setting

Bays in the ED.

21.7.5 Participants and their Roles during production

Students—play themselves as clinicians and provide diagnosis and treatment.

Actors—play patients and clinicians guiding scenario.

Simulation professionals—operate mannequins.

21.7.6 Simulation Resources and Requirements

Extensive simulation professional preparation and rehearsals.

Interactive robotic patient simulation devices.

Simulated ED facility with the appropriate clinical equipment and supplies.

Audio/visual recordings of action in the ED for review phase.

Debriefing arena for replay and analysis of ED action.

21.7.7 Scenario Outline

The ED will see six different patients over 50 minutes. Of the five that enter the ED presenting various signs and symptoms of VHF intoxication, one will not be infected, and one will be "worried-well." The sixth will be a member of the ED that neglects contact precautions.

Patient 1, a robotic simulator, is severely intoxicated with VHF, has a very high fever and profound hemorrhagic shock, and despite all treatment dies 10 minutes after entering the ED. The presence of this patient emphasizes the lethality of VHF.

Patient 2, another robotic simulator, is intoxicated with VHF, is initially treated for fever and hemorrhagic shock, and then proceeds along a roller coaster of temperature spikes and circulatory failure. Final prognosis depends upon treatment. This patient emphasizes the intense vigilance and extensive care required for successful treatment of VHF (Figure 21.1).

Patient 3, a live actor, is intoxicated with VHF, walks into the ED 5 minutes after start of scenario with VHF oral and skin symptoms, is directed to a chair and told to wait. This patient becomes very anxious and disruptive just after observing the death of Patient 1, spits blood (simulated) onto a charge nurse, and should be restrained by students and then removed from the room by the security team. The incorporation of this patient into the scenario emphasizes the potential of the walking wounded to create fear-driven disruption and to spread contamination (Figure 21.2). Redirection of students' attention away from Patient 1 toward Patient 3 allows for surreptitious transformation of the dead Patient 1 into live Patient 4.

Patient 4, the now-reprogrammed robotic simulator that was used for Patient 1, represents a 60-year-old policeman with pre-existing respiratory (asthma) and cardiac diseases (hypertension, coronary artery disease). This patient is not infected with VHF, but the described illnesses and the drugs taken for those illnesses combined with fear make the clinical presentation similar to that of Patient 2. The inclusion of this patient emphasizes the diagnostic challenges of those bioterror agents that produce signs and symptoms similar to those of more common ailments.

Patient 5, a live actor, is a worried-well patient who walks into ED 35 minutes after the start of the scenario. This patient has no physical symptoms at all but is screaming about being poisoned and loudly and persistently demands to be treated. This patient emphasizes the fear-driven disruption by the worried-well and how their vast numbers at

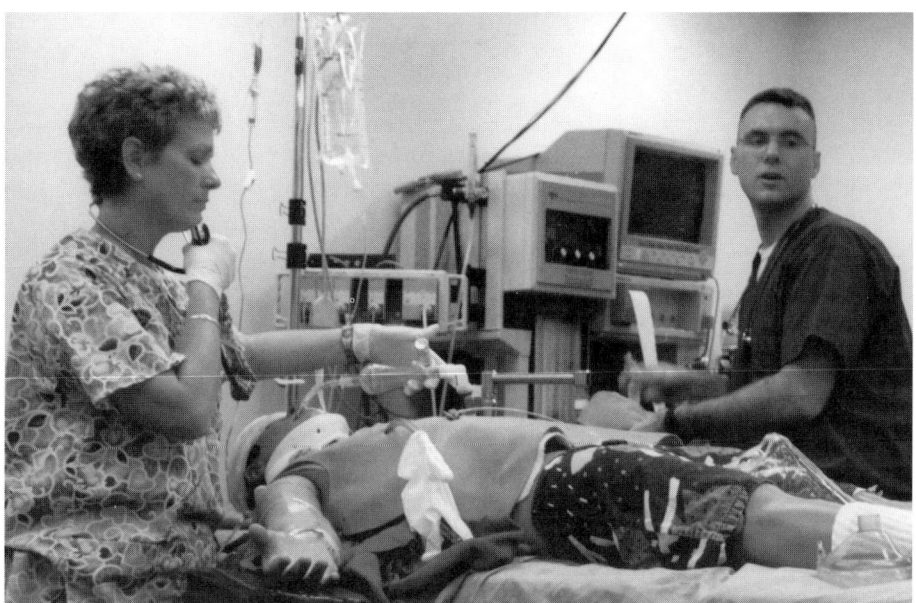

Figure 21.1 Patient #2, portrayed by a robotic patient simulator, receiving extensive invasive treatments by clinicians in the emergency department: intubation, chest tube, and IV access.

treatment facilities must be directed away from patient-care areas.

Patient 6, a live actor, plays a charge nurse who has been working in the ED for the entire scenario, becomes infected from contagious patients, vomits, and then leaves the ED. This actor emphasizes the fact that infectious diseases can contaminate clinical personnel who disregard precautions and fail to protect themselves.

21.8 EXAMPLE 2: Non-clinical Students

Non-clinical students, as a crisies-management team in an EOCC, allocate resources from their treatment facility in response to a SARS-like event.

21.8.1 Students
Disaster Management Team personnel.

21.8.2 Instructor's Teaching Objectives
Familiarization with command, control, communication and collaboration actions, and responsibilities during a facility-wide infection crisis.

21.8.3 Students' Goals
Correctly allocate finite resources to minimize morbidity and mortality during a mass-casualty bio-contamination event.

21.8.4 Setting
Emergency Operations Command Center (EOCC).

21.8.5 Participants and their Roles during production
Students play themselves as non-clinicians and provide non-clinical command and control in response to the event.

Actors and simulation professionals are out-of-sight generators of questions and answers via phone calls and simulated TV news programs (live-interactive or taped).

21.8.6 Simulation Resources and Requirements
Use a real EOCC, or if the actual EOCC is unavailable, stage a simulated EOCC in a conference

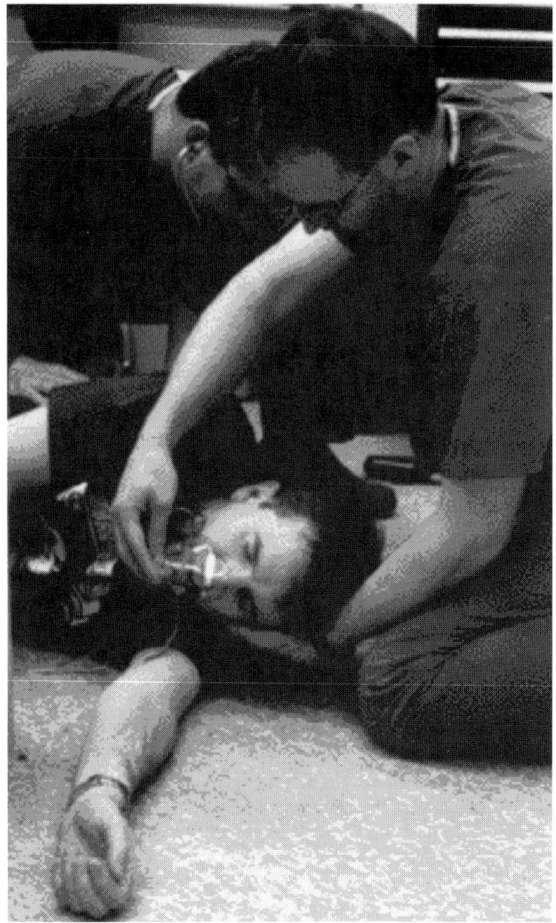

Figure 21.2 Patient #3, portrayed by a human actor, receiving basic non-invasive treatment in the emergency department.

room with sufficient functional devices and props to support the actions called for in the script.

Audiovisual feeds of information to drive scenario

Live telephone calls (interactive)
- Telephones (two per link)
- Telephone callers into the EOCC

Live radio communications (unidirectional but responsive to actions taken by students)
- An actor providing a live "broadcast"
- An EOCC radio wired to acoustically isolated audio studio

Pre-recorded radio broadcasts (unidirectional, indifferent to actions taken by students)
- An audio recorder playing the pre-recorded "broadcast"
- An EOCC radio wired to the remote player of the pre-recorded "broadcast"

A live television feed (unidirectional but responsive to actions taken by students)
- An actor providing a live "broadcast"
- An EOCC television wired to acoustically isolated audio/video studio

Pre-recorded television or video feed (unidirectional, indifferent to actions taken by students)

A television or video monitor wired to the remote player of the pre-recorded "broadcast"

An audiovisual collection of action in the EOCC and transmission to remote telephone actors

Audiovisual recordings of action in EOCC for the review phase

A debriefing arena for replay and analysis of EOCC action

21.8.7 Scenario Outline

Overwhelm decision-making capabilities by introducing unfamiliar demands and by reducing or otherwise compromising resources and by using live and pre-recorded audio and video feeds (telephones, radio, and television) fabricated to drive the scenario.

The specific script content can be a blending of the different types of patients from Example 1 amplified many times and overlaid upon the various physical and functional departments of the treatment facility. For example, the scenario might start early Monday morning with activation of the EOCC because the ED is overwhelmed with all the maintenance personnel who performed routine service over the weekend on the heating-ventilation-and-air-conditioning (HVAC) system in the medical treatment facility. Are their complaints of severe respiratory distress, a mass case of legionnaires' disease, hysteria, industrial action, or something else?

The CDC recommends the following components of preparedness and response in healthcare facilities:

Surveillance and triage
Clinical evaluation
Infection control and respiratory hygiene
Patient isolation and cohorting
Engineering and environmental controls
Exposure reporting and evaluation
Staffing needs and personnel policies
Facility access controls
Supplies and equipment
Communication and reporting

Note that each of these actions map directly to areas of responsibilities of key components of any treatment facility.

21.9 EXAMPLE 3: Clinical and Non-clinical Students

21.9.1 Students

ED and ED augmenters, security, first responders, facilities/maintenance staff, and communications/networks personnel.

21.9.2 Instructor's Teaching Objectives

Familiarization with command, control, communication and collaboration actions required for successful crowd control, decontamination, and triage of mass casualties seeking help and responsibilities during a city-wide bio-crisis.

21.9.3 Students' Goals

Successfully manage the large flow of casualties through the decontamination to securely separate the clean from the dirty, employ clinical judgment to separate the expectant from the treatable, and then provide a secure place for the former while guiding the latter into the ED.

21.9.4 Setting

Parking lot outside the entrance to the ED (see Figure 21.3).

21.9.5 Participants and their Roles during production

Half of the students play themselves, providing crowd control, decontamination, and triage; the other half play casualties seeking treatment inside the ED.

One actor guides the staff of the treatment facility, while another guides the casualties.

21.9.6 Simulation Resources and Requirements

Conference room, with chairs arranged to define five regions of the process:

Dirty Triage
Decontamination
Clean triage
Expectant
Entrance to the ED

Props: Playing cards, blue painters tape, red food coloring, operating-room (OR) caps, audiovisual recordings of action for the review phase, and a debriefing arena for replay and analysis of the action.

21.9.7 Scenario Outline

The casualties will do anything to gain access to the ED in hopes of getting treatment, while the staff of the treatment facility will try to maintain an orderly casualty flow.

First, the participants arrange the chairs into circles representing the five regions listed above. Simple signs should be taped on the chairs to clearly identify the function of each region.

Second, with playing cards, randomly assign half the students to be facility staff (those who receive red cards) and the other half (those who receive black cards) to be casualties. One actor directs the faculty staff to gather round for their "care" instructions, while another asks all the casualties to leave the room to receive their "assault" instructions.

21.9.7.1 Red Rules—told to red players (facility staff) only

All wear a distinctive treatment-facility staff "uniform," such as an OR hat. Those holding

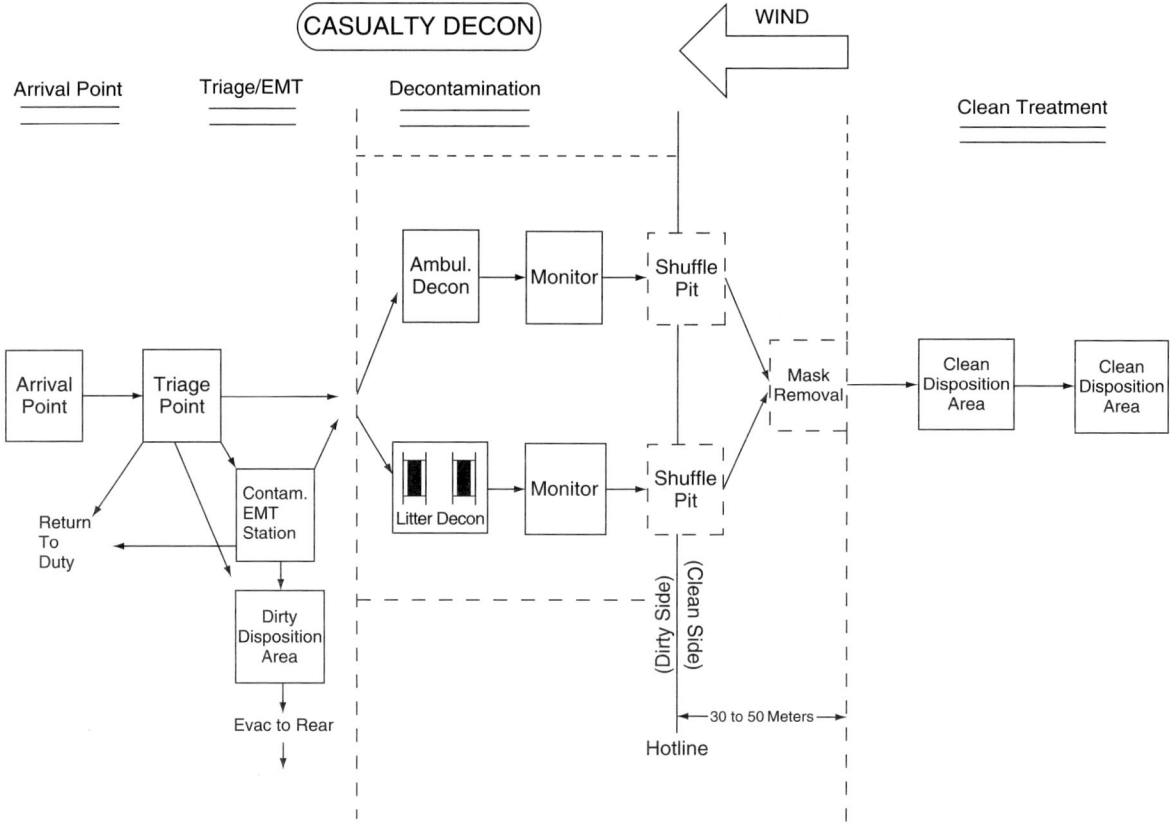

Figure 21.3 Schematic of patient flow through the three distinct and isolated zones of dirty triage, decontamination, and clean triage prior to delivery to the ED for definitive care.

odd-numbered cards (Ace, 3, 5, 7, and 9) are decontamination personnel but can also do security. Those holding *even-numbered cards* (2–10) are clinical (triage and ED) personnel. Those holding *face cards* are security (crowd control). Anyone with *blue tape* must go through decontamination and have the blue tape removed. Decontamination requires the dedicated attention of one decontamination person for 60 seconds. Anyone can go downstream (ED-Triage-Decon-Street) at will. No one is to be allowed upstream from decontamination unless he or she has been decontaminated for 60 seconds. The number of casualties in the ED cannot exceed the number of ED staff.

21.9.7.2 Red Goal

Separate the expectant from the treatable casualties, decontaminate the treatable casualties, and move the treatable casualties into the ED for definitive care.

21.9.7.3 Black Rules—told to black players (casualties) only

Wear no distinctive "uniform." All are to put pieces of *blue tape* on the outside of their clothing, but the tape can be under collars, ties, etc. Any one who agrees can get a drop of red food coloring put onto their tongues (the food coloring looks like blood but washes out with water). Those holding *low-numbered cards* have little or no infection, and some also have *blue tape*. These are the worried-well and the walking wounded. Those holding *high-numbered cards* have more infection and more *blue tape* and ask anyone for help to move toward the ED. Those holding *face cards* are severely infected and have lots of *blue tape*; they collapse before reaching the ED. Those holding *diamonds* are disruptive, distractive, loud, and argumentative and challenge instructions. Those holding *hearts* are sly, sneaky, and quiet and disregard instructions. All should try to contaminate treatment-facility staff through physical contact (i.e., by putting blue tape onto them).

21.9.7.4 Black Goal

Contaminate all treatment-facility staff and draw all clean triage and ED players into decontamination and dirty triage regions.

21.9.7.5 End

The scenario is over when either there is no one left outside the ED to treat, or when there is no one left in the ED to provide treatment.

21.9.8 Review

The *review* focuses upon the difficulties encountered when the individual goal of each casualty (complete safety and cure no matter how severely injured) conflicts with the finite capabilities of the treatment facility and its staff (who can afford to treat only those who with treatment would have a reasonable chance of living).

21.9.9 Replay

Shuffle and deal the cards again, and if necessary, make some adjustments to the rules to allow for more equal balance between *red* and *black*.

21.10 Summary

In the face of a real biodisaster, confidence in one's own competence as well as in the abilities of the rest of the team is a vital prerequisite for any expectation of a successful response. Engaging in scheduled simulated disasters gives treatment-center personnel invaluable learning experiences for improbable but not impossible biodisasters. Disasters can be overwhelming tsunami-like invasions. The product of their great size and very rapid onset characterizes the magnitude of their power for devastation. Formal didactic instruction and on-the-job experiential learning during "normal" situations are inadequate preparations for disasters, especially those that are intentionally created. Simulation, in its many forms, can reveal the gaps in current disaster preparation and can provide methods for exploring various new approaches to fill those gaps.

Reference

1. http://www.nytimes.com/2005/08/02/health/02dent.html?ex=1280635200&en=70fecfef8ea263c&ei=5090&partner=rssuserland&emc=rss

Resources

Disaster Preparation and Response

1. http://www.nbc-med.org/ie40/Default.html—Many PDF text books on medical management of NBC casualties.
2. http://www.bt.cdc.gov/—Many bioterror resources on this web site.
3. http://www.cdc.gov/ncidod/sars/—SARS: What is it, how to treat it, how to prepare healthcare facilities for it.
4. http://www.cdc.gov/ncidod/hip/Blood/Ebola.htm—Viral Hemorrhagic Fever (VHF) in Healthcare Settings.
5. www.emergency.com—Extensive first responder information.
6. www.cbiac.apgea.army.mil—Biological and chemical defense references.
7. http://www.chem-bio.com/resource/1999/cw_irp_cpc_lepo_ems_report.pdf—Chemical protective clothing for law enforcement patrol officers and emergency medical services.
8. http://www.bt.cdc.gov/children/pdf/working/execsumm03.pdf—pediatric WMD.
9. *Fundamentals of Disaster Management: A Handbook for Medical Professionals* Society of Critical Care Medicine Press, ISBN 0-936145-18-8, 2004.
10. Thomas W. McGovern, George W. Christopher, and Edward Eitzen. Cutaneous manifestations of

biological warfare and related threat agents. *Arch Dermatol*, 135: 311–322, 1999.
11. Anthony G. Macintyre, George W. Christopher, Edward Eitzen, Jr. Robert Gum, Scott Weir, Craiig DeAtley, Kevin Tonat, and Joseph A. Barbera. Weapons of mass destruction events with contaminated casualties: effective planning for health care facilities. *JAMA*, 283: 242–249, 2000.
12. Richard Morgan. Dentists prepare to be on front line of civil defense. *New York Times*, August 2, 2005.

Simulation and Disaster Scenarios

13. R. R. Kyle, D. K. Via, R. J. Lowy, J. M. Madsen, A. M. Marty, and P. D. Mongan. Multi-disciplinary approach to teach responses to weapons of mass destruction and terrorism using combined simulation modalities. *Journal of Clinical Anesthesia*, 16(2):152–158, 2004.
14. Simulation and Team Training. *Quality and Safety in Health Care*, Vol 13(1); Oct 2004 (www.qshc.com).
15. David M. Gaba, Kevin J. Fish, and Steven K. Howard. *Crisis Management in Anesthesiology*, Churchill Livingstone, ISBN 0-443-08910-8 (Amazon.com).
16. Robert L. Helmreich, John A. Wilhelm, James R. Klinect, and Ashleigh C. Merritt. Culture, error, and crew resource management. In *Improving Teamwork in Organizations* (E. Salas, C. A. Bowers, and E. Edens eds.), pp. 305–331. Erlbaum, 2001.

Fundamentals of Simulation

17. Paul D. Thacker. Fake worlds offer real medicine: virtual reality finding a role in treatment and training. *JAMA* 290:2107, 11, 12, 2003.
18. Richard Kyle. Technological resources for clinical simulation. In *Simulators in Critical Care and Beyond* (Dunn W. ed.), ISBN 0-936145-15-3. Society for Critical Care Medicine Press, May 2004.
19. Gary Loyd, Carol Lake, and Ruth Greenberg. *Practical Health Care Simulations*, ISBN 1-56053-625-x. Elsevier Mosby Press, June 2004.
20. Lindsey Hensen and Andrew Lee. *Simulators in Anesthesiology Education*, ISBN 0-306-45775-X. Plenum Press, January 1998.
21. Clark Aldrich. *Learning by Doing: A Comprehensive Guide to Simulations, Computer Games, and Pedagogy in e-Learning and Other Educational Experiences*, ISBN 0-7879-7735-7. Pfeiffer, 2005.
22. Karl E. Weick and Kathleen M. Sutcliffe. *Managing the Unexpected—Assuring High Performance in an Age of Complexity*, ISBN 0-7879-6527-9. Jossey-Bass, San Francisco, 2001.
23. Lori K. McDonnell, Kimberly K. Jobe, and R. Key Dismukes. *Facilitating line oriented simulations debriefings: a training manual.* NASA Technical Memorandum 112192 DOT/FAA/AR-97/6, March 1997 (http://www.faa.gov/education_research/training/aqp/library/media/Final_Training_TM.pdf).

22 Hospital Large-Scale Drills

GARRETT HAVICAN

22.1 Introduction

The acute care hospital is in business to treat sick and injured citizens within its municipality and its contiguous communities. The hospital is a repository of clinicians from many disciplines and a consortium of ancillary and diagnostic staff all acting synergistically to achieve the common goal of adding value to precious human life.

As the practice of medicine evolves due to research, new pharmaceutical treatment regimens and technological advances in the field of medicine, the acute care hospital has successfully met these ever-changing needs. Hospitals have proven they are resilient and that they respond to the aforementioned changes appropriately and without undue stress. Many hospital administrators have developed the philosophy of "anticipate, act and adapt" to the substantive changes incurred by the modern day acute care hospital. This adage is all too similar to one of the United States Military mottos, which is to "improvise, adapt and overcome."

Due to the fact that the paradigm is constantly changing in the acute care hospital, it has been challenged with the implementation of certain requirements developed by the Joint Commission on Accreditation of Healthcare Organizations (JCAHO). JCAHO, the primary accrediting body for Acute Care Hospital is a private nonprofit organization whose mission is to "Continuously improve the safety and quality of care provided to the public through the provision of health care accreditation and related services that support performance improvement in health care organizations" [1].

As the oldest and most recognized accrediting agency, JCAHO also acts as a "Clearing House" for the Federal "Center for Medicaid and Medicare Services (CMS)" which administers the Medicare program and works with the States to administer the Medicaid and Child Health programs as well as the "Health Information Portability and Accountability Act (HIPAA)" [2].

Hospitals are extremely reliant upon Medicare and Medicaid reimbursement programs as most of them report that CMS reimbursement accounts for more than half of its overall annual revenue. Therefore, JCAHO compliance and subsequent accreditation is a requirement for the hospital to maintain operations and stay in business. Accredited Hospitals spend countless hours and funds complying with JCAHO standards, preparing for JCAHO visits and identifying process improvement initiatives and strategies to maintain the high standard that JCAHO requires.

One of the most challenging processes required of the acute care hospital under JCAHO is the development and implementation of Emergency Management standards. These standards are required under a specific section in the JCAHO Accreditation Manual dedicated to maintaining a safe and efficient environment, known as the "Environment of Care" standards. The environment of care section identifies seven areas, including Emergency Management, Life Safety, Hazardous Materials and Waste, Security Management, Safety Management, Medical Equipment, and Utility Systems Management. These areas focus on the safety of the patients, the staff and the infrastructure and collaborate with the other standards to assure a safe and efficient healthcare operation.

Under the Emergency Management section, the standard requires the hospitals to initially conduct a "Hazard Vulnerability Analysis (HVA)" which is meant to identify those hazards in the community that a hospital can potentially be subject to; second, the hospitals need to develop an Emergency Management Plan (EMP) and finally, the hospital is required to conduct drills twice annually. The HVA has been a common practice for Local emergency Planning Agencies for years. "The environmental protection agency (EPA) commissioned a national study in 1985 to look at hazardous chemicals and the sources of their release" [3]. Since then, the HVA has been a method utilized by many regulatory agencies including the Occupational Safety and Health Administration (OSHA), the National Institute of Occupational Safety and Health (NIOSH) and the National Fire Protection Association (NFPA). The results of the HVA assist the acute care hospitals in developing the EMP. Based on the identified threats of the external environment and the perceived threats including domestic and international terrorism, the EMP should identify the hospital's role in planning, response to, mitigation and recovery from a large-scale emergency.

Figure 22.1 is an example of a Hazard Vulnerability analysis Matrix.

The EMP is the plan that the acute care hospital utilizes when it is forced with responding to and mitigating a mass-casualty or disaster situation. These plans should be developed to address the overarching response with the identification of an Emergency Operations Center (EOC), the internal "Codes" that are announced to alert the employees required to respond to a disaster and the development of incident-specific annexes that address the responses consistent with the disaster. The EMPs are living documents in that they are constantly being updated and new sections are being added based upon the after action results from a large-scale event including drills and real-life events. It is recommended that the hospital establish an Emergency Management Committee under the auspices of the Environment of Care to plan drills and develop evaluation tools and in a similar manner to examine the results of the evaluations after the drill and make recommendations based on the evaluation findings and improve the EMPs based on these "Best Practices."

22.2 Hospital Drill Planning

Since 2001, JCAHO has required that the hospital perform drills that meet the listed in criteria Figure 22.2.

Hospitals, in general, continue to comply with the JCAHO standards, however, over the past several years, recent natural and terrorist events have added yet another paradigm shift for the acute care hospital. A shift that will require the hospital to ready itself for the likes of "Patient Surge," "Worried and Concerned citizens," "Nerve Agent Exposure," "Radiation illness due to the 'Dirty Bombs,'" "Biological Toxins," "Avian Flu/Pandemic Influenza" and "Incendiary Devices." All were perceived threats in previous HVAs but none truly realized until the onset of the terrorist attacks on New York and Washington DC on September 11, 2001. These attacks not only altered the paradigm, but they unnerved the citizens in the community and proved to the protective services and first responders that we are vulnerable as a nation. The attacks also forced the emergency management professional to focus on "All Hazards" due to the fact that the natural or man-made disaster is much more likely to affect the public and the community infrastructure.

In January 2006, JCAHO will begin to take a closer look at the Hospitals EMPs, how they perform their respective HVAs and how they integrate and collaborate with the resources that are available within the community. JCAHO will evaluate the effectiveness of these plans by assessing the results of scenario-driven drills that the hospitals are required to perform. JCAHO will evaluate the drill's "After Action Reports"(AARs) to identify deficiencies that were uncovered during the drill and a list of objectives established to assure process improvement.

Hospitals are beginning to re-prioritize their emergency preparedness initiatives as well as the development of their drills and exercises.

HAZARD AND VULNERABILITY ASSESSMENT TOOL
NATURALLY OCCURING EVENTS

SCORE	PROBABILITY	SEVERITY = (MAGNITUDE – MITIGATION)					RISK	AVERAGE SCORE
	Likelihood this will occur	HUMAN IMPACT Possibility of death or injury	PROPERTY IMPACT Physical losses & damages	BUSINESS IMPACT Interruption of Services	PREPARED-NESS Preplanning	INTERNAL RESPONSE Time, effectiveness, resources	EXTERNAL RESPONSE Community/ Mutual Aid staff & supplies	Relative threat
	0 = N/A 1 = Low 3 = Moderate 5.5 = High	0 = N/A 1 = Low 3 = Moderate 5.5 = High	0 = N/A 1 = Low 3 = Moderate 5.5 = High	0 = N/A 1 = Low 3 = Moderate 5.5 = High	0 = N/A 1 = HIGH 3 = Moderate 5.5 = LOW OR NONE	0 = N/A 1 = HIGH 3 = Moderate 5.5 = LOW OR NONE	0 = N/A 1 = HIGH 3 = Moderate 5.5 = LOW OR NONE	0–100%
Blizzard	5	2	2	5	1	1	3	49.35%	2.71
Dam Inundation	1.5	2	3	4	5	3	4	58.44%	3.21
Drought	3	2	1	1.5	5	4	5	55.84%	3.07
Epidemic	2	5	3	3	2	3	3	54.55%	3.00
Earthquake	1	3	5	5	5	5	3	70.13%	3.86
Flood, external	3	2	5	3	4	3	3	59.74%	3.29
Hurricane	4	4	5	4	3	3	2	64.94%	3.57
Ice Storm	4	3	3	4	4	3	2	59.74%	3.29
Landslide	1.5	2	3	2	5	4	2	50.65%	2.79
Severe Thunderstorm	5	2.5	2	2.5	4	4	2	57.14%	3.14
Temperature Extremes	5	3	1	2	4	3	4	57.14%	3.14
Tidal Wave	1	5	5	5	5.5	5.5	4	80.52%	4.43
Tornado	2	4	5	4	4	2	2	59.74%	3.29
Volcano	0	0	0	0	0	0	0	0.00%	0.00
Wild Fire	1	3	3	3	4	3	2	49.35%	2.71
								0.00%	0.00

Figure 22.1 Hazard and vulnerability assessment tool. (http://www.osha.gov/dts/osta/bestpractices/html/hospital_firstreceivers.html).

> 1. The hospital tests the response phase of its emergency management plan twice per year, whether in response to an actual emergency or in planned drills.
> 2. Drills are conducted at least four months apart and no more than eight months apart.
> 3. Hospitals that offer emergency services or are community designated disaster-receiving stations must conduct at least one drill a year that includes an influx of volunteers or simulated patients.
> 4. The hospital participates in at least one community-wide practice drill a year (where applicable) relevant to the priority emergencies identified in its hazard vulnerability analysis. The drill assesses the communication, coordination, and effectiveness of the hospitals and community's command structures.
> 5. All drills are critiqued to identify deficiencies and opportunities for improvement.

Figure 22.2 JCAHO Criteria (JCAHO Standard EC 4.20).

The assistance of the federal government through the Department of Health and Human Services (HHS): Health Resources and Services Administration (HRSA), the Centers for Disease Control and Prevention (CDC) and other federal and state funded programs have introduced incentives and reimbursement to hospitals for time spent planning and exercising. The increased attention coupled with the financial incentives backed by federal and state agencies, as well as enhanced scrutiny by regulatory and accrediting bodies makes drill planning and exercise development more of a priority for hospitals.

In the past, hospitals were reliant upon the first response services to respond to and mitigate large-scale disasters. Historically, the local Fire Department is responsible for the on-scene management including decontamination, extrication and fire suppression as the Police Department is responsible for scene protection and evidence collection. The EMS Agent is responsible for the on-scene triage, treatment, and transportation of a victim and is responsible to follow local guidelines to appropriately choose the receiving facility. All of this continues to be true, however, the hospital is beginning to realize that it is not immunized against being the "Scene" itself. Hospital planners consider the "All Hazards" philosophy and theorize that the potential exists that the hospital itself can be the target of a terrorist attack. The hospital can also be "Location 0" for a Pandemic crisis as well as the receiving facility for a patient contaminated with a toxic material at work.

Coming full circle, the hospital emergency planning community considers many different scenarios based upon the results of its HVAs including the man-made and natural disasters in the Nation, terrorist activity and dissemination methods as well as the existence of airborne and blood borne vectors that can cause a pandemic crisis. The identification of the vulnerabilities drives the development of the EMPs. The results of the HVA also prioritize the vulnerabilities from most likely to least likely. The development of a hospital drill considers all of these factors and the hospital emergency planners determine the need to exercise and evaluate a response to a specific vulnerability, the mitigation of this vulnerability and the recovery from the incident. The hospital emergency planner then develops an evaluation tool around each evolution of response and collects the tools when the exercise is over. The evaluation scores and comments are queried and a list of goals and objectives is developed. This list can be measurable (with a numerical value added to each objective) or not. The primary goal of this list of "Lessons Learned" is to continually improve the process of the hospital. Evaluation and process improvement with regard to drills and exercises will be an integral part of the accreditation standards moving forward (Figure 22.3).

Hospitals are now required to think like they are the "First Responders" and that the incident site can very reasonably be within the hospital facility. The business of incident command, decontamination, surge capacity, lock down, and transportation is now a part of the hospital emergency management planning meeting agenda. The EMPs are identifying how the hospital will deal with "All Hazards" incidents and they detail its response, mitigation, and recovery as well as its ability to maintain an incident

Expected responses to be evaluated	Action Taken (Yes/No)	Action Score	Time Score	Time begun	Time completed	Notes
4.0 Hospital Evacuation Policy						
4.1 EOC Activated.	N/A					
4.2 Security will "Lock Down" all entrances.	N/A					
4.3 Appropriate overhead announcements made.						
4.4 Manpower to manage the evacuation gather.						
4.5 The decision is made to identify the closest safest location to evacuate patients to.						
Conklin Building Evacuation						
1.0 Patients directly exposed to the fire/smoke condition moved first.						
1.1 Patients are moved to the opposite side of the floor from the fire/smoke condition.						
1.2 The decision is made to move patients vertically to the second floor in a timely manner.						

Figure 22.3 Evaluation form created by Karyl Burns, RN, PhD; Research Scientist, Hartford Hospital Department of Trauma and Emergency Medicine; 2005.

command center, decontaminate patients and lock-down the facility and its perimeter.

The fire service and other first response agencies have followed an "Incident Command" model for years. Historically, the fire department will maintain the command of the incident and the police department will preserve the integrity and safety of the scene. The EMS Agent will concern itself with the treatment, destination, and transportation based upon the status of the receiving acute care hospital facilities in the area contiguous to the incident. In planning for an emergency, the hospital may have to deal with emergencies that require more resources than they have to provide and for a longer time than they have to give. The senior level administration may or may not be available at the time of the incident to make command decisions and the Supervisor "In-charge" of the hospital when an incident occurs may not have the operational experience necessary to make vital decisions to maintain the operational integrity of the institution. Therefore, the hospital is challenged with identifying a system that will assist in the creation of an incident command model when resources are depleted and the typical administrative positions are unavailable.

Fortunately, there are several models that have been developed to meet these needs and assist in the deployment of an incident command center or EOC in a hospital. These systems identify, through an organizational chart, key leadership positions that need to be filled in order to mitigate the disaster from an operations perspective. However, the positions are ambiguous and can be filled by various members of the hospitals staff. For each one of these positions, a "Job Action Sheet" (Figure 22.4) is written which identifies the immediate, intermediate, and tended needs of a position whether it is the Incident Commander or the Environmental Services Unit Leader. This job action sheet is written to assist a position in making decisions for the first 24 hours of a sustained emergency operations center.

The "Hospital Emergency Incident Command System"(HEICS) is a program that was developed in 1991 by the Orange County Healthcare Agency and funded by the California Emergency Medical Services Authority due to the frequency of natural disasters and how they affect the healthcare system. HEICS is a system of scripted command positions developed for: "Uncomfortable Officials in unfamiliar surroundings, playing uncomfortable roles, making unpopular decisions with inadequate information in far too little time" [4]. To date, HEICS is the most commonly used hospital incident command system in the United States. It is recognized as a "Best Practice" by acute care hospitals across US and plays an integral role in hospital drills and exercises.

When a drill or real emergency takes place, the Hospital uses a set of covert overhead announcements to alert the staff that an emergency exists and how to respond to that specific emergency. Hospital alerts vary from facility to facility which may invoke some confusion, however, employees are taught the emergency codes during employee orientation, are refreshed to the specific codes on an annual basis through competency based education and during the drill activities. Many of the hospitals have developed codes for preparation, full-scale response as well as recovery for an incident on top of the ordinary fire alarms and electrical testing announcements. The codes are kept covert to disguise its intent for the patient and the visitor so as not to invoke unnecessary panic. Employees should practice communicating the intent of the overhead alerts to the inquisitive patient and/or visitor so they are not "caught off guard" and provide too much information that can instill fear or anxiety.

Once activated, the hospital incident command center becomes the central "Hub" of operational activity. The HEICS system supports the concept of interoperability and collaboration, which facilitates the ability to make executive level decisions in an emergent situation. The members of the executive management team and/or their designee assume the role in the incident command center that is most consistent with his/her daily obligations in the institution.

The following organizational chart demonstrates the leadership matrix within the emergency operations center (Figure 22.5).

Mission:	Organize and direct Emergency Operations Center (EOC). Give overall direction for hospital operations and if needed, authorize evacuation.	
Immediate	_____	Initiate the Hospital Emergency Incident Command System by assuming role of Emergency Incident Commander.
	_____	Read this entire Job Action Sheet.
	_____	Put on position identification vest.
	_____	Appoint all Section Chiefs and the Medical Staff Director positions; distribute the four section packets which contain: • Job Action Sheets for each position • Identification vest for each position • Forms pertinent to Section & positions
	_____	Appoint Public Information Officer, Liaison Officer, and Safety and Security Officer; distribute Job Action Sheets. (May be pre-established.)
	_____	Announce a status/action plan meeting of all Section Chiefs and Medical Staff Director to be held within 5–10 minutes.
	_____	Assign someone as Documentation Recorder/Aide.
	_____	Receive status report and discuss an initial action plan with Section Chiefs and Medical Staff Director. Determine appropriate level of service during immediate aftermath.
	_____	Receive initial facility damage survey report from Logistics Chief, if applicable, evaluate the need for evacuation.
	_____	Obtain patient census and status from Planning Section Chief. Emphasize proactive actions within the Planning Section. Call for a hospital-wide projection report for 4, 8, 24 & 48 hours from time of incident onset. Adjust projections as necessary.
	_____	Authorize a patient prioritization assessment for the purposes of designating appropriate early discharge, if additional beds needed.
	_____	Assure that contact and resource information has been established with outside agencies through the Liaison Officer.
Intermediate	_____	Authorize resources as needed or requested by Section Chiefs.
	_____	Designate routine briefings with Section Chiefs to receive status reports and update the action plan regarding the continuance and termination of the action plan.
	_____	Communicate status to chairperson of the Hospital Board of Directors or the designee.
	_____	Consult with Section Chiefs on needs for staff, physician, and volunteer responder food and shelter. Consider needs for dependents. Authorize plan of action.
Extended	_____	Approve media releases submitted by P.I.O.
	_____	Observe all staff, volunteers and patients for signs of stress and inappropriate behavior. Report concerns to Psychological Support Unit Leader. Provide for staff rest periods and relief.
	_____	Other concerns:

Figure 22.4 Emergency incident commander job action sheet (http://www.heics.com/).

Once the incident command center is established and the positions have been determined then the incident commander in conjunction with the other positions in the matrix will make decisions to appropriately manage the disaster. The incident commander for the hospital EOC also sends representatives out to local and state emergency operations centers to act as liaisons and to communicate information between incident command centers. This representative is essential for the hospital and for the community as he/she will facilitate the sharing of resources to assist both entities.

The Large Scale Hospital drill is an excellent opportunity to identify the available resources in the surrounding community and involve them in the exercise process. One of the primary "Lessons Learned" from most large-scale hospital drills is that the hospital is unable to sustain operations without the assistance from the community resources. The ability to communicate with these resources and to plan in advance via a community wide Memorandum

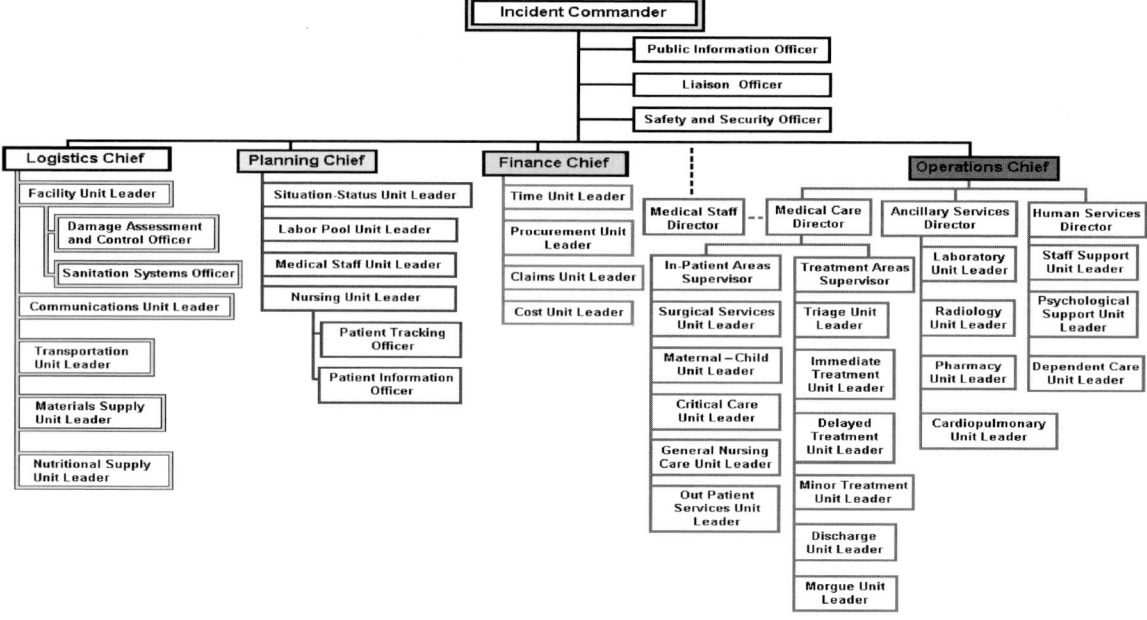

Figure 22.5 HEICS organizational chart.

of Understanding (MOU) or other planning document is essential to ensure the quick and effective mitigation of a large-scale incident.

The large-scale hospital drill is also important from a local emergency planning perspective. The planners in the communities surrounding a major acute care hospital need to consider the size of the hospital population, the lack of essential resources that a hospital does have with regard to security, decontamination, crowd control and communications. It is in the best interest of the community leaders to work with its local acute care hospitals as well as its local, regional, county and state agencies to discuss collaborative responses and develop annexes to highlight specific needs for specific incidents.

22.3 Decontamination

The business of decontamination is not new for the acute care hospital. For years, hospitals that have EDs have been tasked with decontaminating patients who enter through their doors covered in some sort of chemical, biological, or infectious disease agent. The decontamination areas in hospitals were primarily extra rooms near the ED entrance that may or may not have a lead protective lining in the walls and may or may not have a dedicated drain for the run off. These rooms have, at times, doubled as shower stalls for certain patients who may be intoxicated or are very much in need of a shower or to clean the bloody backboards prior to returning them to the EMS providers. The make-up of this decontamination system included a showerhead, a shower curtain and a variety of soap products to assist the individual in decontaminating him or herself. In cases involving unresponsive patients who may be contaminated with an agent, hospitals have performed decontamination procedures in an ED room on a patient gurney and cut off the clothes and rinsed the patient down with bath sponges or towels. Many healthcare workers were unaware of the potential for "Off Gassing" and spread of a bioterrorism agent. The Personal Protective equipment of choice in these situations would historically be the splash-proof hospital gown and a HEPA/N95 or surgical facemask and gloves. The patient's clothes would be handled by the Security Department in most situations and would be locked up in a closet with all of the other patient belongings that the Security Department collected that day. Obviously, over the past several years, the paradigm has yet again shifted. Hospitals now need to take a long, hard look at their decontamination and property collection and storage practices.

Very few hospitals were in the practice of "gross" and "technical decontamination" prior to the events of 9-11-01. Very few hospitals have arranged for a response team of clinical personnel in fully encapsulated suits with Powered Air Purifying Respirators (PAPRs) to respond outside of the ED entrance to greet victims from a potential exposure. In this day and age, the hospital has to learn from lessons of the past and adhere to recommendations from state and federal agencies that are providing funding to enhance emergency preparedness. These recommendations consider the Anthrax attacks from 2001, they assume that a chemical agent is hazardous and that an infectious disease is in imminent danger of life and health and is potentially lethal when transmitted. The practice of "All Hazards" preparedness raises the eyebrow of the clinical practitioner and influences this clinician to make decisions based on the best interest of the Hospital and the staff as well as the patient. Patient care cannot be diligently performed by clinical staff who have been affected with the same agent via patient off-gassing or airborne contamination.

As discussed, the healthcare arena in the post 9–11 world is beginning to consider "All Hazards" and the potentiality of seeing hoards of victims from one single incident. Stories have emerged from incidents such as the Aum shinrikyo's [5]. Sarin gas release in the Tokyo subway system in 1995 and other mass disasters that have introduced contaminated victims into unsuspecting hospitals. Statistics show that the "Psychological Footprint" (Figure 22.6) of patients showing up at ED immediately after a mass-casualty event exceeds the number of medically injured by a factor of 10 or more [6].

The hospital large-scale drill should consider all of these factors, which can lead to a comprehensive scenario that involves multiple disciplines, from multiple departments and external

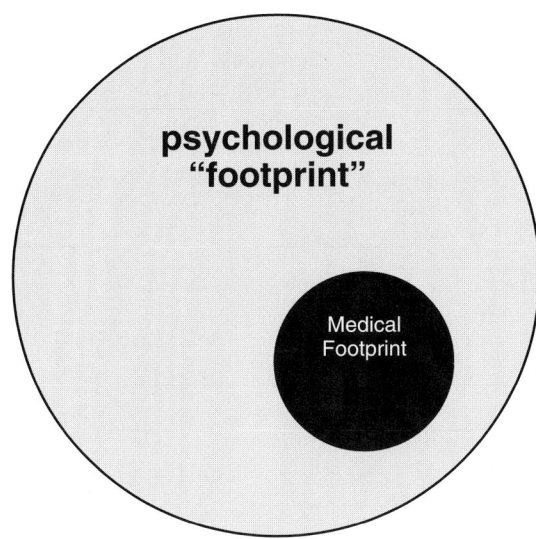

Figure 22.6 Relationship between true casualties and the "worried well."

agencies. The decontamination-specific procedures may require the purchase of additional equipment to perform the decontamination function. This may also force hospitals to enter into an agreement with their local Fire Department or EPA to assist in the decontamination procedures for numerous victims.

In 2005 the Occupational Safety and Health Administrations (OSHA's) released the: "Best Practices for Hospital-Based 1st Receivers of victims from mass-casualty incidents involving the release of hazardous substances" document [7]. "This document is designed to provide hospitals with practical information to assist them in developing and implementing emergency management plans that address the protection of hospital-based emergency department personnel during the receipt of contaminated victims from mass-casualty incidents occurring at locations other than the hospital. Among other topics, it covers victim decontamination, personal protective equipment, and employee training, and also includes several informational appendices." [8].

The hospitals are beginning to conform to the recommendations within this document as it provides a realistic look at the needs of a healthcare facility to maintain the safety and well being of its employees and patients. The purchase of Tyvek® suits as well as loose fitting PAPR hoods are highly recommended for the clinical personnel who are tasked with treating a patient presenting to a hospital with an unknown substance. The hospitals have also utilized funds to purchase decontamination units to assure a greater number of patients decontaminated in a lesser period of time. Many of these decontamination systems are inflatable or made of "PVC" piping to maintain patient modesty, facilitate technical decontamination and expedite patients through the decontamination system.

OSH's "Best Practices" document identifies two zones for the treatment of victims in need of decontamination; a "Hospital Decon Zone" and a "Post-Hospital Decon Zone." The assumption is that the decontamination of possibly contaminated victims will take place in an outside area adjacent to the ED and the staff will don all of the appropriate PPE as recommended by OSHA to manage these patients. The Hospital Decon Zone therefore is the external zone where a full-scale operation is underway and the Post Hospital Decon Zone is the actual ED itself. The lines of demarcation between these two zones are the entrance doors to the hospital ED.

22.4 Drills

Clearly, the hospitals are becoming more and more involved in the practice of incident response as a First Receiver institution. The practice of hosting drills and exercises is becoming ever so important due to the simple fact that hospitals learn from their mistakes. A hospital is not only required by its accrediting body to perform large scale drills, but it is provided incentives to do so by state and federal agencies. It is required to assume safe and efficient means of personal protection and patient care under regulatory bodies such as OSHA and it is sought out by local emergency planning organizations to play an integral role in the local, regional and county response practices.

Hospitals play a key role in the business of drills and exercises. They are also very important members of the world of decontamination, interoperability, and incident management. As time evolves and hospitals become increasingly better at what they do with regard to emergency preparedness initiatives, drills and exercise scenarios will increase in complexity, time commitment and scope. As long as the evaluations are performed in a timely and objective manner and after action reports are submitted to establish recommendations for process improvement, then the acute care hospital is destined to increase its level of preparedness and inevitably assist in the protection of the employee, patient and visitor. The hospital will continue to add value to the community and to the county and state that it resides in and will be a resource for the local planning efforts.

Hospitals will continue to respond to and recover from paradigm shifts and will continue to work together with their partners in the healthcare arena to meet the ever-changing needs of the medical institution.

22.4.1 Examples of Large Scale Hospital Disaster Drills

April 4th, 2005: Top Off III Drill, Hartford Hospital, Hartford, Connecticut

On Monday, April 4th, 2005, Hartford Hospital participated in the nations largest, full-scale international drill called "Top Off 3." Top Off, which is an acronym for "Top Officials," was a multi-state, multi-agency drill that was developed by the federal Department of Homeland Security to examine the "Top Officials" in the United States and their response to an act of terrorism or natural catastrophe. In early 2004, the Federal Government chose Connecticut along with New Jersey, the United Kingdom, and Canada as participants in this unprecedented international exercise.

Connecticut exercised its response to a terrorist release of a chemical agent, its ability to manage casualties from this incident as well as the ability to plan and implement a recovery process. Another unprecedented objective was the inclusion of Connecticut's 32 acute care hospitals and their ability to decontaminate affected patients, manage overload or "surge capacity" and communicate with Department of Public Health (DPH) and other resources to assist in mitigation and recovery. Hartford Hospital played an integral role in the planning, implementation and evaluation of this exercise as a Center of Excellence for Bioterrorism Preparedness and we are proud to have participated in such an important event.

Hartford Hospital responded to the simulated attacks by activating internal emergency response plans, performing decontamination procedures, and collaborating in an EOC to make necessary operational decisions in the event that this was a real emergency. Hartford Hospital worked with the State of Connecticut DPH, the Capitol Region Emergency Planning Committee, and our 14 emergency preparedness partner hospitals in the northern tier of Connecticut for communications and resource allocation.

Overall, Hartford Hospital's response to the Top Off 3 exercise was a success. Clearly, there are specific areas that are in need of improvement, however, the fact that these areas have been identified and will process improvement initiatives will be developed secondary to our findings, adds to its success.

Several weeks prior to Top Off 3, strategic planning meetings were held with several departments to review hospital objectives for the exercise, the respective department's response and barriers that may exist which may hinder that response. All HH Departments directly and/or indirectly involved with the exercise met individually and collaboratively and they include: the Departments of Trauma & Emergency Medicine, Surgery, Hospital Administration, Anesthesia, Fire and Safety, Facilities, Planning, Engineering, Business Development & Community Relations, Telecommunications, Security, MIS, Biomedical Engineering, Bed Management, Materials Management, Pharmacy, Laboratory, Infectious Disease, Occupational Medicine, EMS Education, Nursing, Pastoral Care, and the Institute of Living.

Open information sessions were also held for hospital employees in addition to published articles in the "Rxtra Newsletter" prior to this exercise. Educational programs such as the HEICS and "Toxic Industrial Chemicals (TICS)" and "Toxic Industrial Materials (TIMS)" course were held here at Hartford Hospital in preparation for the Top Off exercise.

The Top Off 3 exercise allowed the various Departments the opportunity to review, test and evaluate their respective plans and how they integrate with the entire facility during an emergency. As mentioned in previous sections, many wonderful recommendations came out of this drill as we move forward into the process improvement initiatives. The following table details the recommendations that were made and the departments that must play an integral role in coordinating this process. Once a department identifies that they are accountable to follow up on a recommendation, they should convene a meeting with key individuals in the institution who will assist them in developing objectives, strategy, and timelines to fulfill these obligations.

All recommendations will be detailed in a progress report format in order to track the improvements. Any recommendation that requires greater resources will be carried over to the After Action Reports for subsequent drills (Figure 22.7).

22.5 Conclusion

The acute care hospital in the post 9–11 era must be cognizant of the fact that the paradigm has changed and that emergency management planning must take a higher priority in the strategy of the organization. The hospital must perform comprehensive HVAs, it must develop or enhance its emergency management plans around the HVAs. The drills that are required twice annually must reflect a realistic scenario based upon the results of the HVA. In planning for the large-scale drill, the hospital must assure that its staff members are trained to the new expectations including donning and doffing personal protective equipment, monitoring and identifying potentially life-threatening hazards, technical and gross decontamination and containment of an incident outside of the hospital facility. Concepts such as "surge capacity," "perimeter control and lockdown," "worried and concerned"

Example After Action Report

#	Recommendation	Coordinating department
1	The decontamination area needs to have a better water supply.	Fire & Safety
2	Communications, especially with Coordinated medical emergency dispatch (C-Med) needs improvement and should be drilled more often.	ED/BT Reg. Planning
3	ED triage team and decontamination personnel need to collaborate and discuss response integration.	ED/Fire & Safety
4	Decontamination should be performed thoroughly prior to patients being allowed in the ED.	Fire Safety
5	There needs to be a greater number of staff members trained in decontamination and donning and doffing PAPRs.	ED/Fire & Safety/ Industrial Hygiene/BT
6	There needs to be a better communication system in the ED, especially between the Attending ED Physician in charge at the time of the emergency and the rest of the staff, representation in the EOC.	ED
7	Communications from area to area (external triage to internal ED) needs to be enhanced as well. The leadership in the ED needs to be well-informed with the most up-to-date information.	ED
8	Identify an alternative location in the plan for family overflow if the Chapel in not sufficient to manage the number or size of the event.	BH/IOL
9	Mechanism to allocate and utilize clinicians that arrive to assist family members or /or families. Plan needs to address where they should report to, who coordinates their activity and assumes accountability.	BH/Security
10	Utilize ED staff/Pastoral Care Staff as a resource to direct social workers for assistance in ED. Perhaps appoint a contact person to coordinate activity.	ED/BH
11	Initial attempts to contact the CTRP, did not have the right phone number and then took some time to get a response back from them.	BHBT Reg. Planning
12	Provide access to a Family assistance center database to determine the patient's location.	HEOC/BH/MIS
13	Determine a specific location of the temporary morgue.	ED/Security/Facilities/IOL
14	Determine a proper location for the Press.	Bus. Devel/PR/Security
15	Insufficient number of two-way radio communications.	Security/Fire/ Comms
16	Battery life on the PAPRs dwindles quickly and needed replaced often.	Industrial Hygiene/BT
17	Need for additional portable radios in EOC with Earpiece.	Comms.
18	EOC telephone lines with lights may have been beneficial to cut down on the noise level.	Comms.

Figure 22.7 The list included a total of 50 recommendations (Hartford Hospital; Hartford Connecticut "After Action Report from Top Off 3," G. Havican, Regional Planning Coordinator).

and "external clinical reception teams" must be addressed within the emergency management plan and tested and evaluated in the large-scale drill.

Evaluations must be created around the emergency management plan and the evaluator must be trained to be objective and follow a matrix of numerically scored sections which will add "weight" to the evaluation instrument. The hospital must discuss said evaluations in its "After Action Reviews" and utilize the results to establish process improvement initiatives to establish "Best Practice" for the institution. The process improvement initiatives and the emergency plans must be reviewed and presented to the JCAHO accrediting agency in the future site visits.

Hospitals must also be aware of the resources in their area and contiguous communities. Planners from the hospitals Environment of Care or Emergency Management committee must collaborate with local emergency planning organizations and develop plans to provide resources to and from hospitals in case of mass disasters.

Hospitals are resilient. Maintaining that resiliency is important to maintain a safe and efficient environment. The practice of large-scale drills and exercises is paramount to continue this safe and well-educated environment. The healthcare worker and administrator of today is responsible for much more than just good patient care. He/She is responsible to maintain the integrity of the organization, to protect the staff and the patients and develop plans to recover from major incidents to resume normal operations.

References

1. http://www.jcaho.org/about+us/jcaho_facts.htm
2. http://www.cms.hhs.gov/about/default.asp
3. http://www.nfpa.org/assets/files/PDF/sup7.pdf
4. http://www.heics.com/
5. http://www.religioustolerance.org/dc_aumsh.htm
6. Katherine Dean. Connecticut's behavioral health crisis response: Integrating Behavioral Health into Response and Recovery, Connecticut Trauma Response & Recovery Program. Department of Mental Health and Addiction Services, Department of Children and Families, Crisis Response, Operations Manual, March 2005, http://155.37.41.133/target/crisis%20 Operational %20Manual%20 3-10-5.doc
7. http://www.osha.gov/dts/osta/bestpractices/firstreceivers_hospital.html
8. http://www.osha.gov/dts/osta/bestpractices/firstreceivers_hospital.html

23 Response to SARS as a prototype for bioterrorism: Lessons in a Regional Hospital in Hong Kong

ARTHUR CHUN-WING LAU, IDA KAM-SIU YIP, MAN-CHING LI, MARY WAN, ALFRED WING-HANG SIT, RODNEY ALLAN LEE, RAYMOND WAI-HUNG YUNG, AND LORETTA YIN-CHUN YAM

23.1 Introduction

Following the boom of the post-war years in the latter half of the twentieth century, the only large-scale infectious disease outbreaks were the influenza pandemics of 1957 and 1968 [1]. Apart from the aged and those with co-morbidities, in whom high morbidity and mortality was recorded, most patients had mild manifestations. With the advent of potent antimicrobial agents, the possible threat of widespread and lethal infections was generally considered minimal, and the world was ill-prepared for the severe acute respiratory syndrome (SARS) outbreak caused by the novel SARS-associated coronavirus (SARS-CoV) in early 2003. SARS wreaked havoc in 29 countries and infected 8422 patients within a short span of a few months [2]. By virtue of its novelty, infectious potential, associated mortality and in particular the lack of proven therapy, SARS-CoV has all the characteristics of a biological agent of choice in bioterrorism. Response to the SARS outbreak can thus serve as a prototype for combating against acts of bioterrorism. We describe our response to this SARS outbreak in the setting of a Hong Kong acute care hospital.

23.2 Recognition of an Impending Outbreak in Hong Kong

On February 11, 2003, the Chinese Ministry of Health reported to the World Health Organization (WHO) 305 cases of an acute respiratory syndrome of unknown etiology, occurring in Southern China between November 16, 2002 and February 9, 2003 [3]. On the same day, the Hong Kong Hospital Authority Head Office (HAHO), which operates 40 public hospitals and delivers over 92% of in-patient services in the territory, convened an Expert Panel on Severe Community-acquired Pneumonia (SCAP) in response to rumors about this infectious condition adjacent to the territory. It aimed to investigate the possibility of a similar situation in Hong Kong, to formulate guidelines for the prevention of its spread, and to require the reporting of all patients presenting with features of SCAP. The Chief of Service (COS) of the Department of Medicine of our institution, Pamela Youde Nethersole Eastern Hospital (PYNEH), which employs over 3500 staff to operate 1829 beds (1219 general beds and 610 psychiatric beds) to serve a population of 750,000 on Hong Kong Island, was appointed to the Panel.

All SCAP patients admitted to the general and medical intensive care units (ICU and MICU) in our institution were reviewed in accordance with this direction. It transpired that etiological diagnosis could be identified in a single patient, a 55-year old Hong Kong gentleman who had made frequent business travels to Shenzhen in the Guangdong Province of Southern China. Admitted on January 22, 2003 to an acute medical ward with respiratory distress and bilateral pneumonia, he was intubated a few hours later in the MICU, but died after 12 days from intractable acute respiratory distress syndrome (ARDS) due to unresolving pneumonia. None of the healthcare workers (HCW) contacting this patient in the general ward and MICU had fallen ill during his stay. His stored sera, checked in May 2003 retrospectively, confirmed SARS-CoV infection, but this case did not provide us with any clues about an impending infectious disease outbreak, nor were there unusual increases in the number of SCAP in Hong Kong throughout the 2003 winter season. At that time, the possible candidate organisms for the pneumonia outbreak in China were thought to be the usual organisms of atypical pneumonia or the avian influenza (H5N1) virus [4]. A new emerging organism did not rank high as etiological agent, and bioterrorism attack with an existing or a genetically engineered virus had not come to mind. The Panel reminded all frontline HCW to take droplet precautions on contacting pneumonia patients. By February 20, 2003, the Chinese authorities had reported to WHO that *Chlamydia pneumoniae* was the likely organism responsible for the recent outbreak of pneumonia [3].

23.3 Recognition of the Outbreak in PYNEH

Another 44-year-old Hong Kong businessman was admitted to an acute medical ward (ward A5) of PYNEH on March 2, 2003 for fever, cough, and sputum for one week. He had also traveled to Guangdong, Southern China on February 22–23, 2003. The White cell count was not elevated, lymphocyte was 1.0×10^9/L, and HIV serology was negative. Chest radiograph (CXR) showed bilateral basal pneumonic infiltrates. He was treated as for community-acquired pneumonia (CAP) and was placed in an open 8-bed cubicle ($42\,m^2$ area) in the ward, with positive pressure ventilation at five air changes per hour (ACH). Because of a report about a fatal case of avian influenza from another hospital in a returnee from China at about the same time [5], for the benefit of doubt our patient was transferred to an isolation room ($13\,m^2$, 8 ACH) on Day 2. After his nasopharyngeal aspirates (NPA) proved negative for influenza A and adenovirus on Day 3, he was moved back to the open cubicle. He then developed diarrhea and CXR continued to deteriorate despite standard antibiotics according to CAP treatment guideline [6]. On Day 6 (March 7, 13 days from symptom onset), he desaturated and was transferred to an isolation room in MICU for non-invasive ventilation (NIV) through a facial mask. On Day 8 (Day 15 from symptom onset), he was intubated because of increasing acute respiratory failure (ARF). Two intubating physicians wore protective garments against contamination by HIV (surgical mask, full-face shield, gown, and gloves), while nurses stood on the side of the bed and wore surgical masks, gown and gloves but not face shields. On Day 14 (March 15, 2003), the World Health Organization (WHO) published the case definition of suspected SARS at the WHO website, which in retrospect matched the presentation of this patient. He died on Day 15 from intractable acute respiratory distress syndrome (ARDS). Subsequent serology against the SARS-CoV was strongly positive. None of the HCW in MICU contracted SARS.

Thirty-two HCW in ward A5 had been exposed to this patient from March 2 to March 7, 2003. On March 9, a nurse from the same ward was admitted with pneumonia and was placed in an isolation room in A5 ward. By March 12, four other HCW from the same ward had requested sick leave due to upper respiratory tract illnesses. As an infectious condition was suspected, all were called back for medical review, blood tests, and CXR. Healthy HCW of the same ward were similarly screened. All CAP patients admitted in the preceding month were reviewed. The patient described above was identified to be the index case and the nurse admitted was his case nurse.

In response to an urgent consultation by the COS of the department, the Chair of Clinical Microbiology of the University of Hong Kong who had managed the contacts of the first local SARS patient (a visiting nephrologist from Guangzhou in Guangdong Province), gave his expert opinion on March 13, 2003. He advised on prescribing levofloxacin to all symptomatic HCW with atypical CAP, and intravenous ribavirin and corticosteroid (to which another HCW contacting the nephrologist had responded) to the only admitted HCW, who by then was in ARF. He concurred with our plan to cohort all pneumonia and suspected cases in one ward and recommended improvement in environmental ventilation. The Hong Kong Department of Health and HAHO were informed of the situation in PYNEH on the same day.

On March 14, all HCW on sick leave plus two others were admitted with progressive atypical pneumonia, including his case medical officer, a nurse, and four supporting staff. Four household contacts of three of the affected HCW, a patient and a visitor of another patient in the same cubicle were admitted over the next two days with the same problem. Three more nurses, including one investigating the outbreak, developed similar illnesses after March 17 and were admitted on March 23–24. These likely represented secondary infections by the first affected HCW before institution of strict droplet and contact precautions [7]. All 16 cases could be traced to this index case, had positive SARS serology subsequently and survived without intubation.

The PYNEH outbreak coincided with a major outbreak in another local hospital, in which 138 HCW contracted SARS from a young pneumonic patient (who had visited "Hotel M") nursed in a general medical ward [8]. It later transpired that the origin of that outbreak was the same nephrologist from Guangzhou who had stayed in this hotel in Hong Kong [9]. The nephrologist and his brother-in-law received treatment and died earlier in another hospital where a smaller nosocomial outbreak had also occurred. The outbreak of SARS in Hong Kong had thus started independently in three hospitals and spread to the community two weeks later.

23.4 Response at the Emergency Room Level

Our emergency room (ER) doctors performed first-line screening and admitting suspected SARS patients according to the prevailing WHO case definitions [10], with advice from pulmonary physicians where indicated. Learning from the experience in Singapore, the ER could effectively screen, treat, and safely discharge the majority of patients using screening questionnaires and a set of admission criteria [11]. The total number of patients screened at ER and admitted as in-patients was 505, including 459 adults and 46 children (Figure 23.1) [41].

23.5 Response at Ward and Department Levels

A total of 90 confirmed SARS cases were eventually treated in our hospital. The first patient was admitted on March 9, and the last was diagnosed on April 28, 2003. By June 13, all SARS patients were discharged from PYNEH. Figure 23.2 shows the number of new SARS patients admitted over time

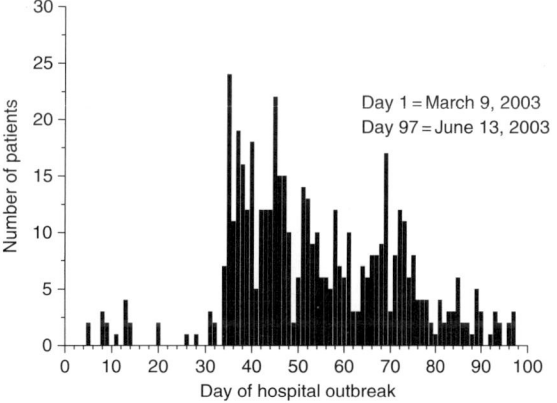

Figure 23.1 Daily number of patients (adults and children) screened at ER and admitted as in-patients to Pamela Youde Nethersole Eastern Hospital during the 2003 SARS outbreak (Total = 505).

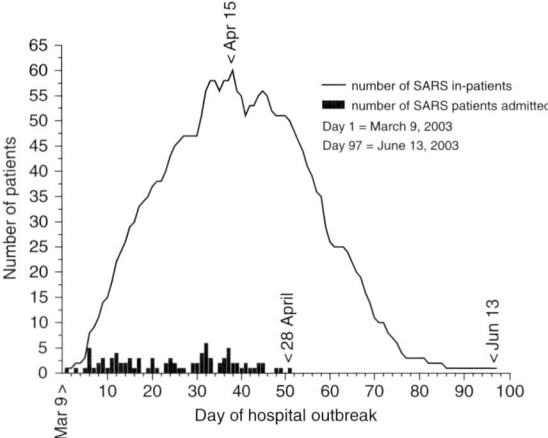

Figure 23.2 The number of new SARS patients admitted over time (Total 90 patients) and the number of confirmed SARS patients in cohort wards each day (peaking at 60 on April 15) during the outbreak.

and the number of confirmed SARS patients in cohort wards each day (peaking at 60 on April 15) during the outbreak. Our strategies to deal with this sudden surge of patients harboring an unknown and highly infectious disease are described.

23.5.1 Infection Control Measures

HAHO has established Infection Control Officers (ICO) in each hospital to head the Infection Control Team (ICT), formulate and enforce the implementation of infection control policies in line with prevailing standards. Guidelines for control against droplet infections have been well-established in Hong Kong hospitals before the occurrence of SARS, in particular for infections which were specified or suspected by ICT to be highly infectious. In general, patients with respiratory tract infections were routinely nursed in general medical wards together with those with other medical problems.

23.5.1.1 Patient cohorting

On receiving the information about the outbreak in ward A5, ICT immediately advised droplet and contact precautions to be implemented. On March 14, 2003, A5 ward became the only pneumonia cohort ward in the hospital, with each of the cubicle and isolation room clearly defined for the screening of new cases with respiratory infection or cohorting of atypical pneumonia cases. With further influx of suspected cases, ward B5 (another medical ward) was designated to be a female cohort ward, with A5 accepting male patients only. Eventually, a total of seven wards were designated for cohorting: five medical wards (two for screening, two for confirmed SARS, and one for convalescent SARS patients to complete the standard course of treatment [12]); as well as one pediatric ward and one SARS ICU.

23.5.1.2 Personal protective equipment (PPE)

HCW in ward A5 initially wore surgical masks only, but as soon as the high infectivity of SARS was recognized, protective gowns, gloves, and N95 respirators were worn during patient care. Hand hygiene was emphasized and safety in the handling of clinical specimens reinforced. The ICT set up different levels of PPE requirements for different clinical areas according to risk stratification (Table 23.1). These rules were enforced until the end of the outbreak. In the early stages, demand on PPE was very high. For peace of mind, some staff further added on their own versions of PPE. To enforce strict infection control policies and to ensure staff safety, HAHO appointed relevant experts to review all PPE with ICT from all hospitals, and only those found to be suitable for the purpose were allowed. Among those rejected were the "barrier man suit" designed against chemical contamination, and the "Stryker T4 protective system" used in operation rooms (OR). A personal air purified particulate respirator (PAPR) system (Airmate®) was used after mid-April during high-risk aerosol generating procedures such as intubation and resuscitation. Consumption and supply of PPE and other essential equipment were closely monitored by administrative services. Two "PPE Complaint Coordinators," a doctor and an administrative staff, were appointed to receive staff feedback.

Table 23.1 Standard provision of protective gear against SARS

Level	Description	Surgical mask	N95 mask	Latex gloves	Protective gown	Protective eye shield	Disposable caps	Shoe cover
1	SARS wards/areas	✓ (indirect patient care)	✓ (direct patient care)	✓	✓	✓	✓	±
2	Acute patient admission	✓	Upon staff special request	✓	✓	✓		
3	Others	✓		✓ (direct patient care)	Gown/apron for splashing like procedure	✓ (splashing like procedure)		

1. Staff should remove all protective gear when leaving the ward.
2. SARS patient should change surgical mask and pajama when leaving the ward.

23.5.1.3 Disinfection and environmental cleanliness

All equipments were cleaned with diluted sodium hypochlorite solution after use in SARS patients. Use of nebulized treatment in all patients was prohibited in light of a report of nosocomial transmission of SARS in another Hong Kong hospital [8]. As many SARS patients had presented with diarrhea, there was a high possibility of oro-fecal spread through contaminated fomites [13]. Additional housekeeping personnel were employed for environmental disinfection with special attention to shared toilet facilities in the wards. In full protective gear, they performed immediate disinfection of the toilet with sodium hypochlorite after its every use by SARS patients. Since SARS could survive for prolonged periods in the environment [14], we submit that this measure had contributed significantly to reduction of nosocomial spread of SARS.

23.5.1.4 Work place re-design and ventilation upgrade

The facilities management team (FMT) worked closely with PCCT and ICT to re-design ward facilities in accordance with infection control requirements. Ward areas were segregated into "clean" or non-infectious from "dirty" or infectious/potentially infectious areas. Separate routings were designed for entry and exit, with dedicated gowning and de-gowning areas, respectively. To reduce unnecessary entry of non-HCW into cohort wards, buffer areas were delineated near the entrances for the delivery of food and other items. Ventilation of staff changing rooms and toilets were upgraded, with the addition of simple showering facilities in every cohort ward in case gross contamination occurred. Nursing care was streamlined to minimize patient contact. CXR were taken with portable machines stationed in the cohort wards. X-ray film cassettes were disinfected between cases. Medical records were prohibited in patient areas, and documentation could only be made after removal of potentially infectious PPE and donning of new and clean PPE. Documents from cohort wards were sent by email and fascimile, and hard copies were avoided.

Hospital wards and operation rooms (OR) in PYNEH had been designed to operate at positive pressure with respect to the surrounding to prevent the ingress of contaminants. Temperature and humidity were closely controlled via a standard heating, ventilation and air-conditioning (HVAC) system. Apart from the OR, a significant proportion of well-mixed room air was re-circulated after filtering and conditioning. As the predominant mode of SARS spread was assumed to be through infectious droplets, the existing HVAC design could not meet infection control requirements. With no clear guidelines for HVAC design for SARS wards and OR, input from ICT and the clinicians were critical toward the modification of engineering and environmental controls. The consensus among all concerned parties in mid-March 2003 was to adopt the isolation room requirements for *Mycobacterium tuberculosis* (TB) [15]. Immediate ventilation improvement works were thus designed and implemented in the SARS wards to provide sufficient air change for dilution and removal of contaminants; to create negative pressure and achieve directional airflow from the clean to the infected areas; and to incorporate local source control to extract contaminants via the shortest possible path and within the shortest time. In retrospect, we strongly believe that this decision had been pivotal to our success in combating SARS and minimizing its nosocomial spread, since air-borne transmission of this disease had been raised by Hong Kong [16] and Canadian [14] researchers to be a real possibility.

In response to the demands of subsequent clinical situations, FMT utilized the same principles to create a negative-pressure OR with unidirectional flow for a SARS patients requiring laparotomy, and temporarily converted the positive-pressure cardiac catheterization laboratory on two occasions for diagnostic and interventional procedures in SARS patients [17,18].

All ventilation improvement works were executed in phases. In Phase 1, frequency of air change was immediately increased on March 13, 2003 from the usual 5 ACH to 6 ACH in all medical wards, and to 7–8 ACH in the SARS cohort ward. Window-type exhaust fans (Figure 23.3) with sound-absorbing hoods were installed, and folding doors were added to segregate the nurse station from patient cubicles. Unidirectional airflow was thus achieved from the corridors outside the SARS ward, through the clean nurse station to patient areas and finally to the window exhaust. Returned air dampers in the HVAC system were closed to achieve 100% fresh air intake. In Phase 2, fan cowls were added to discharge outlets of exhaust fans to reduce fluctuation in performance caused by strong winds (Figure 23.4). In Phase 3, window-type exhaust fans were replaced by heavy-duty ducted exhaust fans with non-return air dampers to achieve 12 ACH. High efficiency particulate air (HEPA) filters were installed at exhaust outlets. Exhaust air ducts were next installed at low level (Figure 23.5) in Phase 4 to create unidirectional airflow from high level supply diffusers through the breathing zone of HCW before passing on to infected patients and then to the low-level exhaust. Air grilles with double deflection supply were adopted to control airflow patterns and

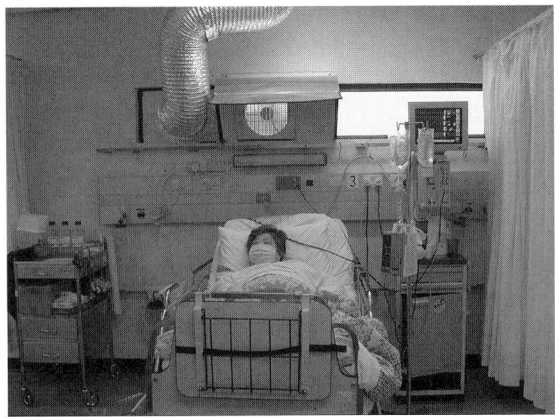

Figure 23.3 Ventilation improvement works (Phases 1–3): Window type exhaust fan and ventilation duct from low level exhaust installed in de-gowning area (not shown) in the SARS ICU.

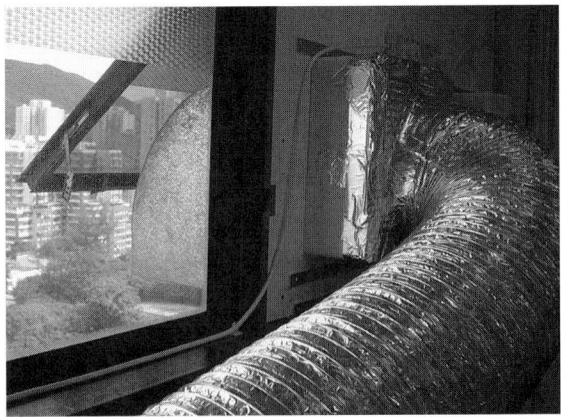

Figure 23.4 Ventilation improvement works (Phases 2–3): Fan cowl covering discharge outlet of window-type exhaust fan to counteract effect of strong winds. The exhaust fan was connected via an air duct to low level exhaust in the de-gowning area (not shown) in the SARS ICU.

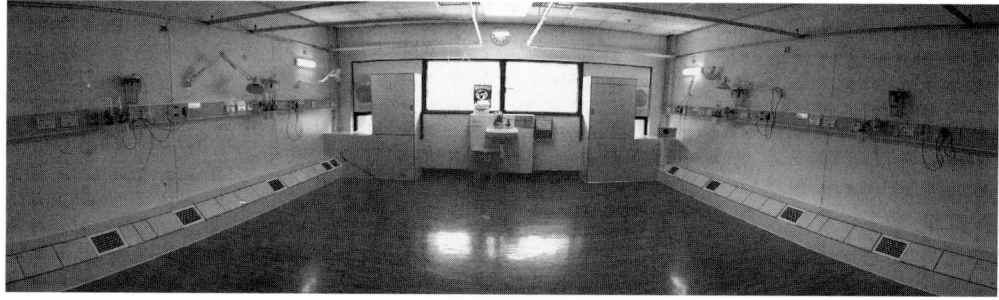

Figure 23.5 Ventilation improvement works (Phase 4): Low level exhaust and back-up window-type exhaust fans in a 6-bed cubicle in a general medical ward.

directions and minimize air turbulence and mixing. Additional HEPA filters were installed at return air grilles to allow air re-circulation in wards with lower infection risks. In the last phase (Phase 5), local source control with adjustable and removable exhaust hoods were installed at both sides of hospital beds (Figure 23.6). Standby exhaust fans were also installed to automatically take over the function of duty fans in case the latter failed.

23.5.2 Staff Deployment and Service Re-organization

The department's Duty Committee devised a staff redeployment plan in case the outbreak should become extended in time and scale. Pregnant HCW were re-deployed to non-SARS wards. Annual and study leaves were cancelled. With further assistance from the FMT, staff quarters and overnight rooms were offered to HCW of cohort wards should they wish to avoid infecting their families. Doctors, nurses, and supporting staff of other departments were deployed to work in non-SARS medical wards. These were still serving 75% of the usual number of patients since PYNEH was designated by HAHO to support another hospital which had been overwhelmed by the sudden influx of SARS patients from its community (the "Amoy Garden cohort") [19]. All non-emergency investigations, procedures and operations in the hospital were stopped. Specialist outpatient clinics, geriatrics day hospital and clinical admission services were reduced. Inter-departmental consultations were stopped unless the conditions were urgent.

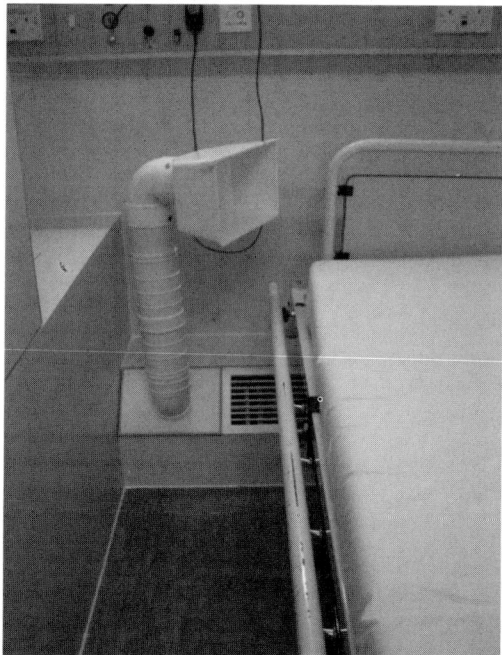

Figure 23.6 Ventilation improvement works (Phase 5): Low level exhaust with local source control device with adjustable and removable hood installed at either side of the head of the bed (only the left side is shown).

23.5.3 Communication Within the Department of Medicine

Both formal and informal channels for staff communication were actively utilized. The COS held meetings with the department 2–3 times a week to transmit important information from HAHO and hospital management, to keep staff up-to-date on the clinical aspects of SARS, progress of outbreak, changing infection control requirements, and clinical and radiographic information toward early identification of this disease. Staff feedback on suggestions and concerns were encouraged and reflected to hospital management where appropriate. The COS frequently appealed to the staff's professionalism and duty of care to patients while assuring them that the risk they were taking for the good of their patients and society were well recognized by the hospital and the department, and all that was possible would be done to protect them and their families [20]. It was later found that anxiety levels were high among front-line HCW in our hospital as in other parts of the world [21]. We have thus learned that, should similar outbreaks ever return, experts must be recruited to the response team to attend to the mental well-being of HCW and supporting staff as well as their family members. Towards this end, integration of mental health care into public health preparedness for infectious outbreaks has been proposed [22].

The department also maintained close contact with HAHO and other hospitals to exchange views about this disease. Training programs and meetings were organized for department staff on infection control and clinical management of SARS, psychosocial care of patients, and communication skills with patients/relatives at times of stress. Meticulous real-time or retrospective documentation was kept at every stage, which facilitated subsequent review for research, reporting, accountability and medico-legal purposes.

23.5.4 Clinical Management

Five members of the Pulmonary and Critical Care team (PCCT, of which the COS was head) took up supervisory roles in SARS wards and SARS ICU throughout the outbreak, assisted later by a geriatrician-cum-pulmonologist. Rotating senior and junior physicians from other medical subspecialties took up front-line roles in the SARS wards. At least two members of the PCCT conducted rounds in each cohort ward twice daily, and the Team discussed patient management together every day to expedite learning and accumulation of experience. A multi-disciplinary team comprising PCCT, ICT, FMT, and administrators was convened and met regularly to plan and monitor different aspects of outbreak response in the light of continuously updated clinical knowledge. Psychiatrists were recruited to manage SARS patients when they developed anxiety and depression and to provide training to staff caring for them.

To keep HCW abreast about the rapidly changing scenario, PCCT developed information sheets containing clinical features, investigation methods, treatment, and prognostic factors, which were frequently updated and distributed to SARS and medical wards. This exercise required PCCT to integrate knowledge gained from various channels in a timely manner, and contributed toward the formulation of a standardized treatment protocol for SARS at an early stage [12]. Our satisfactory treatment outcomes were duly published [23] and efficacy of the protocol was subsequently supported by similar outcomes reported from Taiwan [24].

Encouraged by our observation that non-invasive ventilation (NIV) did not cause SARS transmission when applied in an isolation room with 8 ACH to the index case, we continued to use this ventilatory mode in the early stages of SARS-related ARF. At the same time and unbeknown to us, NIV was totally banned in all other Hong Kong hospitals for fear of nosocomial transmission of SARS. Satisfactory patient outcome was achieved in most of our patients with ARF, however, and no SARS transmission had occurred in over 100 exposed HCW [25]. The efficacy of NIV with avoidance of intubation could be related to two equally beneficial effects: it reduced prevented secondary infection as patients were not intubated, and reduced the chance of SARS transmission to HCW during intubation [26]. The safety of NIV use in our hospital and the possibility that air-borne transmission of SARS could have been possible [14,16] lent full support to the establishment of negative pressure and unidirectional environmental

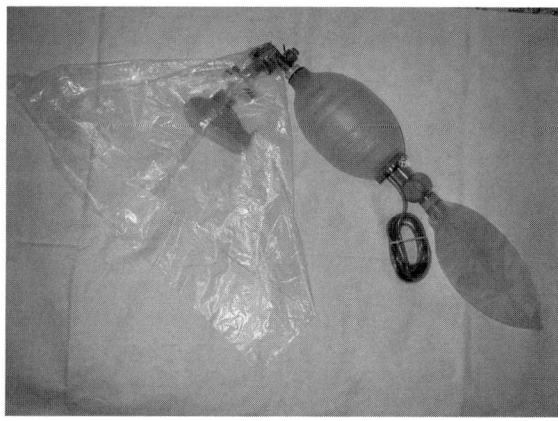

Figure 23.7 Protective device for resuscitation: Bag-valve apparatus with viral-bacterial filter between the bag and the face mask, with plastic shield to cover face shield and patient's face to direct expired air downwards and away from the face of healthcare workers.

ventilation within a few days of the outbreak [42]. We submit that the (still current) recommendations from Canada [27] and the United Kingdom [28] to avoid the use of NIV had not taken into account the utility of improved environmental ventilation in markedly reducing the chance of SARS transmission to HCW.

During resuscitation, we added viral and bacterial filters to ventilator tubings and the bag-valve apparatus, and draped a plastic bag opened on two sides above the face mask to direct expired air to below the patient's face to avoid direct its inhalation by HCW (Figure 23.7) [29]. The department continued a close liaison with the Microbiology Department of the University of Hong Kong, whose team successfully isolated and grew the SARS-CoV [19], and benefited from fruitful advice while also contributing valuable specimens for research.

23.6 Response at Hospital Management Level

Unified command was achieved through an Outbreak Management Team (OMT) headed by the Hospital Chief Executive (HCE), with members comprising General Managers and COS, to oversee all matters related to the outbreak. Daily meetings of HCE in HAHO made major policy decisions to manage the outbreak, followed by OMT meeting in the hospital to ensure swift communication of important corporate messages among all parties involved. Meeting minutes were sent by electronic means to ward managers, department managers and unit heads and posted in the hospital intranet. In addition, weekly summaries of developments were sent to update all Hospital Governing Board members.

23.6.1 Visiting Policy

Visitors to the cohort wards were prohibited, but patients were allowed to freely use their mobile phones for communications with families and responding to enquiries from epidemiologists. Videophones were later installed for visitors in the Patient Resource Center. Visitors were only allowed into the cohort wards under exceptional circumstances, during which their contact information was recorded and the Department of Health notified for medical surveillance. Visitors to acute general wards were similarly prohibited, since rapid diagnosis of SARS was not feasible until very late in the outbreak, and atypical presentation [30] could occur especially in the elderly [31,32]. Visitors were only allowed into the two non-acute wards in which patients had negligible likelihood of SARS. With additional security installed at a single point of entry for the public, surveillance with temperature-taking and completion of designated questionnaires were enforced to facilitate contact tracing. Further security was installed at the entrance to all wards to prevent inadvertent entry of the public from other hospital entrances. Volunteer services and clinical training attachments for medical, nursing and allied health students were suspended.

23.6.2 Reporting Mechanism and e-SARS Registry

In the last week of March 2003, the ICT was assigned by OMT to conduct daily rounds of cohort wards to collect epidemiological and clinical data. All suspected cases fulfilling the case definition were entered into a registry and followed-up daily by the ICT until discharge. Individual registries from 13 acute hospitals were later integrated by HAHO to become an online e-SARS registry, which was later enhanced by the information system of the Hong Kong Police Force designed for criminal tracking and analysis. The resulting linking of clinical information, a smart tracking system and the epidemiological database under the Department of Health served to effectively identify the chain of human transmission of SARS in a timely manner. Because of its efficiency in contact tracing, the e-SARS system had contributed significantly to containment of the outbreak. It was later awarded the Stockholm Challenge Award in 2004 as an innovation in information system which had significant benefit to society [33].

23.6.3 Re-organization of Staff Canteen

Visitors and patients were prohibited from entering the canteen. Signs were put up at the entrance to remind staff not to wear PPE other than a fresh and clean mask, and to clean hands with the alcohol hand sprays provided before food consumption. Close face-to-face interactions were discouraged. All users had to sit facing the same direction, even when having meals together. The number of seats was reduced to increase space between users. Senior staff of the canteen acted as patrol officers to enforce these rules, while members of ICET performed regular spot-checks for non-compliance during peak hours.

23.6.4 Training and Communication Within the Hospital

On March 15, 2003, the first staff forum was jointly held by the COS in Medicine and ICO, a clinical microbiologist and COS in Clinical Pathology. As the outbreak continued, further staff forums were held by the HCE to concentrate on updating staff knowledge about the outbreak, with repeated emphases on the importance of good infection control practices. Many training sessions on this subject were held for HCW, clerical and administrative staff, including lectures and demonstrations on proper gowning and de-gowning of PPE, and safe and effective NPA collection. Training was reinforced by video-viewing at department or workplace level, and display of posters and pamphlets in the most frequented areas of the hospital. Non-hospital personnel recruited by contracted-out services were equally trained by their supervisors. Record of training in the form of signed attendance lists was kept and monitored by the Human Resources Department.

PYNEH set up a "SARS homepage" in the hospital intranet to provide quick and easy reference to all infection control news and guidelines, changes to inpatient services, operation procedures, supporting services, and specialist outpatient services and human resources issues. Staff feedback on all matters related to the SARS outbreak were collected through focus group meetings, designated contact persons ("staff ambassadors") assigned by the Human Resource Department and nursing sections, staff hotlines and suggestion boxes. A designated workplace controller was appointed for every workplace unit to brief staff on a daily basis, or three times a day if shift duty was involved, on issues including hospital updates; reinforcement of infection control measures; a daily bulletin "The SARS Battling Update"; as well as staff sentiment. An administrative staff was designated to handle enquiries from the media and the community.

23.6.5 Administrative Interface
23.6.5.1 Resource prioritization

The PYNEH Administrative Team played a coordinating role to ensure smooth implementation of the response plan. The wide scope of administrative services including general and patient support services; food services management; facilities management; procurement and materials management, is intricately linked to all clinical activities. Material and human resources were prioritized for SARS management. Non-medical wards were converted to medical wards as the latter were turned into cohort wards, with appropriate staff deployments. Resources were appropriately redeployed to purchase PPE, improve environmental ventilation, and employ additional support staff for infection control and security purposes.

23.6.5.2 Implementation of infection control policies at supporting staff level

The ICT's guidelines for standard PPE provision at three levels of clinical areas based on risk assessment were disseminated to all staff involved in patient-related services, including catering, materials transportation, housekeeping, cleansing, security, pest control, repair and maintenance, and medical services. According to a subsequent audit, availability of these guidelines had allayed anxiety and concern of supporting staff, who before had uniformly expressed significantly uncertainty and stress when working in patient care environment. Frequent training sessions on infection control and changes in workflow were held for the supervisors of support staff, who in turn trained and monitored their staff's compliance. As a result, none of the 235 supporting non-HCW staff with SARS patient contact had acquired the disease.

23.6.5.3 Procurement and logistics

Prior to SARS, PPE materials in excess of demand were not stockpiled. By mid-late March 2003, there was a sudden global surge in demand. In-coordination in procurement among local hospitals led to competition for supply. This issue was solved within a week with the introduction of central procurement at HAHO level. PPE procurement and distribution by the supply chain in PYNEH was tightly coupled to ICT guidelines for PPE use in different risk areas. Intensive communications at daily OMT meetings helped foster trust between HCW and procurement staff regarding the guarantee of adequacy of PPE supply. As a result, none of our HCW complained through the media to voice their concern about perceived inadequacy of PPE supply as those in some other hospitals did.

23.6.5.4 Facilities management team (FMT) issues

The central role of FMT and engineering personnel in ventilation improvements to meet the stringent demands of the outbreak has been described. On review, long-standing partnership of the same FMT since the inception of the hospital in 1993, together with a shared culture of trust and cooperation toward patient-centered care, had enabled the achievement of the highest environmental quality at the earliest possible time, enabling treatment perceived to be dangerous by other hospitals (namely NIV) to be carried out for the benefit of patients [25] and in turn protecting staff from exposure to high-risk procedures (namely intubation).

23.7 Further Response at Hospital Authority Head Office (HAHO) Level With Direct Impact on the Department

In Hong Kong, cohorting of SARS patients was instituted in 13 acute hospitals. Similar to Singapore [34], limiting the care of SARS patients to a single designated hospital had been tried locally in late March, but very soon the capacity was so overwhelmed that all acute hospitals had to receive SARS patients. By late March 2003, a "SARS" homepage was established by HAHO in the e-Knowledge Gateway (eKG) of the HA intranet to continuously update all staff on scientific knowledge about this disease.

23.7.1 Infection Control Enforcement Team

To further enhance compliance to infection control policies, HAHO directed the establishment of the Infection Control Enforcement Team (ICET) in every hospital. The objectives were: to convey updated infection control policies on SARS from HAHO to frontline staff; to coordinate operational logistics between hospital administration and frontline departments; to appoint departmental and workplace controllers to enforce and monitor infection control activities at all levels (including staff canteen and relaxation areas); to audit compliance to infection control practices in the workplace; and to report non-compliance to the respective department heads and HCE.

In PYNEH, the chairperson of ICET was elected from among senior non-medical clinicians and this chairperson should report to both HAHO ICET and HCE. Members consisted of senior medical, nursing, administrative staff as well as the ICT. Each wore conspicuous arm-bands for identification and was given the authority to immediately warn or counsel staff on issues related to infection control. The ICET were effective in enhancing compliance to infection control practices among hospital staff, and played an important role towards reduction in the nosocomial transmission of SARS.

23.8 Outbreak Resolution

With two additional HCW who developed breakthrough infection due to non-compliance to infection control measures, a total of 13 HCW among 1300 exposed employees in PYNEH had contracted and recovered from SARS. Four infected HCW transferred from other hospitals also had full recovery. Of the 90 patients confirmed to be suffering from SARS by laboratory criteria [35], 21 (24%) required ICU care and four died. These included the index case and two deaths from concomitant cardiovascular diseases (myocardial infarction and stroke), resulting in the lowest case fatality rate of 3.4% [23] for SARS patients in Hong Kong [8,13,36]. This figure also compared favorably to mortality figures worldwide [37,38]. Apart from the index case, all deaths occurred in patients above the age of 65 years with significant comorbidities [23]. A twice-weekly SARS follow-up clinic was set up in a SARS convalescent ward from April 15 onward, followed by a Post-SARS Clinic under the direction of HAHO. Hong Kong was finally removed from the list of areas with local SARS transmission on June 23, 2003.

23.9 Aftermath

In the aftermath of SARS, the Government of Hong Kong has strengthened our healthcare system to withstand further disease outbreak [39] and potential bioterrorism. Point-to-point communication with Mainland China on outbreak notification was established, together with an electronic web-based platform to report clusters of febrile HCW or patients in hospitals. Facilities in HA hospitals were upgraded to include 530 isolation wards with 1280 isolation beds, and five such wards with 120 isolation beds had been converted in PYNEH. Resources were allocated for training and research in infection control and epidemiology; development of contingency plans; and establishment of a Center for Health Protection (CHP). Conduction of drills based on different clinical scenario further augmented our preparedness against future outbreaks.

23.10 Conclusion

After overcoming the onslaught of SARS, the Hong Kong community has become aware that emerging infections may and can occur at any time. This is further reinforced by the recent avian influenza outbreaks which keep reminding us of this looming threat. In addition, hospitals have to evaluate their levels of preparedness against bioterrorism, which can simulate infectious disease outbreaks. Priority areas for improvement suggested have included community involvement; staff education; improved information technology; disease surveillance; and additional equipment and staff [40]. The experience of our hospital in the SARS outbreak may serve as a prototype for such response in a hospital setting. Under these circumstances, the healthcare system and the community as a whole must join force to combat the common enemy. Multi-dimensional and flexible response plans require strong leadership and clear directions to be effective, but must also take into account human frailties in times of great stress, when every resource is stretched to its utmost limit.

References

1. World Health Organisation (WHO). Communicable disease surveillance and response, Pandemic Influenza Preparedness Planning. Update on 14 March 2005. http://www.euro.who.int/eprise/main/who/progs/csr/cooperation/20050218_1. Accessed on April 19, 2005.
2. World Health Organisation (WHO). Summary table of SARS cases by country, 1 November 2002–7 August 2003. Update on 15 August 2003.

http://www.who.int/csr/sars/country/en/country 2003_08_15.pdf. Accessed on 19 April 2005.
3. World Health Organisation (WHO). WHO issues a global alert about cases of atypical pneumonia. 12 March 2003. http://www.who.int/csr/don/2003_03_12/en/. Accessed April 19, 2005.
4. K. Y. Yuen, P. K. Chan, M. Peiris, D. N. Tsang, T. L. Que, K. F. Shortridge, P. T. Cheung, W. K. To, E. T. Ho, R. Sung, and A. F. Cheng. Clinical features and rapid viral diagnosis of human disease associated with avian influenza A H5N1 virus. Lancet, 351(9101):467–471, 1998.
5. World Health Organisation (WHO). Influenza A(H5N1) in Hong Kong Special Administrative Region of China – Update 2. 27 February 2003. http://www.who.int/csr/don/2003_02_27a/en/. Accessed 19 April 2005.
6. M. S. Niederman, L. A. Mandell, A. Anzueto, J. B. Bass, W. A. Broughton, G. D. Campbell, N. Dean, T. File, M. J. Fine, P. A. Gross, et al. American Thoracic Society (2001) Guidelines for the management of adults with community-acquired pneumonia. Diagnosis, assessment of severity, antimicrobial therapy, and prevention. Am J Respir Crit Care Med, 163: 1730–1754, 2001.
7. W. H. Seto, D. Tsang, R. W. Yung, T. Y. Ching, T. K. Ng, M. Ho, L. M. Ho, and J. S. Peiris; Advisors of Expert SARS group of Hospital Authority. Effectiveness of precautions against droplets and contact in prevention of nosocomial transmission of severe acute respiratory syndrome (SARS). Lancet, 361(9368):1519–1520, 2003.
8. N. Lee, D. Hui, A. Wu, P. Chan, P. Cameron, G. M. Joynt, A. Ahuja, M. Y. Yung, C. B. Leung, K. F. To, S. F. Lui, C. C. Szeto, S. Chung, and J. J. Sung. A major outbreak of severe acute respiratory syndrome in Hong Kong. N Engl J Med. 348(20):1986–1994, 2003. (Epub 2003 Apr 7.)
9. K. W. Tsang, P. L. Ho, G. C. Ooi, W. K. Yee, T. Wang, M. Chan-Yeung, W. K. Lam, W. H. Seto, L. Y. Yam, T. M. Cheung, P. C. Wong, B. Lam, M. S. Ip, J. Chan, K. Y. Yuen, and K. N. Lai. A cluster of cases of severe acute respiratory syndrome in Hong Kong. N Engl J Med, 348(20):1977–1985, 2003. (Epub 2003 Mar 31.)
10. World Health Organisation (WHO). Use of laboratory methods for SARS diagnosis. Updated May 1, 2003. http://www.who.int/csr/sars/labmethods/en/. Accessed April 21, 2005.
11. K. Y. Tham. An emergency department response to severe acute respiratory syndrome: A prototype response to bioterrorism. Ann Emerg Med, 43(1): 6–14, 2004.
12. L. K. So, A. C. Lau, L. Y. Yam, T. M. Cheung, E. Poon, R. W. Yung, and K. Y. Yuen. Development of a standard treatment protocol for severe acute respiratory syndrome. Lancet, 361(9369):1615–1617, 2003.
13. P. L. Ho, X. P. Tang, and W. H. Seto. SARS: hospital infection control and admission strategies. Respirology, 2003, 8 Suppl:S41–S45, 2003.
14. T. F. Booth, B. Kournikakis, N. Bastien, J. Ho, D. Kobasa, L. Stadnyk, Y. Li, M. Spence, S. Paton, B. Henry, B. Mederski, D. White, D. E. Low, A. McGeer, A. Simor, M. Vearncombe, J. Downey, F. B. Jamieson, P. Tang, and F. Plummer. Detection of Airborne Severe Acute Respiratory Syndrome (SARS) Coronavirus and Environmental Contamination in SARS Outbreak Units. J Infect Dis, 2005 May 1;191(9):1472–1477 2005. (Epub 2005 Mar 18.)
15. US Department of Health and Human Services, Centers for Disease Control and Prevention: Guidelines for Preventing the Transmission of Mycobacterium tuberculosis in Health-care Facilities, Oct. 1994.
16. I. T. Yu, Y. Li, T. W. Wong, W. Tam, A. T. Chan, J. H. Lee, D. Y. Leung, and T. Ho. Evidence of airborne transmission of the severe acute respiratory syndrome virus. N Engl J Med, 350(17): 1731–1739, 2004.
17. K. L. Tsui, T. C. Leung, L. Y. Yam, L. K. So, E. Poon, K. C. Lung, and S. K. Li. Coronary plaque instability in severe acute respiratory syndrome. Int J Cardiol, 99(3):471–472, 2005.
18. K. L. Tsui, S. K. Li, M. C. Li, K. K. Chan, T. C. Leung, T. S. Tse, C. K. Chan, K. K. H. Lam, and L. Y. C. Yam. J Invas Cardiol 17: 149–152, 2005.
19. J. S. Peiris, S. T. Lai, L. L. Poon, Y. Guan, L. Y. Yam, W. Lim, J. Nicholls, W. K. Yee, W. W. Yan, M. T. Cheung, V. C. Cheng, K. H. Chan, D. N. Tsang, R. W. Yung, T. K. Ng, K. Y. Yuen; SARS study group. Coronavirus as a possible cause of severe acute respiratory syndrome. Lancet, 361(9366):1319–1325, 2003.
20. M. K. Wynia and L. O. Gostin. Ethical challenges in preparing for bioterrorism: barriers within the health care system (Review). Am J Public Health, 94(7):1096–1102, 2004.
21. L. A. Nickell, E. J. Crighton, C. S. Tracy, H. Al-Enazy, Y. Bolaji, S. Hanjrah, A. Hussain,

S. Makhlouf, and R. E. Upshur. Psychosocial effects of SARS on hospital staff: survey of a large tertiary care institution. *CMAJ*, 170(5):793–798, 2004.
22. R. J. Ursano. Preparedness for SARS, influenza, and bioterrorism. *Psychiatr Serv*, 56(1):7, 2005.
23. A. C. Lau, L. K. So, F. P. Miu, R. W. Yung, E. Poon, T. M. Cheung, and L. Y. Yam. Outcome of coronavirus-associated severe acute respiratory syndrome using a standard treatment protocol. *Respirology*, 9(2):173–183, 2004.
24. G. F. Wang. On corticosteroid therapy of SARS. *Chin Med J*, 42: 682–683, 2003.
25. T. M. Cheung, L. Y. Yam, L. K. So, A. C. Lau, E. Poon, B. M. Kong, and R. W. Yung. Effectiveness of noninvasive positive pressure ventilation in the treatment of acute respiratory failure in severe acute respiratory syndrome. *Chest*, 126(3):845–850, 2004.
26. R. A. Fowler, C. B. Guest, S. E. Lapinsky, W. Sibbald, M. Louie, P. Tang, et al. Transmission of severe acute respiratory syndrome during intubation and mechanical ventilation. *Am J Respir Med Crit Care*, 169:1198–1202, 2004.
27. S. E. Lapinsky, and L. Hawryluck. ICU management of severe acute respiratory syndrome. *Intensive Care Med*, 29:870–875, 2003.
28. W. S. Lim, S. R. Anderson, and R. C. Read on behalf of the SARS guidelines committees of the British Thoracic Society, the British Infection Society and the Health Protection Agency. Hospital management of adults with severe acute respiratory syndrome (SARS) if SARS re-emerges—Updated 10 Feb 2004. Available from http://www.brit.thoracic.org.uk/docs/sars0304.pdf. Accessed April 20, 2004.
29. L. Y. Yam, R. C. Chen, and N. S. Zhong. SARS: ventilatory and intensive care. *Respirology*, 8 Suppl:S31–S35, 2003.
30. K. Y. Chow, C. E. Lee, M. L. Ling, D. M. Heng, and S. G. Yap. Outbreak of severe acute respiratory syndrome in a tertiary hospital in Singapore, linked to an index patient with atypical presentation: epidemiological study. *Brit Med J*, 328:195, 2004. (Epub 2004 Jan 15.)
31. T. T. Tan, B. H. Tan, A. Kurup, L. L. Oon, D. Heng, S. Y. Thoe, X. L. Bai, K. P. Chan, and A. E. Ling. Atypical SARS and *Escherichia coli* bacteremia. *Emerg Infect Dis*, 10:349–352, 2004.
32. A. K. Tee, H. M. Oh, C. T. Lien, K. Narendran, B. H. Heng, and A. E. Ling. Atypical SARS in geriatric patient. *Emerg Infect Dis*, 10:261–264, 2004.
33. http://www.hwfb.gov.hk/policingdisease/SARS-b.htm/
34. G. Gopalakrishna, P. Choo, Y. S. Leo, B. K. Tay, Y. T. Lim, A. S. Khan, and C. C. Tan. SARS transmission and hospital containment. *Emerg Infect Dis*, 10(3):395–400, 2004.
35. World Health Organisation (WHO). Case Definitions for Surveillance of Severe Acute Respiratory Syndrome (SARS) (revised 1 May 2003). http://www.who.int/csr/sars/casedefinition/en/. Accessed April 21, 2005.
36. J. J. Sung, A. Wu, G. M. Joynt, K. Y. Yuen, N. Lee, P. K. Chan, C. S. Cockram, A. T. Ahuja, L. M. Yu, V. W. Wong, and D. S. Hui. Severe acute respiratory syndrome: report of treatment and outcome after a major outbreak. *Thorax*, 59(5):414–420, 2004.
37. C. M. Booth, L. M. Matukas, G. A. Tomlinson, A. R. Rachlis, D. B. Rose, H. A. Dwosh, S. L. Walmsley, T. Mazzulli, M. Avendano, P. Derkach, I. E. Ephtimios, I. Kitai, B. D. Mederski, S. B. Shadowitz, W. L. Gold, L. A. Hawryluck, E. Rea, J. S. Chenkin, D. W. Cescon, S. M. Poutanen, and A. S. Detsky. Clinical features and short-term outcomes of 144 patients with SARS in the greater Toronto area. *JAMA*, 289(21):2801–2809. (Epub 2003 May 6).
38. T. W. Lew, T. K. Kwek, D. Tai, A. Earnest, S. Loo, K. Singh, K. M. Kwan, Y. Chan, C. F. Yim, S. L. Bek, A. C. Kor, W. S. Yap, Y. R. Chelliah, Y. C. Lai, and S. K. Goh. Acute respiratory distress syndrome in critically ill patients with severe acute respiratory syndrome. *JAMA*, 290(3):374–380, 2003.
39. A. Lee, and A. S. Abdullah. Severe acute respiratory syndrome: a challenge for public health practice in Hong Kong. *J Epidemiol Community Health*, 57(9):655–658, 2003.
40. J. K. Murphy. After 9/11: priority focus areas for bioterrorism preparedness in hospitals. J Healthc Manag. 49(4):227–235, 2004.
41. J. C. Ho, G. C. Ooi, T. Y. Mok, J. W. Chan, I. Hung, B. Lam, P. C. Wong, P. C. Li, P. L. Ho, W. K. Lam, C. K. Ng, M. S. Ip, K. N. Lai, M. Chan-Yeung, K. W. Tsang. Impact of severe respiratory syndrome on anxiety levels of frontline health care workers. *Hong Kong Med J*, 10(5):325–330, 2004.
42. E. Poon, K. S. Liu, D. L. Cheong, C. K. Lee, L. Y. Yam, and W. N. Tang. Respiratory syndrome. *Am J Respir Crit Care Med*, 168(12):1449–1456, 2003. (Epub 2003 Aug 28.)

Appendix A   Emergency Preparedness, Response & Recovery Checklist Beyond the Emergency Management Plan

ELISABETH BELMONT, ESQUIRE, BRUCE MERLIN FRIED, ESQUIRE, JULIANNA S. GONEN, ESQUIRE ANNE M. MURPHY, ESQUIRE, JEFFREY M. SCONYERS, ESQUIRE, AND SUSAN F. ZINDER, ESQUIRE*

I. Introduction

Healthcare professionals and organizations are recognized for their central and irreplaceable role in communities, particularly when natural disasters or other emergencies occur. As ordinary citizens may go about their business in the everyday setting, healthcare providers must prepare routinely for a variety of emergency situations that may impair their ability to care for patients on an ongoing basis.[1] Many state laws and regulations require hospitals and other licensed healthcare facilities to engage in emergency planning and drilling.[2] Emergency preparedness, including establishing and maintaining an emergency management plan, also is one of the required seven disciplines of "Management of the Environment of Care" for organizations accredited by the Joint Commission on Accreditation of Healthcare Organizations

---

Source copyright 2004 by American Health Lawyers Association

* The authors wish to express their sincere appreciation to Lori L. Buchsbaum, MPH, who is a J.D. candidate, Winter 2004, at the American University, and Tisha Bai, who is a J.D. candidate, Spring 2005, at George Washington University Law School, for their assistance in preparing this publication. Additionally, the authors wish to thank Lori H. Spencer, Esq. for her willingness to offer her perspective on certain public health law issues. For information about the authors, please see the end of this publication.

[1] The Model State Emergency Health Powers Act addresses a number of issues relating to public health emergencies, including: measures to detect and track potential and existing public health emergencies; declaring a state of public health emergency; special powers of governors and state public health authorities during a state of public health emergency (including control of property and persons); dissemination of information regarding public health emergencies; and planning for such emergencies. See THE CTR. FOR LAW AND THE PUBLIC'S HEALTH AT GEORGETOWN & JOHNS HOPKINS UNIVERSITIES, CTRS. FOR DISEASE CONTROL AND PREVENTION, THE MODEL STATE EMERGENCY HEALTH POWERS ACT (2001) [hereinafter MODEL STATE EMERGENCY HEALTH POWERS ACT (2001)]; THE DRAFT MODEL STATE EMERGENCY POWERS ACT, GUIDELINES FOR CONSIDERATION BY THE STATES (2001), *available at* www.nga.org/cda/files/EmerPowersAct.pdf (last visited Sept. 13, 2004). The preamble to the Draft notes that "[b]ecause each state is responsible for safeguarding the health, security, and well-being of its people, state governments must be able to respond rapidly and effectively to potential or actual public health emergencies." *Id*. at 8. The Model Act therefore "grants specific emergency powers to state governors and public health authorities." *Id*. Because public health laws vary from state to state, some states may consider enacting only certain portions of the Act.

[2] *See* N.Y. COMP. CODES R. & REGS. tit. 10, § 702.7 (2004) (requiring emergency and disaster preparedness for all medical facilities); *see also* WASH. ADMIN. CODE § 246-320-405(5) (2004) (establishing conditions for hospital licensure including implementation of a disaster plan "designed to meet both internal and external disasters").

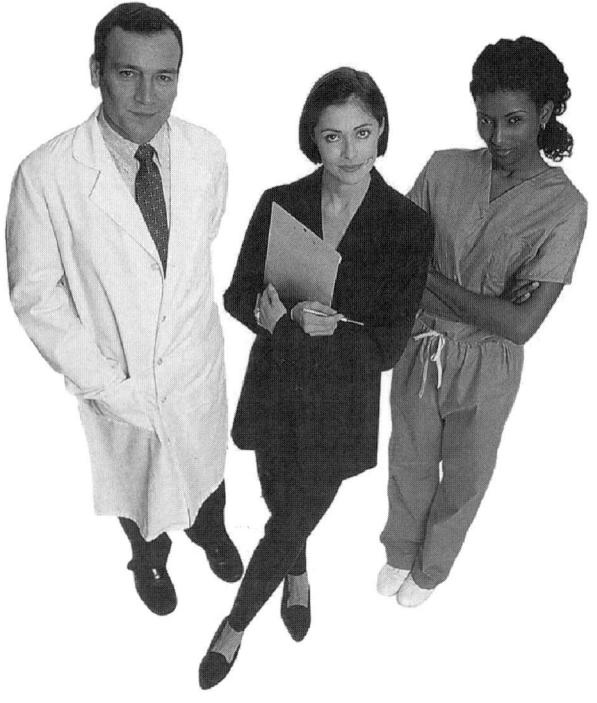

Figure A.1

(JCAHO).[3] Healthcare providers experience unexpected crises in different contexts, ranging from events where no essential hospital services are compromised to a disaster that affects all hospital operations on both large and small scales. Emergency events may be externally triggered (e.g., natural disasters; outbreaks of new, deadly diseases; or vicious acts of terrorism) that result in a massive demand on a healthcare system.

Emergencies also may be entirely institution-based (e.g., a small fire in the data center, a burst pipe in the emergency department, or a hospital-wide labor strike). Regardless of whether emergencies are external or internal to the organization, such events may impair healthcare operations and thereby trigger the implementation of a hospital's emergency management plan and its Incident Command Structure (ICS) or Hospital Emergency Incident Command System (HEICS)[4] response.

For example, Tropical Storm Allison created such an emergency situation for the Memorial Hermann Healthcare System in June 2001, when downtown Houston, TX, and the hospital endured more than twenty inches of rain in a three-day period. The flooding water overwhelmed precautions that had been designed to withstand a 100-year flood; destroyed a pathology laboratory; dispersed medical waste and biohazards; submerged mechanical, electrical, and plumbing systems; damaged communication systems; and required the complete evacuation of the Memorial Hermann Hospital and the Memorial Hermann Children's Hospital.[5]

And, of course, all Americans remember the heroism and professionalism exhibited by healthcare workers in the hours and days after the terrorist attacks in New York, NY, and Washington, D.C., on September 11, 2001. Or consider the example of the North York General Hospital in Toronto, Canada, which experienced a different emergency situation during May and August of 2003, when an outbreak of Severe Acute Respiratory Syndrome (SARS) occurred in

---

[3] *See, e.g.*, JOINT COMM'N ON ACCREDITATION OF HEALTHCARE ORGS., HOSPITAL ACCREDITATION STANDARDS (HAS) Standards EC4.10, EC4.20 (2004) (providing a detailed checklist of required activities and requiring a hospital to conduct drills regularly to test emergency management). *Cf.* NATIONAL FIRE PROTECTION ASS'N, STANDARD 1600 ON DISASTER/EMERGENCY MANAGEMENT AND BUSINESS CONTINUITY PROGRAMS §§ 1.1, 1.2 (2004) (establishing a standard common set of criteria for assessing and implementing emergency and disaster management), *available at* www.nfpa.org/PDF/nfpa1600.pdf (last visited Sept. 13, 2004).
[4] *See* NORTH CAROLINA HOSP. ASS'N, HOSPITAL EMERGENCY INCIDENT COMMAND SYSTEM (1992) (discussing both the Incident Command System and Hospital Emergency Incident Command System disaster response plans).
[5] Juanita F. Romans, *Tropical Storm Allison: The Houston Flood of June 9th, 2001*, 6 THE INTERNET JOURNAL OF RESCUE AND DISASTER MEDICINE (2002), *at* www.ispub.com/ostia/index.php?xmlFilePath=journals/ijeicm/vol6n1/coo.xml (last visited Sept. 14, 2004).

its orthopedic unit.[6] The hospital ultimately had ninety SARS patients, forty-four of them from the hospital's staff. North York General closed its doors to any new patients, and had to find ways to treat those patients who already had or who developed SARS. Hospital staff assumed significant personal risk to treat a new type of disease that affected their friends and colleagues. They did so under extraordinarily difficult circumstances that included a workplace quarantine and the intense scrutiny of a frightened media and populace.[7]

Remember also that, in the summer of 2003, large portions of New England and the mid-Atlantic states suffered power outages as a result of a falling tree limb cutting power lines in Ohio. Community members flocked to hospitals across the region for shelter even as the hospitals were operating on emergency-generator power, canceling elective procedures, and frequently functioning with compromised computer and other systems. As recently as late summer of 2004, four hurricanes devastated the state of Florida, causing the evacuation of local hospitals.

Accordingly, it is vitally important that healthcare providers maintain a constant state of emergency preparedness to ensure appropriate response and recovery within the quickest possible timeframe. Such preparedness encompasses four phases: (i) preparation; (ii) mitigation; (iii) response; and (iv) recovery.[8] Without proper planning, a crisis for the provider may result in unintended consequences involving a potential temporary or permanent business failure, thus adding a crucial community institution to the list of the event's casualties. The purpose of this *Checklist* is to identify the key legal and operational issues arising in an emergency in order to enhance a healthcare provider's emergency preparedness[9] by demonstrating the connection between emergency-planning activities and routine planning, contracting, and operational functions. By considering the following points, a healthcare provider will be in a better position to promote success for the organization as it confronts unexpected events.

This *Checklist* should not be construed as legal advice, however, and does not purport to encompass all possible legal and other issues that may apply in the event of such an emergency situation; each crisis presents its own unique circumstances. Finally, not every crisis will trigger all of the issues identified in this *Checklist*.

Additionally, public health emergencies have the potential for far-reaching effects on the U.S. population at large, and thus pose unique legal and operational issues for local health systems. A public health emergency, as defined in the Model State Emergency Health Powers Act, is an

> occurrence or imminent threat of a health condition caused by bioterrorism or the appearance of a novel or previously controlled or eradicated infectious agent or biological toxin, and poses a high probability of a large number of deaths, serious long-term disabilities, or significant risk of substantial future harm in the affected populations.[10]

The challenges inherent in quickly identifying the disease agent, mode of transmission, and best treatment options significantly affect both the well-being of healthcare workers *and* the daily operations of healthcare facilities. This is true

---

[6] *See* Susan Kwolek, *Lessons Learned from SARS: The Story of North York General Hospital, in* AM. HEALTH LAW. ASS'N, SARS: LEGAL AND RISK MANAGEMENT LESSONS LEARNED FROM TORONTO TO ATLANTA TELECONFERENCE (Nov. 13, 2003).
[7] *Id.*
[8] NATIONAL FIRE PROTECTION ASS'N, *supra* note 3, § 5.1.2.
[9] For additional information relating to operational issues, please see the following websites: Am. Hosp. Ass'n, *Disaster Readiness, at* www.hospitalconnect.com/aha/key_issues/disaster_readiness/index.html (last visited Sept. 10, 2004); Ctrs. for Disease Control and Prevention, Emergency Preparedness and Response, *at* www.bt.cdc.gov (last visited Sept. 10, 2004); Greater New York Hosp. Ass'n (GNYHA), GNYHA Emergency Preparedness Resource Center, *at* www.gnyha.org/eprc (last visited Sept. 10, 2004); Nat'l Disaster Med. Sys., *at* http://oep-ndms.dhhs.gov (last visited Sept. 10, 2004); RAND Ctr. for Domestic and Int'l Health Security, What's New, *at* www.rand.org/health/healthsecurity (last visited Sept. 10, 2004).
[10] MODEL STATE EMERGENCY HEALTH POWERS ACT (2001), *supra* note 1.

particularly in the event that it becomes necessary for the public health authority to assume control of a hospital.

True community-wide emergency preparedness therefore hinges on close coordination and cooperation between public health agencies, healthcare organizations, and their respective legal counsel. Protecting communities from man-made and naturally occurring threats alike requires legal counsel—for both public health agencies and healthcare providers—to establish a clear understanding of legal roles and operational responsibilities of each party, well in advance of any public health emergency. Thi s is important particularly to minimize the loss of lives and reduce the potential economic consequences of these events. To further this goal, the U.S. Centers for Disease Control and Prevention's (CDC's) Public Health Law Program has developed the Community Public Health Legal Preparedness Initiative (Initiative).[11] Through intensive, community-based, one-day workshops, this Initiative aims to build vibrant and enduring partnerships between legal counsel for private and public hospitals, as well as with other healthcare organizations and public health agencies, to enhance the use of law as a tool to advance community health through prevention and health promotion. Resources to facilitate this public health/healthcare partnership are listed in *Appendices D* and *E* of this *Checklist*.

This *Checklist* is organized to reflect the hierarchy established by the ICS structure, which provides a scalable approach to emergency management. The ICS structure offers a model for the immediate (and hopefully short-term) *ad hoc* restructuring of an organization around functional (rather than administrative) lines to better meet the demands of a given emergency situation. ICS identifies key roles within an organization, addresses responsibilities for each role, and assigns individuals and resources to those roles based on their availability as needed during an emergency. The ICS structure is scalable, enabling its use in the full range of emergency situations that may disrupt a healthcare provider's operations. The ICS employs an "Incident Commander" with four "sections" that report to the commander: (i) Operations; (ii) Planning; (iii) Logistics; and (iv) Finance, each with its own "chief."[12]

II. Incident Command (Orange)

The Incident Commander has overall authority and responsibility for operations during an emergency event.[13] The Incident Commander's main job is to allocate resources and ensure safety. Any function not otherwise assigned also is the responsibility of the Incident Commander. In addition to the four identified Incident Command System roles, the Incident Commander has direct reports from the Liaison Officer, Public Information Officer (PIO), Communications Officer, Safety/Security Officer,[14] and Recorder/Transcriber.

A. Emergency Management Plan

It is critical for the organization's personnel and medical staff to be familiar with its emergency management plan and ICS. In particular, personnel and medical staff should be aware of the following:

1. What constitutes a disaster that could trigger the implementation of the organization's emergency management plan and how is a disaster declared by the facility?

---

[11] *See* FIRESCOPE CALIFORNIA, GLOSSARY OF TERMS (ICS 010-1) 11 (1999), *available at* www.firescope.org/ics-pos-manuals/ICS%20010-1.pdf (last visited Sept. 15, 2004) [hereinafter GLOSSARY OF TERMS]. For more information about the Community Public Health Legal Preparedness Initiative and the Workshop Director's Guide, please visit www.phppo.cdc.gov/phlp or contact the CDC Public Health Law Program (Telephone: 770-488-2886, Fax: 770-488-2420; e-mail dreid@cdc.gov).

[12] By custom in the healthcare environment, each of these five key roles (i.e., the Incident Commander and her/his four Chiefs) has an assigned color, as indicated below. *See* NORTH CAROLINA HOSP. ASS'N, *supra* note 4, for an organizational chart showing these four divisions.

[13] FIRESCOPE CALIFORNIA, FIELD OPERATIONS GUIDE (ICS 420-1) 5-2 (2004), *available at* www.firescope.org/ics-big-fog/ICS420-1FOG8x11Cmplt.pdf (last visited Sept. 15, 2004) [hereinafter FIELD OPERATIONS GUIDE].

[14] *See* NORTH CAROLINA HOSP. ASS'N, *supra* note 4.

2. What code is called via the overhead paging system to announce the disaster and trigger implementation of the institution's emergency management plan?
3. Where is the organization's staff to report after an emergency is declared, and how will the organization account for their location? How will staff member locations be recorded (e.g., by sign-in sheet)?
   a. Where is the institution's Command Center primarily located, and under what circumstances might it be moved to an alternate location? Is the Command Center appropriately outfitted, and is it available for immediate use?
   b. What resources in the Command Center might individual staff contribute as part of planning?
      i Are personal contact numbers for relevant staff (e.g., home and cell telephones, personal fax number, e-mail address) available to the Command Center?
      ii Are the personal contact numbers of contacts at governmental offices, sister institutions, and important vendors available to the Command Center?
4. Have the organization's operations personnel been briefed with respect to the personal role and skills of individual staff, and how may those individuals assist an Incident Commander coordinating a response to an emergency?
5. Have personnel and medical staff members been provided with information to enable them to develop family emergency plans, so that they can be confident of their families' safety while they fulfill their obligations to respond during an emergency situation?

B. Command Center

The Command Center is the location from which the response to the emergency will be coordinated. It needs to be located and equipped in such a manner as to facilitate an appropriate response to the disaster, regardless of whether its scope is large or small.

1. Has the institution established a formal Command Center?
2. In choosing a location, has the institution considered what types of emergencies to which the institution will need to respond, so that the center is located in an easily accessible location that is close to the response, but not so close as to risk interfering with it?[15]
3. Is the Command Center connected with the institution's emergency generators?
4. Is it properly equipped with the following resources?
   a. Computers, e-mail, the organization's intranet, Internet access, phones, pagers, radios, and other resources in order to fulfill an institution's communication needs?
   b. Paper, pens, and markers for handwritten communication needs?
   c. Sufficient information about the institution's resources (and made easily accessible and searchable) to enable the functioning of an Incident Commander who may be unfamiliar with the hospital's major relationships and personnel?
   d. Easy access to institutional policies, both those needed for routine operations (e.g., Administration Policy and Procedure Manual, Medical Staff Bylaws) and any policies and procedures that have been adopted in anticipation of an emergency?

---

[15] For example, locating a command center in an emergency room that might have to deal with a mass casualty response may risk pulling people into the Emergency Department who will have administrative but not clinical responsibilities and so may inadvertently interfere with the response.

What mechanism ensures that such policies are always kept up to date? For example, does the Command Center have access to compliance policies with respect to the Health Insurance Portability and Accountability Act (HIPAA) that describe how to respond to inquiries seeking information regarding the location and condition of missing persons who may be patients?
5. Can the Command Center be moved if circumstances require such action?
6. Is the Command Center scalable?
   a. Is it in a single room, or is it in a location that can be expanded?
   b. Is the location accessible to the senior management team?
   c. If the Command Center needs to be expanded, has the institution determined an alternate location? Is that alternate location connected to the emergency generator system?
   d. Is the Command Center (or alternate location) capable of accommodating multiple people who are working multiple phones and computers simultaneously for easy and immediate communication among the ICS officers and Section Chiefs?
   e. Is it close to—but separate from—a personnel staging area, so that the Incident Commander and the Operations Section Chief may easily assign people awaiting instruction, without having these people crowd into the Command Center?
7. Does the Command Center include easy access to community and affiliate resources, including all necessary contact information?

C. Incident Commander

The Incident Commander is the individual who assumes overall authority for the institution's response to the emergency. In an institution that implements a classic ICS structure, the commander role may be filled by almost anyone in the institution who identifies and announces the emergency until such time as someone in an administrative chain of command superior to that person takes over the role of Incident Commander.[16] In a HEICS system, the role of Incident Commander may be filled by individuals who have pre-assigned roles that will automatically slot into the command structure. For example, the organization's chief operating officer may automatically assume command for a hospital-wide emergency; by contrast, the Chief of Engineering may assume command for responding to a broken pipe that floods the hospital's data center. Regardless of whether the Incident Commander is in the institution's organization chart, she is responsible for the response until relieved or the emergency ends.

1. Does the institution's emergency plan call for the implementation of an ICS or HEICS system?
2. If it is an ICS system, are *all* the potential individuals who may declare a disaster and assume command aware of their potential authority?
   a. Are they trained in the emergency management plan?
   b. Do they understand how they may be relieved of responsibility?
3. If an institution uses a HEICS system, are the individuals who may assume command as a result of their roles within the organization aware of their roles and their responsibilities in an emergency? Could the designation of the Incident Commander change, based on the nature of an emergency?
4. If the organization uses a HEICS structure (or other modified ICS structure that preassigns individuals to roles in the incident command structure), is the structure regularly reviewed

---

[16] A classic incident-command response may require an individual who is above the Incident Commander in the organization's standard organization chart to either assume command or become a direct report to the Incident Commander.

when individuals leave (and new individuals join) the organization, and are the assignments updated as needed?

5. Under either an ICS or HEICS of system:
   a. Does the relevant individual know the location of the Command Center and the potential resources in it;
   b. Is that individual familiar with the institution's resources to enable her to gather and assign resources as necessary; and
   c. Does some kind of chart exist that may be populated with names and contacts in order to keep track of the people who are filling the other roles within the command structure?

D. Liaison Officer

The Liaison Officer communicates with external agencies on behalf of the Incident Commander.[17]

1. Has the organization identified those external agencies (e.g., fire, rescue, police, and public health authorities) with which it will need to interact in the event of an emergency?
2. Has the organization compiled contact information for each external agency, and is that contact information available in the Command Center? Is it reviewed on a periodic basis before an emergency occurs to ensure that it is current?
3. Does the contact information include as many different means of communication (e.g., cell telephone, fax, land-line telephone, radio contact information) as possible?
4. Is the Command Center itself set up to be able to use any and all available means of communication?
5. In planning for an emergency, has the organization established appropriate lines of communication with local response agencies, and has it discussed and coordinated the facility's plans with relevant agencies ahead of time?

E. Public Information Officer

The PIO serves as the contact for media inquiries, and coordinates communication between the organization and the public.[18]

1. Does the organization have a designated PIO or media-contact person on call at all times?
2. Does the organization have a policy that all media inquiries must be directed to the PIO or media person on-call?
3. Are the Incident Commander and PIO prepared to make rapid decisions regarding (i) what information to disclose about an organization's particular situation and readiness; (ii) at what times to make such announcements; and (iii) to which media outlets?
4. Has the organization established patient- and family-tracking procedures and mechanisms that will enable the PIO to locate and obtain information on patients that are evaluated and treated during an emergency, as well as to respond appropriately to inquiries?
5. Is the organization equipped with sufficient telephone lines, cell phones, and other resources to communicate quickly and effectively in an emergency situation?
6. Does the Command Center include telephone numbers and other contacts to community media personnel?
7. Has the organization developed HIPAA- and JCAHO-compliant media-consent forms to enable willing and available patients to speak with the media about the facility's response during an emergency? Do such consent forms include an agreement with the media company as required by JCAHO standards?

---

[17] GLOSSARY OF TERMS, *supra* note 11, at 12.
[18] FIELD OPERATIONS GUIDE, *supra* note 13, at 5–3.

8. Has the organization communicated its essential role in emergency response to the community and its political representatives alike, so that the survival of the facility will be a priority consideration that the community and government will take into account after the disaster?

9. Has the organization communicated to donors and other supporters of the organization the essential role that is played by the facility in community emergency response?

F. Communications Officer

The Communications Officer ensures effective communications between the Command Center and the rest of the organization. Emergency events require rapid and accurate communications. Many audiences are involved in communication before, during, and after an event, including: (i) the Command Center and internal response personnel; (ii) staff of the organization; (iii) patients and their families; (iv) other agencies and organizations that are part of the event response; (v) police, fire, military, and other governmental agencies; (vi) the general public; and (vii) donors and other supporters of the organization.

1. How will the organization determine what information should be conveyed to others? Will every-one receive the same information, or will some receive less information than others?

2. How will the organization accommodate staff's desire and need to know about an emergency event from the standpoint of the safety of family members, while ensuring continued staff availability for patients?

3. In the event that external authorities issue orders or assume direction of the organization's response, how will those developments be communicated?

4. Has the organization prepared "template" messages, and made them available in the Command Center, for use in the event of an emergency, to reduce the time needed to distribute messages to staff?

5. How and to whom will any orders to evacuate any portion of the facility, or to terminate services, be communicated?

6. Are all means of communication tested on a periodic basis to ensure readiness for use during an emergency event?

7. Has the organization established, and is the Command Center capable of issuing, multiple alternative means of communication, including telephone calls, overhead announcements, e-mail, intranet and Internet Web postings, meetings, correspondence, handwritten postings, and "runners" assigned to courier handwritten messages?

8. Does the Command Center include contact information for key internal personnel, including individuals who may be away from the facility when an emergency is declared?

G. Safety/Security Officer

Safety and security are essential to incident-response activities. Panic and "mob action" easily can over-whelm an organization unless order is maintained; further, unsafe conditions may put additional lives in jeopardy.

1. Who is responsible for maintaining order during an emergency?

2. What supplies or equipment are needed to maintain order, and are they readily available?

3. Does the organization have the ability to obtain additional security personnel on short notice in the event of an emergency?

4. Is a designated safety officer on call at all times?

5. How will the Incident Commander ensure the safety of individuals participating in emergency response activities (including, without limitation, those engaged in decontamination, crowd control, search and rescue within damaged buildings, or isolation and quarantine)?

6. To ensure the safety of all personnel, does the emergency-response plan call for regular changes of shift (if personnel are available)

to avoid exhaustion and compromised functioning of those in response roles?

7. How will the institution handle community members who may seek shelter in the hospital during an emergency? Is the institution able to designate specific areas for such people? Are these areas away from patient areas, and away from staging and other areas that might interfere with the emergency response? Does the institution have the resources to feed and shelter such people? If not, how would it handle the influx, and where would it send these people? Will it need to contact its local police precinct around this issue?

8. How will the institution handle an influx of individuals seeking relatives who might be unidentified patients?

9. Does the organization have a security plan in place for crowd control and other needed security measures?

H. Recorder/Transcriber

The Recorder/Transcriber maintains records of any actions taken as directed by the Incident Commander, as well as any significant event that may occur during the crisis. The Recorder/Transcriber assures continuous flow of and access to information for Command Center staff.

1. Has the organization provided for a recorder/transcriber in the event of an emergency?

2. How will the records of any incident response be used during debriefing to inform the organization's planning for future readiness?

III. Operations (Red)

The Operations Section Chief reports directly to the Incident Commander, and has responsibility for conducting operations during the emergency.[19] The Operations Section Chief is responsible for whatever services are being provided during the emergency, and frequently oversees a fairly large number of operational leaders responsible for specific areas, such as Decontamination, Emergency Services, Inpatient Services, and the Operating Room.[20] Some key issues facing the Operations Section Chief include the following.

A. Isolation and Quarantine

Government authorities may exercise police powers in an emergency situation, including the isolation of infected individuals and quarantine of healthy individuals who may have been exposed to an infectious agent. For a disease listed in federal Executive Order 13295 as communicable and quarantinable, the U.S. government has jurisdiction to apprehend, detain, and conditionally release individuals to stop its interstate spread or international importation, and need not wait for an interstate spread actually to occur before acting.[21] Thus, it is important for healthcare providers to coordinate isolation and quarantine measures with federal, state, and local authorities.

1. What are the local, regional, state, and national plans for handling a sudden influx of patients who may require decontamination as a result of having been exposed to chemical, biological, or radiological agents?

2. Does the Incident Commander have the authority to implement decontamination, isolation, or quarantine measures? If not, who does? Who needs to be informed in the event that such measures are implemented?

3. Has the organization engaged in isolation or quarantine planning with local and regional public health officials in order to understand what will be expected or demanded if isolation or quarantine is ordered?

---

[19] *See* NORTH CAROLINA HOSP. ASS'N, *supra* note 4.
[20] FIELD OPERATIONS GUIDE, *supra* note 13, at 7–2.
[21] 42 U.S.C. § 264 (2004).

4. Is the organization familiar with the plans of all such authorities, and has it coordinated its emergency planning with these authorities?

5. Do procedures exist to identify incoming patients who may require decontamination or isolation? Are staff members trained in them, and is appropriate equipment available to conduct such procedures? How is the safety of staff ensured in the event that a patient requires decontamination or isolation?

6. What plans exist for placing, observing, and caring for individuals subject to isolation or quarantine? Do local officials plan to utilize hospitals or other private facilities for these purposes in an emergency?

7. What legal procedures are required to implement isolation or quarantine of individuals or groups?

8. If a patient is admitted to a hospital, how will isolation and quarantine orders be delivered to the patient during her stay? What constitutes valid orders for isolation or quarantine? Does the organization have a system for receiving and recording any such orders?

9. Is the organization at risk if it implements an isolation or quarantine order issued without a court hearing?

10. Are a court hearing and court order required for the imposition of isolation or quarantine measures? Is an order that is issued without a hearing valid?

11. If a hearing is necessary for a hospital patient who is subject to an isolation or quarantine order, how will the hearing be conducted?

12. Can local, regional, or state agencies provide either legal indemnification or an opinion of counsel regarding the liability of healthcare providers for cooperating with isolation or quarantine orders?

13. How will facilities be compensated for their additional expenses incurred and revenue lost if they are designated as isolation or quarantine facilities? What documentation will be required to make claims for expenses and lost revenues relating to an isolation or quarantine event?

14. Following an isolation or quarantine event, what entity will compensate facilities for their costs of recovery, and what will be the basis for such compensation? What documentation will be required to make claims for these costs of recovery?

15. Who, if anyone, is financially responsible for lost wages due to an order of quarantine or isolation? Who is responsible for compensating a healthcare worker who is sent home by her employer following an exposure? In what way does the answer to this question change if the person is ordered into home quarantine by public health authorities? How does the answer change if the person experienced exposure in a work environment, rather than in a home environment or while traveling abroad?

16. Is it possible for facilities to employ workplace-quarantine measures? Can an employee be quarantined at home outside of working hours (i.e., permitted to leave the home only to go to work)?

17. Who is financially responsible for the costs of isolation or quarantine in a hospital that occurs pursuant to a public health order? What is the response going to be if a third-party payor determines that care for a particular illness is not covered, or is no longer medically necessary, and refuses to pay?

18. Who is responsible for enforcing isolation and quarantine orders? (For example, if a patient must be physically detained in isolation, who will ensure the patient stays there?)

B. Patient Diversion Issues

In an emergency, the normal flow of patients to and among healthcare providers almost certainly will be interrupted. See *Appendix A* for a discussion of the applicability of the Emergency Medical

Treatment and Active Labor Act (EMTALA)[22] in the event of a major public health emergency.

1. How will the determination be made that the organization's emergency-response plan (or the community emergency-response plan) should be implemented (e.g., whether an official declaration is necessary)? Has a threshold number of cases been established to require the triggering of the plan? What occurs if the plan appears to conflict with an organization's own legal or other obligations? What happens if the community has not developed an emergency-response plan? Does the institution have its own plan?
2. Does the organization have in place a full range of transfer agreements to provide for the emergency transfer of patients whose medical conditions are beyond the scope of its services? If the organization is a tertiary care facility, does it have in place transfer agreements with other community providers under which the tertiary care facility will receive patients in an emergency?
3. Do the organization's transfer agreements with any long term care facilities address the immediate return of hospitalized residents in the event of an emergency situation requiring an evacuation of patients?
4. Do the organization's routine files, as well as its Command Center records, include (in readily accessible locations) the list of such community and affiliate resources, including a description of the potential resources and appropriate contact information, for easy reference by the incident-command staff in an emergency?
5. Has the organization planned for partial or complete closure (including partial or complete evacuation) of the facility in the event of an emergency?
6. Does the organization have an established protocol for closure of the facility to incoming patients as the result of an emergency?
7. Has the organization identified all parties who need to receive notice of any closure, including other providers, ambulance companies, agencies responsible for triage and patient allocation in an emergency, first responders, and regulatory or licensing authorities?
8. Is the organization a participant in the National Disaster Medical System (NDMS), under which hospital beds are made available to the Department of Homeland Security for use in the federal medical response to major emergencies and declared disasters? If so, what are the organization's responsibilities within the NDMS program?
9. Is the organization's process for closure or diversion compliant with the organization's obligations under EMTALA, and with state or local rules and orders of public health officials? Will the organization continue to provide for screening examinations and required stabilizing care within its available resources at all times it remains in operation?
10. Has the Centers for Medicare & Medicaid Services (CMS) issued any emergency guidance? What should hospitals do in the interim between the arrival of patients and the issuance of CMS guidance, as this could lead to treatment differences before and subsequent to such an issuance?
11. May patients be directed to the organization by a governmental authority, including a public health, police, or military official, overriding the organization's EMTALA duties? If so, is the Command Center equipped to receive documentation of the order or direction? In the alternative, has the Incident Commander created appropriate records of the directions received?

---

[22] *See generally* Emergency Medical Treatment and Active Labor Act, 42 U.S.C. § 1395dd (2004).

12. What is the institution's threshold response in such situations (e.g., any initial evaluation provided; immediate diversion to designated facility; patients presenting with symptoms covered by emergency-response situation, as well as other symptoms)?
13. Can medical-screening exam procedures be altered due to concerns over contamination (e.g., performed outside)?
14. Will response differ by acuity of circumstances (e.g., mass disaster vs. intermittent flow of affected patients)?
15. How will EMTALA compliance be demonstrated and/or documented in the event that an emergency-response plan is implemented?
16. Does the organization have a contingency plan if a potentially exposed patient presents, but the case must first be evaluated by law enforcement or public health? Does this constitute an "undue delay" under EMTALA?
17. What is facility's obligation, if a patient is diverted elsewhere, to ensure that patient transfer is effectuated?
18. Have state or local authorities made declarations that will protect the organization in circumstances where an emergency is not "national," and therefore does not trigger protection from sanctions in the regulations?
19. If the facility in question is the designated treatment facility, how are existing patients handled? What happens once capacity is reached? Does the designated facility have a memorandum of understanding (MOU) or mutual-aid agreement with other facilities, or with state or local government?
20. Has there been a presidential declaration of emergency that suspends EMTALA obligations? Will some or all EMTALA obligations be suspended or waived in the event of a local emergency in the absence of a federal or local declaration?[23]

C. Patient Tracking and Placement

In a mass-casualty event, organizations may be over-whelmed with a sudden influx of patients. It is essential for facilities to both track and be able to report on these patients.

1. Does the organization have an identified triage area for large numbers of incoming patients?
   a. Has the organization identified secondary triage site(s) if its original triage site becomes overwhelmed by an influx of patients?
   b. Is the organization able to staff and supply such site(s)?
   c. If the organization utilizes secondary sites, might they be separated by purpose (e.g., all patients needing decontamination in one area, those not needing decontamination into another)?
   d. Are such secondary site(s) separate from staging areas for any human resources and other resources?
   e. Can the triage zone accommodate decontamination procedures, if needed?
2. Have tracking forms and other tools been made readily available in the emergency department and in the Command Center to permit manual tracking of incoming patients?
3. Does the organization have a method (and the necessary paper forms and supplies) for recording patient medical information when patient volume or other conditions do not permit the use of computerized systems? Does the organization have a plan to record manually gathered information into computer systems when conditions permit?
4. Where will a large number of incoming patients be housed? What portions of the facility can be converted to patient care on short notice?

---

[23] To date, CMS has not stated this explicitly, but it is important to note that policy in this area is evolving.

5. If a large number of incoming patients require isolation due to contamination or infectious disease, where will they be placed? Who will care for them, and what protective equipment, supplies, or facility changes will be needed?
6. Does the organization have an identified area for family members and other concerned individuals to obtain information about patients at the facility? Has it identified needed resources for such individuals, including food and water, as well as emotional and spiritual counselors?
7. Has the organization trained the emergency department and other relevant staff in techniques of triage? Does the organization provide emotional and spiritual support for front-line staff engaged in triage and treatment?

D. Reporting Requirements

Each state has its own requirements for reporting communicable diseases and conditions to either local or state health departments who, in turn, report information to the CDC. Some local jurisdictions also may have communicable-disease reporting requirements. The time and manner of reporting likely will vary among jurisdictions and among diseases. Some state laws on communicable-disease reporting may bestow immunity on some individuals making such reports.

1. Has the organization identified the communicable-disease reporting laws for state or local jurisdictions?
2. Are those responsible for making the reports aware of the timeframes and procedures for reporting each type of communicable disease? (Particular attention should be paid to those communicable diseases that are identified as "Category A" critical biological agents—anthrax, botulism, plague, smallpox, tularemia, and viral hemorrhagic fevers).
3. Has the organization's staff been informed of confidentiality requirements whenever reporting of communicable diseases to any government agency is mandated by law?
4. Has the organization assessed the availability of legal immunity for a person making such a report?
5. Has the organization distributed guidelines to personnel and medical staff describing permissible uses and disclosures of protected health information for public health and other reporting purposes under HIPAA?[24]

E. Personnel Issues

In addition to their role as providers of healthcare services, healthcare institutions also are employers. In this context, healthcare institutions must comply with myriad state and federal laws. In the event of an emergency, institutional personnel of all varieties will be called upon to perform various functions, both within and outside of their typical scope of duties. Preparing for and dealing with the aftermath of a crisis will involve an array of duties not only to the public and individual patients, but to the institution's employees as well. Although the laws and regulations discussed in this section apply specifically to the employment relationship between healthcare

---

[24] *See generally* Health Insurance Portability and Accountability Act of 1996, Pub. L. No. 104–191, 110 Stat. 1936 (codified as amended in scattered sections of 26, 29, and 42 U.S.C.) (establishing guidelines for confidentiality issues). The Department of Health and Human Services has issued a Privacy Rule that provides comprehensive Federal protection for the privacy of health information. Standards for Privacy of Individually Identifiable Health Information, 65 Fed. Reg. 82,462, 82,596 (Dec. 28, 2000) (codified at 45 C.F.R. pts. 160, 164). The Privacy Rule recognizes that various agencies and public officials will need protected health information (PHI) to deal effectively with a bioterrorism threat or emergency. To facilitate the communications that are essential to a quick and effective response to such events, the Privacy Rule permits covered entities to disclose needed information to public officials in a variety of ways. Covered entities may disclose PHI without the individual's authorization to a public health authority acting as authorized by law in response to a bioterrorism threat or public health emergency. 45 C.F.R. § 164.512(b) (2004). The Privacy Rule also permits a covered entity to disclose PHI to public officials who are reasonably able to prevent or lessen a serious and imminent threat to public health or safety related to bioterrorism.

institutions and their employees, it is important to note that some providers and other personnel work as independent contractors rather than as employees. Institutions should consider the effects of independent-contractor status with respect to the ability to use certain personnel in the event of an emergency, particularly if such individuals have relationships with more than one institution. Moreover, public-sector healthcare institutions also must bear in mind liability issues that might arise under various civil-rights statutes.[25]

1. *General Considerations.* In developing an emergency management plan, organizations should consider the following personnel-related issues.
    a. Have the institution's employees received materials and training on the development of personal emergency plans for themselves and their families? Do employees' families understand that, in an emergency, their personal emergency plans may need to be initiated without the employees (or with them only calling into a designated contact), as they may be required to stay at the facility and assist in the facility's response? Do they have enough information about family emergency plans to feel confident that their family will be safe during the emergency so they can focus on their responsibilities?
    b. Has the institution identified multiple safe staging areas for groups of employees, outside of the primary emergency-response areas, so that they can be assigned as needed? Have the locations of the staging areas been communicated to employees?
    c. Does the institution have a mechanism that ensures that employees are only released to return home if they are not needed, and if the institution believes that the employee may safely leave the premises? Has the institution developed mechanisms that will enable it to learn of unsafe conditions that would interfere with employees and others exiting the institution (e.g., closed roads, bridges, and mass-transit problems)?
    d. Has the institution made provision for emergency emotional, spiritual, psychological, and potentially psychiatric support to its employees who are dealing with the personal effects of the emergency? Does it have a plan to employ a triage or other mechanism in such a situation?
    e. Has the institution anticipated providing some long-term, post-response support to its employees in the event of a major disaster? Does it have the internal resources to do so, or would it need to go to another organization or agency? If it needs to go elsewhere, does it know where to go?
    f. If an independent contractor has any of its employees performing responsibilities onsite at the institution, has that contractor set up a mechanism to locate and safeguard its employees? Do such employees have a central place to gather and sign in?
    g. Does the institution know who the independent-contractor employees are, and where they would gather in an emergency in case it needs to call upon their expertise (e.g., a contractor providing routine on-site staffing and management for an institution's data center)? Does the institution know who to contact at the independent contractor's office to get those individuals resourced appropriately in an emergency?
    h. Does the independent contractor know what the institution's expectations are with respect to the use of contractor employees in an emergency?
    i. Has the independent contractor trained or drilled its employees in their responsibilities to the institution in an emergency?
2. *Workers' Compensation.* State workers'-compensation laws could be implicated if an employee contracts an illness on the job during the course of a public health emergency. This

---

[25] *See generally* 42 U.S.C. § 1983 (2004).

most likely will occur among first responders, law enforcement, and healthcare workers. Emotional distress due to fear of exposure generally is compensable under these rules. In an emergency, healthcare workers may experience injuries while rendering aid during the crisis. Workers' compensation also may be available for such injuries, depending on the activity causing the injury and the worker's job duties during the emergency. Where the injury involves a disease for which a vaccine or medication is available, the application of worker's compensation may depend on whether the person undertakes voluntary vaccinations or medical treatment. Finally, because workers'-compensation laws vary significantly among the states, it is necessary to consult the workers'-compensation laws of the jurisdiction in question.

a. Has the organization reviewed workers'-compensation statutes and regulations for the appropriate jurisdiction?
b. Has the organization identified the potential liability for injuries, medical expenses, retirement benefits, and disability benefits incurred by the participation of employees and volunteers during an emergency?
c. Has the organization determined whether other federal or state benefit programs may apply or, alternatively, may bar submission of a claim (e.g., if state laws constitute an exclusive remedy) regarding certain disaster or disaster-preparedness situations?
d. Has the applicable jurisdiction(s) established any compensation programs specific for certain activities (e.g., vaccination), and is coverage different for employees as opposed to volunteers?
e. Does a "no-fault" compensation program apply?
f. Has the organization identified the availability of workers' compensation and/or other forms of financial support for persons unable to return to work because of an isolation/quarantine order?
g. How will the organization address any potential legal liability for implementing "working" quarantine policies for essential service personnel?
h. If an employee is quarantined, but is asymptomatic, is the employee entitled to compensation for the time spent in quarantine?
i. Is the institution prepared for workers'-compensation claims, which may be filed months or years after the actual emergency event, claiming that the event and the event response negatively affected employees' physical or psychological health?

3. *Other Compensation and Wage/Hour Issues.* Similar to other employers, healthcare institutions are subject to federal regulations that pertain to employee compensation and hours.[26] In addition, organizations must comply with specific labor, compensation, and general employment laws relating to healthcare workers. For example, some states have enacted measures banning mandatory overtime for nurses and other healthcare professionals.[27] Meeting these obligations could present a significant challenge in the face of a major public health emergency, involving a redefinition of the work day, work week, and/or overtime. Some states are considering mandating the continuation of wages if employees are kept from work due to isolation or quarantine (policies that might be considered akin

---

[26] Please *see* discussion regarding the Fair Labor Standards Act in Section III(F)(5) of this *Checklist*, which is the text accompanying notes 42–43.
[27] *See* Ann E. Rogers et al., *The Working Hours of Hospital Staff Nurses and Patient Safety*, 23 HEALTH AFF. 202, 203 (2004); ME. REV. STAT. ANN. tit. 26, § 603(5) (2003) (stating that any nurse "who is mandated to work more than 12 consecutive hours" in the event of an unforeseen emergent circumstance "must be allowed as least 10 consecutive hours of off-duty time immediately following the worked overtime"); *see also* OR. REV. STAT. § 441.166 (2003); N.J. STAT. ANN. § 34:11–56a34 (2004).

to jury duty). Such measures might enhance compliance by reducing individuals' fears of lost income, and also afford protection for the rest of the workforce.
  a. Would discharging an employee who is absent because she is subject to quarantine be deemed illegal as a public-policy violation?
  b. What is the outcome if extended hours required of healthcare workers run up against legal limits on the hours that physicians and nurses can work consecutively?
  c. Will payment be provided for temporary lodging, meals, or other incidental expenses?
  d. How will payroll and benefits be maintained?
4. *Credentialing Issues, Including Disaster Privileges.* Issues may arise regarding whether a hospital or healthcare entity may allow outside medical personnel to assist regular staff during an emergency due to existing medical-privileges requirements. JCAHO requires hospitals to establish a procedure for verifying credentials and granting privileges during and after a disaster,[28] and has established procedures for doing so. In addition, at the federal level, the Secretary of the Department of Health and Human Services is required to establish a system for advance registration of health professionals to provide for verification of credentials, licenses, accreditations, and hospital privileges when such professionals volunteer during a public health emergency.[29]
  a. Has the appropriate state or local jurisdiction adopted regulations regarding the use of disaster privileges during an emergency situation? Do such regulations provide immunity for granting or denying such disaster privileges, or for providing care after being granted such privileges?
  b. Does the chief executive officer (CEO), medical staff president, or another official have the option to grant disaster privileges pursuant to JCAHO standards? Does the institution have a document that delegates this responsibility to the Incident Commander as the designee if the designated official is not physically available during the disaster?
  c. Who has been designated in writing to grant disaster privileges? Has the organization specified such individual's duties, as well as a mechanism to manage the activities of healthcare practitioners who receive disaster privileges (and to readily identify such individuals)? Will the designated individual treat the verification process as a high priority? Is this position identified in the emergency management plan and/or otherwise accessible to the Incident Commander in an emergency?
  d. Does the medical staff have a mechanism to initiate the verification process of the credentials and privileges of individuals who receive disaster privileges as soon as the immediate situation is under control?
  e. Are the organization's disaster and emergency-privileging processes consistent with the process established under the medical staff bylaws for granting temporary privileges to fulfill an important patient-care need? If not, is an amendment to the medical-staff bylaws contemplated and/or needed?
  f. Has the appropriate jurisdiction established procedures regarding credentials? Does the appropriate jurisdiction allow an expedited and/or different process for verifying that the person practicing has the proper credentials when in an emergency situation? Are immunity protections associated

---

[28] JOINT COMM'N ON ACCREDITATION OF HEALTHCARE ORGS., *supra* note 3, at Standard MS 4.10.
[29] Public Health Security and Bioterrorism Response Act of 2002, Pub. L. No. 107–188, § 107, 116 Stat. 594, 608 (codified as amended at 42 U.S.C. § 247d–7b).

with the credentialing process available during an emergency?
            g. Are "request for staff privileges" forms for collecting credentials data available in the Command Center?
    5. *Use of Licensed Professionals Outside Their Scope of Practice.* The use of licensed professionals outside their normal scopes of practice, or using non-licensed professionals to perform tasks that would typically require a license, may raise legal issues. Some states may have statutes that specifically authorize such practices, or allow certain licensed professionals (e.g., physicians) to delegate certain tasks to others while providing supervision. Additionally, emergency-management statutes or other public health emergency-preparedness laws may allow the governor of a state (or another designated individual, e.g., a state agency director) to suspend certain statutes to authorize such activities during a crisis.
        a. Do the appropriate local and state jurisdictions allow for medical staff to delegate their authority during an emergency situation? If so, to what extent?
        b. Does legal authority exist to suspend professional-licensure requirements during a major disaster? If so, who has that authority? Does the institution know how that decision would be communicated to it during an emergency?
    6. *Use of Licensed Professionals from Other States.* Issues may arise relating to using licensed professionals from other states to assist in responding to an emergency. The National Emergency Management Association has published a model law, entitled *The Emergency Management Assistance Compact (EMAC)*;[30] most states have entered into this compact. Article V of *EMAC* provides that whenever (i) any person holds a license, certificate, or other permit issued by any *EMAC*-participating state evidencing qualifications for professional, mechanical, or other skills, and (ii) when such assistance is requested by the receiving party state, such person shall be deemed to be licensed, certified, or permitted by the state requesting assistance to render aid involving such skill to meet a declared emergency or disaster.[31] It also is possible that state professional-regulatory and/or emergency-management statutes address these issues.
        a. Has the organization's state adopted *EMAC* or other measures that address the use of licensed professionals from other jurisdictions during an emergency?
        b. Does the organization know what limitations and conditions the governor of the state may prescribe when issuing an order pursuant to *EMAC* or other statutory provisions? Do *EMAC* or other state statutory provisions confer immunity on licensed professionals from other jurisdictions in an emergency?
        c. Does the organization know if licensed medical personnel employed by federal agencies are permitted to assist during an emergency, and is their ability to practice in an emergency contingent upon the state's licensure requirements?

---

[30] *See* Emergency Mgmt. Assistance Compact (EMAC), EMAC Emergency Management Assistance Model Legislation, *at* www.emacweb.org/EMAC/About_EMAC/Model_Legislation.cfm (last visited Sept. 11, 2004).

[31] *Id.* at art. V. It should be noted that Article VI of EMAC provides that

> Officers or employees of a party state rendering aid in another state pursuant to this compact shall be considered agents of the requesting state for tort liability and immunity purposes; and no party state or its officers or employees rendering aid in another state pursuant to this compact shall be liable on account of any act or omission in good faith on the part of such forces while so engaged or on account of the maintenance or use of any equipment or supplies in connection therewith. Good faith in this article shall not include willful misconduct, gross negligence, or gross recklessness.

F. Statutory and Regulatory Considerations

As part of their emergency-management planning, organizations should evaluate the implications of the following laws and regulations.

1. *Occupational Safety and Health Act* (OSHA).[32] OSHA applies to most private-sector employers. It is enforced by the Occupational Safety and Health Administration (also known as OSHA) within the U.S. Department of Labor (DOL).[33] The Act contains a "General Duty Clause" requiring employers to furnish a place of employment free from recognized hazards likely to cause death or serious physical harm. OSHA sets work-place standards for safety and for various toxic/chemical exposures.
   a. Does the emergency present a hazardous working condition triggering OSHA obligations and attendant employee protections? (In some circumstances, employees are permitted to refuse to work in the face of real danger of death or injury.)
   b. Has OSHA promulgated guidelines for diseases, toxic or chemical exposures, or similar health hazards involved in the emergency?[34] Are any such guidelines being contemplated?

2. *Family and Medical Leave Act* (FMLA).[35] The FMLA requires employers with fifty or more employees to allow eligible employees to take up to twelve weeks of unpaid leave in a twelve-month period for a serious health condition (among other reasons).[36] A "serious health condition" is defined as an illness, injury, impairment, or physical or mental condition that involves inpatient care or continuing treatment by a healthcare provider.[37] Some states have analogous provisions, some of which are more generous than the federal law.
   a. Does FMLA cover an employee who is an asymptomatic patient subject to quarantine or isolation?
   b. Does FMLA cover an employee's family member who is an asymptomatic patient subject to quarantine or isolation?
   c. Would a major emergency requiring the participation of all available personnel potentially excuse noncompliance with FMLA, except for those employees with absolute medical needs?

3. *Americans with Disabilities Act* (ADA).[38] The ADA creates a variety of duties applicable to employers with regard to disabled employees. It prohibits discrimination against individuals with disabilities who are otherwise qualified for a job, and it limits pre-employment inquiries. A "disability" is defined as "a physical or mental impairment that substantially limits one or more of the major life activities of such individual."[39] The ADA applies to employers with fifteen or more employees, and is enforced by the federal Equal Employment Opportunity Commission (EEOC).[40] Healthcare organizations and others must consider the following issues in an emergency, given the nature of an institution's physically impaired employees for whom it might previously have provided an ADA accommodation.

---

[32] Occupational Health and Safety Act of 1970, 29 U.S.C. § 651 (2004).
[33] For a further discussion of the Occupational Health and Safety Administration, see Occupational Health and Safety Admin, U.S. Dep't of Labor, *at* www.osha.gov (last visited Sept. 25, 2004).
[34] *See* OCCUPATIONAL HEALTH AND SAFETY ADMIN., U.S. DEP'T OF LABOR, INFORMATION REGARDING SEVERE ACUTE RESPIRATORY SYNDROME (SARS) (establishing guidelines for healthcare workers, laboratories, and airlines dealing with SARS), *at* www.osha.gov/dep/sars/index.html (last visited Sept. 14, 2004).
[35] Family Medical Leave Act, 29 U.S.C. §§ 2601–2654 (2004).
[36] *Id.* §§ 2611–2612.
[37] *Id.* § 2611.
[38] Americans with Disabilities Act, 42 U.S.C. § 12101 (2004).
[39] *Id.* § 12102.
[40] *Id.* § 12111.

a. Do the individuals need any special considerations in ensuring that they:
   - Are located properly at the beginning of an emergency;
   - Can go to (or be brought to) a staging area for contribution to the response;
   - Contribute to the response, and not somehow get in the way of it; and
   - Can safely return to their offices (and responsibilities), and/or home, after the response?
b. Would it constitute disability discrimination to fire an employee kept out of work due to quarantine or isolation? Does such a decision depend on the employee's disease condition?
c. Do any of the organization's employees have a disability that will require special assistance in the event of an evacuation? Is the organization's evacuation plan consistent with the needs and special requirements of each of its employees and medical staff members?
d. An employer may reject a job applicant with a disability, or terminate an employee with a disability, for safety reasons if the person poses a direct threat (i.e., a significant risk of substantial harm to self or others) without violating the ADA. This might cover an adverse-employment decision with regard to an employee subject to isolation or quarantine due to exposure and the risk of infection. Could a bona fide emergency convert an accommodation that normally is a reasonable one into an undue hardship?
e. What should be the organization's response where employee absenteeism mounts due to the stress of a particular emergency situation, and employees claim that they are suffering from post-traumatic stress disorder? Can such employees' essential job functions be accommodated at home?

4. *National Labor Relations Act* (NLRA).[41] The NLRA provides legal protection for employees engaging in "protected concerted" activity, and governs the relationship among unions, employees, and employers. The NLRA is enforced by the National Labor Relations Board (NLRB), and governs most private-sector employers.
   a. Has the organization addressed special emergency circumstances (e.g., overtime, lost wages, work rules, duty to bargain, grievances) ahead of time in existing collective-bargaining agreements? If not, will such issues be addressed during the next renewal of collective bargaining agreements?
   b. What is the role of union stewards in an emergency situation?

5. *Fair Labor Standards Act* (FLSA).[42] This federal statute establishes minimum-wage, maximum-hour, and overtime requirements. It requires that all non-exempt employees working over forty hours a week receive overtime pay at a rate of one and one half times the regular rate. Hospitals and other healthcare institutions are covered employers under the FLSA. The FLSA is enforced by the Wage and Hour Division within the Employment Standards Administration of the DOL.
   a. Does time spent in mandatory quarantine count toward the calculation of compensable hours worked?
   b. In the event of a major emergency requiring all available personnel to work extended hours, could the good-faith provisions of the Portal to Portal Act[43] excuse noncompliance with economically burdensome overtime requirements (particularly

---

[41] National Labor Relations Act, 29 U. S. C.§§ 151–169 (2004).
[42] 29 U.S.C. § 201 (2004).
[43] *See* 29 U.S.C. § 251 (2004).

where much of the emergency services provided might well be without any reimbursement or payment)?

IV. Planning (Blue)

The Planning Section Chief anticipates the course of events over the relevant time horizon, and makes plans to ensure continued smooth operation of the facility.[44] At the initiation of an emergency, the Planning Section Chief assesses staffing needs, calls in off-duty staff, arranges for transportation of those who need it, establishes a labor pool, and other related tasks. Once a longer period becomes the relevant planning horizon, the Planning Section Chief shifts from a focus on the "next several hours" to an emphasis on "the next several days" as emergency operations commence and stabilize. Eventually, the Planning Section Chief prepares for the demobilization or "standing down" of the organization from the emergency. But planning activities go well beyond the activities of a Section Chief during an emergency. Planning is the heart of good emergency response, and it is found in all activities engaged in by the organization for its daily operations. Emergency planning weds the knowledge that an emergency will occur with the routine management activities the institution conducts.

A. Corporate Governance

It is important that an appropriate chain of succession is established in the event that key players are unavailable during an emergency situation.

1. Has the organization established a chain of command?
2. Has a process been established that ensures continuous command-and-control functions at all times and by appropriate individuals?
3. Are documentation requirements established for an individual who asserts command responsibilities during an emergency?
4. Is it clear within the emergency-management plan and other documents how an incident commander is identified? Is the incident commander's authority with respect to the administrative commander (e.g., the CEO) identified in the documentation, and understood by those who might assume incident command and/or maintain administrative authority over the institution?
5. Has the organization's board of directors ratified the chain of command, and is documentation to that effect on file in the Command Center?
6. Are senior leaders trained in their expected emergency-response roles, as well as in alternative roles they may be expected or required to assume during an event?
7. Has the organization drilled for the activation of the Command Center during evening, night, and weekend shifts?
8. Have specific departments drilled in their potential responsibilities? In addition to emergency department drills, has the senior-management team drilled together? Have other departments (e.g., finance, human resources) been included in the drills?

B. Hazard Vulnerability Analysis

It is important for each organization to conduct a Hazard Vulnerability Analysis (HVA). In an HVA, the organization identifies the foreseeable risks it faces, classifies them as "high" or "low" likelihood, and assesses their potential effect on the organization. What results is a prioritization of emergencies to plan for, enabling the organization to devote its attention to the high-likelihood, high-effect risks.

1. Who is charged with the preparation of the HVA (e.g., a member of senior management, the facilities department, a committee)?
2. If the charged individual is not a member of senior management, have members of the senior management team provided their input?

---

[44] FIELD OPERATIONS GUIDE, *supra* note 13, at 8–3.

3. Where is the HVA located? Has a copy been included in the institution's emergency-management manual?
4. Does the organization's senior management understand the major issues identified as part of the analysis, and do these issues inform the facility's documentation and contracting processes?
5. Does the HVA include the possibility of responding to terrorism and the so-called "CNBC" (i.e., concussive, nuclear, biological, and chemical) events, as well as the differing effects each might have on the ability of the facility to respond?
6. Is the organization located in a potential terrorist target area? If so, does the organization need to stockpile certain mission-critical supplies, and is it keeping track of its incurred expenses in doing so?
7. Does the HVA and the institution's other emergency plans contemplate whether and how the emergency could limit access to (and from) the institution for patients, employees, and vendors?
    a. Are critical roads and transit points subject to their own risks (e.g., earthquakes), or are they targets for terrorist attacks?
    b. Do such ingress/egress thoroughfares run by locations that may need to limit their own access in an emergency and beyond (e.g., past police headquarters or governmental buildings)?
    c. Does the organization understand how long a threatened closure may last (e.g., during the emergency; during the cleanup; permanently)?
    d. Based on the length of possible closure, how might the closure affect both the response to the emergency and the eventual recovery from it?
8. Have the institution's vendors been apprised of the possible limitations of access to the facility, and can they contribute to any necessary work-around strategy to ensure the delivery of supplies and equipment to the facility?

C. Community-Support, Affiliation, and Transfer Agreements

Healthcare providers often are parties to myriad community-support, affiliation, or transfer agreements. Such agreements can be a source of support during a crisis situation.

1. Does the facility participate in community or industry organizations that may provide support, or to which the facility may need to contribute, during an emergency in the community? Is the contact information for these organizations readily accessible to the Command Center?
2. Is the facility part of a larger healthcare system upon whose resources it can call (or to whose resources the facility may need to contribute) in an emergency?
    a. Are such potential emergency contributions (i.e., resources of system members to other system members) described in any document or other agreement? For instance, in an emergency, will other facilities assist the organization by sending staff, supplies, and/or equipment?
    b. If the facility generally is a stand-alone facility, can agreements be implemented with other community providers (perhaps even with potential competitors) for emergency assistance?
    c. How will these contributions be compensated?
3. Is the institution part of a regional association that can coordinate resources and response among facilities?
    a. Will the communication lines with any such association be clear, even in an emergency?
    b. Is the institution confident that the association will address the institution's unique concerns relating to its patient population, location, and available resources?
4. Does the organization have mutual-assistance pacts with other facilities that may be able to supply needed personnel, supplies, or equipment? Are such mutual-assistance agreements

specific to the organization (e.g., does a pediatric hospital have access to pediatric ventilators in an emergency)?

D. Vendor Agreements

The institution's mission-critical[45] vendor agreements should provide for the vendor's assistance in planning for and responding to an emergency.

1. As part of the contracting process, has the institution discussed with its potential vendors the outcome of its HVA?
2. Is the vendor aware of the potential risks that are of particular concern to the institution?
3. Have contract discussions addressed any expectations between the parties about vendor response and/or assistance in an emergency?
4. Has the organization sought and included input from the vendor(s) in developing the institution's disaster-recovery plans?
5. Does the institution have the leverage to demand a priority response in an emergency? Should it attempt to negotiate such a priority anyway?
6. Have any expectations been discussed with respect to compensation for additional emergency services and/or goods? (The parties may decide legitimately to leave the agreement silent on this point, or may go into depth about this issue.)
7. Does the vendor understand that the institution expects that the vendor will show up in an emergency and that the parties will discuss the compensation after the disaster, but that the consideration will not reflect a mark-up in the negotiated consideration purely because of the emergency?
    a. Could access to the institution be interrupted, disrupting the flow of services and/or goods to the institution in a disaster?
    b. Will the institution have access to alternative suppliers of services and/or goods (e.g., food)?
8. Is the contract clear that a disaster at the institution's location will not necessarily relieve the vendor of its obligations?
9. Does a disaster experienced by the *vendor* at its location relieve the vendor of all contractual obligations, or would it instead trigger the vendor's obligation to implement its own disaster-recovery plan in addition to the disaster-recovery plan of the institution?
10. If a disaster interferes with the provision of the underlying services for a certain period of time (e.g., notwithstanding an involved disaster-recovery plan, the institution's software applications are unable to process its data for thirty days after the disaster), may the institution terminate the underlying agreement?

E. Documentation

Documentation of a healthcare institution's operational, financial, and administrative activities is important for many purposes. Nevertheless, documentation in patient charts, for example, may be less complete than usual when providers are responding to an emergency situation. This may pose a legal vulnerability for healthcare providers. During an emergency situation, documentation also may be particularly important for insurance-reimbursement and grant purposes if grants are made available based on what was done (and adequately documented) during the emergency. If documentation is insufficient, then an organization can lose track of patients, symptoms and diagnoses, and loved ones because the organization is not following its usual systems.

1. Is a triage tagging system in place that determines the triage classification of each person who is evaluated and treated in the emergency department?

---

[45] Mission-critical items are not limited to clinical issues such as medical supplies. Mission-critical items may include food-service agreements, software agreements for billing applications, and other items important to the organization's operation.

2. Does the organization have a system of documentation sufficient for tracking of patients and communication with healthcare providers?
3. Is the documentation in the chart sufficient to demonstrate that the standard of care was met, as well as to enable continuity of care?
4. If the institution relies on a computer registration system that may be unavailable during portions of an emergency event, can the institution print out blank screens (i.e., template information-entry screens providing the prompts for information that can be manually recorded on hard-copy) prior to or during the emergency, so that demographic, insurance, and other information elements usually captured by the computer system electronically can still be captured (if only by hand) and then backloaded into the computer system once the crisis has passed? Similarly, if the organization's information technology (IT) system fails temporarily, is a process in place to document critical entries in a patient's medical record by hand, and ultimately to transfer them to the electronic system when it is again functional?
5. Does the system of the documentation in place during emergencies meet requirements for insurance reimbursement, subsequent loans, funding from the Federal Emergency Management Agency (FEMA), payor funding, and/or other emergency funding?
6. Is the documentation sufficient to comply with reporting obligations to licensing agencies?
7. How will the organization's payroll records accurately capture the significant overtime provided in an emergency?
8. Are any supplies that are given out to the community or government authorities appropriately documented for subsequent reimbursement?
9. Do any state-statutory immunity provisions apply to recordkeeping during an emergency?
10. Have disaster funds been secured by proper declarations from the President, the governor, the Secretary of Agriculture, and/or the Secretary of Commerce as appropriate? (*see Section VI(D), Declaration of an Emergency or Major Disaster, and Securing Disaster Funds*).

F. Physical Plant and Facilities

It is important for a healthcare organization to assess any potential vulnerabilities with its physical plant and facilities, as well as to take appropriate measures to ensure the continuation of utilities, IT systems, communications, and other services necessary to maintain its operations.

1. If an IT system is judged to be mission-critical, is it on the electrical backup systems? Are the computers that need to access the system also on the backup systems?
2. What are the institution's emergency power capabilities? Are there any issues in accessing the emergency power if a mass blackout is caused for any reason?
3. Can the institution access portable generators? Might the placement of a portable emergency generator cause any street and/or zoning issues? Have the organization's personnel been trained in the proper operation of emergency generators?
4. Has the organization assessed potential vulnerabilities relating to the physical location of individual departments (e.g., placement of a data center in a basement location that may be subject to flooding)?

G. Civil Liability

When designing an emergency-preparedness plan for a healthcare institution, it is likely that questions or concerns will be raised regarding the potential civil liability of healthcare entities or personnel who respond to an emergency. It is possible that state-statutory immunity provisions may apply to such situations. Immunity provisions may be found in state "Good Samaritan," emergency-management, or other statutes.

1. Does the appropriate jurisdiction(s) provide exemption from civil liability for emergency care as provided in a Good Samaritan act, emergency-management laws, or other statutes?
2. Has the organization's medical staff and allied health practitioners been apprised of the applicable statutes, and of their liabilities and immunities during an emergency situation?

V. Logistics (Yellow)

The Logistics Section Chief arranges for the needed support to operations, including delivery of food and other supplies; assessment and safe use of the facility, if in question (e.g., following an earthquake or explosion); and equipping of rooms and alternate-care sites if evacuation or relocation becomes necessary.[46]

A. Personnel

In an emergency situation, some staff will need to remain on duty in order to maintain the continued functioning of the organization and provide patient care, while others may need to be released or evacuated. Plans should be in place to mobilize needed personnel while effectively moving non-essential staff away from the institution.

1. Who is responsible for notification of an emergency situation to the organization's employees and members of its medical staff? How is such notification carried out?
2. Are staging areas assigned for specific groups of employees?
3. Do the relevant employees know where those staging areas are?
4. How are the staging areas for off-campus locations (e.g., clinics, physicians, and back offices) coordinated?
5. How will the institution ensure that adequate personnel will be deployed, but not so many that the institution becomes overrun dealing with personnel instead of patients?
6. How is the information about available personnel at these off-campus locations communicated to the Incident Commander?
7. What occurs if one of the off-campus locations has its own demand for additional personnel to respond to the crisis? Does the institution's management plan contemplate a response from multiple locations?
8. Have issues of food and rest been contemplated in choosing the staging areas?
9. Is the institution prepared to provide places of rest for employees who are unable to return home (e.g., cots, physician examination tables, unoccupied beds and administrative offices, local motel rooms)?
10. Are these places of rest separate from patient-care areas?
11. If employees will need to overstay their shift, is adequate food available onsite to feed them? If not, will the facility's usual food suppliers be able to access the institution in an emergency, or will the hospital need to seek alternate suppliers (e.g., local restaurant(s))?
12. How will the institution handle employees' need to contact their families?
13. Do the employees have family emergency plans in place?
14. How will the institution handle employees who need/demand to leave in order to safeguard their own families?
15. What occurs if certain employees demand to leave, but it may be unsafe to do so? How will the institution obtain information about the surrounding streets? How will it convey that information to its employees?
16. How will adequate staffing during the crisis be ensured? Does the organization have an

---

[46] FIELD OPERATIONS GUIDE, *supra* note 13, at 9–3.

emergency- or contingency-staffing plan in the event that personnel either are unable or unwilling to report to work? Is the organization aware of state-specific laws and regulations affecting personnel overtime or extended shifts?[47]

17. How will the institution communicate to those of its employees who were not at the facility at the start of the crisis that they should/should not try to report to the facility?

18. How will the institution handle bringing personnel to the facility if the usual means of access is interfered with by the event (e.g., a blizzard or flood)?

19. How will the organization ensure the availability of contract or leased healthcare practitioners (who may have relationships with other institutions) during the emergency situation? Does the independent-contractor or employee-leasing agreement(s) contemplate alternative-staffing arrangements in the event of an emergency? Do such agreements clearly delineate what duties the organization can require of contracted or leased employees during an emergency situation?

20. How will documentation of employee and contract healthcare practitioner overtime be documented, and how will such personnel records be protected?

21. How will the institution account for an employee who could not get to work and/or was not needed to respond (e.g., will the time away from the individual count as paid time off, or will her wages be docked)? What labor agreements may influence the thinking around this issue, and what do they say about it?

22. How will the institution demobilize its employees from their response?

23. Will some or all employees need to be debriefed in the aftermath of the emergency event?

24. Is an evacuation plan in place? Does the evacuation plan involve movement to particular sites? What assumption of liability does the institution assume when effecting such an evacuation?

B. Information Technology Infrastructure and Software Applications

An organization's agreements relating to IT infrastructure and software applications should take into account emergency-response needs.

1. Do the institution's software licenses specifically authorize the regular backup of relevant software and the data, as well as the loading of the software in test, backup, and disaster-recovery environments to protect the applications and data?

2. What, if any, redundancy is built into the institution's IT infrastructure?

3. Has the choice of the location of the institution's data center taken into account issues such as the age of the building's underlying infrastructure, access to emergency generator power, access to air conditioning, and related concerns, as well as the critically of the applications to be run out of the center?

4. Will the IT emergency plan be effective in a "minor" disaster (e.g., a cut power line or data-center flood) that is not primarily or initially an institution-wide issue?

5. Does the institution have in place disaster-recovery sites and plans for its software applications?
   a. Are its software applications and data backed up on a regular basis?

---

[47] Note that state laws may limit mandatory overtime. *See, e.g.*, WASH. REV. CODE § 49.28.140 (2004). State laws may also limit nurse-to-patient staffing ratios. *See, e.g.*, CAL HEALTH & SAFETY CODE § 1276.4 (2004); *see also* ACCREDITATION COUNCIL FOR GRADUATE MEDICAL EDUCATION (ACGME), COMMON PROGRAM REQUIREMENTS § VI (2003), *available at* www.acgme.org/DutyHours/dutyHoursCommonPR.pdf (last visited Sept. 25, 2004).

b. If the organization's software applications generally are run on-site, is its disaster-recovery site located off-site (or vice versa)?
c. Have the advantages and disadvantages of the locations of the organization's primary software-operations and disaster-recovery sites been taken into account in the various contracting processes?
d. If the institution's software applications are run in a Web-based or remote-computing mode, is the vendor's disaster-recovery plan accessible to the institution, and has the institution reviewed that plan?
e. Based upon the review of the remote vendor's disaster plan, is it necessary for the organization to separately contract for a disaster-recovery site for that application, or can the primary agreement be considered to include a disaster-recovery component?
f. If the institution is relying upon the disaster-recovery plans of the remote vendor, will the institution be notified of any changes to that plan?
g. Does the institution have the negotiating leverage necessary to require its consent to any changes in the vendor's disaster-recovery plan? Does the institution have the expertise to exercise effectively its consent over a remote vendor's disaster-recovery plan, or is it better to rely on the vendor's expertise in the particular instance?

C. Developing Emergency Plans for IT Services

In preparing for emergencies, an organization's goal should be to maintain continuity of critical IT services during and following the emergency, and to have in place a disaster-recovery plan that allows IT services to be re-established as quickly as possible.

1. What are the organization's critical IT services?
   a. How long can the organization afford to be without such IT services from the perspective of safety, cost, and other relevant considerations? (In other words, what is the organization's risk threshold for various IT functions?)
   b. Does the facility's emergency plan currently address maintaining continuity of IT services and recovery of IT services?
   c. For IT services provided in-house (if any), what type of backup systems does the facility have in place (e.g., redundant or "fail over" systems, personnel, skill sets; off-site data storage; off-site backup operations)?
   d. Has the facility identified potential failures in its IT operations?
   e. Has the facility developed detailed procedures for mitigating each of the potential failures?
   f. What plans does the facility have in place for ensuring that necessary IT personnel are available during and following emergencies?
   g. Has the facility established plans for communicating with key IT personnel (including vendor personnel) in case of an emergency, and for ensuring that they can communicate with each other?
   h. Has the facility tested its emergency plans and mitigation procedures at least annually?
   i. Have the vendor's personnel participated in the emergency planning, mitigation procedures, and drills?
2. For outsourced IT services, what additional issues require consideration by healthcare organizations?
   a. What IT issues can/will the facility handle in the event of an emergency?
   b. What issues does the organization expect its IT vendor(s) to handle?
   c. Do the facility's IT vendor(s) have emergency plans in place?
   d. Do these plans specifically ensure that the facility's IT services will be maintained during an emergency?

e. Has the facility coordinated its emergency IT plans with those of its vendor(s)?
f. Are the IT vendor's emergency plans addressed in the contract between the facility and the vendor?
g. Has the facility established plans for communicating and coordinating with its IT vendor(s) in the event of an emergency?
h. Are these communication and coordination plans incorporated into the contract between the facility and the vendor?

D. Mitigation of ISP Failure

A specific element for consideration in relation to the facility's emergency IT planning is how to maintain Internet Service Provider (ISP) service during and following an emergency.

1. Does the facility maintain two separate ISP relationships in the event that one ISP fails? Does the organization prefer to have the second ISP arranged as a back-up service (in which case it will only be activated if the primary ISP fails), or does the facility wish to maintain two fully functioning ISPs at all times?
2. Does the organization maintain a service-level agreement with its ISP provider(s) that guarantees immediate service if the facility experiences problems with the ISP? Does the agreement include a provision specifying the service that the organization expects to receive during and following an emergency?

E. Maintaining a Hot or Cold Site

The organization will need to decide whether to maintain a "hot site" for some or all IT services (either directly or through an IT vendor). A hot site is a physical location to which the facility can move its data operations and communications in the event of an emergency. The hot site will be configured to the facility's specifications, with computers, printers, Internet services, and work stations for staff. The hot site maintains the same data as is maintained at the facility, either through regular backups or through real-time synchronization. In case of an emergency, a hot site will allow the facility to restore operations within hours or days, depending on the level of service purchased. A cold site, by contrast, generally does not allow for immediate restoration of data operations and communications. A cold site usually consists of pre-arranged contracts for the lease of computers, equipment, and space in an emergency, as well as off-site storage of data tapes. Although a cold site is a less expensive option, it will take more time for that site to become fully operational. The choice of whether to maintain a hot site, cold site, or some combination of the two, will depend on the facility's need to immediately restore data operations and communications in an emergency. Conducting a business analysis or HVA can help determine the facility's capacity to handle "downtime" in its data operations and communications, and guide the selection of backup services and facilities.

1. For how long can the facility afford to be without its IT services?
2. How serious is the effect of having the facility's IT services unavailable?
3. Has the facility conducted a business analysis regarding the effects of losing its IT services, or is loss of IT services included in the HVA?
4. How much is the facility willing to spend to ensure that the continuity of IT services is maintained (e.g., on a real-time basis; on a delayed-response basis)?
5. Does the facility's IT vendor(s) maintain hot or cold sites that will be used to protect the facility's IT services?
6. Would it be less expensive to contract with an IT vendor to provide the facility with hot site or cold site backup, as opposed to contracting for the backup system directly?

VI. Finance (Green)

The Finance Section Chief makes arrangements to ensure the organization's continued financial health, from recording the cost of emergency response to arranging credit for needed supplies and coordinating financial arrangements for emergency operations, such as costs associated with relocating patients from an evacuated building.

A. Cash Flow

Regardless of whether they are operated on a for-profit or nonprofit basis, healthcare institutions depend upon regular cash flow to remain operational. The majority of income for most healthcare institutions comes from patient insurance reimbursement (either private or government-sponsored). An emergency may interrupt the usual revenue cycle, either due to loss of the institution's computer system or a more general local or regional event.

Accordingly, the continued financial operations of a hospital are dependent primarily on an ability to document and bill for services provided during an emergency in a manner that closely approximates the documentation that is used for usual operations.

1. Does the institution's emergency-management planning establish how to conduct billing when the computer system (or other infrastructure components) is compromised? Can personnel print out blank screens from the computer system, complete them by hand, and then back-load the data entry once the crisis passes?
2. If full documentation for billing purposes is not available, are methods for recordkeeping sufficient to retroactively establish services rendered, either (i) for purposes of billing third-party payors who would accept billing based on such records and/or (ii) claims under business-inter-ruption insurance policies and/or governmental grant programs?
3. Are potential recordkeeping methods varied to enable a confirmation of services through multiple records?
4. To the extent that the institution needs to provide goods and supplies to other responders, has the institution determined how it will keep track of what has been provided, and at what cost, in order to obtain subsequent reimbursement from the party who received the goods or services (or from some other source)? Are the tools necessary to track such outgoing items (including, but not limited to, a pen and paper) available to the Logistics Section Chief in during a response?

B. Patient Insurance Coverage

Healthcare organizations should review third-party payor agreements, as well as examine what other funding sources may exist to cover treatment rendered to patients during an emergency situation.

1. Do private health-insurance policies provide for coverage for treatment mandated by public health authorities (e.g., in the case of isolation)?
    a. Is such treatment covered by a private payor, Medicaid, Medicare, or the Federal Employees Health Benefits Program (FEHBP)?
    b. Can a determination of medical necessity by a public health authority trump a determination to the contrary by a private payor?
    c. Are prior authorization/precertification requirements waived in the event of a major disaster or emergency?
    d. Do payor agreements contain a *force majeure* clause that references epidemics or other public health emergencies as excluded events?
    e. Are Medicare Disproportionate Share (DSH) payments[48] or other similar funds available to cover the costs of this treatment if private-payor coverage falls short?
    f. Can institutions address these issues in provider agreements with health plans?
2. What other funding sources are available to the institution?
    a. Is business-interruption insurance available?
    b. Does the county or state have funds to compensate an institution if private coverage is insufficient?

---

[48] *See* 42 C.F.R. §§ 412.106, 447.272(c)(2) (2004).

c. Are federal funds available for any of the following:
- Bioterrorism preparedness appropriations (and, if received, can the organization set aside these funds for cash-flow interruption in an emergency);
- New CMS funds appropriated in the Medicare Modernization Act for hospitals to aid hospitals providing uncompensated care; and/or
- Post-event appropriations?

d. Can the institution create a new funding stream through patient surcharges or other mechanisms?

e. Are Red Cross funds available?

f. If the institution is designated as an isolation or quarantine facility, are there plans (on a federal and/or state level) to provide compensation to facilities if revenues are adversely affected?

C. Institutional Insurance Coverage

Managing risk is an important part of ensuring continued viability and protection in the event of an unexpected occurrence for any business, including the provision of healthcare. (For additional information on terrorism and natural-disaster risk management, please see *Appendix B*.) Insurance plays a vital role in the management of risk by providing a mechanism for spreading that risk. Insurance allows businesses to accept what would otherwise be unacceptable risk.

1. Does the organization review its insurance coverage on a periodic basis?
   a. What is the current level of coverage? What coverage is available? What are the institution's deductibles?
   b. Is the organization subject to minimum-coverage requirements for the different types of insurance?
   c. How should the institution determine appropriate coverage levels? What resources/tools are available to aid assessment of risk/vulnerability?
   d. What causes of loss are covered by the institution's policy? Are distinctions made between differing causes of loss (e.g., natural disaster vs. terrorism vs. naturally occurring bio-incident)? Must the emergency be publicly declared in order to make a claim under the insurance, or may other crises that trigger an interruption of one or more operations generate a claim?
   e. Does the institution have a copy of the policy in an easily accessible location? Can the Finance Section Chief locate a copy in an emergency?
   f. When was the institution's policy last reviewed? Does the institution have a policy in place for how often its coverage is reviewed?
   g. What documentation is required to file a claim?
   h. Have appropriate steps been taken to identify and protect vital records (e.g., are copies of important records kept off-site, or in a safe place where they may be accessed easily following an emergency)? Are vital insurance records stored in a fireproof cabinet?

2. What property insurance is available?
   a. What method will be used to value the insured property?
   b. How does the institution's insurer evaluate preventive/mitigating action?
      - Does the policy allow for reduced premiums if preventative measures are taken?
      - Does the policy require mitigation of known risks?
   c. Are recent improvements or additions insured? Must the organization notify the insurer to cover such improvements?
   d. What costs are covered (e.g., repair to pre-disaster condition; rebuilding; relocation costs)? Have sublimits that may apply in an emergency been established (e.g., flood or earthquake limits)? Are these limits adequate for recovery from a catastrophe, or will additional resources be required?

3. What liability insurance coverage is available?
   a. Could the institution be held liable to third parties for contributing to loss by failing to take appropriate protective measures or for negligence (e.g., failure to take appropriate measures to prevent the spread of infection within the facility; failure to provide adequate evacuation routes)?
   b. What are the limits to the institution's liability coverage? If the limits are determined on a per-occurrence basis, how is an "occurrence" defined in the policy?
   c. Should the institution consider an umbrella policy (i.e., excess liability insurance) to protect it in the event of a large catastrophic loss?
4. What business-interruption insurance is available?
   a. How will the organization's lost business income be measured? What documentation is required to establish a loss?
   b. Does the organization's policy specify a time period for coverage, or is it covered until operations resume?
   c. Is the organization covered if the business loss is not a result of insurable peril such as a fire?
      - For example, Loss of business income as a result of evacuation in response to civil authority in the event of a bioterrorist attack?
      - For example, Loss of business income due to supplier interruption?
   d. What costs are covered?
      - For example, Premium prices paid in order to maintain minimal operations or facilitate recovery; salaries; other operating expenses?
      - For example, workers' compensation; health and life insurance costs?

D. Declaration of an Emergency or Major Disaster, and Securing Disaster Funds

Large-scale emergencies[49] and major disasters[50] are declared by the President of the United States, upon request from the governor(s) of the affected state(s), and must "be based on a finding that the [emergency or major] disaster is of such severity and magnitude that effective response is beyond the capabilities of the State and the affected local governments and that Federal assistance is necessary."[51] Less-serious disasters can be declared by the Small Business Administration (SBA), which coordinates disaster assistance for businesses.[52] Business can apply for several types of disaster-assistance loans (including pre-disaster mitigation loans), depending on the nature of the disaster and the amount of damage suffered.[53] Disaster assistance for individuals is coordinated through FEMA.[54]

1. Has the President of the United States declared an emergency or major disaster, triggering federal response mechanisms (including SBA and FEMA)?

---

[49] An "Emergency" for purposes of obtaining federal funding, is defined as "any occasion or instance for which, in the determination of the President, Federal assistance is needed to supplement State and local efforts and capabilities to save lives and to protect property and public health and safety, or to lessen or avert the threat of a catastrophe in any part of the United States." 42 U.S.C. § 5122(1) (2004).

[50] For purposes of obtaining federal funding, a major disaster is defined as "any natural catastrophe (including any hurricane, tornado, storm, high water, wind-driven water, tidal wave, tsunami, earthquake, volcanic eruption, landslide, mudslide, snowstorm, or drought), or, regardless of cause, any fire, flood, or explosion, in any part of the United States, which in the determination of the President causes damage of sufficient severity and magnitude to warrant major disaster assistance under this chapter to supplement the efforts and available resources of States, local governments, and disaster relief organizations in alleviating the damage, loss, hardship, or suffering caused thereby." *Id.* § 5122(2).

[51] *Id.* § 5170.

[52] *See* U.S. Small Business Admin., Understanding How Disaster Declarations Are Made, *at* www.sba.gov/disaster_recov/basics/declarations.html (last visited Sept. 20, 2004) [hereinafter Understanding How Disaster Declarations Are Made].

[53] *See* 15 U.S.C. § 636(b) (2004).

[54] *See id.* § 636(b)(1)(C); Understanding How Disaster Declarations Are Made, *supra* note 52.

2. Has the SBA declared a disaster, triggering the SBA disaster-loan program?
3. Is the organization located in the declared emergency or disaster area?
   If yes, is it located in a declared county or an adjacent county? (This may affect the type of SBA loan for which the business is eligible.)
4. What type of assistance does the organization seek from state and federal agencies?
   a. Is short-term aid (e.g., supplies, personnel, debris removal, technical assistance) required? (This type of assistance is coordinated through FEMA.)
   b. Are long-term loans necessary? (Loans are coordinated through the SBA.)
   c. Are federal equipment, supplies, facilities, personnel, and other resources indicated?
   d. Is technical and advisory assistance to state or local governments needed?
   e. Are medicine, food, and consumables needed? Will additional relief be required from disaster-assistance organizations?
   f. Are debris or wreckage removal; search and rescue; emergency medical care; emergency shelter; provision of food, water, and other essential needs; temporary facilities for schools and essential community services; demolition of unsafe structures; dissemination of public information; or technical advice necessary?
   g. Are other hazard-mitigation efforts warranted?
   h. Are repair, restoration, and/or replacement of damaged facilities indicated?
   i. Is establishment of temporary emergency-communications systems desirable?
5. Is the institution considered a "large" or "small" business by federal standards? Large businesses are eligible for SBA Physical Disaster Business Loans,[55] but not Economic Injury Disaster Loans or Pre-Disaster Mitigation Loans[56] Small businesses are eligible for all three types of loans.[57]
6. Is the institution eligible for loans from other sources that can be used for disaster assistance? If yes, then the business may not be eligible for SBA disaster-assistance loans.[58]

For additional information on securing federal disaster funds, see *Appendix C*.

VII. Recovery: Ending Emergency Operations

This *Checklist* should provide legal counsel with the necessary tools to assist healthcare providers in preparing for an emergency, and in facilitating the return of the organization from emergency operations to normal status as quickly as possible. The Planning Section Chief will spend considerable time planning for the transition back to routine activities, including demobilization of any additional resources implemented during the crisis. This recovery constitutes the fourth and final stage of emergency preparedness. The Recovery phase includes: implementing any necessary repairs; granting furloughs to staff who responded to the emergency; returning patients to previously closed units; submitting applications for available emergency relief funding; and similar steps.

It is important to ensure that the organization has adequate staffing and resources to resume its ongoing operations.

---

[55] U.S. Small Business Admin., Physical Disaster Business Loans, *at* www.sba.gov/disaster_recov/loaninfo/phydisaster.html (last visited Sept. 20, 2004) [hereinafter Physical Disaster Business Loans]; *see also* 13 C.F.R. § 123.200(a) (2004).
[56] 13 C.F.R. § 121.302 (2004).
[57] *Id.* § 123.200(a); *see* Physical Disaster Business Loans, *supra* note 55; U.S. Small Business Admin., Economic Injury Disaster Loans For Small Business, *at* www.sba.gov/disaster_recov/loaninfo/ecoinjury.html (last visited Sept. 20, 2004) [hereinafter Economic Injury Disaster Loans For Small Businesses]; U.S. Small Business Admin., Pre-Disaster Mitigation Loan Program, *at* www.sba.gov/disaster_recov/loaninfo/pre_disaster_mitigation.html (last visited Sept. 20, 2004) [hereinafter Pre-Disaster Mitigation Loan Program].
[58] 13 C.F.R. §§ 123.101(c), 123.201(a) (2004).

Finally, debriefing from the emergency is an important step to obtain input with regard to "lessons learned" for use in the event of future crises. Administrative and clinical personnel alike should participate in debriefing the event, and the information gathered during debriefing, and those gleaned from the records kept in the Command Center, should form the basis for the next round of preparation and mitigation—the first two phases of emergency planning. In this way, successfully concluding the response to (and recovery from) an emergency creates the opportunity for further improvement in readiness in anticipation of the unknown but inevitable next emergency.

VIII. Selected Resources

1. Mark A. Rothstein, et al., Inst. for Bioethics, Health Pol'y and Law, Univ. of Louisville Sch. of Med., Quarantine and Isolation: Lessons Learned from SARS, A Report to the Centers for Disease Control and Prevention (Nov. 2003).
2. Lawrence Gostin, Georgetown Univ. Law Center, The Model State Emergency Health Powers Act: Public Health and Civil Liberties in a Time of Terrorism (2002 Working Paper Series in Public Law and Legal Theory and Law and Economics, Working Paper No. 346504, 2003).
3. GAO Report to Congressional Committees, Hospital Preparedness: Most Urban Hospitals Have Emergency Plans but Lack Certain Capacities for Bioterrorist Response, GAO-03-924 (Aug. 2003).
4. Joint Commission on Accreditation of Healthcare Organizations, Health Care at the Crossroads: Strategies for Creating and Sustaining Community-wide Emergency Preparedness Systems (2003).
5. Department of Health and Human Services, Centers for Disease Control and Prevention, Public Health Guidance for Community-Level Preparedness and Response to Severe Acute Respiratory Syndrome, Supplement A Command and Control (Jan. 8, 2004).
6. Emergency Management Institute, U.S. Fire Administration, Department of Homeland Security, National Incident Management System (NIMS), An Introduction, at http://training.fema.gov/EMIWeb/IS/is700.asp (last visited Sept. 9, 2004); North Carolina Hospital Association, Hospital Emergency Incident Command System, at www.ncha.org/public/docs/bioterrorism/HEICS.pdf. (last visited Sept. 9, 2004).
7. National Fire Protection Association (NFPA) 1600 Standard on Disaster/Emergency Management and Business Continuity Programs (2004) at www.nfpa.org.

Appendix A.A

Application of EMTALA During a Major Public Health Emergency

Recent events have raised questions regarding whether a provider's obligations under the Emergency Medical Treatment and Active Labor Act (EMTALA)[59] might be modified or waived in the event of a major public health emergency.[60] On November 8, 2001, the Centers for Medicare & Medicaid Services (CMS) issued an informal policy statement in response to hospitals' inquiries regarding the extent of their EMTALA obligations following the fall 2001 anthrax incidents.[61] Up to

---

[59] Emergency Medical Labor and Active Treatment Act, 42 U.S.C. § 1395dd (2004).
[60] Sara Rosenbaum & Brian Kamoie, *Finding a Way Through the Hospital Door: The Role of EMTALA in Public Health Emergencies*, 31 J.L. MED. & ETHICS 590, 591 (2003).
[61] Letter from Director, Survey and Certification Group, Ctrs. for Medicare and Medicaid Servs., to Regional Administrators, State Survey Agencies (Nov. 8, 2001) (Question and Answer Relating to Bioterrorism and the Emergency Medical Treatment and Labor Act), *available at* www.cms.hhs.gov/medicaid/survey-cert/110801.asp (last visited Sept. 20, 2004) [hereinafter Letter to Regional Administrators].

that point, administrative and case law involving EMTALA had not contemplated public health emergencies. The statute itself contains no suggestion that its obligations would vary in the face of a community-wide emergency; nevertheless, when such events began to seem more likely, concerns and questions arose.[62] Although it reiterated to some extent the continued application of EMTALA's obligations, the 2001 CMS letter suggested that there was an exception to the stabilization requirement if a community response plan is in place.[63] Moreover, the letter indicated that a hospital's initial screening obligation might be limited if a community-response plan designated certain facilities to handle particular categories of patients in a bioterrorism situation, and if the hospital in question is not such a designated facility.[64]

The Public Health Security and Bioterrorism Preparedness and Response Act of 2002[65] articulated a more formal policy regarding EMTALA obligations in an emergency situation. The legislation authorized the Secretary of the Department of Health and Human Services (DHHS) to waive sanctions for EMTALA violations when the violations when the violation comes from an inappropriate transfer of an unstable patient in public health emergency circumstances (as defined by a presidential declaration). This potential limitation on EMTALA obligations during a public health emergency is more circumscribed than what the 2001 CMS letter suggested, as it does not indicate a reduction in the screening obligation (nor does it eliminate private individuals' right of action).

The final EMTALA rule promulgated on September 9, 2003,[66] also addressed public health emergency situations. Similar to the 2001 CMS letter and the 2002 Public Health Security and Bioterrorism Preparedness and Response Act, this final rule did not answer definitely the question regarding the extent of EMTALA obligations in a crisis situation. The preamble to the rule references the 2001 CMS letter, and notes that the final rule adds a public health emergency provision to the EMTALA regulations.[67] The new provision states that "sanctions under EMTALA for an inappropriate transfer during a national emergency do not apply to a hospital with a dedicated emergency department located in an emergency area.... In the event of such an emergency, CMS would issue appropriate guidance to hospitals."[68]

CMS Interpretive Guidelines issued to State Survey Agency Directors on May 13, 2004,[69] seemed to restate the position taken in the 2001 CMS letter. Referencing the new regulatory provision implemented with the 2003 final rule,[70] the guidelines state that, in the event of a national emergency or crisis, if state or local governments have implemented community-response plans designating certain facilities to

---

[62] New indications that hospitals are not adequately prepared for bioterrorism or similar incidents have heightened such concerns. *See* JOINT COMM'N ON ACCREDITATION OF HEALTHCARE ORGS., HEALTH CARE AT THE CROSSROADS: STRATEGIES FOR CREATING AND SUSTAINING COMMUNITY-WIDE EMERGENCY PREPAREDNESS SYSTEMS, *available at* www.jcaho.org/about+us/public+policy+initiatives/emergency+preparedness.pdf (last visited Sept. 20, 2004); U.S. GENERAL ACCOUNTING OFFICE, HOSPITAL PREPAREDNESS: MOST URBAN HOSPITALS HAVE EMERGENCY PLANS BUT LACK CERTAIN CAPACITIES FOR BIOTERRORISM RESPONSE, GAO-03-924, at 1 (Aug. 2003), *available at* www.gao.gov/new.items/d03924.pdf (last visited Sept. 25, 2004).
[63] Letter to Regional Administrators, *supra* note 61.
[64] *Id.*
[65] Public Health Security and Bioterrorism Preparedness and Response Act of 2002, Pub. L. No. 107–188, 116 Stat. 594 (codified as amended in scattered sections of 7, 21, 29, 38, 42, 47 U.S.C.).
[66] Clarifying Policies Related to the Responsibilities of Medicare-Participating Hospitals in Treating Individuals With Emergency Medical Conditions, 68 Fed. Reg. 53,222 (Sept. 9, 2003) (to be codified at 42 C.F.R. pts. 413, 482, 489).
[67] *Id.* at 53,257.
[68] *Id.*
[69] Letter from Director, Survey and Certification Group, Ctrs. for Medicare and Medicaid Servs., to State Survey Agency Directors (May 13, 2004) (Revised Emergency Medical Treatment and Labor Act (EMTALA) Interpretive Guidelines), *available at* www.cms.hhs.gov/medicaid/survey-cert/sc0434.pdf. (last visited Sept. 25, 2004) [hereinafter Letter to State Survey Agency Directors].
[70] 42 C.F.R. § 489.24(a)(2) (2004).

handle particular categories of patients, then hospitals in the area that are not designated facilities must still provide a medical screening exam, but may then transfer patients in those categories to a designated facility without triggering EMTALA sanctions.[71]

The Project Bioshield Act of 2004, signed into law on July 21 of that year, contains a brief provision relating to EMTALA's screening obligations, allowing the DHHS Secretary to waive standard EMTALA requirements, and allow for "the direction or relocation of an individual to receive medical screening in an alternate location pursuant to an appropriate State emergency preparedness plan."[72]

Appendix A.B
Risk-Management Considerations
Terrorism Risk Management

Individuals and businesses typically purchase insurance coverage from direct insurers. Direct insurers write the policies, collect the premiums, and pay claims to the insured. Reinsurers, on the other hand, provide some protection from exposure for direct insurers by acting as insurance for the direct insurers. Following the attacks on September 11, 2001, the majority of the property and liability loss was passed on to reinsurers. As a result, reinsurers began excluding terrorism risk from their policies, which led direct insurers to begin taking similar actions. Currently, state insurance regulators *require* direct insurers to offer terrorism risk insurance. Reinsurers, who are not regulated by state insurance commissioners, however, are not required to provide reinsurance for terrorism risk, creating a major weakness in the support structure of the insurance industry.

In late 2002, the Terrorism Risk Insurance Act[73] (TRIA) was enacted. The act's enumerated purposes are "to address market disruptions, ensure the continued widespread availability and affordability of commercial property and casualty insurance for terrorism risk, and to allow for a transition period for the private markets to stabilize and build capacity while preserving State insurance regulation and consumer protections."[74] The Act's "make available" provision found in § 103(c) requires all entities that meet the act's definition of insurer to "make available" in their "property and casualty insurance policies, coverage for insured losses resulting from an act of terrorism."[75] This coverage cannot differ materially in form from coverage applicable to losses arising from other events.

The Terrorism Risk Insurance Program places the federal government in the role of reinsurer.[76] However, several limitations apply. Under the act, the federal government only reimburses insurers for a portion of their "insured losses"[77] resulting from certified "acts of terrorism."[78] The "act of terrorism" must meet specific requirements including commission "by individual(s) on behalf of any foreign person or foreign interest, as part of an effort to coerce the U.S. civilian population or to influence the policy or affect the conduct of the U.S."[79] Thus, acts of domestic terrorism are excluded.

---

[71] Letter to State Survey Agency Directors, *supra* note 69, at 31.
[72] Project Bioshield Act of 2004, Pub. L. No. 108-276 § 8, 118 Stat. 835, 864 (codified as amended at 42 U.S.C. § 1320b-5).
[73] Terrorism Risk Insurance Act of 2002, Pub. L. No. 107–297, 116 Stat. 2322 (codified in scattered sections of 12, 15, 28 U.S.C.).
[74] *Id.* § 101(b), 116 Stat. at 2323.
[75] *Id.* § 103(c), 116 Stat. at 2327.
[76] The Federal "reinsurance" is 90% of covered losses that exceed an insurer's deductible. This share is subject to an annual industry aggregate limit of $100 billion. The insurer's deductible is based on an insurance company's earned premiums from the previous calendar year. *Id.* § 103(e)(1)(A), 116 Stat. at 2328.
[77] The Act defines "insured loss" as any loss resulting from an "act of terrorism." Terrorism Risk Act of 2002 § 102(5), 116 Stat. at 2325.
[78] Under the Act, the "act of terrorism" must be certified as such by the Secretary of the Treasury, in concurrence with the Secretary of State and the Attorney General. 31 C.F.R. § 50.5(b) (2004).
[79] Additionally, the act must "be a violent act or an act that is dangerous to human life, property, or infrastructure;" must occur in the United States or abroad in the case of air carriers, vessels, or missions; and must result in damages in excess of $5 million. *Id.* An act cannot be certified if it occurs in the course of a "war declared by Congress" (except for workers' compensation coverage). *Id.*

Although the act's definition of "insured loss" does not exclude losses from nuclear, biological, or chemical perils, losses resulting from certified acts of terrorism involving those perils are only covered "if the coverage for those perils is provided in the primary or excess property and casualty policy issued by [the institution's] insurer."[80] The act does not prohibit an insurer from excluding coverage for nuclear, biological, or chemical perils if the same exclusions are also applied to losses arising from events other than acts or terrorism, and if the exclusion is permitted by state law.[81] Although TRIA temporarily[82] ensures the availability of some coverage for losses due to terrorism, the act is not comprehensive even in the limited terrorism-risk insurance arena.

Natural-Disaster Risk Management

Recent focus has been on emergencies resulting from acts of terrorism. Historically, however, disasters *not* related to terrorism have been the primary cause of public health emergencies. Natural disasters (e.g., earthquakes, floods, hurricanes, and tornadoes) may have a devastating effect on businesses. According to the Insurance Information Institute, more than 30% of businesses never reopen following closure due to hurricane, tornado, flood, or other disaster.[83]

Commercial-property insurance and business-interruption insurance typically will provide the two main sources of protection for the institution in the event of a natural disaster. Property insurance will cover the cost of damage repairs, while business-interruption insurance will cover the loss of business income.

Two types of business-interruption coverage are available: named perils and all-risk policies. The former provides protection only for specifically named perils, while the latter provides coverage for all perils *except* those specifically excluded. The two types of insurance generally are purchased as a package, and the same perils will be covered under both policies. It is important to note that two common exceptions to property insurance are earthquake and flood damage.

Coverage for these events typically can be added for additional fees. In fact, in certain areas, flood insurance may even be required.[84] Ensuring adequate insurance coverage is an important means to survival following disaster.

Appendix A.C

Securing Disaster Funding

Disaster assistance for businesses is coordinated through the Small Business Administration (SBA).[85] In order to qualify, the business must be in a declared disaster area.[86] Two types of disaster declarations activate SBA disaster-assistance efforts: Presidential Declaration and

---

[80] Interpretive Letter from Jeffrey S. Bragg Executive Director of Terrorism Risk Insurance Program, to Mr. D. (Mar. 24, 2004), *available at* www.treasury.gov/offices/domestic-finance/financial-institution/terrorism-insurance/pdf/redactedci.pdf (last visited Sept 20, 2004).
[81] *Id.*
[82] *See* Terrorism Risk Insurance Act of 2002, Pub. L. No. 107-297, § 108, 116 Stat. 2322, 2336. (stating that the Terrorism Risk Insurance Act of 2002 will terminate in December 2005).
[83] Press Release, Insurance Information Institute, Can Your Business Survive a Natural Disaster? Advance Planning, Proper Insurance are Essential (Apr. 13, 2004), *available at* www.iii.org/media/updates/press.736350/ (last visited Sept. 20, 2004).
[84] Flood insurance is underwritten by the National Flood Insurance Program, which is managed by the Mitigation Division of the Federal Emergency Management Agency. In areas deemed by the National Flood Insurance Program to be at high risk for flooding, flood insurance is a prerequisite to obtaining secured financing to buy, build, or improve structures. *See* Fed. Emergency Mgmt. Agency, *Flood Hazard Mapping, Insurance Professionals and Lenders, at* www.fema.gov/fima/nfip.shtm (last visited Sept. 21, 2004); Fed. Emergency Mgmt. Agency, *Mitigation Division, at* www.fema.gov/fima/ (last visited Sept. 27, 2004); NAT'L FLOOD INSURANCE PROGRAM, PROGRAM DESCRIPTION, MANDATORY FLOOD INSURANCE PURCHASE REQUIREMENT 29 (Aug. 1, 2002), *available at* www.fema.gov/doc/library/nfipdescrip.doc (last visited Sept. 21, 2004).
[85] *See* U.S. Small Business Admin., *About Small Business Administration, at* www.sba.gov/aboutsba/index.html (last visited Sept. 21, 2004).
[86] *See* 13 C.F.R. §§ 123.2-123.3 (2004); Understanding How Disaster Declarations Are Made, *supra* note 52.

SBA Declaration.[87] A Presidential Declaration is made when damages are significant. In the case of a Presidential Declaration, "SBA offers physical and economic injury loans in the declared counties and economic injury (EI) loans only in contiguous counties. ...If the damages are less extensive the Governor can ask for a SBA declaration."[88] Two types of SBA declarations may be made: Physical Disaster Declaration and Economic Injury Declaration. The SBA makes three types of disaster-assistance loans to business,[89] and individual assistance is coordinated through FEMA.

1. *Physical Disaster Business Loans.* These loans cover uninsured physical damages.[90] Any business located in a declared disaster area that incurred damage during the disaster may apply for a loan to help repair or replace damaged property (e.g., real property, machinery, equipment, fixtures, inventory, and leaseholds) to its pre-disaster condition.

2. *Economic Injury Disaster Loans.* These loans are provided to small businesses located in a declared disaster area that suffer substantial economic injury, regardless of *physical* damage.[91] "Small businesses and small agricultural cooperatives that have suffered substantial economic injury resulting from a physical disaster or an agricultural production disaster designated by the Secretary of Agriculture may be eligible for the SBA's Economic Injury Disaster Loan Program. Substantial economic injury is the inability of a business to meet its obligations as they mature and to pay its ordinary and necessary operating expenses."[92]

3. *Pre-Disaster Mitigation Loans.* These low-interest, fixed-rate loans are made to small businesses for mitigation measures to protect business property from damage that may be caused by future disasters.[93] "A mitigation measure is something done for the purpose of protecting real and personal property against disaster-related damage. Examples of mitigation measures include retaining walls, sea walls, grading and contouring land, elevating flood-prone structures, relocating utilities, and retrofitting structures against high winds, earthquakes, floods, wild-fires, or other disasters."[94] The Pre-Disaster Mitigation Loan program is a pilot program designed to support FEMA's Pre-Disaster Mitigation Program. Loans are made available to businesses which propose mitigation measures that conform to the priorities and goals of the community in which the business is located (as defined by FEMA).

4. *Individual Disaster Assistance.*[95] Disaster assistance for individuals is coordinated through FEMA. Individuals apply for most assistance directly through FEMA. To apply for SBA loans, individuals who are homeowners or renters must first register with FEMA to obtain a FEMA Registration ID number. FEMA generally establishes local Disaster Recovery Centers to coordinate assistance. After an application for assistance is received, the damaged property is inspected to verify the loss.[96] The deadline for most individual-assistance programs is sixty days following the president's declaration of a

---

[87] *See* 13 C.F.R. § 123.3; Understanding How Disaster Declarations Are Made, *supra* note 52.
[88] Understanding How Disaster Declarations Are Made, *supra* note 52.
[89] 13 C.F.R. § 123.5 (2004).
[90] *See id.* §§ 123.200-123.204; Physical Disaster Business Loans, *supra* note 55.
[91] *See* www.sba.gov/disaster_recov/loaninfo/ecoinjury.html; 13 C.F.R. 123.300–123.303.
[92] Economic Injury Disaster Loans For Small Businesses, *supra* note 57.
[93] *See* 13 C.F.R. § 123.400; Pre-Disaster Mitigation Loan Program, *supra* note 57.
[94] Pre-Disaster Mitigation Loan Program, *supra* note 57.
[95] *See* Fed. Emergency Mgmt. Agency, Individual Assistance Programs, *at* www.fema.gov/rrr/inassist.shtm (last visited Sept. 21, 2004).
[96] *See* Fed. Emergency Mgmt. Agency, Help After a Disaster 4 (May 2004), *at* www.fema.gov/pdf/about/process/help_after_disaster_english.pdf (last visited Sept. 27, 2004).

major disaster.[97] Affected individuals may apply for disaster aid consisting of:

- Disaster housing;[98]
- Funding for housing repairs and replacement of damaged items needed to make homes habitable;[99]
- Disaster grants to cover necessary expenses not covered by insurance and other aid programs, including replacement of personal property, transportation, medical care, dental care, and funeral expenses;[100]
- Low-interest disaster loans for repair or replacement of homes, automobiles, clothing, or other damages personal property (loans are administered through the Small Business Administration);[101]
- Crisis counseling;[102]
- Disaster-related unemployment assistance;[103]
- Legal aid and assistance with income tax, Social Security, and veteran's benefits;[104] and
- Hazard mitigation.[105]

Appendix A.D

Directories of State and Territorial Public Health Directors, State Public Health Legal Counsel, and CDC Emergency-Preparedness Contacts

1. Directory of State and Territorial Public Health Directors, *updated version available at* www.statepublichealth.org/index.php.

2. Directory of State Public Health Legal Counsel, *updated version available at* www.phppo.cdc.gov/od/phlp.

3. Emergency Preparedness Contacts: Centers for Disease Control and Prevention, *updated information available at* www.cdc.gov/nceh/emergency/default.htm.

Appendix A.E

Selected Public Health Emergency-Preparedness Standards and Plans

1. Smallpox Response Plan and Guidelines (V3.0), Executive Summary and Sections A-F, *full and updated version available at* www.bt.cdc.gov/agent/smallpox/prep/index.asp#responseplanning.

2. Public Health Guidance for Community-Level Preparedness and Response to Severe Acute Respiratory Syndrome (V2/3), Supplement C: Preparedness and Response in Healthcare Facilities, *full and updated version available at* www.cdc.gov/ncidod/sars/guidance/C/index.htm.

3. Pandemic Influenza Preparedness Plan, Executive Summary, *full and updated version available at* www.hhs.gov/nvpo/pandemicplan/.

---

[97] Fed. Emergency Mgmt. Agency, *Region IV, Ten Days Remain for Disaster Aid*, Oct. 16, 1998, *at* www.fema.gov/regions/iv/1998/r4_095.shtm (last visited Sept. 21, 2004).
[98] *See* 42 U.S.C. § 5174(b) (2004).
[99] *Id.* § 5174(c).
[100] *Id.* § 5174(e).
[101] Fed. Emergency Mgmt. Agency, *supra* note 95.
[102] 42 U.S.C. § 5183 (2004).
[103] *Id.* § 5177(a).
[104] *See* Fed. Emergency Mgmt. Agency, *supra* note 95
[105] *Id.*

Appendix B   Model Hospital Mutual Aid Memorandum of Understanding[1]

I. Introduction and Background

As in other parts of the nation, (name of city, county, and or state served by MOU) is susceptible to disasters, both natural and man-made, that could exceed the resources of any individual hospital. A disaster could result from incidents generating an overwhelming number of patients, from a smaller number of patients whose specialized medical requirements exceed the resources of the impacted facility (e.g., hazmat injuries, pulmonary, trauma surgery, etc.), or from incidents such as building or plant problems resulting in the need for partial or complete hospital evacuation.

II. Purpose of Mutual Aid Memorandum of Understanding

The mutual aid support concept is well established and is considered "standard of care" in most emergency response disciplines. The purpose of this mutual aid support agreement is to aid hospitals in their emergency management by authorizing the Hospital Mutual Aid System (H-MAS). H-MAS addresses the loan of medical personnel, pharmaceuticals, supplies, and equipment, or assistance with emergent hospital evacuation, including accepting transferred patients.

This Mutual Aid Memorandum of Understanding (MOU) is a voluntary agreement among the hospital members, (name of hospital association or council) or (list hospitals party to MOU), for the purpose of providing mutual aid at the time of a medical disaster. For purposes of this MOU, a *disaster* is defined as an overwhelming incident that *exceeds the effective response capability* of the impacted health care facility or facilities. An incident of this magnitude will almost always involve (name of local) emergency management agency and (name of local) public health department. The disaster may be an "external" or "internal" event for hospitals and *assumes that each affected hospital's emergency management plans have been fully implemented.*

This document addresses the relationships between and among hospitals and is intended to augment, not replace, each facility's disaster plan. The MOU also provides the framework for hospitals to coordinate as a single H-MAS community in actions with (name of local) management agency, (name of local) public health department, and emergency medical services during planning and response. This document does not replace but rather supplements the rules and procedures governing interaction with other organizations during a disaster (e.g., law enforcement agencies, the local emergency medical services, local public health department, fire departments, American Red Cross, etc).

By signing this Memorandum of Understanding each hospital is evidencing its intent to abide by the terms of the MOU in the event of a medical disaster as described above. The terms of this MOU are to be incorporated into the hospital's emergency management plans.

---

[1] *The American Hospital Association is grateful to the District of Columbia Hospital Association, who developed the original MOU from which this model is adapted.*

III. Definition of Terms

Command Post	An area established in a hospital during an emergency that is the facility's primary source of administrative authority and decision-making.
Clearinghouse	A communication and information center that has H-MARS network capabilities allowing for the immediate determination of available hospital resources at the time of a disaster. The clearinghouse must be operational 24 hours a day and requires daily maintenance. The clearinghouse does not have any decision-making or supervisory authority but merely collects and disseminates information, and performs regular radio checks of the H-MARS system.
Donor Hospital	The hospital that provides personnel, pharmaceuticals, supplies, or equipment to a facility experiencing a medical disaster. Also referred to as the patient-receiving hospital when involving evacuating patients.
H-MAS	Hospital Mutual Aid System
H-MARS	Hospital Mutual Aid Radio System—The primary communication system used by hospitals to communicate during an emergency.
Impacted Hospital	The hospital where the disaster occurred or disaster victims are being treated. Referred to as the recipient hospital when pharmaceuticals, supplies, or equipment are requested, or as the patient-transferring hospital when the evacuation of patients is required.
Medical Disaster	An incident that exceeds a facility's effective response capability or cannot appropriately resolve solely by using its own resources. Such disasters will very likely involve the (name of local) emergency management agency and (name of local) public health department and may involve loan of medical and support personnel, pharmaceuticals, supplies, and equipment from another facility, or, the emergent evacuation of patients.
Partner ("Buddy")	The designated facility that a hospital communicates with as a facility's "first call for help" during a medical disaster (developed through an optional partnering arrangement).
Patient-Receiving Hospital	The hospital that receives transferred patients from a facility responding to a disaster. When patients are evacuated, the receiving facility is referred to as the patient-receiving hospital. When personnel or materials are involved, the providing hospital is referred to as the donor hospital.
Patient-Transferring Hospital	An impacted facility. The hospital that evacuates patients to patient-receiving facility in response to a medical disaster. Also referred to as the recipient hospital when personnel and materials are moved to the facility.
Participating Hospitals	Health care facilities that have fully committed to H-MAS.
Recipient Hospital	The impacted facility. The hospital where disaster patients are being treated and has requested personnel or materials from another facility. Also referred to as the patient-transferring hospital when evacuating/transferring patients from the facility during a medical disaster.

IV. General Principles of Understanding

1. *Participating Hospitals*: Each hospital designates a representative to attend the (name of organization) Hospital Mutual Aid System meetings and to coordinate the mutual aid initiatives with the individual hospital's emergency management plans. Hospitals also commit to participating in H-MAS exercises and maintaining their radio links to H-MARS.

2. *Partner Hospital Concept*: Each hospital has the option of linking to a designated partner or "buddy" hospital as the hospital of 'first call for help' during a disaster. The hospitals comprising each partner-network should develop, prior to any medical disaster, methods for coordinating communication between themselves, responding to the media, and identifying the locations to enter their buddy hospital's security perimeter.

3. *Implementation of Mutual Aid Memorandum of Understanding*: A health care facility becomes a participating hospital when an authorized administrator signs the MOU. During a medical emergency, only the authorized administrator (or designee) or command center at each hospital has the authority to request or offer assistance through H-MAS. Communications between hospitals for formally requesting and volunteering assistance should therefore occur among the senior administrators (or designees) or respective command centers.

4. *Command Center*: The impacted facility's command center is responsible for informing the clearinghouse of its situation and defining needs that cannot be accommodated by the hospital itself or any existing partner hospital. The senior administrator or designee is responsible for requesting personnel, pharmaceuticals, supplies, equipment, or authorizing the evacuation of patients. The senior administrator or designee will coordinate both internally, and with the donor/patient-accepting hospital, all of the logistics involved in implementing assistance under this Mutual Aid MOU. Logistics include identifying the number and specific location where personnel, pharmaceuticals, supplies, equipment, or patients should be sent, how to enter the security perimeter, estimated time interval to arrival and estimated return date of borrowed supplies, etc.

5. *Clearinghouse*: Each hospital will participate in an annual H-MAS exercise that includes communicating to the clearinghouse a set of data elements or indicators describing the hospital's resource capacity (see appendices). The Clearinghouse will serve as an information center for recording and disseminating the type and amount of available resources at each hospital. During a disaster drill or emergency, each hospital will report to the Clearinghouse the current status of their indicators. (For a more detailed account of the Clearinghouse's responsibilities, see "Clearinghouse Requirements.") Hospitals also participate in daily radio checks performed by the Clearinghouse.

6. *Hospital Indicators*: A set of hospital resource measures that are reported to the Communication Center during a disaster drill or actual disaster. The indicators are designed to catalogue hospital resources that could be available for other hospitals during a disaster.

7. *Documentation*: During a disaster, the recipient hospital will accept and honor the donor hospital's standard requisition forms. Documentation should detail the items involved in the transaction, condition of the material prior to the loan (if applicable), and the party responsible for the material.

8. *Authorization*: The recipient facility will have supervisory direction over the donor facility's staff, borrowed equipment, etc., once they are received by the recipient hospital.

9. *Financial and Legal Liability*: The recipient hospital will assume legal responsibility for the personnel and equipment from the donor hospital during the time the personnel,

equipment and supplies are at the recipient hospital. The recipient hospital will reimburse the donor hospital, to the extent permitted by federal law, for all of the donor hospital's costs determined by the donor hospital's regular rate. Costs includes all use, breakage, damage, replacement, and return costs of borrowed materials, for personnel injuries that result in disability, loss of salary, and reasonable expenses, and for reasonable costs of defending any liability claims, except where the donor hospital has not provided preventive maintenance or proper repair of loaned equipment which resulted in patient injury. Reimbursement will be made within 90 days following receipt of the invoice.

10. *Patient-accepting hospitals assume the legal and financial responsibility for transferred patients upon arrival into the patient-accepting hospital.*

11. *Communications*: Hospitals will collaborate on the H-MARS radio communication system to ensure a dedicated and reliable method to communicate with the Clearinghouse and other hospitals. The back-up conference call landline telephone system may be used as a semi-secure system for discussing sensitive information.

12. *Public Relations*: Each hospital is responsible for developing and coordinating with other hospitals and relevant organizations the media response to the disaster. Hospitals are encouraged to develop and coordinate the outline of their response prior to any disaster. The partner hospitals should be familiar with each other's mechanisms for addressing the media. The response should include reference to the fact that the situation is being addressed in a manner agreed upon by a previously established mutual aid protocol.

13. *Emergency Management Committee Chairperson*: Each hospital's Emergency Management Committee Chairperson is responsible for disseminating the information regarding this MOU to relevant hospital personnel, coordinating and evaluating the hospital's participation in exercises of the mutual aid system, and incorporating the MOU concepts into the hospital's emergency management plan.

14. *Hold Harmless Condition*: The recipient hospital should hold harmless the donor hospital for acts of negligence or omissions on the part of the donor hospital in their good faith response for assistance during a disaster. The donor hospital, however, is responsible for appropriate credentialing of personnel and for the safety and integrity of the equipment and supplies provided for use at the recipient hospital.

V. General Principles Governing Medical Operations, the Transfer of Pharmaceuticals, Supplies or Equipment, or the Evacuation of Patients

1. *Partner hospital concept*: Each hospital has the option of designating a partner or *buddy* hospital that serves as the hospital of "first call for help" (see lists under Clearinghouse Function). During a disaster, the requesting hospital may first call its pre-arranged partner hospital for personnel or material assistance or to request the evacuation of patients to the partner hospital. The donor hospital will inform the requesting hospital of the degree and time frame in which it can meet the request.

2. *Clearinghouse*: The recipient hospital (patient-transferring hospital) is responsible for notifying and informing the Clearinghouse of its personnel or material needs or its need to evacuate patients and the degree to which its partner hospital is unable to meet these needs. Upon the request by the senior administrator or designee of the impacted hospital, the Clearinghouse will contact the other participating hospitals to determine the availability of additional personnel or material resources, including the availability of beds, as required by the situation. The recipient hospital will be informed as to which hospitals

should be contacted directly for assistance that has been offered. The senior administrator (or designee) of the recipient or patient-transferring hospital will coordinate directly with the senior administrator (or designee) of the donor or patient-accepting hospital for this assistance.

3. *Initiation of transfer of personnel, material resources, or patients*: Only the senior hospital administrator or designee at each hospital has the authority to initiate the transfer or receipt of personnel, material resources, or patients. The senior administrator (or designee) and medical director, in conjunction with the directors of the affected services, will make a determination as to whether medical staff and other personnel from another facility will be required at the impacted hospital to assist in patient care activities.

Personnel offered by donor hospitals should be limited to staff that are **fully accredited or credentialed in the donor institution**. No resident physicians, medical/nursing students, or in-training persons should be volunteered. In the event of the evacuation of patients, the medical director of the patient-transferring hospital will also notify the (name of local) fire department of its situation and seek assistance, if necessary, from the emergency medical services. (Name of local) fire department will be requested to notify the (name of local) emergency management agency and the (name of local) public health department.

VI. Specific Principles of Understanding

A. Medical Operations/Loaning Personnel

1. *Communication of request*: The request for the transfer of personnel initially can be made verbally. The request, however, must be followed up with written documentation. This should ideally occur prior to the arrival of personnel at the recipient hospital. The recipient hospital will identify to the donor hospital the following:
   a. The type and number of requested personnel.
   b. An estimate of how quickly the request is needed.
   c. The location where they are to report.
   d. An estimate of how long the personnel will be needed.

2. *Documentation*: The arriving donated personnel will be required to present their donor hospital identification badge at the site designated by the recipient hospital's command center. The recipient hospital will be responsible for the following:
   a. Meeting the arriving donated personnel (usually by the recipient hospital's security department or designated employee).
   b. Confirming the donated personnel's ID badge with the list of personnel provided by the donor hospital.
   c. Providing additional identification, e.g., "visiting personnel" badge, to the arriving donated personnel.

   The recipient hospital will accept the professional credentialing determination of the donor hospital but only for those services for which the personnel are credentialed at the donor hospital.

3. *Supervision*: The recipient hospital's senior administrator or designee, (the command center) identifies where and to whom the donated personnel are to report, and professional staff of the recipient hospital supervise the donated personnel. The supervisor or designee will meet the donated personnel at the point of entry of the facility and brief the donated personnel of the situation and their assignments. If appropriate, the "emergency staffing" rules of the recipient hospital will govern assigned shifts. The donated personnel's shift, however, should not be longer than the customary length practiced at the donor hospital.

4. *Legal and financial liability*: Liability claims, malpractice claims, disability claims, attorneys'

fees, and other incurred costs are the responsibility of the recipient hospital. An extension of liability coverage will be provided by the recipient facility, to the extent permitted by federal law, insofar as the donated personnel are operating within their scope of practice. The recipient hospital will reimburse the donor hospital for the salaries of the donated personnel at the donated personnel's rate as established at the donor hospital if the personnel are employees being paid by the donor hospital. The reimbursement will be made within ninety days following receipt of the invoice.

The Medical Director of the recipient hospital will be responsible for providing a mechanism for granting emergency credentialing privileges' for physician, nurses and other licensed health care providers to provide services at the recipient hospital.

5. *Demobilization procedures*: The recipient hospital will provide and coordinate any necessary demobilization procedures and post-event stress debriefing. The recipient hospital is responsible for providing the donated personnel transportation necessary for their return to the donor hospital.

B. Transfer of Pharmaceuticals, Supplies or Equipment

1. *Communication of Request*: The request for the transfer of pharmaceuticals, supplies, or equipment initially can be made verbally. The request, however, must be followed up with a written communication. This should ideally occur prior to the receipt of any material resources at the recipient hospital. The recipient hospital will identify to the donor hospital the following:
   a. The quantity and exact type of requested items.
   b. An estimate of how quickly the request is needed.
   c. Time period for which the supplies will be needed.
   d. Location to which the supplies should be delivered.

The donor hospital will identify how long it takes for them to fulfill the request. Since response time is a central component during a disaster response, decision and implementation should occur quickly.

2. *Documentation*: The recipient hospital will honor the donor hospital's standard order requisition form as documentation of the request and receipt of the materials. The recipient hospital's security office or designee will confirm the receipt of the material resources. The documentation will detail the following:
   a. The items involved.
   b. The condition of the equipment prior to the loan (if applicable).
   c. The responsible parties for the borrowed material.

The donor hospital is responsible for tracking the borrowed inventory through their standard requisition forms. Upon the return of the equipment, etc., the original invoice will be co-signed by the senior administrator or designee of the recipient hospital recording the condition of the borrowed equipment.

3. *Transporting of pharmaceuticals, supplies, or equipment*: The recipient hospital is responsible for coordinating the transportation of materials both to and from the donor hospital. This coordination may involve government and/or private organizations, and the donor hospital may also offer transport. Upon request, the receiving hospital must return and pay the transportation fees for returning or replacing all borrowed material.

4. *Supervision*: The recipient hospital is responsible for appropriate use and maintenance of all borrowed pharmaceuticals, supplies, or equipment.

5. *Financial and legal liability*: The recipient hospital, to the extent permitted by federal law, is responsible for all costs arising from the use, damage, or loss of borrowed pharmaceuticals, supplies, or equipment, and for liability claims arising from the use of borrowed supplies and equipment, except where the donor hospital has not provided preventive maintenance or

proper repair of loaned equipment which resulted in patient injury.
6. *Demobilization procedures*: The recipient hospital is responsible for the rehabilitation and prompt return of the borrowed equipment to the donor hospital.

C. Transfer/Evacuation of Patients

1. *Communication of request*: The request for the transfer of patients initially can be made verbally. The request, however, must be followed up with a written communication prior to the actual transferring of any patients. The patient-transferring hospital will identify to the patient-accepting hospital:
   a. The number of patients needed to be transferred.
   b. The general nature of their illness or condition.
   c. Any type of specialized services required, e.g., ICU bed, burn bed, trauma care, etc.
2. *Documentation*: The patient-transferring hospital is responsible for providing the patient-receiving hospital with the patient's complete medical records, insurance information and other patient information necessary for the care of the transferred patient. The patient-transferring hospital is responsible for tracking the destination of all patients transferred out.
3. *Transporting of patients*: The patient-transferring hospital is responsible for coordinating and financing the transportation of patients to the patient-receiving hospital. The point of entry will be designated by the patient-receiving hospital's senior administrator or designee. Once admitted, that patient becomes the patient-receiving hospital's patient and under care of the patient-receiving hospital's admitting physician until discharged, transferred or reassigned. The patient-transferring hospital is responsible for transferring of extraordinary drugs or other special patient needs (e.g., equipment and blood products) along with the patient if requested by the patient-receiving hospital.
4. *Supervision*: The patient-receiving hospital will designate the patient's admitting service, the admitting physician for each patient, and, if requested, will provide at least temporary courtesy privileges to the patient's original attending physician.
5. *Financial and Legal Liability*: Upon admission, the patient-receiving hospital is responsible for liability claims originating from the time the patient is admitted to the patient-accepting hospital. Reimbursement for care should be negotiated with each hospital's insurer under the conditions for *admissions without precertification requirements* in the event of emergencies.
6. *Notification*: The patient-transferring hospital is responsible for notifying both the patient's family or guardian and the patient's attending or personal physician of the situation. The patient-receiving hospital may assist in notifying the patient's family and personal physician.

D. Clearinghouse Function

The H-MARS provides the means for the hospitals to coordinate among themselves, and as a unit to integrate with (name of local) emergency management agency, (name of local) public health department, police, and emergency medical services during a disaster event.

The clearinghouse serves as the data center for collecting and disseminating current information about equipment, bed capacity and other hospital resources during a disaster (see appendices). The information collected by the Communication Center is to be used only for disaster preparedness and response.

In the event of a disaster or during a disaster drill, hospitals will be prepared to provide the communication center the following information:

1. The total number of injury victims your emergency department can accept, and if possible, the number of victims with minor and major injuries

2. Total number of operating beds *current available to accept patients* in the following units:
   - general medical (adult)
   - general surgical (adult)
   - general medical (pediatric)
   - general surgical (pediatric)
   - obstetrics
   - cardiac intensive care
   - neonatal intensive care
   - pediatric intensive care
   - burn
   - psychiatric
   - subacute care
   - skilled care beds
   - operating suites

3. The number of items *currently available for loan or donation* to another hospital:
   - respirators
   - IV infusion pumps
   - dialysis machines
   - hazmat decontamination equipment
   - MRI
   - CT scanner
   - hyperbaric chamber
   - ventilators
   - external pacemakers
   - atropine
   - kefzol

4. The following number of personnel *currently available for loan* to another hospital:
   Physicians
   - Anesthesiologists
   - Emergency Medicine
   - General Surgeon
   - OB-GYN
   - Pediatricians
   - Trauma Surgeons

   Registered Nurses
   - Emergency
   - Critical Care
   - Operating Room
   - Pediatrics

   Other Personnel
   - Maintenance Workers
   - Mental Health Workers
   - Respiratory Therapists
   - Plant Engineers
   - Security Workers
   - Social Workers
   - Others as indicated

E. Partner Hospital Concept (Optional)

Each "paired" hospital should standardize a set of contacts to facilitate communications during a disaster.

The procedural steps in the event of a disaster are as follows:

1. Determine the total number of patients the emergency department and hospital can accept, and if possible, the total number of patients with major and minor injuries.

2. Impacted hospital contacts partner hospital to determine availability of beds, equipment, supplies, and personnel. (Contacts secondary partner hospital if primary hospital is unable to meet needs.)

3. Impacted hospital contacts the clearinghouse and notifies the center of its needs, how they are being met, and any unmet needs.

4. At the request of the impacted hospital, the clearinghouse will contact other hospitals to alert them to the situation and to begin an inventory for any possible or actual unmet needs.

Appendix B.1: Primary Data Collection Form

In the event of an emergency, record the time of communication, the total number of injury victims the receiving hospital can accept, and, if possible, the number of major and minor injury victims the hospital can accept.

Date: _____

Page No.: _____

Hospitals (list abbreviated name of each member hospital)	Time	Total Number of Patients	Minor Injuries[a]	Major Injuries[b]	Comments

[a] *Minor injury victims*: Those expected to be treated and released or require very little medical/hospital resources.
[b] *Major injury victims*: Those expected to require admission and/or significant medical/hospital resources (operating room, critical care, extensive orthopedics intervention, etc.).

Appendix B.2a: Secondary Data Collection Form[a]

If time or need permits, request the following information from the donating hospital.

Hospital Name: _____

Person completing form: _____

Date: _____   Time: _____

Number of open/available beds		Total available to donate	
General medical (adult)		Respirators	
General surgical (adult)		IV Infusion Pumps	
General medical (pediatric)		Dialysis Machines	
General surgical (pediatric)		Hazmat Decontamination Equipment	
Obstetrics		MRIs	
Cardiac ICU		CT Scanners	
NICU		Hyperbaric Chamber	
PICU		Ventilators	
Burn		external pacemakers	
Psychiatric		atropine	
Trauma		kefzol	
OR Suites			
Skilled Nursing & Subacute Care			

[a] During an actual disaster or disaster drill, hospitals should complete the above form with the most current information available and have this information ready for dissemination to (name of local) emergency management agency, fire department, requesting hospitals, and the H-MARS clearinghouse.

Appendix B.2b: Secondary Data Collection Form[a]

Hospital Name: _____

Person completing form: _____

Date: _____   Time: _____

Physician	Number of personnel currently available to loan/donate to partner hospital[a]
Anesthesiology	
Emergency medicine	
General surgeon	
General medicine	
OB-GYN	
Pediatrician	
Trauma surgeon	
Other as indicated	
Registered nurses	
Emergency	
Critical care	
Operating room	
Pediatrics	
Other as indicated	
Other personnel	
Maintenance workers	
Mental health workers	
Respiratory therapists	
Plant engineers	
Security personnel	
Social workers	
Other as indicated	

[a]During an actual disaster or disaster drill, hospitals should complete the above form with the most current information available and have this information ready for dissemination to (name of local) emergency management agency, fire department, requesting hospitals, and the H-MARS clearinghouse.

Appendix C   Protecting Building Environments from Airborne Chemical, Biological, or Radiological Attacks

DEPARTMENT OF HEALTH AND HUMAN SERVICES, CENTERS FOR DISEASE CONTROL AND PREVENTION, NATIONAL INSTITUTE FOR OCCUPATIONAL SAFETY AND HEALTH

Scope

This document identifies actions that a building owner or manager can implement without undue delay to enhance occupant protection from an airborne chemical, biological, or radiological (CBR) attack. The intended audience includes building owners, managers, and maintenance personnel of public, private, and governmental buildings, including offices, laboratories, hospitals, retail facilities, schools, transportation terminals, and public venues (for example, sports arenas, malls, coliseums). This document is not intended to address single-family or low-occupancy residential housing (less than five family units). Higher risk facilities such as industrial facilities, military facilities, subway systems, and law enforcement facilities require special considerations that are beyond the scope of this guide.

The likelihood of a specific building being targeted for terrorist activity is generally difficult to predict. As such, there is no specific formula that will determine a certain building's level of risk. Building owners must make their own decisions about how to reduce their building's risk to a CBR attack. These decisions may be aided by a comprehensive building security assessment. Many government and private organizations have identified resources that provide insight into building security assessments. The reference list at the end of this document will help the reader obtain this information.

No building can be fully protected from a determined individual who is intent on releasing a CBR agent. The recommendations in this guide will not preclude injuries or fatalities in the event of a CBR release. However, facility owners and managers can transform their buildings into less attractive targets by increasing the difficulty of introducing a CBR agent, by increasing the ability to detect terrorists before they carry out an intended release, and by incorporating plans and procedures to mitigate the effects of a CBR release. Some of the references listed in the back of this document can provide information on how to recognize if a CBR release has occurred. These recommendations focus on airborne releases of CBR agents[a] in quantities capable of being easily transported by a few individuals. Protection from other types of attacks such as explosions, building collapses, and water supply contamination require much different measures and are not addressed in this document.

The recommendations set forth in this document are not intended to be a minimum requirement that every building owner and manager should implement for every building. Rather, the decisions concerning which protective measures should be implemented for any building should be based on several factors, including the perceived risk associated with the building and its tenants, engineering and architectural feasibility, and cost.

---

[a] *Note*: References to a release of CBR agent in this document will always refer to an airborne CBR release.

Background

Terrorism events have increased interest in the vulnerability of U.S. workplaces, schools, and other occupied buildings to CBR threats. Of particular concern are the airflow patterns and dynamics in buildings, specifically in the building heating, ventilating, and air-conditioning (HVAC) systems. These systems can become an entry point and a distribution system for hazardous contaminants, particularly CBR agents. Building owners need reliable information about how they can (1) modify their buildings to decrease the likelihood or effects of a CBR incident and (2) respond quickly and appropriately should a CBR incident occur. Comprehensive guidance is needed in several areas, including:

- How to modify existing buildings for better air protection and security.
- How to design new buildings to be more secure.
- What plans building managers should prepare in advance to help them make effective decisions in the midst of a CBR incident.

Preparatory Recommendation—Know Your Building

While more comprehensive guidance is being developed, this document focuses on the shorter-term goals of identifying those protective actions that you can take immediately. But it recognizes that some recommendations may not be feasible for you or in all situations.

In initiating any plan to modify building system design or operation, an important first step is to understand these systems: How were they intended to operate? How do they currently operate?

Getting to know your building may best be handled by conducting a walk-through inspection of the building and its systems, including the HVAC, fire protection, and life-safety systems. During this inspection, compare the most up-to-date design drawings available to the operation of the current systems.[b] This step may require, or benefit from, the assistance of qualified outside professionals. Without this baseline knowledge, it is difficult to accurately identify what impact a particular security modification may have on building operation. While it is important to understand how the existing building systems function, the systems need not operate per design before you implement security measures. A *partial* list of items to consider during your building walk-through includes:

- What is the mechanical condition of the equipment?
- What filtration systems are in place? What are their efficiencies?
- Is all equipment appropriately connected and controlled? Are equipment access doors and panels in place and appropriately sealed?
- Are all dampers (outdoor air, return air, bypass, fire and smoke) functioning? Check to see how well they seal when closed.
- How does the HVAC system respond to manual fire alarm, fire detection, or fire-suppression device activation?
- Are all supply and return ducts completely connected to their grilles and registers?
- Are the variable air volume (VAV) boxes functioning?
- How is the HVAC system controlled? How quickly does it respond?
- How is the building zoned? Where are the air handlers for each zone? Is the system designed for smoke control?
- How does air flow through the building? What are the pressure relationships between zones? Which building entryways are positively or negatively pressurized? Is the building connected to other buildings by tunnels or passageways?
- Are utility chases and penetrations, elevator shafts, and fire stairs significant airflow pathways?

---

[b] *Note*: If sufficient questins or surprises arise from the building walk-through, an independent evaluation by a qualified HVAC professional should be used to establish a useful baseline.

- Is there obvious air infiltration? Is it localized?
- Does the system provide adequate ventilation given the building's current occupancy and functions?
- Where are the outdoor air louvers? Are they easily observable? Are they or other mechanical equipment accessible to the public?
- Do adjacent structures or landscaping allow access to the building roof?

Specific Recommendations

The recommendations can be divided into four general categories: (1) things not to do; (2) physical security; (3) ventilation and filtration; and (4) maintenance, administration, and training. Some of these items, such as securing mechanical rooms, may be started prior to your completing the recommendations in the "Know your building" section. Items within each of the four categories are listed in the order of priority. Items considered to be highly critical are identified by "*" next to the number. As you review these recommendations, consider their potential implications upon the contract language necessary for existing and future service contracts. A brief discussion of the four categories and some commonly considered recommendations follow.

Things not to do

More than anything else, building owners and managers should ensure that any actions they take do not have a detrimental effect on the building systems (HVAC, fire protection, life safety, etc.) or the building occupants under normal building operation. Some efforts to protect the building from a CBR attack could have adverse effects on the building's indoor environmental quality. Building owners and managers should understand how the building systems operate and assess the impact of security measures on those systems.

*1. *Do not permanently seal outdoor air intakes.* Buildings require a steady supply of outdoor air appropriate to their occupancy and function. This supply should be maintained during normal building operations. Closing off the outdoor air supply vents will adversely affect the building occupants and likely result in a decrease in indoor environmental quality and an increase in indoor environmental quality complaints.

*2. *Do not modify the HVAC system without first understanding the effects on the building systems or the occupants.* This caution directly relates to the recommendation that building owners and managers should understand the operation of their building systems. If there is uncertainty about the effects of a proposed modification, a qualified professional should be consulted.

*3. Do not interfere with fire protection and life safety systems. These systems provide protection in the event of fire or other types of events. They should not be altered without guidance from a professional specifically qualified in fire protection and life safety systems.

Physical Security

Preventing terrorist access to a targeted facility requires physical security of entry, storage, roof, and mechanical areas, as well as securing access to the outdoor air intakes of the building HVAC system. The physical security needs of each building should be assessed, as the threat of a CBR attack will vary considerably from building to building. For example, the threat to a large corporate headquarters may be considered greater than the threat to a small retail establishment. Some physical security measures, such as locking doors to mechanical rooms, are low cost and will not inconvenience the users of the building. These types of measures can be implemented in most buildings. Other physical security measures, such as increased security personnel or package X-ray equipment, are more costly or may inconvenience users substantially. These measures should be implemented when merited after consideration of the threat and consequences of a terrorist attack. Building owners and managers should be familiar with their buildings and understand what assets require protection and what characteristics about the building or its occupants make it a potential target. By first assessing the vulnerabilities of facilities, building owners and managers can address physical security in an effective manner. While the identification and resolution of building vulnerabilities will be specific to each building, some physical security actions are applicable to many building types. These include:

*1. *Prevent access to outdoor air intakes.* One of the most important steps in protecting a building's indoor environment is the security of the outdoor air intakes. Outdoor air enters the building through these intakes and is distributed throughout the building by the HVAC system. Introducing CBR agents into the outdoor air intakes allows a terrorist to use the HVAC system as a means of dispersing the agent throughout a building. Publicly accessible outdoor air intakes located at or below ground level are at most risk—due partly to their accessibility (which also makes visual or audible identification easier) and partly because most CBR agent releases near a building will be close to the ground and may remain there. Securing the outdoor air intakes is a critical line of defense in limiting an external CBR attack on a building.

Relocate outdoor air intake vents. Relocating accessible air intakes to a publicly inaccessible location is preferable. Ideally, the intake should be located on a secure roof or high sidewall. The lowest edge of the outdoor air intakes should be placed at the highest feasible level above the ground or above any nearby accessible level (i.e., adjacent retaining walls, loading docks, handrail) (Figure C.1). These measures are also beneficial in limiting the inadvertent introduction of other types of contaminants, such as landscaping chemicals, into the building.

Extend outdoor air intakes. If relocation of outdoor air intakes is not feasible, intake extensions can be constructed without creating adverse effects on HVAC performance. Depending upon budget, time, or the perceived threat, the intake extensions may be temporary or constructed in a permanent, architecturally compatible design (Figure C.2). The goal is to minimize public accessibility. In general, this means *the higher the extensions, the better*—as long as other design constraints (excessive pressure loss, dynamic and static loads on structure) are appropriately considered (Figure C.3). An extension height of 12 feet (3.7 m) will place

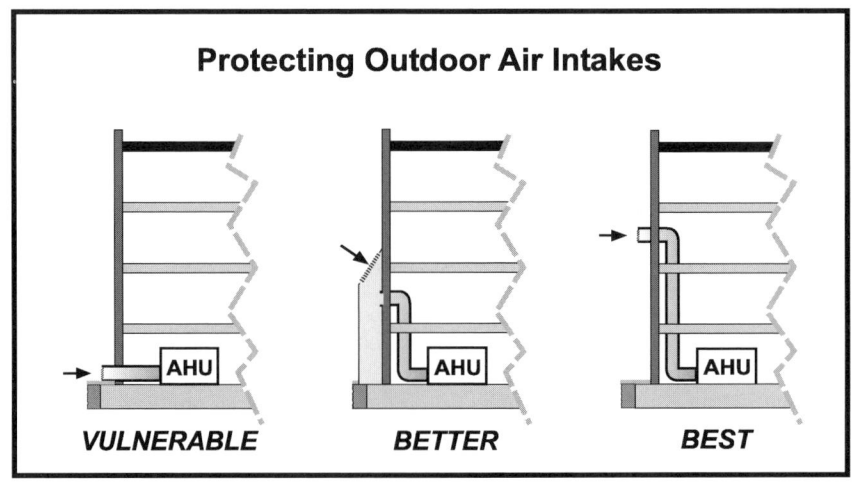

Figure C.1

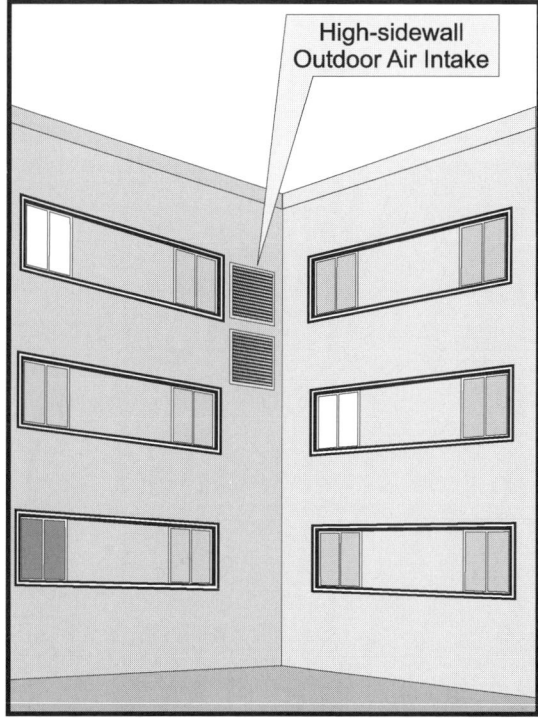

Figure C.2

the intake out of reach of individuals without some assistance. Also, the entrance to the intake should be covered with a sloped metal mesh to reduce the threat of objects being tossed into the intake. A minimum slope of 45° is generally adequate (Figure C.4). Extension height should be increased where existing platforms or building features (i.e., loading docks, retaining walls) might provide access to the outdoor air intakes.

Establish a security zone around outdoor air intakes. Physically inaccessible outdoor air intakes are the preferred protection strategy. When outdoor air intakes are publicly accessible and relocation or physical extensions are not viable options, perimeter barriers that prevent public access to outdoor air intake areas may be an effective alternative. Iron fencing or similar see-through barriers that will not obscure visual detection of terrorist activities or a deposited CBR source are preferred. The restricted area should also include an open buffer zone between the public areas and the intake louvers. Thus, individuals attempting to enter these protected areas will be more conspicuous to security personnel and the public. Monitoring the buffer zone by physical security, closed-circuit television (CCTV), security lighting, or intrusion detection sensors will enhance this protective approach.

*2. *Prevent public access to mechanical areas.* Closely related to the relocation of outdoor air intakes is the security of building mechanical areas. Mechanical areas may exist at one or more locations within a building. These areas provide access to centralized mechanical systems (HVAC, elevator, water, etc.), including filters, air handling units, and exhaust systems. Such equipment is susceptible to tampering and may subsequently be used in a CBR attack. Access to mechanical areas should be strictly controlled by keyed locks, keycards, or similar security measures. Additional controls for access to keys, keycards, and key codes should be strictly maintained.

*3. *Prevent public access to building roofs.* Access to a building's roof can allow ingress to the building and access to air intakes and HVAC equipment (e.g., self-contained HVAC units, laboratory or bathroom exhausts) located on the roof. From a physical security perspective, roofs are like other entrances to the building and should be secured appropriately. Roofs with HVAC equipment should be treated like mechanical areas. Fencing or other barriers should restrict access from adjacent roofs. Access to roofs should be strictly controlled through keyed locks, keycards, or similar measures. Fire and life safety egress should be carefully reviewed when restricting roof access.

4. *Implement security measures, such as guards, alarms, and cameras to protect vulnerable areas.* Difficult-to-reach outdoor air

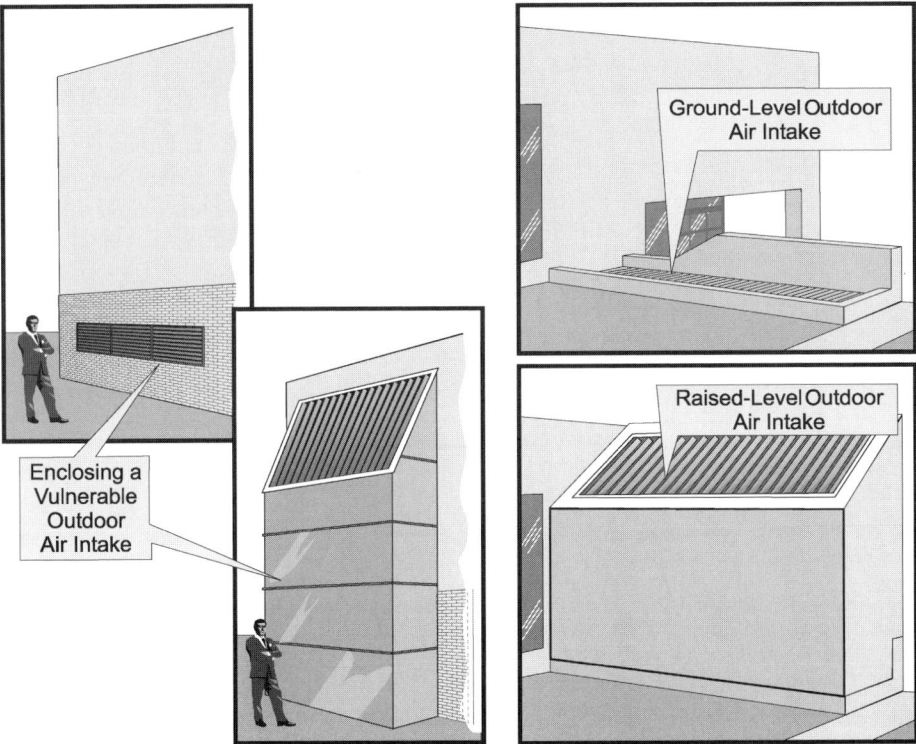

Figure C.3

intakes and mechanical rooms alone may not stop a sufficiently determined person. Security personnel, barriers that deter loitering, intrusion detection sensors, and observation cameras can further increase protection by quickly alerting personnel to security breaches near the outdoor air intakes or other vulnerable locations.

5. *Isolate lobbies, mailrooms, loading docks, and storage areas.* Lobbies, mailrooms (includes various mail processing areas), loading docks, and other entry and storage areas should be physically isolated from the rest of the building. These are areas where bulk quantities of CBR agents are likely to enter a building. Building doors, including vestibule and loading dock doors, should remain closed when not in use.

To prevent widespread dispersion of a contaminant released within lobbies, mailrooms, and loading docks, their HVAC systems should be isolated and the areas maintained at a negative pressure relative to the rest of the building, but at positive pressure relative to the outdoors. Physical isolation of these areas (well-sealed floor to roof-deck walls, sealed wall penetrations) is critical to maintaining the pressure differential and requires special attention to ensure airtight boundaries between these areas and adjacent spaces. In some building designs (those having lobbies with elevator access, for example), establishing a negative pressure differential will present a challenge. A qualified HVAC professional can assist in determining if the recommended isolation is feasible for a given building. In addition, lobbies, mailrooms, and loading docks should not share a return-air system or return pathway (e.g., ceiling plenum) with other

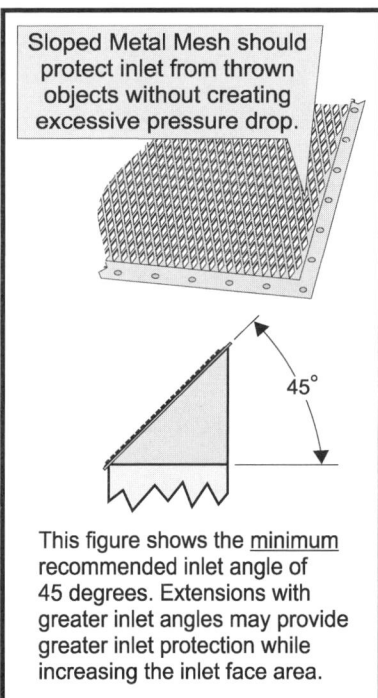

Figure C.4

areas of the building. Some of these measures are more feasible for new construction or buildings undergoing major renovation.

Building access from lobby areas should be limited by security checks of individuals and packages prior to their entry into secure areas. Lobby isolation is particularly critical in buildings where the main lobbies are open to the public. Similar checks of incoming mail should also occur before its conveyance into the secure building areas. Side entry doors that circumvent established security checkpoints should be strictly controlled.

6. *Secure return air grills.* Similar to the outdoor-air intake, HVAC return-air grills that are publicly accessible and not easily observed by security may be vulnerable to targeting for CBR contaminants. Public access facilities may be the most vulnerable to this type of CBR attack. A building-security assessment can help determine, which, if any, protective measures to employ to secure return-air grills. Take caution that a selected measure does not adversely affect the performance of the building HVAC system. Some return-air grill protective measures include (1) relocating return-air grills to inaccessible, yet observable locations, (2) increasing security presence (human or CCTV) near vulnerable return-air grills, (3) directing public access away from return-air grills, and (4) removing furniture and visual obstructions from areas near return air-grills.

7. *Restrict access to building operation systems by outside personnel.* To deter tampering by outside maintenance personnel, a building staff member should escort these individuals throughout their service visit and should visually inspect their work before final acceptance of the service. Alternatively, building owners and managers can ensure the reliability of pre-screened service personnel from a trusted contractor.

8. *Restrict access to building information.* Information on building operations—including mechanical, electrical, vertical transport, fire and life safety, security system plans and schematics, and emergency operations procedures—should be strictly controlled. Such information should be released to authorized personnel only, preferably by the development of an access list and controlled copy numbering.

9. *General building physical security upgrades.* In addition to the security measures for HVAC and other building operations described earlier, physical security upgrades can enhance the overall security of a building. A building or building complex might have security fencing and controlled access points. Some buildings such as museums are, by their very nature, openly accessible to the public. However, even in these buildings, areas such as mechanical rooms need to remain off-limits to unauthorized individuals. Unless the building is regarded as open to the general public, owners and managers should consider

not allowing visitors outside the lobby area without an escort. Layered levels of security access should be considered. For example, entry to a hospital's patient care areas could be less strict than to hospital laboratories, and successively more strict for other areas, such as ventilation control rooms. Physical security is of prime concern in lobby areas.

Ventilation and Filtration

HVAC systems and their components should be evaluated with respect to how they impact vulnerability to the introduction of CBR agents. Relevant issues include the HVAC system controls, the ability of the HVAC system to purge the building, the efficiency of installed filters, the capacity of the system relative to potential filter upgrades, and the significance of uncontrolled leakage into the building. Another consideration is the vulnerability of the HVAC system and components themselves, particularly when the facility is open to the public. For buildings under secure access, interior components may be considered less vulnerable, depending upon the perceived threat and the confidence in the level of security.

*1. *Evaluate HVAC control options.* Many central HVAC systems have energy management and control systems that can regulate airflow and pressures within a building on an emergency response basis. Some modern fire alarm systems may also provide useful capabilities during CBR events. In some cases, the best response option (given sufficient warning) might be to shut off the building's HVAC and exhaust system(s), thus, avoiding the introduction of a CBR agent from outside. In other cases, interior pressure and airflow control may prevent the spread of a CBR agent released in the building and/or ensure the safety of egress pathways. The decision to install emergency HVAC control options should be made in consultation with a qualified HVAC professional that understands the ramifications of various HVAC operating modes on building operation and safety systems.

Depending upon the design and operation of the HVAC system and the nature of the CBR agent release, HVAC control may not be appropriate in all emergency situations. Lobbies, loading docks, and mailrooms might be provided with manually operated exhaust systems, activated by trained personnel to remove contaminants in the event of a known release, exhausting air to an appropriate area. In other instances, manipulation of the HVAC system could minimize the spread of an agent. If an HVAC control plan is pursued, building personnel should be trained to recognize a terrorist attack quickly and to know when to initiate the control measures. For example, emergency egress stairwells should remain pressurized (unless they are known to contain the CBR source). Other areas, such as laboratories, clean rooms, or pressure isolation rooms in hospitals, may need to remain ventilated. All procedures and training associated with the control of the HVAC system should be addressed in the building's emergency response plan.

*2. *Assess filtration.* Increasing filter efficiency is one of the few measures that can be implemented in advance to reduce the consequences of both an interior and exterior release of a particulate CBR agent. However, the decision to increase efficiency should be made cautiously, with a careful understanding of the protective limitations resulting from the upgrade. The filtration needs of a building should be assessed with a view to implementing the highest filtration efficiency that is compatible with the installed HVAC system and its required operating parameters. In general, increased filter efficiency will provide benefits to the indoor environmental quality of the building. However, the increased protection from CBR aerosols will occur only if the filtration efficiency increase applies to the particle size range and physical state of the CBR contaminant. It is important to note that particulate air filters are used for biological and radiological particles and are not effective for gases and vapors typical of chemical attacks. These types of compounds require adsorbent filters (i.e., activated carbon or other sorbent-type media) and result in substantial initial and recurring costs.

Upgrading filtration is not as simple as merely replacing a low-efficiency filter with a higher efficiency one. Typically, higher efficiency filters have a higher pressure loss, which will result in some airflow reduction through the system. The magnitude of the reduction is dependent on the design and capacity of the HVAC system. If the airflow reduction is substantial, it may result in inadequate ventilation, reductions in heating and cooling capacity, or potentially frozen coils. To minimize pressure loss, deep pleated filters or filter banks having a larger nominal inlet area might be feasible alternatives, if space allows. Also, high-pressure losses can sometimes be avoided by using prefilters or more frequent filter change-outs. Pressure loss associated with adsorbent filters can be even greater.

The integrity of the HVAC system's filter rack or frame system has a major impact upon the installed filtration efficiency. Reducing the leakage of unfiltered air around filters, caused by a poor seal between the filter and the frame, may be as important as increasing filter efficiency. If filter bypass proves to be significant, corrective actions will be needed. Some high-efficiency filter systems have better seals and frames constructed to reduce bypass. During an upgrade to higher efficiency filters, the HVAC and filtration systems should be evaluated by a qualified HVAC professional to verify proper performance.

While higher filtration efficiency is encouraged and should provide indoor air quality benefits beyond an increased protection from CBR terrorist events, the overall cost of filtration should be evaluated. Filtration costs include the periodic cost of the filter media, the labor cost to remove and replace filters, and the fan energy cost required to overcome the pressure loss of the filters. While higher efficiency filters tend to have a higher life cycle cost than lower efficiency filters, this is not always the case. With some higher efficiency filter systems, higher acquisition and energy costs can be offset by longer filter life and a reduced labor cost for filter replacements. Also, improved filtration generally keeps heating and cooling coils cleaner and, thus, may reduce energy costs through improvements in heat transfer efficiency. However, when high-efficiency particulate air (HEPA) filters and/or activated carbon adsorbers are used, the overall costs will generally increase substantially.

3. *Ducted and non-ducted return air systems.* Ducted returns offer limited access points to introduce a CBR agent. The return vents can be placed in conspicuous locations, reducing the risk of an agent being secretly introduced into the return system. Non-ducted return air systems commonly use hallways or spaces above dropped ceilings as a return-air path or plenum. CBR agents introduced at any location above the dropped ceiling in a ceiling plenum return system will most likely migrate back to the HVAC unit and, without highly efficient filtration for the particular agent, redistribute to occupied areas. Buildings should be designed to minimize mixing between air-handling zones, which can be partially accomplished by limiting shared returns. Where ducted returns are not feasible or warranted, hold-down clips may be used for accessible areas of dropped ceilings that serve as the return plenum. This issue is closely related to the isolation of lobbies and mailrooms, as shared returns are a common way for contaminants from these areas to disperse into the rest of the building. These modifications may be more feasible for new building construction or those undergoing major renovation.

4. *Low-leakage, fast-acting dampers.* Rapid response, such as shutting down an HVAC system, may also involve closing various

dampers, especially those controlling the flow of outdoor air (in the event of an exterior CBR release). When the HVAC system is turned off, the building pressure compared to outdoors may still be negative, drawing outdoor air into the building via many leakage pathways, including the HVAC system. Consideration should be given to installing low leakage dampers to minimize this flow pathway. Damper leakage ratings are available as part of the manufacturer's specifications and range from ultra-low to normal categories. Assuming that you have some warning prior to a direct CBR release, the speed with which these dampers respond to a "close" instruction can also be important. From a protective standpoint, dampers that respond quickly are preferred over dampers that might take 30 seconds or more to respond.

5. *Building air tightness.* Significant quantities of air can enter a building by means of infiltration through unintentional leakage paths in the building envelope. Such leakage is of more concern for an exterior CBR release at some distance from a building, such as a large-scale attack, than for a directed terrorist act. The reduction of air leakage is a matter of tight building construction in combination with building pressurization. While building pressurization may be a valuable CBR-protection strategy in any building, it is much more likely to be effective in a tight building. However, to be effective, filtration of building supply air must be appropriate for the CBR agent introduced. Although increasing the air tightness of an existing building can be more challenging than during new construction, it should still be seriously considered.

Maintenance, Administration, and Training

Maintenance of ventilation systems and training of staff are critical for controlling exposure to airborne contaminants, such as CBR agents.

*1. Emergency plans, policies, and procedures. All buildings should have current emergency plans to address fire, weather, and other types of emergencies. In light of past U.S. experiences with anthrax and similar threats, these plans should be updated to consider CBR attack scenarios and the associated procedures for communicating instructions to building occupants, identifying suitable shelter-in-place areas (if they exist), identifying appropriate use and selection of personal protective equipment (i.e., clothing, gloves, respirators) and directing emergency evacuations. Individuals developing emergency plans and procedures should recognize that there are fundamental differences between chemical, biological, and radiological agents. In general, chemical agents will show a rapid onset of symptoms, while the response to biological and radiological agents will be delayed.[c] Issues such as designated areas and procedures for chemical storage, HVAC control or shutdown, and communication with building occupants and emergency responders, should all be addressed. The plans should be as comprehensive as possible, but, as described earlier, protected by limited and controlled access. When appropriately designed, these plans, policies, and procedures can have a major impact upon occupant survivability in the event of a CBR release. Staff training, particularly for those with specific responsibilities during an event, is essential and should cover both internal and external events. Holding regularly scheduled practice drills, similar to the common fire drill, allows for plan testing, as well as occupant and key staff rehearsal of the plan, and increases the likelihood for success in an actual event. For protection systems in which HVAC control is done via the energy management and control system, emergency procedures should be exercised periodically to ascertain that the various control options work (and continue to work) as planned.

---

[c] *Note*: Additional information on CBR agents may be found via the references at the end of this document.

*2. *HVAC Maintenance staff training.* Periodic training of HVAC maintenance staff in system operation and maintenance should be conducted. This training should include the procedures to be followed in the event of a suspected CBR agent release. Training should also cover health and safety aspects for maintenance personnel, as well as the potential health consequences to occupants of poorly performing systems. Development of current, accurate HVAC diagrams and HVAC system labeling protocols should be addressed. These documents can be of great value in the event of a CBR release.

*3. *Preventive maintenance and procedures.* Procedures and preventive maintenance schedules should be implemented for cleaning and maintaining ventilation system components. Replacement filters, parts, and so forth should be obtained from known manufacturers and examined prior to installation. It is important that ventilation systems be maintained and cleaned according to the manufacturer's specifications. To do this requires information on HVAC system performance, flow rates, damper modulation and closure, sensor calibration, filter pressure loss, filter leakage, and filter change-out recommendations. These steps are critical to ensure that protection and mitigation systems, such as particulate filtration, operate as intended.

Conclusions

Reducing a building's vulnerability to an airborne chemical, biological, or radiological attack requires a comprehensive approach. Decisions concerning which protective measures to implement should be based upon the threat profile and a security assessment of the building and its occupants. While physical security is the first layer of defense, other issues must also be addressed. Preventing possible terrorist access to outdoor air intakes and mechanical rooms and developing CBR-contingent emergency response plans should be addressed as soon as possible. Additional measures can provide further protection. A building security assessment should be done to determine the necessity of additional measures. Some items, such as improved maintenance and HVAC system controls, may also provide a payback in operating costs and/or improved building air quality. As new building designs or modifications are considered, designers should consider that practical CBR sensors may soon become available. Building system design features that are capable of incorporating this rapidly evolving technology will most likely offer a greater level of protection.

While it is not possible to completely eliminate the risk of a CBR terrorist attack, several measures can be taken to reduce the likelihood and consequences of such an attack. Many of the recommendations presented here are ones that can be implemented reasonably quickly and cost effectively. Many are applicable to both new construction and existing buildings, although some may be more feasible than others. Building owners and managers should assess buildings by looking first for those items that are most vulnerable and can be addressed easily. Additional measures should be implemented as feasible. The goals are to make your building an unattractive target for a CBR attack and to maximize occupant protection in the event that such an attack occurs.

For Additional Information

Several organizations have developed guidance to assist building owners and operators in addressing issues related to building security and CBR terrorist attacks. Many other organizations have guidance that addresses security needs and disaster response plans for events such as fire, natural disasters, and bomb threats. While this latter guidance may not specifically address the terrorist threat to HVAC systems, readers may find portions of the information beneficial in establishing their own building's emergency response plans.

The following list is not all-inclusive. Available guidance is updated regularly as additional organizations and evolving technologies identify new protective recommendations.

Organization	Reference or Link	Description
National Institute for Occupational Safety and Health (NIOSH)	http://www.cdc.gov/NIOSH/homepage.HTML	Health and Safety guidance, publications, and training information.
Centers for Disease Control and Prevention (CDC)	http://www.cdc.gov/	Health guidance for CBR agents.
U.S. Army Corps of Engineers (USACE)	http://BuildingProtection.sbccom.army.mil/basic/ *Protecting Buildings and Their Occupants from Airborne Hazards*	Document presents a variety of ways to protect building occupants from airborne hazards.
U.S. Environmental Protection Agency (EPA)	http://www.epa.gov/iaq/largebldgs/baqtoc.html *Building Air Quality: A Guide for Building Owners and Facility Managers*	Provides procedures and checklists for developing a building profile and performing preventive maintenance in commercial buildings.
	http://www.epa.gov/iaq/schools/*Indoor Air Quality (IAQ) Tools for Schools Kit*	Provides procedures and checklists for developing a building profile and performing preventive maintenance in schools.
U.S. General Services Administration (GSA)	http://hydra.gsa.gov/pbs/pc/facilitiesstandards/*Facility Standards for the Public Buildings Service (PBS-P100)*	Establishes design standards and criteria for new buildings, major and minor alterations, and work in historic structures for the Public Building Service. Also provides information on conducting building security assessments.
Central Intelligence Agency	http://www.cia.gov/cia/publications/cbr_handbook/cbr-book.htm *Chemical, Biological, Radiological Incident Handbook*	Unclassified document describing potential CBR events, recognizing potential CBR events, differences between agents, common symptoms, and information for making preliminary assessments when a CBR release is suspected.
Lawrence Berkeley National Laboratory	http://securebuildings.lbl.gov	Web site with advice for safeguarding buildings against chemical or biological attack.
Federal Facilities Council (FFC)	http://www4.nas.edu/cets/ffc.nsf/web/chemical_and_biological_threats_to_buildings?OpenDocument	Online notes and presentations from FFC seminar on chemical and biological threats to buildings.

Organization	URL / Resource	Description
American Institute of Architects (AIA)	http://www.aia.org *Building Security Through Design*	An AIA resource center that offers architects and others, up-to-date, in-depth material on building security issues.
American Society of Heating Refrigerating and Air-Conditioning Engineers (ASHRAE)	http://www.ashrae.org/ *Risk Management Guidance for Health and Safety under Extraordinary Incidents*	Draft report provides recommendations for owners and managers of existing buildings.
American Society for Industrial Security	http://www.asisonline.org/	Locates security specialists and provides the *Crises Response Resources* link to find information related to terrorism and building security.
Building Owners and Managers Association	http://www.boma.org/emergency/	Information on emergency planning and security assessments.
	http://www.boma.org/pubs/bomapmp.htm *How to Design and Manage Your Preventive Maintenance Program*	Recommendations to effectively manage and maintain a building's systems. (Information for purchasing only.)
International Facility Management Association (IFMA)	http://www.ifma.org/	Information on security-related training courses.
National Institute of Building Sciences (NIBS)	www.wbdg.org *Whole Building Design Guide*	Internet site featuring security-related design information.

Appendix C.A
Interagency Workgroup on Building Air Protection

Kenneth Stroech, Chair	White House Office of Homeland Security
William Blewett	U.S. Army
Ed Dailide	Naval Facilities Engineering Command
Gary S. Earnest	National Institute for Occupational Safety and Health
Elissa Feldman	U.S. Environmental Protection Agency
John Girman	U.S. Environmental Protection Agency
George Glavis	U.S. Department of State
Michael G. Gressel	National Institute for Occupational Safety and Health
Robert Kehlet	Defense Threat Reduction Agency
Kenneth R. Mead	National Institute for Occupational Safety and Health
Rudy Perkey	Naval Facilities Engineering Command
Andrew Persily	National Institute of Standards and Technology
Laurence D. Reed	National Institute for Occupational Safety and Health
Rich Sextro	Lawrence Berkeley National Laboratory
Mary Smith	U.S. Environmental Protection Agency
Patrick F. Spahn	U.S. Department of State
John Talbott	U.S. Department of Energy
John R. Thompson, Jr.	Defense Advanced Research Projects Agency
Robert Thompson	U.S. Environmental Protection Agency
Jeanne Trelogan	U.S. General Services Administration
Debra Yap	U.S. General Services Administration

Appendix C.B
Research Team on Building Vulnerabilities

Team Leader
Laurence D. Reed

Team Members
Centers for Disease Control and Prevention-NIOSH:

James S. Bennett, Ph.D.	Kenneth F. Martinez
Andrew Cecala	Kenneth R. Mead
Keith Crouch, Ph.D.	R. Leroy Mickelsen
Kevin Dunn	Ernest Moyer, Ph.D.
Gary S. Earnest, Ph.D.	John W. Sheehy, Ph.D.
Michael G. Gressel, Ph.D.	Anthony Zimmer, Ph.D.
Paul A. Jensen, Ph.D.	

Sandia National Laboratories:
Richard Griffith, Ph.D.

Agency for Toxic Substances and Disease Registry:
Robert Knowles

Appendix D   Develop a Mitigation Plan (FEMA)

Overview

The hazard identification and risk assessment described in Phase 2 will determine what facilities and systems in your jurisdiction are at highest risk. In Step 1 of Phase 3, you will develop goals and objectives for the protection of these assets to prevent or avoid an attack and to reduce losses in the event an attack occurs. Step 2 discusses the issues unique to identifying and prioritizing mitigation actions for terrorism and technological hazards. These actions primarily focus on creating a resilient, protective built environment. Step 3 highlights special considerations in developing an implementation strategy. Step 4 summarizes the important components to include in your terrorism and technological hazard mitigation plan. Cross-references are made to *Developing the Mitigation Plan: Identifying Mitigation Actions and Implementation Strategies* (FEMA 386-3).

> **Goals** are general guidelines that identify what you want to achieve. They are usually long-term in nature.
>
> **Objectives** define measurable strategies or implementation steps to attain a goal. They are shorter in range and more specific than goals.

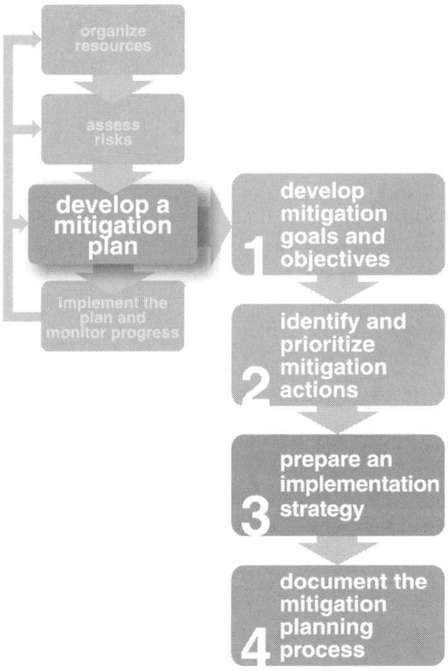

Step 1: Develop Mitigation Goals and Objectives

The process for developing the mitigation goals and objectives that will shape your implementation strategy is the same whether you are addressing natural or manmade hazards. As discussed in *Developing the Mitigation Plan: Identifying Mitigation Actions and Implementation Strategies* (FEMA 386-3), you will review the risk assessment and loss estimation findings to identify assets at greatest risk. Manmade risk information should be combined with the findings for natural hazards to create a comprehensive picture of your community or state's vulnerabilities to both natural and manmade hazards. Your terrorism and technological disaster mitigation goals, as with those for natural disasters, should strive to protect lives and property, reduce the costs of disaster response, and minimize disruption to the community or state following a disaster. See *Developing the Mitigation*

Figure D.1

Plan for more details on formulating and prioritizing your goals.

> **Goals and objectives** help determine where efforts and resources should be focused to maximize the effectiveness of mitigation-related activities. Whenever possible, mitigation goals and objectives should be multi-hazard in nature in order to provide the most comprehensive protection to your community or state. In addition to brainstorming, the planning team can identify additional goals and objectives in the following ways:
>
> - **Review existing plans.** Review existing mitigation, comprehensive, and emergency plans, building upon and/or modifying existing initiatives to maximize coordination between plans and minimize conflicts and duplication of effort. To the extent possible, existing plans should be used to address the special problems posed by technological and other manmade hazards rather than generating new, stand-alone documents.
> - **Solicit public opinions.** Including the community in identifying goals and objectives will help ensure buy-in when mitigation actions are selected, and both the media and the Internet can be valuable communication tools. There are a number of methods for gauging public opinion:
>   - Establish working groups or advisory committees
>   - Hold town hall meetings
>   - Administer surveys
>   - Hold facilitated meetings with community representatives
>
> While all of these methods can be effective on their own, it may be advantageous to combine multiple strategies, such as surveys and town hall meetings, in order to obtain the advantages of both a structured questionnaire as well as a free-flowing discussion.

> **Sample Mitigation Goals and Objectives for Terrorism and Technological Hazard Mitigation**
>
> **Goal 1: Reduce the community's risk of exposure to hazardous materials.**
>
> Objective 1: Install security measures at the anhydrous ammonia transfer and storage facility.
> Objective 2: Increase the level of security of the facility using landscape design, lighting, and vehicle barriers.
> Objective 3: Assess feasibility of hardening product storage and handling infrastructures.
>
> **Goal 2: Protect the community's water supply.**
>
> Objective 1: Install security measures at the city water treatment plant.
> Objective 2: Secure all remote pump facilities.
> Objective 3: Monitor for radiological, biological, and chemical contaminants.
>
> **Goal 3: Ensure that the city government has reliable communications systems.**
>
> Objective 1: Update the telecommunications capabilities of city government offices.
> Objective 2: Create redundant/backup capability for landline telephone system.
> Objective 3: Develop off-site backup of information technology systems.
>
> **Goal 4: Reduce risk to critical government facilities.**
>
> Objective 1: Increase vehicle standoff distance from the Emergency Operations Center.
> Objective 2: Restrict parking and vehicle access to the underground parking garage at City Hall.

Step 2: Identify and Prioritize Mitigation Actions

Once you have developed goals and objectives for mitigation, you should identify specific actions to help you achieve them. As you consider mitigation options, keep in mind that attacks and accidents are functions of human activity, and the risk of such events is a characteristic of the target itself rather than of its geographic location. Clearly, there are areas in most communities where the chances of an attack or accident are considerably different from other parts of the jurisdiction—higher at industrial parks and critical facilities than in suburban residential neighborhoods, for example—but there is no such thing as a definable "terrorism zone" or "accident district" in the same sense as there are identifiable floodplains and seismic fault lines. Thus, it is not effective to protect people, buildings, and systems from manmade hazards by simply relocating them as one could for some natural disasters.

Rather than removing potential victims from the hazard, then, mitigation strategies for manmade hazards focus primarily on creating a built environment that is difficult to attack, resilient to the consequences of an attack or accident, and protective of its occupants should an incident occur. This can be accomplished through target hardening and other actions. Additional actions such as public awareness and education initiatives are not discussed in this guide but should be considered when formulating your mitigation strategy.

Target hardening actions range from small-scale projects, such as installing security fencing around an HVAC system's air intake, to community-wide initiatives, such as altering land use patterns to require buffer zones around campuses of high-risk buildings. Also, while some actions are highly specific in nature and function, others can meet multiple goals. For example, designing a building to resist the force of a bomb blast will also offer protection from windstorms, and requiring buffer zones around critical facilities can help meet open space requirements and protect wetlands. The planning team is encouraged to take advantage of these complementary approaches whenever possible.

Taking Advantage of Existing Processes, Strategies, and Tools

Some actions and techniques used for mitigating natural hazards may also provide protection against manmade hazards, such as:

Earthquake mitigation techniques that provide structural strengthening of buildings may help resist impact/explosion effects of bombs. Examples of such techniques include adding steel moment frames, shear walls, cross bracing, stronger floor systems, walls reinforced with shotcrete/fiber materials, columns reinforced with fiber wraps/steel jackets, tension/shear anchors, vibration dampers, and strengthening or providing additional detailing of the building's connections.

Fire mitigation techniques may help protect facilities against the effects of bombs and incendiary attacks. Examples of such techniques include improved sprinkler systems, increased use of fireproofing and/or fire-resistant materials, redundant water supplies for fire protection (day-to-day and alternative), and site set-backs.

High wind mitigation techniques that provide building envelope protection and structural strengthening may also help mitigate against impact/explosion effects of bombs. Examples of such techniques include openings using windows with impact-resistant laminated glazing, improving connections and the load path of the building, and adding/reinforcing shear walls.

Terrorism mitigation is becoming an integral part of multi-hazard mitigation, in process and often in practice. Additionally, an action that addresses the fullest possible spectrum of natural and manmade hazards will likely show the most cost-effectiveness.

Target hardening actions draw from a wide variety of disciplines, all of which, as discussed in Phase 1, should be represented on (or at least accessible to) the mitigation planning team. Potential hardening techniques and strategies are numerous, and a listing of every possible action lies beyond the scope of this guidance. The list of potential actions provided below gives an overview of the techniques and strategies available. The Library in Appendix C contains references to many sources of information on these topics. The following section will discuss special considerations when evaluating actions to meet your goals and objectives.

> **The planning team** should draw on all available sources of expertise when selecting specific actions, keeping in mind the overall objectives of maximizing opportunities for multi-hazard mitigation; promoting sustainability through choosing socially, economically, and environmentally beneficial solutions; supporting preparedness, response, and recovery; and ensuring cost-effectiveness.

Terrorism and Technological Hazard Mitigation Actions

The list of actions below is by no means exhaustive or definitive; rather, it is intended as a point of departure for identifying potential mitigation techniques and strategies in your community or state.

Site Planning and Landscape Design

- Implement Crime Prevention Through Environmental Design (CPTED)
- Minimize concealment opportunities in landscaping and street furniture, such as hedges, bus shelters, benches, and trash receptacles
- Design grounds and parking facilities for natural surveillance by concentrating pedestrian activity, limiting entrances/exits, and eliminating concealment opportunities
- Separate vehicle and pedestrian traffic
- Implement vehicle and pedestrian access control and inspection at perimeter (ensure ability to regulate flow of people and vehicles one at a time)
- Design site circulation to minimize vehicle speeds and eliminate direct approaches to structures
- Incorporate vehicle barriers such as walls, fences, trenches, ponds/basins, plantings, trees, sculptures, and fountains into site planning and design
- Ensure adequate site lighting
- Design signage for simplicity and clarity
- Locate critical offices away from uncontrolled public areas
- Separate delivery processing facilities from remaining buildings
- Maintain access for emergency responders, including large fire apparatus
- Identify and provide alternate water supplies for fire suppression
- Eliminate potential site access through utility tunnels, corridors, manholes, etc.

Architectural and Interior Space Planning

- Collocate/combine staff and visitor entrances; minimize queuing in unprotected areas
- Incorporate employee and visitor screening areas into planning and design
- Minimize device concealment opportunities such as mailboxes and trash receptacles outside screened areas
- Prohibit retail activities in non-secured areas
- Do not locate toilets and service spaces in non-secured areas
- Locate critical assets (people, activities, systems) away from entrances, vehicle circulation and parking, and loading and maintenance areas

- Separate high-risk and low-risk activities
- Separate high-risk activities from areas accessible to the public
- Separate visitor activities from daily activities
- Separate building utilities from service docks, and harden utilities
- Locate delivery and mail processing facilities remotely or at exterior of building; prevent vehicles from driving into or under building
- Establish areas of refuge; ensure that egress pathways are hardened and discharge into safe areas
- Locate emergency stairwells and systems away from high-risk areas
- Restrict roof access
- Ensure that walls, doors, windows, ceilings, and floors can resist forced entry
- Provide fire- and blast-resistant separation for sprinkler/standpipe interior controls (risers) and key fire alarm system components
- Use visually open (impact-resistant, laminated glass) stair towers and elevators in parking facilities
- Design finishes and signage for visual simplicity

Structural Engineering

- Create blast-resistant exterior envelope
- Ensure that structural elements can resist blast loads and progressive collapse
- Install blast-resistant exterior window systems (frames, security films, and blast curtains)
- Ensure that other openings (vents, etc.) are secure and blast-resistant
- Ensure that mailrooms are secure and blast-resistant
- Enclose critical building components within hardened walls, floors, and ceilings

Mechanical Engineering

- Locate utility and ventilation systems away from entrances, vehicle circulation and parking, and loading and maintenance areas
- Protect utility lifelines (water, power, communications, etc.) by concealing, burying, or encasing
- Locate air intakes on roof or as high as possible; if not elevated, secure within CPTED-compliant fencing or enclosure
- Use motorized dampers to close air intakes when not operational
- Locate roof-mounted equipment away from building perimeter
- Ensure that stairways maintain positive pressure
- Provide redundant utility and ventilation systems
- Provide filtration of intake air
- Provide secure alternate drinking water supply

Electrical Engineering

- Locate utility systems and lifelines away from entrances, vehicle circulation and parking, and loading and maintenance areas
- Implement separate emergency and normal power systems; ensure that backup power systems are periodically tested under load
- Locate primary and backup fuel supplies away from entrances, vehicle circulation and parking, and loading and maintenance areas
- Secure primary and backup fuel supply areas
- Install exterior connection for emergency power
- Install adequate site lighting
- Maintain stairway and exit sign lighting
- Provide redundant telephone service
- Ensure that critical systems are not collocated in conduits, panels, or risers
- Use closed-circuit television (CCTV) security system

Fire Protection Engineering

- Ensure compliance with codes and standards, including installation of up-to-date fire alarm and suppression systems
- Locate fire protection water supply system critical components away from entrances, vehicle circulation and parking, and loading and maintenance areas
- Identify/establish secondary fire protection water supply
- Install redundant fire water pumps (e.g., one electric, one diesel); locate apart from each other
- Ensure adequate, redundant sprinkler and standpipe connections
- Install fire hydrant and water supply connections near sprinkler/standpipe connections
- Supervise or secure standpipes, water supply control valves, and other system components
- Implement fire detection and communication systems
- Implement redundant off-premises fire alarm reporting
- Locate critical documents and control systems in a secure yet accessible place
- Provide keybox near critical entrances for secure fire access
- Provide fire- and blast-resistant fire command center
- Locate hazardous materials storage, use, and handling away from other activities
- Implement smoke control systems
- Install fire dampers at fire barriers
- Maintain access to fire hydrants
- Maintain fire wall and fire door integrity
- Develop and maintain comprehensive pre-incident and recovery plans
- Implement guard and employee training
- Conduct regular evacuation and security drills
- Regularly evaluate fire protection equipment readiness/adequacy

Security

- Develop backup control center capabilities
- Secure electrical utility closets, mechanical rooms, and telephone closets
- Do not collocate security system wiring with electrical and other service systems
- Implement elevator recall capability and elevator emergency message capability
- Implement intrusion detection systems; provide 24-hour off-site monitoring
- Implement and monitor interior boundary penetration sensors
- Implement color closed-circuit television (CCTV) security system with recording capability
- Install call boxes and duress alarms
- Install public and employee screening systems (metal detectors, x-ray machines, or search stations)

Parking

- Minimize off-site parking on adjacent streets/lots and along perimeter
- Control all on-site parking with ID checks, security personnel, and access systems
- Separate employee and visitor parking
- Eliminate internal building parking
- Ensure natural surveillance by concentrating pedestrian activity, limiting entrances/exits, and eliminating concealment opportunities
- Use transparent/non-opaque walls whenever possible
- Prevent pedestrian access to parking areas other than via established entrances

Prioritize Mitigation Actions

When prioritizing natural hazard mitigation actions, a benefit-cost analysis is generally conducted for each proposed action. Several factors are considered, including:

- Cost(s) of the mitigation action;
- Dollar value of risk reduction (i.e., loss of life, structure, content, and function) each time the hazard occurs (discussed in detail in *Understanding Your Risks: Identifying Hazards and Estimating Losses* [FEMA 386-2]);
- Frequency with which the benefits of the action will be realized (i.e., frequency of hazard occurrence); and
- Time value of money (i.e., the fact that benefits and costs in the future are worth less than benefits and costs today).

These factors are then combined by calculating the net present value of aggregate future benefits and costs over the life span of the action. For more details, see *Using Benefit-Cost Analysis in Mitigation Planning* (FEMA 386-5).

> **While many benefits can be achieved** through implementing mitigation actions, planners should be sensitive to potential negative impacts as well. For example, altering traffic patterns may increase commute times and distances, and reducing on-street parking may impact retail activity. Such considerations can be pivotal in determining the feasibility, viability, and potential for success of mitigation planning initiatives.

Three challenges arise when applying this benefit-cost framework to terrorism and technological disaster mitigation actions: (1) the probability of an attack or frequency of the hazard occurrence is not known; (2) the deterrence rate may not be known; and (3) the lifespan of the action may be difficult to quantify.

First, the frequency factor is much more complex in the case of manmade hazards than for natural hazards. While it is possible to estimate how often many natural disasters will occur (for example, a structure located in the 100-year floodplain is considered to have a 1 percent chance of being flooded in any given year), it is very difficult to quantify the likelihood of a terrorist attack or technological disaster. Quantitative methods to estimate these probabilities are being developed but have not yet been refined to the point where they can be used to determine incident probability on a facility-by-facility basis. Therefore, the planning team must use a qualitative approach based on threat and vulnerability considerations to estimate the relative likelihood of an attack or accident rather than the precise frequency. Such an approach is necessarily subjective but can be combined with quantitative estimates of cost-effectiveness (the cost of an action compared to the value of the lives and property it saves in a worst-case scenario) to help illustrate the overall risk reduction achieved by a particular mitigation action.

> **It is possible to determine** fairly accurately how effective mitigation efforts will be in preventing damages from a given type of attack. The performance of many security and mitigation actions can be modeled using established engineering techniques. For example, structural engineers can determine how a hardening action will protect a building's envelope. Naturally, the effectiveness of actions that rely on personnel or complex hardware can be more difficult to ascertain. For example, what is the probability that a security guard will fall asleep or that lightning will disable a perimeter sensor system?

Second, the deterrence or preventative value of an action cannot be calculated if the number of incidents it averts is not known. Deterrence in the case of terrorism may also have a secondary impact in that once a potential target is hardened, a terrorist may turn to a less protected facility—changing the likelihood of an attack for both targets.

Third, the lifespan of a mitigation action presents another problem when carrying out a benefit-cost analysis for terrorism and technological hazards. Future benefits are generally calculated for a natural hazard mitigation action in part by estimating the number of times the action will perform successfully over the course of its useful life. However, some protective actions may be damaged or destroyed in a single manmade attack or accident. For example, blast-resistant window film may have performed to 100% effectiveness by preventing injuries from flying glass, but it may still need replacement after one "use." Other actions, such as a building setback, cannot be "destroyed" or "used up" per se. This is in contrast to many natural hazard mitigation actions, where the effectiveness and life span of a structural retrofit or land use policy are easily understood and their value over time quantifiable.

Step 3: Prepare an Implementation Strategy

As stated in the Foreword, this how-to guide assumes that your community or state is engaged in a natural hazards mitigation planning process and is intended to serve as a supplemental resource to help you address the unique risks associated with terrorism and technological hazards. If you have incorporated terrorism and technological hazards into a well-managed process, the implementation strategies and tools you use should enable you to effectively reduce your community or state's vulnerability to manmade disasters as well. *Developing the Mitigation Plan* (FEMA 386-3) provides more details on preparing an implementation strategy.

Step 4: Document the Mitigation Planning Process

The mitigation plan for manmade hazards will be based on the risk assessment conducted in Phase 2 and will include a comprehensive strategy to address the mitigation priorities developed in Phase 3, Step 2. This information, which should be integrated into the natural hazard mitigation plan, should include:

> **Ideally, terrorism and technological hazards will be incorporated into your existing mitigation plan;** a single comprehensive plan is generally easier to manage and implement than a collection of stand-alone documents. However, some information may be of such high sensitivity that it should not be included in publicly available mitigation planning documents. Examples of such information include vulnerability studies of critical infrastructure and data on security plans and systems. This material should be treated as an addendum to the mitigation plan so that it is still part of the plan, but access to it can be controlled. For guidance on protecting sensitive information, see Phase 4, Consideration 1, Community Interest and Information Sensitivity.

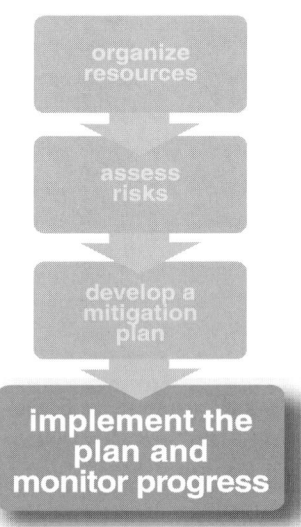

Figure D.2 Phase 4.

- A summary of the planning process, including the sequence of actions taken and a list of the team members and stakeholders who participated;
- The results of the risk assessment and loss estimation;
- Mitigation goals and objectives aimed at reducing or avoiding the effects of manmade hazards;
- Mitigation actions that will help the community or state accomplish the established goals and objectives; and
- Implementation strategies that detail how the mitigation actions will be implemented and administered.

The hazard mitigation plan should serve as the focal point and basis for mitigation decisions for *all* hazards—natural and manmade. As such, it should be written so that anyone who reads it can gain an understanding of current and future hazards and risks as well as the community's or state's intended solutions to those problems.

Appendix E Medical Examiner/Coroner Guide For Mass Fatality Management of Chemically Contaminated Remains

DEPARTMENT OF JUSTICE, OFFICE OF JUSTICE PROGRAMS, OFFICE OF STATE & LOCAL DOMESTIC PREPAREDNESS
DEPARTMENT OF DEFENSE, US ARMY SOLDIER AND BIOLOGICAL CHEMICAL COMMAND, IMPROVED RESPONSE PROGRAM

The Chief Medical Examiner/Coroner (CME) role is to create an infrastructure that can process a large number of contaminated remains, as well as accommodate integrating supporting assets into the response effort (Figure E.1).

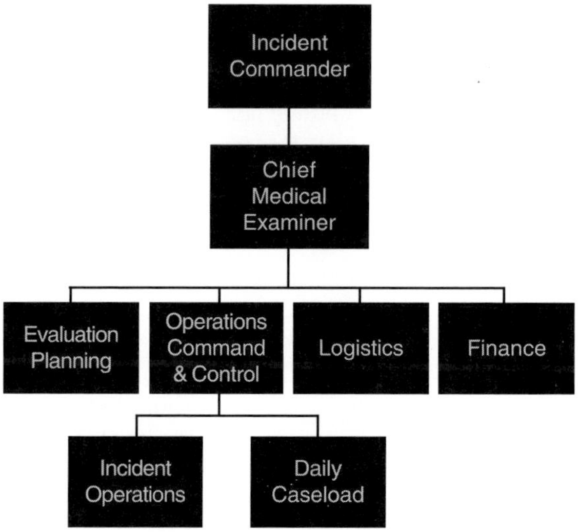

Figure E.1 Mass Fatality Incident Command.

The Emergency Manager (EM) role is to provide coordination between the Medical Examiner/Coroner (ME/C) and county, state, and federal assets to support the Me/C in processing remains in a Mass Fatality Incident (MFI).

Managing the Incident Site

1. **Obtain Information from Incident Commander (IC).**
   - Type of incident and possible hazards.
   - Type of chemical agent.
   - Estimated number of remains.
   - Location of scene and accessibility to remains.
   - Location of incident command post.
2. **Form a team to evaluate the specific incident.**
   - Form an evaluation team with Medical Examiner (ME/C), Hazmat technicians, Law Enforcement and other relevant agencies and prepare to enter the scene.
   - Check required level of Personal Protective Equipment (PPE). ME/C should have two 2-person groups (primary/backup) that can operate in Level A PPE.

- During evaluation:
  - Determine issues (e.g., fragmentation, difficult excavation).
  - Take initial pictures of site.
  - Determine total number of remains and their location.
  - Determine initial number of cases for autopsy.
3. **Plan incident specific operations with appropriate agencies** (e.g., Law Enforcement, Disaster Mortuary Operational Response Team (DMORT), Emergency Manager, and Department of Public Health)
   - Coordinate security requirements for remains processing with Incident Commander.
   - Determine morgue requirements and location: Holding Morgue and Temporary Morgue.
     - Try to co-locate Mass Fatality Management functions in close proximity to one another.
   - Determine decontamination solvents and safe handling procedures based on the specific agent.
   - Establish criteria for autopsy based on ME/C capability and Law Enforcement evidence requirements.
   - Determine chemical monitoring method and procedures, monitoring location and who will perform the monitoring.
     - To obtain accurate chemical vapor concentration reading, monitor bodies at the same temperature that they will be processed.
   - Create infrastructure to process remains (see processing flow of contaminated remains diagram on the back of this guide).
     - Establish who, what, when, where, and how for each function of Remains Processing.
     - Personnel must continue to wear PPE until remains are verified clean by chemical agent monitoring.
   - Evaluate requirements for embalming based on incident circumstances.
   - Establish effective communications between Holding Morgue, Temporary Morgue, Family Assistance Center (FAC), and the ME/C Headquarters.
   - Avoid 24-hour operations when possible.
4. **Assemble necessary resources**
   - See Resource Management.

Resource Management

1. **Personnel.**
   - Determine and assemble personnel who can operate in PPE and assist in the response effort.
   - Determine and assign responsible jurisdiction's ME/C personnel to supervisory positions.
   - Form teams with local ME/C and law enforcement for each function.
   - Determine if additional non-ME/C personnel are needed and assign task to each.
   - Establish shifts/breaks with PPE limitations in mind.
   - Coordinate water/hydration stations.
   - Establish support for ME/C staff (e.g., Critical Incident Stress Management (CISM)).
2. **Assemble other agencies according to established plan.**
   - Local agencies: HazMat teams, funeral home directors, surrounding ME/Cs, local forensic labs, public health department, etc.
   - State agencies: Department of Environment, National Guard, public health department.
   - Federal agencies: Disaster Mortuary Operational Response Team (DMORT), Federal Emergency Management Agency (FEMA).
   - Military agencies: Joint Task Force—Civil Support.
   - Volunteer agencies: American Red Cross (ARC).
3. **Assemble equipment according to established plan.**
   - Appropriate level of PPE for personnel.
   - Waterproof durable tracking tool.

- Decontamination line/equipment for Holding and Temporary Morgues.
- Refrigerated trucks for temporary storage/transportation.
- Ventilation fans.
- Storage containers for personal effects.
- Tents/structure to keep remains from public view.
- Embalming station to include final rinse station (based on incident specific decision).
- Additional remains pouches and duct tape.
- Additional evidence collection containers (e.g., new paint cans).

Remains Processing

1. **Recovery.**
   - Determine who will perform the recovery of remains.
   - Determine and assign team leaders and members as per plan.
     - Assign tasks to each agency assisting in the recovery.
     - Determine what order personnel will enter scene to perform tasks, between the ME/C and Law Enforcement.
     - Use waterproof durable tracking/triage tag for remains and personal effects.
   - Triage remains—autopsy or external examination.
   - Take photographs of remains (i.e., where they were found) to facilitate identification and evidence collection.
   - Consider establishing temporary cold storage if the holding morgue is not able to process remains quickly.

2. **Holding Morgue.**
   - Establish private area at the incident site to perform.
     - Evidence collection.
     - Initial external evaluation.
     - Initial ID check.
     - Removal and tagging of personal effects—separate into durable and non-durable items.
   - Determine:
     - If law enforcement is needed to help identify evidence.
     - If ME/C needs to perform additional procedures as part of the external evaluation (e.g., chemical agent body swab, clothing samples).
   - Obtain:
     - Refrigeration storage units/vehicles based on situation.
     - Bulk storage for personal effects (e.g., 55-gallon drums).
     - New/unused paint cans to store evidence.
   - Establish area to perform decontamination.
     - Water and bleach/detergents for decon (Figure E.2).
     - Can incorporate detailed decon and monitoring remains to verify clean.
     - Mitigate contaminated water run-off.
     - Use double remains pouches—first sealed with duct tape.

3. **Transportation and Storage.**
   - Obtain refrigerated vehicles (e.g., trucks or railroad cars).
     - Do not stack remains (use shelving units).
     - Do not place remains higher than waist level of handlers.
   - Use of available storage facility in accordance with established plan.

4. **Morgue Operations.**
   - Determine if all morgue operations can be centralized in one location or if it must be decentralized into several smaller locations.
   - Establish morgue flow.
     - Perform detailed decontamination and monitoring if remains are not previously verified clean.
     - Perform autopsy on designated remains.
     - Perform external examination on all remains.
     - Perform identification procedures.
     - If embalming remains, perform final rinse after embalming procedures.

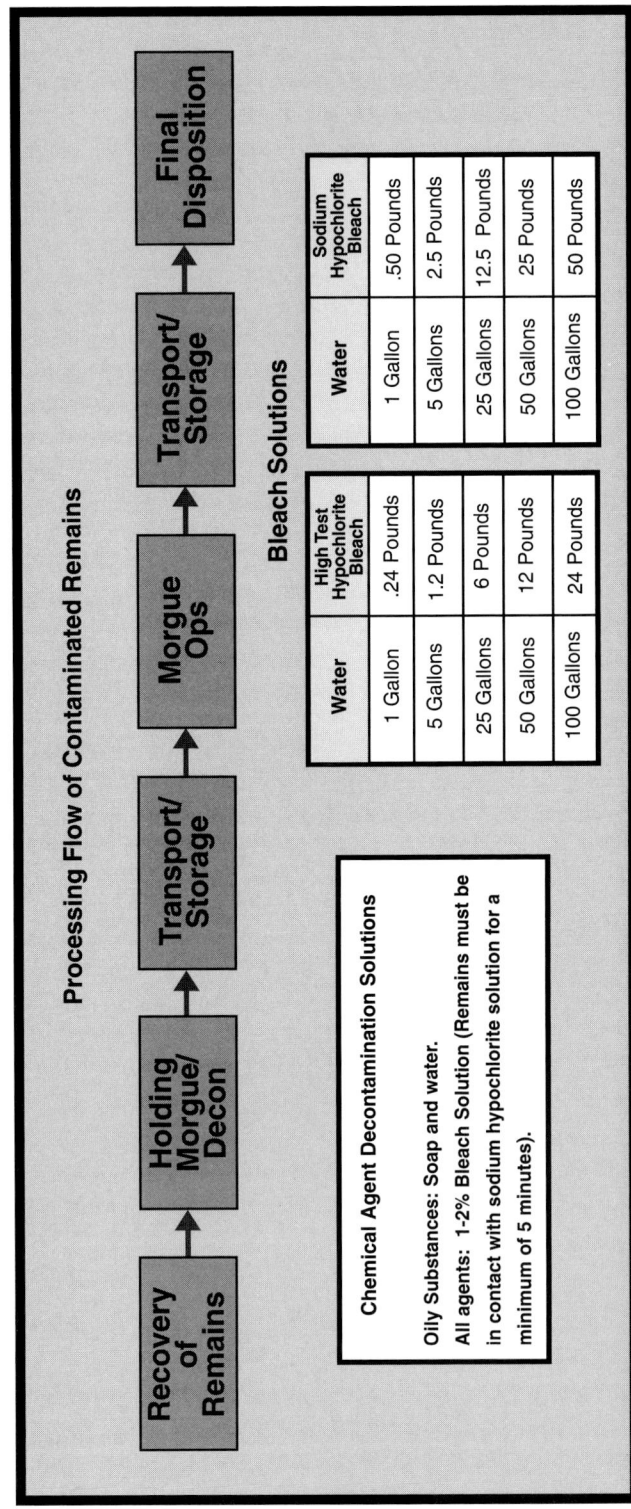

Figure E.2 Processing Flow of Contaminated Remains.

5. **Final Disposition.**
   - Determine location for storage until final disposition.
   - Determine if a public health hazard exists.
   - Return of remains to family:
     - Traditional burial.
     - Sealed casket burial.
     - Voluntary cremation.
   - Government sponsored disposition.
     - Government burial.
     - Cremation.

Additional Coordination

1. **Participate in establishing the Family Assistance Center (FAC).**
   - Convey FAC requirements to the Emergency Manager:
     - Determine specific role of the ME/C at the FAC.
     - Determine who will oversee FAC (e.g., Public Health, American Red Cross).
     - Hotline/help-line for notification and identification process.
     - Location should be in reasonable proximity to Temporary Morgue.
     - Coordinate information dissemination to family and Public Information Officer (PIO).
     - Need for multiple religious leader support.
     - Address if and when personal effects may be released.

2. **Maintain managing the daily caseload.**
   - Add additional shifts to handle incident remains so that original staff can focus on daily caseload.
   - Keep incident and daily caseloads separate.

3. **Establish security for all aspects of the Mass Fatality Incident.**
   - To include all aspects of the incident operation, the daily caseload and the FAC.

4. **Determine financial issues.**
   - Determine if incident is considered a presidential declared disaster.
   - Track all activities and expenses.

Websites

SBCCOM—www2.sbccom.army.mil/hld
DOJ—www.ojp.usdoj.gov/osldps
Office of Victims of Crime—www.ojp.usdoj.gov/ovc
DMORT—www.dmort.org
National Transportation and Safety Board—www.ntsb.gov

Appendix F Systems and Communications Security During Recovery and Repair

C. WARREN AXELROD

During disasters, when all information systems and communications staff are focused on system recovery and repair, computer and communications facilities and information and network resources are critically vulnerable. Security procedures are often ignored, and security controls are often not in place. This chapter presents guidelines for the data security administrator, who must ensure that security and integrity of data and facilities are not further compromised during the recovery and repair of systems and communications networks.

Many organizations assign resources to primary security controls and contingency planning, but few plan beyond the initial recovery process. As information technology (IT) systems become larger, more dispersed, and increasingly linked together over local area and wide area networks (LANs and WANs) and such public networks as the Internet, they become not only more critical to organizations but also more vulnerable to abuse. The occurrences of abuse and disaster are becoming more frequent and are having greater impact as system size, distribution, and interconnections increase. As a result, secondary backup measures and further protection during the recovery process are becoming more critical as well as more complex. Yet, data security during system backup and disaster recovery is not usually addressed by most corporate contingency plans.

Computer systems and communications networks are most vulnerable to breaches in security during backup and disaster recovery activities, in particular. In addition, standard backup measures, such as creating multiple copies of data, programs, passwords, encryption keys, and procedures, and storing these copies at a second location, expose systems to even greater risk of information leaks and security breaches.

Security systems traditionally focus on controlling access to secured facilities, computer software, data, and communications networks. Very little attention is paid to recovering, repairing, and preventing further damage to the security system itself. In some circumstances, fixing a damaged security system first, thereby preventing continuing damage, may be more important than recovering systems and data that remain vulnerable to further damage. After all, restoring a system and network makes little sense when the source of the initial breach is still active. However, circumstances do exist in which the systems and networks are so critical that they must be restored as quickly as possible despite the risk of subsequent breaches.

In this chapter, both the backup of security systems and security procedures during backup and recovery are discussed.

Security and Recovery Basics

Computers and communications networks can be protected by applying the following six basic security functions: avoidance, deterrence, prevention, detection, recovery, and correction. The first three functions address the need to restrict access and limit the authority to have access; the last three are responses to unauthorized intrusions, abuse, or destruction of assets.

These security functions can be defined as follows:

- *Avoidance*. Removal or elimination of any threat to assets, the protection or removal of threatened assets from actual or potential danger, and not creating surplus vulnerable assets.
- *Deterrence*. Discouragement of action that threatens system security. Publicizing disciplinary actions previously taken or that will be taken if such actions are discovered.
- *Prevention*. Implementation of measures to protect assets from security breaches and from intentional or accidental misuse.
- *Detection*. Implementation of means to recognize potential threats to asset. Monitoring the computer and network environment to determine whether such a threat is imminent, is in process, or has already breached the preventative measures. Detection can include raising an alarm in event of a security breach.
- *Recovery*. Effort to return the system and networks to an operating condition.
- *Correction*. Introduction of new measures or improvement of existing measures to avoid, deter, or to prevent recurrences of security breaches and misuse of or damage to the computer systems and communications networks.

Data security systems should protect the following three major areas of vulnerability: access, misuse, and damage. Each area can be briefly described as follows:

- *Access*. The gaining of entry, physically or electronically, to computer resources, including software, data, the IT facility, or the communications network.
- *Misuse*. The manipulation of computer and network assets in a manner outside of or detrimental to the interests of the organization, whether or not any specific damage resulted.
- *Damage*. The modification or destruction of physical or logical computer and network assets.

In summary, the goal of computer and network security systems is to prevent unauthorized access to IT and communications systems and facilities. If such access does occur, misuse of or damage to the computer and communications assets must be prevented. If, despite such precautions, access is gained and damage occurs, it is necessary to recover the systems and networks from the intrusion and violation of assets and to take action to prevent recurrence.

Control of Access, Misuse, or Damage

Some security functions relate specifically to access control and are directed at preventing unauthorized intrusion. However, misuse and damage can result from a variety of causes, each of which may require different preventative measures and recovery procedures. Misuse or damage can be caused by either intentional misbehavior, negligence, or accident. Based on the six-stage breakdown of security functions previously outlined, Figure F.1 shows which security functions are effective for controlling access and which work to limit misuse and damage.

As shown in Figure F.1, the only security function that can be used to control authorized access is detection. That is, no preventative measures are taken if access is detected and observed to be legitimate. However, for unauthorized access, all available security control should be applied. If unauthorized access is detected, backup security should be implemented to prevent the potential recurrence of similar unauthorized access. As a simple example, if current security access codes, such as passwords, are used by someone not authorized to use the system, the codes should be changed immediately, and authorized users should be informed of the change. If users are responsible for changing their own passwords, they should be notified to make immediate changes.

Appendix F 377

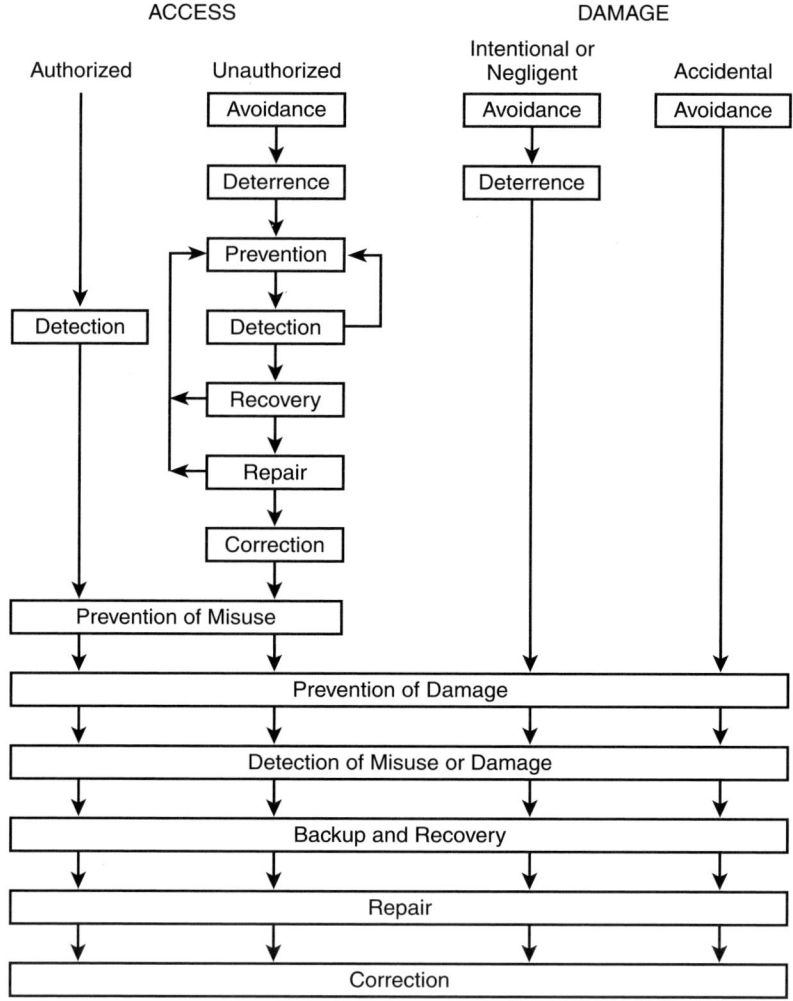

Figure F.1 Measures for controlling access, misuse, and damage.

It should be noted that in Figure F.1 an additional step, repair, has been added to the sequence of security functions. When unauthorized access is detected, after invoking security measures to prevent further similar intrusions, an attempt should be made to recover from the intrusion and to repair or replace damaged or compromised security controls. As an extreme example, if attempted physical access results in an injured guard and a damaged door, it is necessary to replace the guard and repair the door to restore access security. Correction, as shown in Figure F.1, is different from repair in that it involves changing preventative measures to make them more effective rather than fixing existing measures.

Avoidance and deterrence of damage refers to cases in which the damage is caused by an event other than access, such as a fire in the electrical wiring, a burst pipe causing a flood, or an earthquake. Securing a facility against such damage involves such activities as equipment and facility inspections and worker training. To secure a system against intentional damage or accidental damage caused by negligence, all the avoidance measures should be taken. In addition, it is important to deter any actions that might result in physical damage.

Once access has been gained, whether authorized or not, misuse must be prevented. If misuse is not prevented, it must be at least limited so that it does not cause serious damage. Similarly, potential system abusers should be aware of disciplinary actions, and nonconformance to security guidelines should be noted and eliminated. Preventive measures against misuse and damage generally include access restrictions to systems, networks, and facilities, restrictions on potentially damaging activities (e.g., smoking or keeping open flames), the use of non-flammable and waterproof materials, the locating of computers and network equipment in secured areas, and the installation of protective devices (e.g., surge protection devices and automatic cut-off valves). It should be noted that, in cases of system and network recovery, the deadline requirements for returning the systems and networks to operation may dictate that recovery is only feasible if backup systems, networks, or facilities are available.

Security During Backup

Once access, misuse, or damage is detected and the organization begins backup, recovery, and repair, security procedures should be followed to:

- Prevent further access, misuse, and damage due to continuance of the initial intrusion or cause of damage.
- Prevent access, misuse, and damage during the vulnerable backup and recovery processes.
- Prevent access, misuse, and damage during the repair process.
- Ensure that security controls do not unduly hinder the backup, recovery, and repair processes.

Prevention During Recovery

After the detection of unauthorized access, misuse, or damage, the highest priority of the data security administrator should be stemming further violations or abuses of the computer systems and networks, with the proviso that human safety should not be compromised. For example, if a fire is detected, the first consideration should be the evacuation of personnel to safety. Immediately after personnel safety is ensured, an attempt should be made to extinguish the fire, but only if the persons doing so are not at risk or are authorized fire fighters.

In the case of detecting unauthorized access to a system or network, the first step is to disconnect unauthorized users from the system, unless apprehension of the perpetrators would be hindered or more harm would be caused to the organization than by allowing continued access. More harm would be caused, for example, if the entire system or network were shut down to stop further unauthorized access—depriving authorized users from performing their work.

The data security administrator should determine whether prevention of further intrusion and abuse is more harmful than continuation of the adverse practice. Because a decision made under such immediate pressure could easily be the wrong one, the rules of action should be carefully specified in advance and strictly enforced during an event. Because it is frequently during the initial moments of an emergency that decisions are most critical, rehearsals, simulations, and other training techniques are a crucial part of such contingency planning.

Security During Recovery

When the source of abuse has been halted and the situation has been stabilized, recovering the system and facility begins. This may be achieved either on site or at off-site backup facilities.

Physical Access. Because backup and recovery frequently involves non-employees (e.g., fire fighters, messengers, or service engineers) the data security administrator should ensure surveillance of such persons while they are on the premises or handling confidential information. Alternatively, security may be achieved if only authorized persons are allowed access to sensitive areas of information. This may be done by designating emergency personnel in advance. Ironically, emergency surveillance is often conducted by temporarily employing unknown security guards who are unfamiliar with the environment.

Transfer of Data. Transferring confidential, valuable information (e.g., magnetic tapes, reports, or disk packs) to backup sites and returning these media, plus any new information created at the backup site, presents many opportunities for corruption or theft of information. Backup and recovery often necessitate the use of more vulnerable public communications networks, rather than more secure, private data communications networks so that exposures have to be anticipated and the preventative actions taken.

Examples of various approaches to achieving security during backup and recovery are listed in Table F.2 and are discussed in detail in the following sections.

Physical Access Control. Physical access at the primary and backup sites and access to information and materials in transit can be controlled by retaining reliable security guard service. Temporary security services should be selected in advance, and their references should be checked carefully to avoid hurried, reactive decisions. Unreliable guard service can negate many of the security controls of backup and recovery. At the same time, contingency access procedures should be developed at both primary and backup sites and for primary and backup communications network facilities, and authorized employees and the guard service should be familiar with these procedures. If electronic entry systems are employed, an alternative method for gaining access should

Table F.2 Backup and recovery security procedures

Security control	Backup and recovery procedure
Physical Access	
Guards—on site	Contract for guard service in advance and preassign employees to guard duty.
Guards—in transit	Contract in advance with secured transportation service for relocating media and equipment.
Electronic card entry system	Provide emergency batter backup for security systems dependent upon electricity and provide for manual override system invoked by authorized personnel. Set up contingency access procedures in advance.
Voice and data communications networks	Provide security on contingency lines and equipment equivalent, if possible, to primary networks.
Logical Access	
Passwords	Ensure that existing system passwords can be used on backup systems or issue special contingency passwords. Ensure that changes to the primary system are reflected in the contingency system.
Security software	Provide comparable and compatible security software and contingency systems.
Dial-up procedures	Provide contingency dial-up numbers for authorized personnel. Pre-specify contingency call-back numbers if the system is designed to hand up and call the user back. Set up equipment and software and specify telephone numbers in advance.
Network security	Ensure that network security measures (e.g., encryption for data, scrambling for voice) are compatible with the backup systems and that changes to the primary system are reflected in the contingency system.

be provided in case the electronic systems are disabled.

Communications Security. Backup communications networks should be armed with security controls. Securing of backup networks is often more difficult than for primary networks, because backup communications lines are often public. Communications backup procedures should accommodate the need to inform users of new changes in dial-up procedures, encryption keys, and communications log-on procedures, when appropriate, and other necessary contact information.

Securing data over public communications carriers can include encryption, error detection codes, positive Acknowledgment, or echoplexing. These methods verify message integrity but do not control access. The retention of encryption capability is an issue particularly during the recovery process because it means making the required encryption keys available at multiple locations and ensuring that the mechanisms are in place to transfer host or client locations without compromising the security effected by encryption.

Logical Access Controls. It is imperative either to update access passwords and procedures on the backup copies of the system or to have a means of informing users of their backup passwords in case the backup system is activated. Backup passwords should be distributed in the same secure manner as primary passwords. In addition, the security software for the backup system must be continually updated. It would compound a disaster if, after a successful move to a backup site, users were unable to gain access to the system because the security software was not compatible with the primary system or had not been updated to reflect changes in the primary systems and networks.

In summary, specific security measures to ensure continuing system integrity should be appended to every recovery procedure.

Special Security Provisions

The efficiency and effectiveness of the recovery process can be compromised if the same security measures designed to protect the systems and networks under normal operation are implemented during recovery. Security measures must be designed specifically for contingency situations. These security controls must allow for the unusual and urgent requirements of a recovery environment yet still offer protection during a very vulnerable situation.

The most fundamental and significant aspects of security during the recovery phase are that security controls appropriate in normal situations do not work best during disaster recovery and that special provision must be made in the security procedures to account for such differences. As a simple example, many data centers do not allow system programmers to gain physical access to the computers and prevent applications programmers from having access to production systems. However, during a disaster, a programmer may be critical to effecting a specific recovery. The security procedures must allow for certain individuals to have, in emergency situations, controlled privileged access that may not be available to them under normal operating conditions.

Security During Repair and Correction

Frequently, when a disaster has passed and the risk to systems and networks has been reduced, there is a tendency to relax security and repair procedures. Repair and reconstruction often proceeds without the diligence and concentration afforded the recovery process; however, major dangers can result from such relaxation.

First, if another damaging event occurs before the completion of the repair and correction process, the organization may be left without backup or primary systems and networks. Whereas it is improbable that two independent, damaging events will occur in rapid succession, the repair process itself can pose added risk (e.g., welding or high-voltage electrical repair work can increase the risk of fire or further electrical outages). Also, some events have anticipated potential subsequent effects, such as aftershocks from an earthquake or structural damage from a fire or flood resulting in the shifting or collapse of a building.

Second, the repair process usually involves persons (e.g., contractors, electricians, vendors' technicians) who are not familiar with normal, daily operations. The probability of security breaches and abusive or damaging actions increases because of these individuals. A conflict frequently arises between the urgency in repairing damage and the need to plan and control the repair and reconstruction process carefully. Because many types of damage are difficult to predict, setting up contingency plans is impractical or infeasible for any but the most likely incidents. For example, most facilities have procedures for fire prevention and control and for personnel evacuation. Planning for repairs following a fire is often done only after an event when the extent of the damage is known. Much confusion can be eliminated, however, if some simple procedures are followed, such as keeping an up-to-date list of names and telephone numbers for all relevant vendors, contractors, suppliers, and employees. On the other hand, preparation for repair and reconstruction for very rare events, such as a chemical spill, might be handled after the event rather than planned in advance. Basic contingency arrangements, such as ensuring that a full set of floor plans and equipment and network layouts is stored at another location, should be made.

A reasonable procedure is to make preliminary plans for repairing damage caused by the most likely events, but planning for repairing improbable types of damage does not make sense. Even less justifiable is planning for reconstruction before the event, although names and telephone numbers of contractors and related services should be retained on site. However, special security procedures should be followed during the repair process.

Recommended Course of Action

Risks to computer system and network integrity—through security breaches, misuse, and damage—are amplified considerably after such abuses occur, when the IT and communications environment is in a vulnerable state. Therefore, guarding against further abuses is especially important during the recovery and repair phases following the initial problem. The first line of defense is to ensure that there are fall-back procedures and resources in the event that the primary security system is damaged or otherwise compromised. This helps prevent subsequent breaches. If damage to the computer systems and communications networks occurs despite all precautions, and a recovery and repair process is initiated, security controls, based on those outlined in Table F.2, should be implemented during the recovery and repair process.

Appendix G Altered Standards of Care in Mass-Casualty Events

HEALTH SYSTEMS RESEARCH, INC.

Executive Summary

Background and Purpose

The events of September 11, 2001 and subsequent anthrax attacks underscored the need for U.S. health care organizations and public health agencies to be prepared to respond to acts of bioterrorism and other public health emergencies. Much has been accomplished in the past several years to improve health system preparedness. Many States and health care organizations and systems have developed preparedness plans that include enhancing surge capacity to respond to such events.

Many of these plans assume that even in large-scale emergencies, health care will be delivered according to established standards of care and that health systems will have the resources and facilities needed to support the delivery of medical care at the required level. However, it is possible that a mass casualty event—defined, for the purpose of this paper, as an act of bioterrorism or other public health or medical emergency involving thousands, or even tens of thousands, of victims—could compromise, at least in the short term, the ability of local or regional health systems to deliver services consistent with established standards of care. Therefore, it is critically important to identify, plan, and prepare for making the necessary adjustments in current health and medical care standards to ensure that the care provided in response to a mass-casualty event results in as many lives being saved as possible.

To address this extremely important issue, in August 2004, a meeting of a number of the foremost experts in the fields of bioethics, emergency medicine, emergency management, health administration, health law and policy, and public health was convened by the Agency for Healthcare Research and Quality (AHRQ) and the Office of the Assistant Secretary for Public Health Emergency Preparedness (OASPHEP) within the U.S. Department of Health and Human Services (DHHS). These experts were joined by highly knowledgeable representatives from key Federal agencies and professional and other health organizations (see Appendix G.I for a complete list of participants). The purposes of this meeting were to:

- Examine how current standards of care might need to be altered in response to a mass casualty event in order to save as many lives as possible.

Funding to support the Altered Standards of Care in Mass Casualty Events report was provided by the U.S. Department of Health and Human Services, Agency for Healthcare Research and Quality, under Contract No. 290-04-0010.
The authors of this report are responsible for its content. No statement in the report should be construed as an official position of theAgency for Healthcare Research and Quality or the U.S. Department of Health and Human Services.
This document is in the public domain and may be used and reprinted without permission except those copyrighted materials noted, for which further reproduction is prohibited without the specific permission of copyright holders.

- Identify what planning, guidance, and tools are needed and what related issues need to be addressed to ensure an effective health and medical care response to a mass-casualty event.
- Recommend specific action that will begin to address the needs of Federal, State, regional, community, and health systems planners on this critically important subject.

Consistent with these purposes, the panel of experts was asked to address the following questions:

- What do planners need to know to develop plans that provide an effective health and medical care response to a mass-casualty event?
- What key principles should guide the planning for a health and medical response to a mass-casualty event?
- What important issues must be considered and addressed in planning for the provision of health and medical care in a mass-casualty event?
- What information, tools, models, and other resources are available to address the needs of planners?
- What other steps might be undertaken to move toward effective planning for such an event?

This paper summarizes the deliberations and recommendations of the expert panel.

Key Findings

The key findings that emerged from the experts' discussion of the provision of health and medical care in a mass casualty event are summarized below. These findings are discussed in greater detail in Chapters G.2 and G.3.

- The goal of an organized and coordinated response to a mass-casualty event should be to maximize the number of lives saved.
- Changes in the usual standards of health and medical care in the affected locality or region will be required to achieve the goal of saving the most lives in a mass-casualty event. Rather than doing everything possible to save every life, it will be necessary to allocate scarce resources in a different manner to save as many lives as possible.
- Many health system preparedness efforts do not provide sufficient planning and guidance concerning the altered standards of care that would be required to respond to a mass-casualty event.
- The basis for allocating health and medical resources in a mass casualty event must be fair and clinically sound. The process for making these decisions should be transparent and judged by the public to be fair.
- Protocols for triage (i.e., the sorting of victims into groups according to their need and resources available) need to be flexible enough to change as the size of a mass-casualty event grows and will depend on both the nature of the event and the speed with which it occurs.
- An effective plan for delivering health and medical care in a mass casualty event should take into account factors common to all hazards (e.g., the need to have an adequate supply of qualified providers available), as well as factors that are hazard-specific (e.g., guidelines for making isolation and quarantine decisions to contain an infectious disease).
- Plans should ensure an adequate supply of qualified providers who are trained specifically for a mass casualty event. This includes providing protection to providers and their families (e.g., personal protective equipment, prophylaxis, staff rotation to prevent burnout, and stress management programs).
- A number of important nonmedical issues that affect the delivery of health and medical care need to be addressed to ensure an effective response to a mass casualty event. They include:
    - The authority to activate or sanction the use of altered standards of care under certain conditions.
    - Legal issues related to liability, licensing, and intergovernmental or regional mutual aid agreements.

- Financial issues related to reimbursement and other ways of covering medical care costs.
- Issues related to effective communication with the public.
- Issues related to populations with special needs.
- Issues related to transportation of patients.
• Guidelines and companion tools related to the development of altered standards of care in a mass casualty event are needed by, and would be extremely useful to, preparedness planners at the Federal, State, regional, community, and health systems levels.

Recommended Action

The expert panel offered recommendations for action that could be undertaken to support planning an effective response to a mass casualty event. The list of recommendations is not meant to be comprehensive, but it provides a starting point for further discussion. These ideas suggest that a collaborative approach should be taken when developing next steps. Both government and private organizations have unique roles and important contributions to make in moving forward. The panel's recommendations include:

- Develop general and event-specific guidance for allocating scarce health and medical care resources during a mass casualty event.
- Develop and implement a process to address nonmedical (i.e., finance, communication, etc.) issues related to the delivery of health and medical care during a mass-casualty event.
- Develop a comprehensive strategy for risk communication with the public before, during, and after a mass-casualty event.
- Identify, analyze, and consider modification of Federal, State, and local laws and regulations that affect the delivery of health and medical care during a mass-casualty event.
- Develop practical tools, such as searchable databases, for verifying credentials of medical and other health personnel prior to and onsite during a mass-casualty event.
- Create strategies to ensure health and medical leadership and coordination for the health and medical aspects of system response during a mass-casualty event.
- Continue and expand efforts to train providers and others to respond effectively in a mass-casualty event.
- Develop and support a research agenda specific to health and medical care standards for a mass casualty event.
- Develop a *Community-Based Planning Guide for Mass Casualty Care* to assist preparedness planners in their efforts.
- Identify and support States, health systems, communities, and regions to develop mass casualty health and medical care response plans based on the *Planning Guide*; share their results widely.

Chapter G.1   Introduction

Overview

The events of September 11, 2001 and subsequent anthrax attacks underscored the need for U.S. health care organizations and public health agencies to be prepared to respond to acts of bioterrorism and other public health emergencies. Much has been accomplished in the past several years to improve health system preparedness. Many States and health care organizations and systems have developed preparedness plans that include enhancing surge capacity to respond to such events.

Most of these plans assume that even in large-scale emergencies, health care will be delivered according to established standards of care and that health systems will have the resources and facilities needed to support the delivery of medical care at the required level. However, it is possible that a mass-casualty event—defined, for the purpose of this paper, as an act of bioterrorism or other public health or medical emergency involving thousands, or even tens of thousands, of victims—could compromise, at least in the short term, the ability of local or regional health systems to deliver services consistent with established standards of care. Therefore, it is critically important to identify, plan, and prepare for making the necessary adjustments in current health and medical care standards to ensure that the care provided in response to a mass-casualty event results in as many lives being saved as possible.

To address this extremely important issue, in August 2004, a meeting of a number of the foremost experts in the fields of bioethics, emergency medicine, emergency management, health administration, health law and policy, and public health was convened by the Agency for Healthcare Research and Quality (AHRQ) and the Office of the Assistant Secretary for Public Health Emergency Preparedness (OASPHEP) within the U.S. Department of Health and Human Services (DHHS). These experts were joined by highly knowledgeable representatives from key Federal agencies and professional and other health organizations (see Appendix G.1 for a complete list of participants). The purposes of this meeting were to:

- Examine how current standards of care might need to be altered in response to a mass-casualty event in order to save as many lives as possible.
- Identify what planning, guidance, and tools are needed and what related issues need to be addressed to ensure an effective health and medical care response to a mass-casualty event.
- Recommend specific action that will begin to address the needs of Federal, State, regional, community, and health systems planners on this critically important subject.

Consistent with these purposes, participants were asked to address the following questions:

- What do planners need to know to develop plans that provide an effective health and medical care response to a mass-casualty event?
- What key principles should guide the planning for a health and medical response to a mass-casualty event?
- What important issues must be considered and addressed in planning for the provision of health and medical care in a mass-casualty event?
- What information, tools, models, and other resources are available to address the needs of planners?
- What other steps might be undertaken to move toward effective planning for such an event?

This White Paper summarizes the deliberations and recommendations of this group of experts. Chapter G.2 provides these experts' assessment of the need to develop and plan for the possible implementation of altered standards of care in response to a mass-casualty event. Chapter G.3 then outlines a framework and set of principles that can guide the development of strategies for adjusting the manner in which health and medical care is delivered in a mass-casualty event to maximize the number of lives saved. Chapter G.4 identifies an important set of related issues that must be addressed if these strategies are to be as effective as possible in achieving their goal. And, finally, Chapter G.5 presents the experts' recommendations concerning the action steps to be taken to help States, communities, health systems, and providers to be prepared to respond to a mass-casualty event in ways that save as many lives as possible.

Chapter G.2 Health and Medical Care Delivery in a Mass-Casualty Event

Health and Medical Care Standards in the Context of a Mass-Casualty Event

Substantial work has already been done and continues to be undertaken throughout the country to improve the ability of health systems to respond to acts of terrorism or other public health emergencies. Much of the planning in this area focuses on increasing the surge capacity of affected delivery systems through the rapid mobilization and deployment of additional resources from the community, State, regional, or national levels to the affected area. However, few of these plans specifically address a situation in which the delivery system is unable to respond (even if only temporarily) according to established standards of care due to the scope and magnitude of a mass-casualty event.

A key issue upon which the experts agreed is that the goal of the health and medical response to a mass-casualty event is to save as many lives as possible. There is consensus that, to achieve this goal, health and medical care will have to be delivered in a manner that differs from the standards of care that apply under normal circumstances. This issue is not addressed in a comprehensive manner in many preparedness plans.[1] Finally, the experts also agreed that for health and medical care delivered under these altered standards to be as effective as possible in saving lives, it is critically important that current preparedness planning be expanded to explicitly address this issue and to provide guidance, education, and training concerning these altered care standards.

Standards of health and medical care, broadly defined, address not only what care is given, but to whom, when, by whom, and under what circumstances or in what places. A comprehensive set of standards for health and medical care specifies the following:

What—what types of interventions, clinical protocols, standing orders, and other specifications should be used in providing health and medical care?

To whom—which individuals should receive health and medical care according to their condition or likelihood of response?

When—with what urgency should health and medical care be provided?

By whom—which individuals are certified and/or licensed to provide care within a defined scope of practice and other regulations?

Where—what facility and system standards (prehospital, hospital, alternate care site, etc.) should be in place for the provision of health and medical care?

Under normal conditions, current standards of care might be interpreted as calling for the allocation of all appropriate health and medical resources to improve the health status and/or save the life of each individual patient. However, should a mass-casualty event occur, the demand for care provided in accordance with current standards would exceed system resources. In a small

---

[1] In preparation for the expert meeting, information and a sample of existing triage protocols and preparedness models were collected and reviewed. A brief summary of that review is provided in Appendix G.II.

rural hospital, 10 victims from a local manufacturing accident might be considered a mass casualty event. In a metropolitan area, several hundred victims would be manageable within system resources. In an event involving thousands of victims, preserving a functioning health care system will require a move to altered standards of care. It may also be necessary to create both pre-hospital operations and alternate care sites to supplement hospital care.

The term "altered standards" has not been defined, but generally is assumed to mean a shift to providing care and allocating scarce equipment, supplies, and personnel in a way that saves the largest number of lives in contrast to the traditional focus on saving individuals. For example, it could mean applying principles of field triage[2] to determine who gets what kind of care. It could mean changing infection control standards to permit group isolation rather than single person isolation units. It could mean limiting the use of ventilators to surgical situations. It could mean creating alternate care sites from facilities never designed to provide medical care, such as schools, churches, or hotels. It could also mean changing who provides various kinds of care or changing privacy and confidentially protections temporarily.

Hypothetical Scenarios Illustrating Changes in the Delivery of Care in Response to a Mass Casualty Event

Two hypothetical mass casualty scenarios were developed by the panel of experts to help illustrate specific ways in which care standards would have to change in response to a mass casualty event (see Figure G.1). The first scenario involves the simultaneous explosion of multiple dirty bombs in a metropolitan area. The second scenario involves the release of a biological agent. The use of these two scenarios facilitates the examination of the impacts and implications of two serious events that differ in nature and occur at different velocities. For example, the explosive scenario would produce

---

Two mass casualty scenarios were developed by the panel of experts to help identify how care delivered at the event scene or pre-hospital setting, hospital, and alternate care sites would vary from care provided under normal circumstances.

Scenario 1. Multiple, simultaneous explosions
A series of multiple dirty bombs have been set off simultaneously throughout a large metropolitan subway system. The city's hospitals also have been targeted and approximately 40 percent of the hospitals are no longer operational. There are an estimated 10,000 victims.

Scenario 2. Biological agent release
A highly lethal communicable biological agent with a set but initially unknown incubation period has been released in a heavily populated area. Diagnosis is dependent on laboratory tests. Medical staffs are required to use personal protection equipment. Treatment requirements include patient isolation and the use of ventilators; however, the impact and effectiveness of treatment is unknown.

Figure G.1 Two Mass-casualty scenarios used to identify anticipated changes to care delivery.

---

a large number of casualties upon detonation and place an immediate demand on all aspects of the health care system. The biological scenario would develop more slowly, with its peak impact occurring at the end of an unknown incubation period.

The examination of these scenarios revealed that the explosive and biological terrorism mass casualty scenarios are likely to share common elements, but also raise issues that are specific to the nature of each event and the speed with which the event places demands on the health care system. The following discussion highlights these common elements. Event-specific issues for each scenario appear in Figures G.2 and G.3 and are organized by setting (scene [or pre-hospital], hospital, and alternate care sites).

Changes in Care Delivery Common to Two Scenarios

At their peaks, both the explosive and biological mass casualty scenarios are likely to involve the following:

---

[2] The term triage refers to the process of sorting victims according to their need for treatment and the resources available.

> **Scenario 1:** A series of multiple dirty bombs have been set off simultaneously throughout a large metropolitan subway system. The city's hospitals also have been targeted and approximately 40 percent of the hospitals are no longer operational. There are an estimated 10,000 victims.

In addition to the changes common to both scenarios described in this report, the following additional changes in medical care delivery may occur under this scenario.

Pre-hospital

- Physicians most likely will not be at the scene. Emergency medical services and other first responders will perform triage.
- Anyone at the scene who can help may need to act as "medical staff."
- Triage protocols currently used (e.g., START, JumpSTART) may not apply, given magnitude of the event.
- Buses and other forms of nonmedical transportation may have to be used to supplement emergency transport systems.
- With an insufficient number of usual pre-hospital treatments and supplies, such as spineboards and immobilization equipment or the need to respond quickly, ambulatory victims may have to walk or self-transport to the nearest facility or hospital.

Hospital

- Even if a hospital is among those still functioning, it may experience water, heating and cooling, electricity shortages, and communication problems.
- Reserved medical supplies and equipment may not arrive quickly enough from national and regional resources, such as the Strategic National Stockpile, given the velocity of the event.
- The provider-patient relationship may be interrupted. Providers may have service-specific assignments rather than patient group assignments (e.g., they would perform all intravenous infusions rather than provide all aspects of care for a group of patients).
- The hospital may need to exercise strict control of access to and from the hospital and diversion of ambulatory victims to alternate care sites. The emergency department should be protected in order to care for more critically injured victims (i.e., those who cannot walk to the hospital) who will arrive later.
- Decontamination practices will change, so that only gross decontamination (e.g., removal of clothes) is performed.
- Only lifesaving surgeries will be performed, and initial surgical care will aim to stabilize the patient. When more resources become available, additional surgery to fully treat injuries can occur.
- The practice of ordering only the supplies needed for immediate use means that limited supplies will run out quickly. This situation will be compounded by same vendor/resource dependence. It will also be compounded by an event requiring large amounts of specialized supplies or care. Examples include mass casualty events involving mostly children (substantial pediatric supplies needed) or demand for burn beds and related care.

Alternate Care Sites

- Ambulatory patients will be redirected to alternate care sites within or outside of the hospital, such as the hospital cafeteria or a nearby school, to be re-triaged and receive care for minor injuries.

Figure G.2 Changes Specific to Care Delivery in a Multiple Explosion (Scenario 1).

- *Triage efforts that will need to focus on maximizing the number of lives saved.* Instead of treating the sickest or the most injured first, triage would focus on identifying and reserving immediate treatment for individuals who have a critical need for treatment and are likely to survive. The goal would be to allocate resources in order to maximize the number of lives saved. Complicating conditions, such as underlying chronic disease, may have an impact on an individual's ability to survive.

- *Triage decisions that will affect the allocation of all available resources across the spectrum of care*: from the scene to hospitals to alternate care sites. For example, emergency department access may be reserved for immediate-need patients; ambulatory patients may be diverted to alternate care sites (including nonmedical

> **Scenario 2:** *A highly lethal communicable biological agent with a set but initially unknown incubation period has been released in a heavily populated area. Diagnosis is dependent on laboratory tests. Medical staff are required to use personal protection equipment. Treatment requirements include patient isolation and the use of ventilators; however, the impact and effectiveness of treatment is unknown.*

In addition to the changes common to both scenarios described in this report, the following additional changes in medical care delivery may occur under this scenario.

Pre-hospital

- There will be no initial "scene" in a biological event. Pre-hospital activity related to triage, diagnosis, and case identification, will be done at physicians' offices, community health centers, emergency departments, and even pharmacies.
- Communication among providers will be important in order to develop a coordinated understanding of the symptoms and a systematic approach to treatment that is consistent with coordinated planning.
- Public health/epidemiological surveillance, including data mining from disparate sources (such as over-the-counter medication purchases, work/school absenteeism, etc.) may be useful in outbreak analysis and epidemiological projection.
- Emergency medical services may be used to transport victims to specific quarantine or isolation locations and other alternate care sites.

Hospital

- The emphasis will be on prevention and contagion control, as well as treatment, depending on staff and resources available. Victims who are conclusively diagnosed as infected will be isolated. Group isolation may be necessary.
- "Suspected" exposure patients will be quarantined. If laboratory tests and other diagnostic tools are not available, these patients may be treated based on histories reported and physician clinical judgment.
- Staff shortages are likely at all hospitals due to concerns about exposure to the infection. A recent survey suggests that as many as 50 percent of hospital workers may not show up for work during a bioterrorism event.
- Protection of all staff and their families, such as prophylaxis, will be needed to help ensure adequate staffing (including nonmedical staff such as housekeeping and dietary staff).
- "Early treaters/responders" will have to be quarantined and treated as if they have been exposed to the biological agent. Their quarantine will have a negative impact on provider supply.
- Demand for pharmaceuticals is likely to outstrip the supply. Both experimental and expired drugs may have to be used.
- Initially, standards of care initially may improve for the first wave of patients, but as the number of victims increases, standards could degrade.

Alternate Care Sites

- Alternate care sites will be used for triage and distribution of vaccines or other prophylactic measures, as well as for quarantine, minimum care, and hospice care.

Figure G.3 Changes Specific to Care Delivery in a Biological Event (Scenario 2).

space, such as cafeterias within hospitals, or other nonmedical facilities) where "lower level" hospital ward care or quarantine can be provided. Intensive or critical care units may become surgical suites and regular medical care wards may become isolation or other specialized response units.

- *Needs of current patients, such as those recovering from surgery or in critical or intensive care units; the resources they use will become part of overall resource allocation.* Elective procedures may have to be cancelled, and current inpatients may have to be discharged early or transferred to another setting. In addition, certain lifesaving efforts may have to be discontinued.

- *Usual scope of practice standards that will not apply.* Nurses may function as physicians, and physicians may function outside their specialties. Credentialing of providers may be granted on an emergency or temporary basis.

- *Equipment and supplies that will be rationed and used in ways consistent with achieving the ultimate goal of saving the most lives* (e.g., disposable supplies may be reused).
- *Not enough trained staff.* Staff will be scared to leave home and/or may find it difficult to travel to work. Burnout from stress and long hours will occur, and replacement staff will be needed. Some scarce and valuable equipment, such as ventilators, may not be used without staff available who are trained to operate them.
- *Delays in hospital care due to backlogs of patients.* Patients will be waiting for scarce resources, such as operating rooms, radiological suites, and laboratories.
- *Providers that may need to make treatment decisions based on clinical judgement.* For example, if laboratory resources for testing or radiology resources for x-rays are exhausted, treatment based on physical exam, history, and clinical judgement will occur.
- *The psychological impact of the event on providers.* Short- and long-term stress management measures (e.g., Critical Incident Stress Management programs) are essential for providers and their families.
- *Current documentation standards that will be impossible to maintain.* Providers may not have time to obtain informed consent or have access to the usual support systems to fully document the care provided, especially if the health care setting is damaged by the event.
- *Backlog in processing fatalities.* It may not be possible to accommodate cultural sensitivities and attitudes toward death and handling bodies. Numbers of fatalities may make it difficult to find and notify next of kin quickly. Burial and cremation services may be overwhelmed. Standards for completeness and timeliness of death certificates may need to be lifted temporarily.

Based on a review of the health and medical care issues presented by these two scenarios, the panel of experts identified a need for more guidelines to ensure a systematic approach to decisionmaking in mass casualty events. Guidelines should take into account and be scaleable to the size, nature, and speed of the event, so that they can guide the following decisions:

- How to ensure and protect an adequate supply of trained providers and support staff.
- How to triage patients into groups by the nature of their condition, probability of success of interventions/treatment, and consideration of resources available.
- How to maintain infection control and a safe care environment.
- How to use and reuse common supplies and equipment, such as gloves, gowns, and masks.
- How to allocate scarce clinical resources of a general nature, such as beds, surgery capability, and laboratory and other diagnostic services.
- How to allocate scarce and highly specialized clinical resources, such as decontamination units, isolation units, ventilators, burn beds, and intensive and critical care units.
- How to treat specific conditions, including how to make best use of available pharmaceuticals.
- How to protect health care providers and support staff and their families.
- How to modify documentation standards to ensure enough information to support care and obtain reimbursement without posing an undue administrative burden.
- How to manage excessive fatalities.

As illustrated in these scenarios, the occurrence of a mass-casualty event will require significant changes in the way in which health and medical care is delivered under extraordinary circumstances. The panel of experts was quite clear in its view that if the health care system is to be successful in saving as many lives as possible, planning, education, and training efforts should be focused on the development and implementation of appropriate altered standards of care in response to a mass-casualty event. A framework and set of principles to guide work in this area were developed by the panel and are presented in the next chapter.

Chapter G.3 Framework and Guiding Principles When Planning for Health and Medical Care in a Mass Casualty Event

Framework

The expert panel suggested that a framework for planning should take into account the ways in which response to a mass-casualty event is both similar to and different from responses to current surge capacity issues in health care facilities. The goal is to devise a framework that is applicable to both ordinary ("daily routine") and extraordinary situations. To this end, they recommended that plans for a medical care response to a mass casualty event should:

- Be compatible with or capable of being integrated with day-to-day operations.
- Be applicable to a broad spectrum of event types and severities.
- Be flexible, to permit graded responses based on changing circumstances.
- Be tested, to determine where gaps in the framework exist.

A model reflecting the concept of a graded response that is sensitive to changing circumstances was shared with the panel and is depicted in Figure G.4. This matrix illustrates how the release of a biological agent resulting in mass casualties would require that health and medical care standards be altered over time as the disease progresses within the population and demands on the health system grow. The disease progresses from a pre-release state (upper left) through death, at each stage placing greater demands on the system, and thus requiring increasing alterations in standards. This staged model approach allows for the development of care guidelines for each stage that are consistent with the overall goal of maximizing the number of lives saved.

Although Figure G.4 is based on a disease model, this graded response could be adapted easily to other types of mass-casualty events (e.g., chemical releases or explosions) by compressing the stages according to the magnitude and velocity of the event. High magnitude, high velocity events will require the system to adopt altered standards more quickly than smaller or slower-developing events. However, it is also important to recognize that as the impact of the event wanes and resources become more available, it may be possible to return to established standards of care used in normal situations.

Guiding Principles for Developing Altered Standards of Care to Respond to a Mass Casualty Event

In addition to offering suggestions for a framework for the development of plans to respond to a mass casualty event, the expert panel also articulated five principles that should steer the development of such guidelines. Incorporating these five principles will ensure that standards of care are altered sufficiently to respond to issues arising from a mass-casualty event.

Level of Standards → / Stage of Disease in the Population	Normal Medical Care Standards	Near Normal Medical Care Standards (alternate sites of care, use of atypical devices, expanded scope of practice)	Focus on Key Lifesaving Care (cannot offer everyone highest level of care but can offer key lifesaving care)	Total System/ Standards Alteration (questions asked about who gets access to what resources)
Pre-release of agent	✓			
Release responses	✓	✓		
Symptomatic		✓	✓	
Illness			✓	✓
Death			✓	✓

Figure G.4 How Health and Medical Care Standards May Have to Be Modified in a Mass-Casualty Event by Stage of Disease in the Population. (Source: Dr. Michael Allswede, University of Pittsburgh, UPMC Health System)

Principle 1: In planning for a mass casualty event, the aim should be to keep the health care system functioning and to deliver acceptable quality of care to preserve as many lives as possible.

Adhering to this principle will involve:

- Allocating scarce resources in order to save the most lives.
- Developing a basis for the allocation of resources that is fair, open, transparent, accountable, and well understood by both professionals and the public.
- Ensuring, to the possible extent, a safe environment for the provision of care, and placing a high priority on infection control measures, and other containment processes.

Principle 2: Planning a health and medical response to a mass casualty event must be comprehensive, community-based, and coordinated at the regional level.

Effective planning should:

- Be done at the facility level. However, facility-level planning alone is not sufficient.
- Integrate facility-level planning into a regional systems approach.
- Involve a broad array of public and private community stakeholders.[3]

---

[3] These stakeholders include: emergency management agencies, police and fire departments, emergency medical services, ambulance and other transport providers, health departments and community health centers, hospitals, ambulatory care centers, private physician offices, medical examiners, nursing homes, health centers, mental health services, morticians, and others. They also may include schools, churches, hotels, businesses, and other organizations that can provide space for alternate care facilities and cooperate in the preplanning required to activate such sites.

- Begin with the agreement on shared responsibility among all partners in the planning process. It is not adequate for individual institutions and systems to have emergency response plans unless those plans are coordinated into a single unified response system.
- Be consistent. Planning also should be integrated with Federal, State and local emergency plans.

Principle 3: There must be an adequate legal framework for providing health and medical care in a mass casualty event.

An adequate legal framework for providing health and medical care in a mass-casualty event would do the following:

- Include a designation of the authority to declare an emergency and implement temporary alterations in standards of care.
- Define the conditions for temporary modification of laws and regulations that govern medical care under normal conditions.
- Be simple, clear, and easy to communicate to providers and the public.
- Be flexible enough to accommodate the demands of events that vary in size and velocity, such as an explosive or biological event.

Principle 4: The rights of individuals must be protected to the extent possible and reasonable under the circumstances.

The rights of individuals must be protected to the extent possible and reasonable:

- In establishing and operationalizing an adequate legal framework for the delivery of care.
- In determining the basis on which scarce resources will be allocated.
- When considering limiting personal freedom through quarantine or isolation as well as the conditions for release.
- When privacy and confidentiality may have to be breached.

Principle 5: Clear communication with the public is essential before, during, and after a mass-casualty event.

To manage expectations and educate the public about the impact of an event, whom to call for information, where to go for care, and what to expect, the following points should be kept in mind:

- The public should be brought into the discussion during the early stages of planning so that citizens develop a clear understanding of concepts such as rationing of resources.
- Public understanding and acceptance of plans are essential to success.
- Messages should be consistent and timely at all stages.
- Official health and medical care messages should be delivered through public media by a local physician whom the public perceives to have knowledge of the event and the area, a representative of the Centers for Disease Control and Prevention (CDC), or the Surgeon General, depending on the level of communication necessary.
- Spokespersons at all levels—local, State, regional, and Federal—should coordinate their messages.
- It may be necessary to vary the modes of communication according to the type of information to be communicated, the target audience for which it is intended, and the operating condition of media outlets, which may be directly affected. Variations that illustrate this point but that do not reflect expert discussion include the need to use languages other than English and the need to use alternatives to usual media outlets in the affected area. Also, national audience messages would be less detailed and specific than messages to the affected area.

Chapter G.4 The Larger Context: Important Related Issues

The expert panel emphasized that, for health systems and providers to respond effectively to a mass casualty event, a number of important legal, policy, and ethical issues related to altered standards of care must be addressed before such an event occurs. These issues are discussed below.

The Authority to Activate the Use of Altered Standards of Health and Medical Care

It is important to establish clear authority to activate the use of altered standards of health and medical care. The following questions pertain:

- What circumstances will trigger a call for altered standards of care?
- Who is authorized to make that call, and at what level (site, community, region, State, or Federal) should the call be made?
- Under what legal statutory authority, should the call be made?
- Once the call is made, who assumes responsibility for directing emergency actions?
- What is the relationship of otherwise autonomous institutions to the incident management system?

Generally, when a decision exceeds the authority of a particular organization or region, responsibility for the decision moves to the next level of decisionmaking and authority. Nonetheless, it is advisable that State and local jurisdictions empower local decisionmakers to act before Federal or other outside assistance arrives. Some decisions may emanate from public officials at higher levels of authority, such as the mayor, governor, or president, whereas clinical decisions will need to come from health and medical professionals closer to the event.

While decisions made by those closer to the event may trigger a move to altered standards of care, policies that support the move to altered standards must be put in place by the highest levels of authority necessary. For example, during a mass casualty event, a hospital may decide that the demand for medical care has exceeded the hospital's ability to provide care under normal standards. This decision will require a move to expanded functions for staff (e.g., nurses may perform some physician duties). In this case the decision to move to altered standards of care emanates from the clinical level. However, it is important that the appropriate higher level of authority has put in place the policies, such as provisions allowing the modification of State scope of practice laws that support the decision and empower the hospital's nurses or other health care staff to provide an expanded level of care.

Examples of existing resources that offer starting points for addressing questions of authority are described in the accompanying exhibits. One is a draft checklist developed by the American Bar Association for State and local government attorneys to prepare for possible disasters (Figure G.5). Another is the Model State Emergency Health Powers Act (Figure G.6). A third is draft executive orders developed in Colorado that create a legal framework for an emergency and address a variety of legal issues (Figure G.7).

Legal and Regulatory Issues

The organization and delivery of health care is highly regulated. In a mass-casualty event, it is likely that some provisions for temporary

> Questions of authority are addressed by the "Draft Checklist for State and Local Government Attorneys To Prepare for Possible Disasters" prepared by the Task Force on Emergency Management and Homeland Security of the State and Local Government Law Section, American Bar Association (March 2003).
>
> The checklist includes lists of questions pertaining to authority in general, authority for surveillance, and intergovernmental joint powers agreements. It also addresses public information, administrative and fiscal issues, contracting, personnel, and liability.
>
> For more information, see http://www.abanet.org/statelocal/disaster.pdf

Figure G.5 Draft checklist for state and local government attorneys to prepare for possible disasters.

> The Model State Emergency Health Powers Act (Model Act) grants specific emergency powers to State governors and public health authorities in the event of a large public health emergency. The Model Act was developed for the Centers for Disease Control by The Center for Law and the Public's Health at Georgetown and Johns Hopkins Universities to ensure an effective response to large-scale emergency health threats while protecting the rights of individuals. It provides a broad set of powers for an entity called the Public Health Authority.
>
> As it may relate to altered standards of care, the Model Act provides that a declaration of an emergency activates the disaster response and recovery aspects of State, local, and interjurisdictional disaster emergency plans. There is no mention of local-level involvement. The Public Health Authority is empowered to take control over facilities (health care and other) and "materials," such as food, fuel, clothing and other commodities, and roads. It may control health care supplies by rationing resources; establishing priority distribution to health care providers, disaster response personnel and mortuary staff; and establishing a general distribution to all others. It may establish and enforce quarantine and other infection control measures.
>
> The following provisions of the Model Act have provoked considerable discussion among public health scholars and practitioners:
>
> - *Quarantine*. "Special Powers" of the Public Health Authority apply to: performing physical examinations, necessary tests, and/or vaccination. Any person refusing examination, tests, or vaccination may be isolated or quarantined. These sections (601, 603) have been subject to media and public scrutiny. States have designed widely differing solutions. However, the Model act has helped to modernize State laws on quarantine and encourages greater consistency among State laws regarding quarantine provisions.
> - *Liability*. Health care providers are not held liable for any civil damages, except in cases where they are found to be negligent in treating or in failing to provide treatment. This includes out-of-State health care providers for whom relevant permits to practice have been waived by the Public Health Authority. The Model Act also explicitly states that except in cases of gross negligence or willful misconduct, the State (and the State and local officials specified in the act) is not liable for any property damage, death, or injury incurred as a result of complying with the Act (§804(a)).
> - *Compelling Provider Participation*. The Model Act states (§608 (a)) that the Public Health Authority can compel in-State health care providers to assist in vaccination, testing, treatment, or examination of an individual as a licensure condition.
> - *Other Provisions*. Other provisions of the Model Act include the use of otherwise protected private medical information, public information obligations, access to mental health services and personnel, compensation for private property (calculated according to nonemergency eminent domain procedures) and reimbursement for health care supplies.
>
> For more information, see http://www.publichealthlaw.net/Resources/Modellaws.htm

Figure G.6 Model state emergency health powers act.

modification of regulatory requirements at all levels of government will be necessary. At the present time, uncertainty about legal issues, particularly liability, may be creating a reluctance to anticipate and plan for a mass-casualty event that would require altered health and medical care standards. As mentioned earlier, it is important to establish clear authority to activate altered standards of medical care. Alternatives may include enhancing or modifying a number of laws and

> Colorado has chosen to plan for disaster emergencies by using draft executive orders to create a legal framework for an emergency and address a variety of legal issues. These orders are summarized in this exhibit.
>
> - *Executive Order 0.0 Declaring a State of Disaster Emergency Due to Criminal Acts of Biological Terrorism.* This executive order declares a disaster emergency of an epidemic type. The Governor's Expert Emergency Epidemic Response Committee would meet and advise the governor that an emergency exists. The governor would then issue this order, which is good for 30 days and sets the stage for other orders directing specific actions to meet the emergency.
> - *Executive Order 1.1 Ordering Hospitals to Transfer or Cease the Admission of Patients to Respond to the Current Disaster Emergency.* In directly authorizing hospitals to cease admissions and transfer patients, this order permits hospitals to determine on their own without central guidance whether they have reached their capacity to examine and treat patients. It further grants immunity from civil or criminal liability to those hospitals, physicians, and emergency service providers who act in good faith to comply with the executive order. The order takes the position that the Emergency Medical Treatment and Labor Act (EMTALA) requirements do not preempt this order.
> - *Executive Order 2.0 Concerning the Procurement and Taking of Certain Medicines and Vaccines Required to Respond to the Current Disaster Emergency.* This order authorizes the seizure of certain named drugs from public and private outlets listed in the State's pharmacy statutes, and embargoes the supply of those drugs. At the same time, it exempts from seizure those supplies that certain facilities are required to keep on hand for the chemoprophylaxis of their employees. It provides for keeping records of drugs embargoed and for compensating the outlets at the cessation of the emergency.
> - *Executive Order 3.0 Concerning the Suspension of Certain Statutes and Regulations to Provide for the Rapid Distribution of Medication in Response to the Current Disaster Emergency.* This order implements Colorado's Strategic National Stockpile Plan and suspends certain pharmacy statutes to facilitate the rapid distribution of medicines and vaccines in response to an emergency epidemic. The order further authorizes named officials to direct listed health care providers to participate in this effort and explicitly permits the limited participation in that effort by nonmedical personnel. The order is not intended for application in response to a chemical event.
> - *Executive Order 4.0 Concerning the Suspension of Physician and Nurse Licensure Statutes to Respond to the Current Disaster Emergency.* This order permits physicians and nurses who hold a license in good standing in another State, or who hold an unrestricted but inactive Colorado license, to practice under the supervision of a Colorado-licensed physician during the emergency, provided they do so without charge to the State or any individual patient or victim. This order would permit more physicians and nurses to be available to treat infected persons during the emergency.
> - *Executive Order 5.0 Concerning the Suspension of Certain Licensure Statutes to Enable More Colorado Licensed Physician Assistants and Emergency Medical Technicians to Assist in Responding to the Current Disaster Emergency.* Under normal conditions, physician assistants (PAs) and emergency medical technicians (EMTs) licensed in Colorado can practice only in association with or under the supervision of physicians by prior agreement. This order permits PAs and EMTs to practice under the supervision of any licensed physicians in order to afford treatment to the greatest number of infected individuals. The PAs, EMTs, and physicians involved are granted immunity from civil or criminal liability if they act in good faith to meet the terms of the order.
> - *Executive Order 6.0 Concerning the Isolation and Quarantining of Individuals and Property in Response to the Current Disaster Emergency Epidemic.* This order empowers the Colorado Department of Public Health and Environment to establish, maintain, and enforce isolation (of infected individuals) and quarantine of (exposed individuals) as needed to protect the public health in an epidemic situation. It further grants similar powers to local boards of health to combat infectious disease epidemics.
> - *Executive Order 7.0 Ordering Facilities to Transfer or Receive Patients with Mental Illness and Suspending Certain Statutory Provisions to Respond to the Current Disaster Emergency.* This order permits the transfer of mentally ill persons from a designated facility to some other facility as necessary to treat them for the infectious disease causing the epidemic. It further specifies requirements related to required services and use of identifying personal information, and provides for immunity from civil or criminal liability for any facility acting in good faith under the order.
> - *Executive Order 8.0 Concerning Suspension of Certain Statutes Pertaining to Death Certificates and Burial Practices in Response to the Current Disaster Emergency.* This order suspends the statutory timing requirements for filing death certificates and authorizes the executive director of the Colorado Department of Public Health and Environment to direct the disposition of dead bodies in a manner that will protect the public health.

Figure G.7 Colorado's approach to planning for disaster emergencies—executive orders.

regulations pertaining to the delivery of health and medical care in normal conditions. The level of authority necessary to modify laws and regulations during a mass-casualty event will correspond with whether they are Federal, State, regional, or local laws. However, in all cases, it is important to make all providers and institutions aware of the established legal framework and authority to modify laws and regulations, so that responders to a mass-casualty event will know which laws do and do not apply in a given situation.

To the extent possible, existing laws and other mechanisms should be used to the fullest and should not impede the process of planning for a mass-casualty event. It is therefore important to examine existing State public health laws, licensing/certification laws, interstate emergency management compacts and mutual aid agreements, and other legal and regulatory arrangements to determine the extent to which they meet potential new threats. Any waivers granted are likely to be targeted to the affected area for a temporary and specified period of time. In the case of a mass-casualty event involving a communicable agent that moves from region to region, it will be important to have flexibility to extend or expand such waivers.

Some of the Federal, State, and local laws and regulations that govern the delivery of health and medical care under normal conditions may need to be modified or enhanced in the case of a mass casualty event. These include laws to: ensure access to emergency medical care; protect patient privacy and confidentiality of medical information; shield medical providers and other rescuers from lawsuits; govern the development and use of health and medical facilities; and regulate the number of hours health and medical providers can work as well as the conditions in which they work. Relevant laws include but are not limited to the following:

- Emergency Medical Treatment and Active Labor Act (EMTALA).
- Health Insurance Portability and Accountability Act (HIPAA).
- Federal Volunteer Protection Act.
- Good Samaritan Law.

Additional types of laws and regulations that relate to the delivery of health and medical care include:

- 80-hour work week rule for medical residents.
- Occupational Safety and Health Administration and other workplace regulations.
- Building codes and other facility standards.
- Publicly funded health insurance laws (including Medicare, Medicaid, and the State Children's Health Insurance Program).
- Laws pertaining to human subject research.
- Laws and regulations governing the use and licensure of drugs and devices.

In developing a comprehensive plan for the delivery of health and medical care during a mass casualty event, it is important to consider mechanisms to allow for legal, regulatory, or accreditation adjustments in the following areas:

- *Liability of providers and institutions for care provided under stress with less than a full complement of resources.* The plan may have to provide for "hold harmless" agreements or grant immunity from civil or criminal liability under certain conditions.
- *Certification and licensing.* Although it is important to ensure that providers are qualified, it is also important to have flexibility in granting temporary certification or licenses for physicians, nurses, and others who are inactive, retired, or certified or licensed in other States.
- *Scope of practice.* It may be necessary to grant permission to certain professionals on a temporary and emergency basis to function outside their legal scope of practice or above their level of training.
- *Institutional autonomy.* If organizations and institutions cede their authority in order to participate in a unified incident management system in a crisis, the plan may have to address the legal implications for those organizations.
- *Facility standards.* Standards of care that pertain to space, equipment, and physical facilities may have to be altered in both traditional medical care facilities and alternate care sites that are created in response to the event.
- *Patient privacy and confidentiality.* Provisions of HIPAA and other laws and regulations that require signed releases and other measures to ensure privacy and confidentiality of a patient's medical information may have to be altered.

- *Documentation of care.* Minimally accepted levels of documentation of care provided to an individual may have to be established, both for purposes of patient care quality and as the basis for reimbursement from third-party payers.
- *Property seizures.* Provisions may have to be made to take over property, including facilities, supplies, and equipment, for the delivery of care or to destroy property deemed unsafe.
- *Provisions for quarantine or mass immunization.* In anticipation of biological event, the plan will have to address the establishment and enforcement of isolation, quarantine, and mass immunization and provisions for release or exception.

Financial Issues

Preparing for and providing health and medical care during a mass-casualty event could result in large financial losses for all involved organizations, if issues surrounding the financing of such preparation and care are not addressed. Concern about financial resources and reimbursement for health and medical care provided during a mass-casualty event applies to all providers, organizations, and sites, including governmental and nongovernmental, not for profit and for profit. It includes concern about costs of the following:

- Providing care in traditional medical settings, alternate care sites and pre-hospital care settings.
- Creating alternate care sites in settings such as schools, neighborhood centers, or hotels.
- Training providers.
- Staging drills.
- Repairing physical plant damage.

One potential source of disaster relief is the Stafford Act (Public Law 93-288). However, financing from the Federal government must be supplemented by funds from other public as well as private organizations. In preparing a comprehensive plan, it may be very valuable for planners to include financial management experts from the participating organizations, such as hospital systems. In addition formal mutual aid agreements or other contracts should be developed in advance to document relationships, expectations, and requirements related to obtaining emergency reimbursements. On the patient side, issues of financial access, such as requiring proof of insurance, apply. This concern is closely related to legal issues of documentation for reimbursement. It is not likely that providers will be able to maintain documentation practices beyond what is considered minimally adequate to support treatment; altered standards of documentation for reimbursement purposes may have to be defined.

Communicating with the Public

Comprehensive plans for responding to a mass-casualty event include strategies for communicating with the public before, during, and after an event, as follows:

- Prior to the occurrence of a mass-casualty event, the goal should be to educate the public about:
  - Signs and symptoms of chemical, biological, radiological, and other exposures.
  - Appropriate self-care responses.
  - Appropriate use of health and medical care.
  - What to expect from the health care system in the event of a mass casualty incident.
- During a mass-casualty incident, the goal should be to:
  - Provide information to the public about the status of the response.
  - Give consistent messages about when and where to seek care.
  - Manage expectations regarding the delivery of health and medical care.
  - Provide guidance on how to obtain information about the status of missing persons.
- Following a mass-casualty incident, the goal should be to provide ongoing information to the public about:
  - Signs and symptoms of sequelae of exposure to toxic agents and post-traumatic stress.

- Who to call for information.
- Where to go for help.

Clear communication with the public is an essential part of a health and medical response to a mass-casualty event. In order to deliver clear and appropriate messages before, during, and after a mass-casualty event, it is important to consider a number of issues:

- Providing consistent and regular messaging, preferably through a single spokesperson with professional (medical) credibility, is highly desirable.
- Conveying clinical information requires particular care to assure that a lay audience can understand it.
- Distinguishing between political and professional messages is essential.
- Making provisions for communication in languages other than English may be necessary.

Strategies for public communication can be built from effective models of risk communication in use today for natural disasters, such as hurricanes and earthquakes. They should reflect and be tied to our long history of civil defense and other preparedness efforts dating as far back as World War II and the Cold War.

Ensuring an Adequate Supply of Health Care Providers

One of the key components of an effective health and medical care response is ensuring adequate supplies of a broad array of qualified responders and providers who are available and willing to serve in a mass-casualty event. This is likely to involve the following:

- Recruiting from retired or currently unemployed but qualified volunteer providers within the community and State.
- Making use of reserve military medical and nursing providers and other responders, as well as an expanded group of providers, such as veterinarians, dentists and dental auxiliary providers, pharmacists, and health professional students.
- Modifying State certification and licensing requirements to allow out-of-State providers to practice on a temporary basis.
- Modifying State regulations on a temporary basis to broaden scope of practice standards among various trained providers.
- Reallocating providers from nonemergency care and nonemergency sites to emergency response assignments and from unaffected regions to affected regions (this will involve identifying skill sets of each practitioner group [e.g., paramedics, nurse midwives, etc.], so as to optimize reassignment potential).
- Creating and training a pool of nonmedical responders to support health and medical care operations.
- Making adequate provisions to protect providers (and their families) who serve in mass casualty event situations to ensure their willingness to respond.
- Developing systems for the advance registration and credentialing of clinicians to augment health care personnel needs during a mass casualty event.

Provider Training and Education Programs

Adopting altered standards of care, even temporarily, will have a significant impact on health care delivery operations and therefore on the needs of providers for training and education to serve in those circumstances. Planners should not assume that individual providers will know how to deliver appropriate care in a mass-casualty event, but rather should develop or identify training programs to ensure a knowledgeable and systematic, coordinated response effort.

A wide array of preparedness training has been designed and is being delivered throughout the country. Some of the training has been evaluated for effectiveness. In the absence of a national clearinghouse for training for all providers and conditions, it is not possible to provide a complete picture of what is available and effective. General principles that might guide the development and identification of effective training include the following:

- Training should be competency based.
- Training should be ongoing.
- Training should be provided to all responders, including nonmedical personnel and potential community volunteer responders, as well as primary care providers in office and clinic settings.
- Training should be based on the doctrine of daily routine, which assumes that providers will do best what they do most often, but anticipate extension and expansion of provider roles.
- Training should be provided on a just-in-time basis only where appropriate, especially if it differs from daily routine.
- Training should be specific to the role a person is likely to play in a mass casualty event (e.g., clinic nurses and nurse aides may need training in burn care).
- Training should be specific to the conditions of performance (type of hazard, type of site) and involve opportunities to practice new skills through simulation and other mechanisms.
- Training should be effective, as demonstrated by evaluations and trainee performance.
- Training should be made available to all potential traditional and non-traditional providers, including veterinarians, dentists and dental auxiliary providers, pharmacists and health professional students.

A beginning list of the types of training needed by all responders and providers in pre-hospital, hospital, and alternate care sites includes but is not limited to the following:

- General disaster response, including an introduction to altered standards of care and how the move to such standards may affect triage and treatment decisions as well as facility conditions.
- Legal and ethical basis for allocating scarce resources in a mass casualty event.
- Orientation on how an incident management system would work in a mass casualty event.
- How to treat populations with special needs (e.g., children and elderly persons).
- How to recognize the signs and symptoms of specific hazards and a trend of similar types of signs and symptoms.
- How to treat specific conditions.
- How to recognize and manage of the effects of stress on themselves and their patients.

Finally, as components of preparedness training are defined, they should be incorporated into the original training for each provider group. For example, if paramedics are expected to participate in mass immunizations or assist in emergency departments, it would be desirable that they get basics on immunization and sterile technique in their original training.

Protection of Health Care Providers and Facilities

It is important for planners to consider the following to ensure the protection of health care providers:

- Personal protective equipment, prophylaxis, and other protections that enable them to work safely.
- Training specific to provider responsibilities and to the nature of the event.
- Adequate rotation of staff to prevent burnout and errors due to fatigue.
- Freedom from threats of malpractice (see earlier discussion of legal issues).
- Mental health support during and following stressful situations (e.g., Critical Incident Stress Management).
- Care and support for health care providers' families.

A related concern is to protect the integrity and safety of existing health care facilities (e.g., hospitals, the providers who work there, and the patients who are already under care) at the time a mass-casualty event occurs. The protection of alternate care sites created in response to a mass casualty event would also be important. A plan to protect health care facilities might include steps to ensure the following:

- Current patients and facility staff do not become secondary victims.
- Contaminated victims are not permitted to enter "clean" treatment areas.
- Facilities may utilize temporary security procedures, such as lockdowns, to enforce safety.
- Decontamination processes in all care settings are adequate.
- Noncritically ill patients are safely relocated to other facilities, if needed.

Caring for Populations with Special Needs

It is essential that plans for the delivery of health and medical care in a mass casualty event address how the special needs of several groups within the general population can be met. These needs may vary from providing for alternate means of decontamination for babies and other nonambulatory persons, to having translators available at intake centers, to providing mental health assessment resources within the health care setting. Involving organizations and services designed to serve groups with special needs under normal conditions may be a successful approach. As mentioned earlier, a victim's underlying medical condition may affect their survivability, and therefore may be considered negatively in triage. In some cases resources may be diverted away from adults to children because of their greater life expectancy.

Populations recognized as having special needs in a mass casualty event include but may not be limited to the following:

- *Children.* The unique physiology and wide variation in physical and cognitive development by age within childhood requires that triage personnel be trained in pediatric triage standards and other pediatric assessment protocols (e.g., JumpSTART); family care and adult care be available in pediatric settings; appropriately-sized supplies, equipment and medication doses be available; and safe use of decontamination procedures be ensured. Provisions for treating children whose parents are not present and for treating parents who will not leave their children are important considerations.
- *Persons with physical or cognitive disabilities.* As under normal standards of care, provisions to accommodate the special disability-related needs of some persons are important aspects of the organization of care. These are likely to include issues of physical access to and within care sites, alternative and safe decontamination procedures, enhanced communication, and issues involving informed consent.
- *Persons with preexisting mental health and/or substance abuse problems.* Preexisting mental health and substance abuse conditions are known to exacerbate an individual's ability to cope with physical and emotional trauma. Provisions should be made for screening and direction to appropriate services as part of triage or other assessment protocols.
- *Frail or immunocompromised adults and children.* Individuals in these groups who are victims may require adjustments in treatment regimens and special monitoring, but these adjustments will be made within the context of any overriding goal to maximize lives saved.
- *Non-English speakers.* Local and regional planning may have to take into account the need for communication tools in languages other than English. Although printed materials of a general nature may be prepared in advance, printed materials and signs will not be an adequate response for those who cannot read any language. An additional challenge may be present if undocumented individuals fear discovery and reprisal if they come forward for health care in a mass casualty event. Involvement of formal and informal networks,

organizations, and media outlets that serve non-English speaking groups is essential.

Transportation of Patients

Addressing issues related to the transportation of patients during a mass casualty event is also important. Roads may be blocked and the emergency transport system will not be adequate to meet the need. Issues to consider include the following:

- Who will accompany patients, since health and medical personnel may be needed elsewhere?
- How should all available public and private transport, including public and school buses, taxis, and limousines, be mobilized?
- What kind of prior agreements can be established to ensure this mobilization can occur?

Chapter G.5   Recommended Action Steps

Several recommendations for action related to planning a health and medical care response to a mass casualty event are identified below. The list of recommendations is not meant to be comprehensive, but it provides a starting point for discussion. These ideas suggest that a collaborative approach should be taken when developing next steps; both government and private organizations have unique roles and important contributions to make in moving forward.

Step 1: Develop general and event-specific guidance for allocating scarce health and medical care resources during a mass casualty event.

Public and private organizations, including professional societies, should develop guidance in specific areas related to allocating scarce clinical resources. Examples include but are not limited to the following:

- Triage guidelines and measures for specific types of events.
- Allocation guidelines for scarce resources, such as ventilators, burn beds, or surgical suites.
- Guidance for the triaging and treatment of children, specifically the ways in which altered standards of care might differ for a pediatric population.

Step 2: Develop and implement a process to address nonclinical issues related to the delivery of health and medical care during a mass-casualty event.

Examples of non-clinical issues include but are not limited to the following:

- Alternative ways to establish authority to move to altered standards of health and medical care in a mass casualty situation.
- Alternative ways to ensure an adequate legal framework, including liability, certification and licensing, and mutual aid agreements for the provision of health and medical care in a mass casualty event.
- Alternative ways to resolve issues of finance and reimbursement issues related to the provision of health and medical care in a mass casualty event.

Step 3: Develop a comprehensive strategy for risk communication with the public before, during, and after a mass casualty event.

Experts agreed that a unified strategy and tools for public communication around mass casualty risk and health and medical care response are indicated. Part of the challenge is to craft credible messages that the public will perceive as immediately relevant and important to their daily lives without causing undue alarm. Such a strategy should take the form of anticipatory guidance. Messages should be developed collaboratively with various stakeholders (such as the American Hospital Association, the Joint Commission on the Accreditation of Health Care Organizations, and others), that should also participate in their dissemination.

Specific ideas and suggestions made regarding public communication include but are not limited to the following:

- Continue and expand CDC training of journalists to cover health events as a means to partner effectively with the media in reaching the public.

- Find effective ways to communicate clinical information to lay audiences.
- Utilize primary care providers and local public health departments, especially nurses, in getting out agreed-upon messages in local communities on a one to one basis.
- Provide a communications capability at the level of the individual facility as well as through joint information centers.
- Include communications internal to health care facilities and among system components, such as hospitals and alternate care sites, in communications strategies.
- Build on the HANS (Health Alert Network System), part of CDC's emergency alert system, to develop an overall communication strategy.

Step 4: Identify, analyze, and consider modification of Federal, State, and local laws and regulations that may affect the delivery of health and medical care during a mass casualty event.

As part of an effort to develop a legal framework for providing health and medical care in a mass casualty situation, an effort should be made to create a compendium of laws and regulations at the Federal, State and local levels that affect the delivery of health and medical care. This compendium of laws and regulations would facilitate the creation of an adequate legal framework for moving to altered standards of care when necessary. It would identify the following:

- The responsible parties for each law or regulation (local, State or Federal government).
- Circumstances when each law or regulation can be modified.
- Specific ways each law or regulation could be modified on a temporary basis.

Step 5: Develop means for verifying credentials of medical and other health personnel prior to and on-site during a mass casualty event.

In disaster situations, individuals who claim to be qualified providers and who want to volunteer their services typically approach health care facilities. In order to be able to make use of such resources, facility and incident managers need to have tools and methods, such as searchable databases, for verifying credentials. Efforts are underway at both the State and Federal levels to address this need. Emergency Systems for Advance Registration of Volunteer Health Care Personnel (ESAR-VHP), as outlined in the Public Health Security and Bioterrorism Preparedness and Response Act of 2002 (Public Law 107-188), as well as the Medical Reserve Corps credentialing efforts, and other State-developed systems are examples of tools that could be useful in this regard.

Step 6: Create strategies to ensure health and medical leadership and coordination for the health and medical aspects of system response during a mass casualty event.

Experience in developing preparedness strategies suggests there is a need to assure high-level health and medical leadership at the system and regional levels. For some systems and regions, this may involve creating a designated Medical Disaster Specialist or a role with comparable responsibilities to coordinate the health and medical aspects of system response. The expertise required ensuring appropriate health and medical leadership in a mass casualty event includes the following:

- Knowledge about how and when to initiate altered standards of care.
- Knowledge and skill to facilitate communication and provide the link between the medical care system and overall incident response.
- Knowledge and skill to provide disaster-related medical leadership in a system of community

or region, including all aspects of medical preparedness and response.
- Knowledge and skill to provide leadership for training.
- Knowledge of and the ability to match hospital and system-specific resources to interventions in a crisis.
- Knowledge of surge plans, resources, and techniques for that particular region/city.
- Knowledge and skill in developing resource-sharing agreements, such as regional travel teams and memoranda of understanding, with adjacent areas.

Step 7: Continue and expand efforts to train providers and others to respond effectively in a mass casualty event.

A wide range of provider training is needed to ensure an effective health and medical response to a mass-casualty event. Training needs include, but are not limited to:

- General disaster response, including an introduction to altered standards of care and how the move to such standards may affect triage and treatment decisions as well as facility conditions.
- Legal and ethical basis for allocating scarce resources in a mass-casualty event.
- Orientation to how an incident management system would work in a mass-casualty event.
- How to treat children and other groups who may need special equipment or modified approaches to care.
- How to recognize the signs and symptoms of specific hazards.
- How to treat specific conditions.
- How to recognize and manage of the effects of stress on themselves and their patients.

General principles to guide the design of effective training programs are included in Chapter 4.

Step 8: Develop and support a research agenda specific to health and medical care standards for mass casualty events.

Ideas for research related to health and medical care standards for mass-casualty events are listed below. The focus of these suggested studies should be on practical application, testing, and sharing of promising practices.

- Examine how different combinations of resources, signs/symptoms, and response to treatment may affect the numbers of lives that can be saved. A better understanding of survivability is especially important in developing criteria for the allocation of scarce treatment resources.
- Analyze or develop models to predict how much injury or illness can be prevented under different kinds of mass casualty scenarios. A better understanding of achievable reductions in injury and illness is important to setting goals for a system under stress.
- Examine international models and other real-world experiences of health and medical care delivery for evidence of what happens when "usual" rules are suspended or impossible to maintain. Other models and experiences may include specific disaster experiences (e.g., the Madrid train bombing and suicide bombings in Israel), as well as countries whose health systems operate daily with mildly, moderately, or severely constrained resources compared with the U.S. health care system. The focus of the research might be on methods for and outcomes of rationing scarce resources under different conditions.
- Evaluate all aspects of demonstrations and mock mass-casualty events, such as "TOPOFF 3" and other drills, to find and address weak points in the system.
- Conduct research on effective risk communication with the public.
- Identify ways to share promising and tested practices in resource sharing (e.g., mutual aid

agreements in St. Louis, Louisiana, New York City, and New Jersey).

Step 9: Develop a community-based planning guide for mass casualty care.

Experts agree that local and regional planners need a resource to assist them in enhancing surge capacity plans so that they include situations involving mass-casualty events. A *Community-Based Planning Guide for Mass Casualty Care* could be developed that includes guidelines, principles, templates, and examples of promising or tested practices for addressing the many and varied aspects of this task, whether the focus is site-specific, local, regional, or statewide. Although some tools and resources exist that could be incorporated into a *Planning Guide*, others—including guidelines for the allocation of scarce resources during a mass-casualty event—have yet to be fully developed or evaluated. It is important that the *Planning Guide* not be prescriptive, but rather offer suggestions and identify tools and resources that may be useful in guiding triage and the allocation of scarce resources.

Step 10: Identify and support states, health systems, and regions to develop mass casualty and health and medical care response plans based on the Planning Guide and to share their results widely.

A number of practice-oriented "centers of excellence" could be supported in their efforts to build on surge capacity planning to prepare for a health and medical response to mass-casualty events. The goal would be to move beyond specific elements of a plan limited to facilities, such as hospitals, to create a health and medical care response plan that is coordinated among its participants and with the overall emergency response system for the system or region. A central expectation of this approach is that the supported centers would develop and implement plans based on the *Planning Guide* and serve as demonstrations whose results would be widely shared with peers around the country.

Appendix G.A Final Participant List: Expert Meeting on Mass Casualty Medical Care,

August 3-4, 2004, The Hotel George, Washington, DC

Mr. Mark Ackermann
Senior Vice President and Chief Corporate Services Officer
Saint Vincent's Catholic Medical Centers

Michael Allswede, D.O.
Associate Professor of Emergency Medicine
Section Chief, Special Emergency Medical Response, Emergency Medical Services
Department of Emergency Medicine
University of Pittsburgh

Sherlita Amler, M.D., M.S., FAAP
Terrorism Medical Officer
Division of Injury and Disability Outcomes and Programs
National Center for Injury Prevention and Control
Centers for Disease Control and Prevention
U.S. Department of Health and Human Services

Knox Andress, R.N.
Weapons of Mass Destruction Response Coordinator and 2004 Chair
Emergency Preparedness Committee
Emergency Nurses Association
CHRISTUS Schumpert Health System

Joshua Bobrowsky, M.P.H.
Director, Preparedness Policy
Association of State and Territorial Health Officials

Lieutenant Commander Sumner L. Bossler, Jr.
U.S. Public Health Service
Senior Public Health Analyst
Division of Health Care Emergency Preparedness
Special Programs Bureau
Health Resources and Services Administration
U.S. Department of Health and Human Services

Ms. Shayne Brannman
Special Assistant
Office of the Assistant Secretary for Public Health Emergency Preparedness
U.S. Department of Health and Human Services

Stephen V. Cantrill, M.D., FACEP
Associate Director
Department of Emergency Medicine
Denver Health Medical Center

Arthur L. Caplan, Ph.D.
The Emanual and Robert Hart Professor of
  Bioethics
Chair, Department of Medical Ethics
Director, Center for Bioethics
University of Pennsylvania

Mr. Joseph L. Cappiello
Vice President
Accreditation Field Operations
Joint Commission on Accreditation of Health
  Organizations

Robert G. Claypool, M.D.
Deputy Chief Medical Officer
Office of the Assistant Secretary for Public
  Health Emergency Preparedness
U.S. Department of Health and Human Services

Janice Doyle, R.N., M.S.N.
Nurse Specialist
Bethel School District
National Association of School Nurses

Lieutenant Colonel Rhonda Earls, M.S.N.,
  C.N.M.
United States Army Fellow
Office of the Assistant Secretary for Public
  Health Emergency Preparedness
U.S. Department of Health and Human Services

Mr. Michael Feeser
Program Analyst
Office of Plans, Policy and Preparedness
U.S. Department of Veterans Affairs

Michael Fraser, Ph.D.
Deputy Executive Director
National Association of Country and City
  Health Officials

Edward J. Gabriel, M.P.A., A.E.M.T.-P.
Deputy Commissioner of Preparedness
Office of Emergency Management
City of New York

Commander Valerie Jensen, R.Ph.
U.S. Public Health Service
Senior Regulatory Project Manager
Drug Shortage Program
Center for Drug Evaluation and Research
Food and Drug Administration
U.S. Department of Health and Human Services

Brian Kamoie, J.D., M.P.H.
Assistant Research Professor
Department of Health Policy and
Department of Health Services Management
  and Leadership
School of Public Health and Health Services
George Washington University

Sharon Katz, M.P.A.
Acting Associate Director for Planning, Policy
  and Evaluation
Office of Terrorism Preparedness and
  Emergency Response
Centers for Disease Control and Prevention
U.S. Department of Health and Human Services

Ann R. Knebel, R.N., DNSc.
Captain, U.S. Public Health Services
Senior Program Manager
Office of Public Health Emergency Preparedness

Lieutenant Colonel William J. Kormos, Jr.
National Disaster Medical System Liaison
  Officer
Office of the Assistant Secretary of Defense
  Health Affairs/Personnel and Readiness
Force Health Protection and Readiness
U.S. Department of Defense

Mr. Kurt Krumperman
Vice President for Federal Affairs and
  Strategic Initiatives
Rural/Metro Corporation
American Ambulance Association Liaison to
  DHS/HHS for Disaster Preparedness

David Markenson, M.D.
Deputy Director
National Center for Disaster Preparedness
Mailman School of Public Health
Columbia University

Angela Martinelli, D.N.Sc., R.N., CNOR
Commander, U.S. Public Health Service
Office of Force Readiness and Deployment (OFRD) Room 117
U.S. Department of Health and Human Services

Robert J. McNellis, M.P.H., P.A.-C.
Director
Clinical Affairs and Education
American Academy of Physician Assistants

The Honorable Dan K. Morhaim, M.D.
Member, Council of State Governments
Delegate, Maryland House of Delegates

Jerry L. Mothershead, M.D., FACEP
Member, American College of Emergency Physicians
Senior Medical Advisor
Medical Readiness and Response Group
Battelle Memorial Institute
Battelle Eastern Science and Technology Center

Mr. Edward Peloquin
Domestic Preparedness Coordinator
New Jersey Association of Non-Profit Homes for the Aging

Sally Phillips, R.N., Ph.D.
Director, Bioterrorism Preparedness Research Program
Center for Primary Care, Prevention, and Clinical Partnerships
Agency for Healthcare Research and Quality
U.S. Department of Health and Human Services

Rosamond Rhodes, Ph.D.
Professor, Medical Education
Director, Bioethics Education
Mount Sinai School of Medicine

Lewis Rubinson, M.D., Ph.D.
Fellow, Center for Biosecurity
University of Pittsburgh Medical Center

Ms. Roslyne Schulman
Senior Associate Director
Department of Policy Development
American Hospital Association

Elizabeth A. Simpson, J.D.
Deputy General Counsel
MedStar Health, Inc.

Mr. Larry Smith
Vice President for Risk Management
MedStar Health, Inc.

Mark S. Smith, M.D.
Chair, Department of Emergency Medicine
Washington Hospital Center
Georgetown University School of Medicine

Leslee Stein-Spencer, R.N., M.S.
Chief, Division of Emergency Medical Services and Highway Safety
Illinois Department of Public Health

Lew Stringer, M.D.
Senior Medical Advisor and Director
Response Division
U.S. Department of Homeland Security

Eric M. Wassermann, M.D.
Senior Medical Advisor
Office of the Assistant Secretary for Public Health Emergency Preparedness
U.S. Department of Health and Human Services

Betsy Weiner, R.N., Ph.D., B.C., FAAN
Assistant Director
International Nursing Coalition for Mass Casualty Education
School of Nursing
Vanderbilt University

HSR Staff

Health Systems Research, Inc.
1200 18th Street, NW, Suite 700
Washington, DC 20036
Phone: (202) 828-5100
Fax: (202) 728-9469

Lawrence Bartlett, Ph.D., Facilitator
Director
E-mail: lbartlett@hsrnet.com

Rilla Murray, Dr.PH.
Project Director
E-mail: rmurray@hsrnet.com

Appendix G.B Preliminary Review of Selected Emergency Response Protocols and Models

A preliminary review of a number of triage protocols and preparedness models was conducted prior to the expert meeting to assess the extent to which these documents provided explicit guidance on the issue of altered standards of care in the context of a mass casualty event. Brief summaries of the review of several field triage protocols and the Modular Emergency Medical System (MEMS) are presented below.

Field Triage Protocols

One category of altered standards of care focuses on specific methods for field triage. In a mass casualty situation of any magnitude, methods of triage, or sorting victims according to their condition and resources available, are used to identify and, if possible, move to immediate treatment those who are most likely to survive or can benefit the most from treatment. Thus, triage standards address who receives care and when care is provided or the urgency with which it is provided. Triage is performed most often by first responders.

Triage begins in the field if there is a fixed event site; however, it also occurs within care settings, such as hospitals and alternate care sites, where individual victims may present themselves for care independent of organized responses. Secondary triage also may be necessary within a facility, such as a hospital, as demands on the system grow.

Several well-established standards for triage are currently in use.[1-5] Triage systems include START; JumpSTART (a pediatric modification to START); START, then SAVE; MASS; and others. Each system seeks to establish a small number of categories among victims that indicate the urgency with which they should be treated. Colors are often used to represent the categories—for example, red (immediate care); yellow (delayed); green (ambulatory and minor injuries); and black (dead and/or "expectant).

The adequacy of the triage system used depends on the nature of the event and the population affected. For example, systems such as START and JumpSTART are trauma-oriented and may be effective in an explosive event. Traditional epidemic approaches to triage, considered more appropriate for biological events, sort infected patients into three categories: susceptible individuals, infected individuals, and removed individuals (by successful immunization, recovery, or death).

These standards have the impact of allocating resources for patient care. The standards are relevant to pre-hospital, hospital, and alternate care sites and to a situation where resources are constrained and demand is so great that rationing is required. While most systems offer detailed clinical measurements of status for triage purposes, they do not, by definition, provide actual clinical protocols for the treatment that would follow.

Modular Emergency Medical System

Another type of standard that is pertinent to this discussion is one that addresses the organization of care and provides a context in which triage and medical care guidelines would be used. The Modular Emergency Medical System (MEMS) offers a comprehensive plan of operations and standards for responding to a mass casualty event of such size that alternate care delivery sites would be required.

MEMS emerged in response to Title IV of The Defense against Weapons of Mass Destruction Act of 1996 (Public Law 104–201). The law required that the Secretary of Defense develop and carry out a program to improve the responses of Federal, State, and local agencies to emergencies involving biological and chemical weapons. In response, the U.S. Department of Defense (DOD) created the Biological Warfare Improved Response Program. DOD then invited the Departments of Health and Human Services (DHHS), Energy (DOE), and Agriculture (USDA), and the Federal Emergency Management Agency (FEMA), the Federal Bureau of Investigation (FBI) and

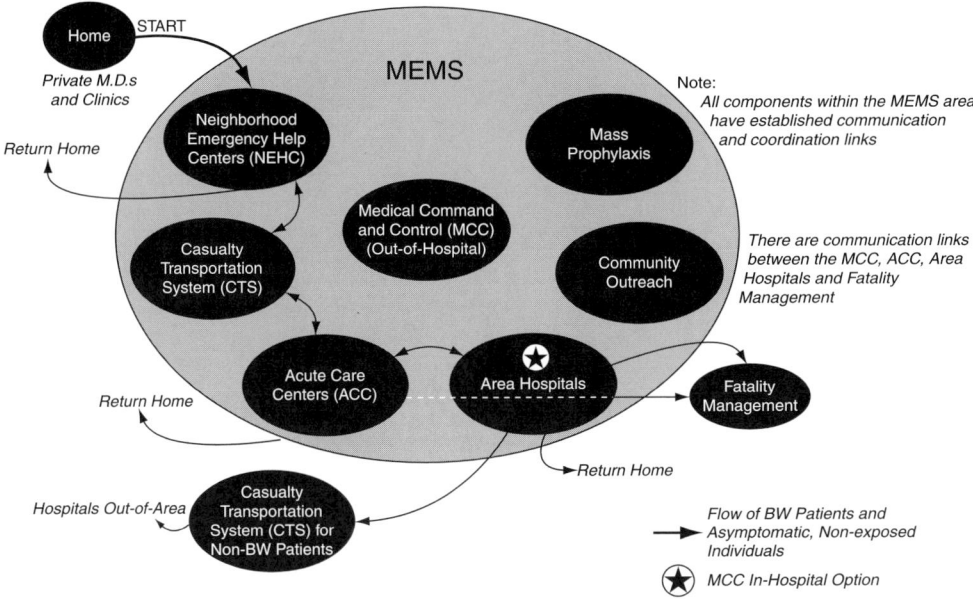

Figure G.8 Operation of the modular emergency medical system (MEMS). (Source: U.S. Army Soldier and Biological Chemical Command. Modular Emergency Medical System: Expanding Local Healthcare Structure in a Mass Casualty Incident. June 2002. Retrieved Aug. 17, 2004, from http://accem.org/pdf/mems_copper_book.pdf)

the Environmental Protection Agency (EPA), as well as emergency responders and managers from multiple States and local communities, to participate.

MEMS offers detailed standards for a system of care that can be expanded and contracted in modular units as the need arises. It provides a framework for the organization of care, particularly for setting up predetermined, special-use alternate care sites. Thus, MEMS answers the questions of what general kinds of care are provided and where (alternate site standards). In specifying the staffing required for alternate care sites, MEMS also addresses who will provide care. One of the underlying assumptions in MEMS is that resources will be brought in or created within the area most affected by the mass casualty event. Figure G.8 on the following page graphically depicts the operation of MEMS.

References

1. J.F. Wackerle. Disaster planning and response. *N Eng J Med*, 324:815–821, 1991.
2. L. Romig. The "JumpSTART" Rapid Pediatric Triage System. Available at: www.jumpstarttriage.com
3. M. Benson, K.L. Koenig, and C.H. Schultz. Disaster Triage. START, then SAVE—A New Method of Dynamic Triage for Victims of a Catastrophic Earthquake. *Prehospital and Disaster Medicine*, 11(2), 1996
4. MEDDAC Non-Commissioned Office Development Program. *Emergency Management Planning* slide presentation. Fort Carson, CO. Available at:http://evans.amedd.army.mil/herd/ncopd/EMP%20ODP.ppt. Accessed December 2004.
5. F.M. Burkle. Mass casualty management of a large-scale bioterrorist event: an epidemiological approach that shapes triage decision. *Emergency Med Clin N Am*, 20:409–436, 2002

Appendix H Surge Hospitals: Providing Safe Care in Emergencies

Executive Summary

After Hurricane Katrina slammed into the Gulf Coast in late August 2005 followed closely by Hurricane Rita, the health care community quickly mobilized to provide care to thousands of people who were caught in the storms' paths. Because the hurricanes and subsequent flooding caused the same sort of devastation to many local health care facilities as it did to other types of buildings in the region, the disaster forced many health care organizations to set up temporary facilities called "surge hospitals" in places such as shuttered retail stores, athletic arenas, and veterinary hospitals. The surge hospitals, so-called because they are designed to treat a surge in the number of patients needing care, contained triage, treatment, and sometimes even surgical capabilities. These temporary facilities were established to serve as a stopgap measure to provide medical care until the area's health care organizations could reopen. The severity of the damage that was done to the region's health care facilities has brought the health care community's responsibility for planning, building, and operating effective surge hospitals into focus. As this disaster has shown, health care organizations may be forced to provide care at surge hospitals for an extended period of time due to the damage sustained to their permanent facilities during catastrophic events. This reality challenges the Joint Commission to consider implementing a minimum set of standards to ensure that care provided at surge hospitals is safe and of high quality. Should the development of these standards move forward, the Joint Commission would seek input from groups that have extensive knowledge of surge hospitals, such as the Texas A&M University System Health Science Center. (Representatives of this organization were involved in establishing and operating the surge hospital described in Case Study 5, which begins on p. 21.)

It is crucial that health care organizations understand what surge hospitals are and how they can plan for and establish them, including whom they should work with to do so. Hurricanes Katrina and Rita have shown us that having plans to "surge in place," meaning expanding a functional facility to treat a large number of patients after a mass casualty incident, is not always sufficient in disasters because the health care organization itself may be too damaged to operate. Where outside of its own walls does a health care organization go to expand its surge capacity? Who should be involved in planning, establishing, and operating surge hospitals? This paper provides the answers to these questions and offers real-life examples of how surge hospitals were established on the Gulf Coast.

Introduction

A familiar concept to health care organizations, *surge capacity* is a health care system's ability to expand quickly beyond normal services to meet an increased demand for medical care [1]. *Surge hospitals* have been defined as facilities designed to supplement existing hospitals in the case of an emergency [2].

Because many health care organizations' ability to *surge in place*, meaning the capability to expand the surge capacity of a functioning health care facility, is limited, health care organizations need to have plans for increasing surge capacity which include the establishment of temporary surge

---

[1] Source: © 2006 by the Joint Commission on Accreditation of Healthcare Organizations

hospitals. It is critical that health care organizations (in concert with community leadership) initiate pacts with other organizations such as medical centers, schools, hotels, veterinary hospitals, and/or

> "Few, if any, hospitals in America today could handle 100 patients suddenly demanding care. There is no metropolitan area, no geographically contiguous area, that could handle 1,000 people suddenly needing advanced medical care in this country right now."
>
> Source: U.S. Congress. Senate. Committee on Government Affairs. *FEMA's Role in Managing Bioterrorist Attacks and the Impact of Public Health Concerns on Bioterrorism Preparedness.* 107th Cong., 1st sess., July 23, 2001. Testimony of Tara J. O'Toole, M.D., M.P.H., Johns Hopkins Center for Civilian Biodefense Studies.

convention centers to establish locations for the off-site triage of patients as well as for acute care during an emergency. Hospitals and other health care organizations must develop communitywide response plans that integrate their capacities into a single, organized response. Communications and data sharing that link health care organizations to local and state public health agencies are critical to this process.

In truth, no single model exists for the surge hospital. Today's health care leaders must examine the various types of surge hospital facilities that have been used to respond to emergencies and build their plans based on the needs of the community as well as the resources available to the organization.

Goal of this publication

This publication provides information to health care planners at the community, state, and federal level about what surge hospitals are, the kind of planning they require, how they can be set up, and who should be responsible for their establishment and operation. The case studies at the end of this paper describe how surge hospitals along the Gulf Coast were established and operated, providing a real-life perspective on the importance of creating safe surge hospitals after disasters strike as well as on the challenges that go along with providing care under these makeshift conditions.

Acknowledgments

We would like to extend our gratitude to the following people, both of whom were instrumental in writing this publication:

Pam Brick
Freelance Writer
Paul K. Carlton, Jr., M.D., FACS
Lt. General, USAF (Ret.)
Director, Office of Homeland Security
Texas A&M University System Health Science Center

Using surge hospitals to respond to emergencies

Positioning a hospital emergency room near the site of every potential disaster is impossible, yet a patient with serious injury needs to be transported to surgery within the "golden hour" after the injury occurs for the best chances of survival. Health care planners have developed a number of innovative ways that a surge hospital can respond to this need. These solutions include opening shuttered hospitals or closed wards in an existing facility, temporarily using buildings in the community to obtain greater surge capacity, transporting mobile medical facilities to the site, installing portable medical or surgical units near the emergency, and using these types of portable facilities to augment hospital capacity. Agreements for use of these facilities should, if possible, be made in advance to expedite the delivery of care in a worst-case scenario. A description of the different kinds of surge hospitals follows.

Types of surge hospitals
Shuttered hospitals or closed wards
The Agency for Healthcare Research and Quality (AHRQ), a branch of the U.S. Department of Health and Human Services (DHHS), offers guidance on using closed hospitals to expand surge capacity in an emergency. The agency recommends

two occasions when the use of a shuttered facility is warranted: mass casualty events and cases where quarantines must be instituted to guard against transmission of an infectious agent or communicable disease. Any institution contemplating the use of a closed hospital to expand surge capacity should ideally engage in advance planning to thoroughly assess the facility, although it must be acknowledged that in many cases the urgency of a situation often calls for swifter action. The best approach might be for an existing hospital or other health care organization to acquire the shuttered hospital as a satellite of the medical center so that patient services such as pharmacy and laboratory can be extended to the satellite. Whether the site is a shuttered hospital, or, as is described in Sidebar 1 below, a closed hospital ward, the first staff to enter the facility should be an environmental crew that would clean the facility to ensure that the water, air, and general environment are sanitary and adequate for their intended use.

Sidebar 1. An example of "surging in place"—opening a closed hospital ward

Baton Rouge's largest public health hospital, the 200-bed Earl K. Long Medical Center, is a facility that provides care to the indigent: the poor, the uninsured, the frail elderly, and prisoners from the city's four jails. This hospital's method of increasing surge capacity to treat victims of Hurricane Katrina was to open several closed wards within the hospital. This step expanded its capacity by 200 beds, effectively doubling the hospital in size. Jimmy Guidry, M.D., state health officer of Louisiana and medical director for Louisiana's Department of Health & Hospitals (DHH), made the decision to open the wards, using the strategy of "surging in place" to increase the hospital's surge capacity.

Facilities of opportunity

"Facilities of opportunity" are nonmedical buildings that, because of their size or proximity to a medical center, can be adapted into surge hospitals. These facilities may include sites such as veterinary hospitals, convention centers, exhibition halls, empty warehouses, airport hangars, schools, sports arenas, or hotels. Health care organizations can designate such nearby buildings and equip them to handle an overflow of patients. Sometimes a medical facility designed for another purpose, such as a day surgery center, can quickly adapt into a surge hospital with minimal cost and effort.

Mobile medical facilities

Another type of surge hospital is the mobile surge hospital, such as an 18-wheeler truck fitted with state-of-the-art surgical and intensive care units that can rapidly deploy to the scene of an emergency. These mobile intensive care units typically have six beds and their surgical units contain pre-op and post-op recovery areas, a centralized nursing station, and clean and soiled utility rooms. An additional advantage is that these facilities can be used not only for disaster management but also as portable clinics offering preventive services to rural or otherwise underserved areas. These dual-use facilities have been referred to as *Thursday hospitals* because they can be used for patient care in one given location on a certain day of the week (such as on a Thursday) and can be used in other locations the rest of the week, while remaining available for other purposes of disaster response at all times.

Portable facilities

An additional answer to the surge capacity problem is the portable, mobile medical facility that can be set up quickly and be ready to be used to provide care in a few hours. Such units, commonly known as *hospitals in a box*, are fully equipped, self-contained, turnkey systems designed to be set up near mass casualty events to treat the most severely wounded as soon as possible. One soon-to-be-available protoype, the Advanced Surgical Suite for Trauma Casualties (ASSTC), is a highly mobile, lightweight, self-contained surgical facility that has both military and civilian uses. It can be set up in less than 30 minutes and is stored in a 5ft. × 5ft. × 10ft. box. Supply cabinets in the unit can be stockpiled with medications and equipment tailored to the specific situation.

Project ER One

Project ER One is a prototypical emergency care facility developed by Washington Hospital Center in Washington, D.C., and conceived as a chemical- and bioterrorism-ready mass casualty facility. Intended as a model for all new emergency departments constructed in the nation, ER One features the following emergency-ready elements to enable a rapid response in disaster-stricken communities:

Treatment areas designed to thwart cross-contamination and cross-infection
Modular scalability to serve many patients on a daily basis and then expand for larger numbers in minutes
An educational training center that can also serve as a planning hub for neighboring health care organizations and for handling non-conventional threats
State-of-the-art computer information system that can track patients and patient records in real time
The ability to share encrypted data with sanctioned medical, public safety, military, and governmental agencies
A laboratory for research and development in bioterrorism and similar events

ER One embodies the hallmark principles of the surge facility, which include dual use, scalability, and modularity. During phase one of the project, design specifications were developed for the emergency facility at Washington Hospital Center. The Phase II design study will put the phase one findings into operation at the hospital center.

Planning for, establishing, and operating surge hospitals

When planning for the potential use of a surge hospital, health care institutions need to consider their definition of *surge capacity* as more than just the number of available hospital beds. Instead, they need to think about their ability to handle a public health emergency by examining two additional types of resources inside their institutions: staffing and equipment. Organizations also need to investigate pharmaceutical reserves in local pharmacies so they can have a ready supply of needed medications that last until additional supplies arrive from the Strategic National Stockpile (see p. 7 for a detailed description of the Strategic National Stockpile). In addition, communications systems and information technology should be in place so that the organization can communicate with both internal staff and outside agencies. Another fundamental part of the planning process is the connectivity with community leaders and planning organizations to ensure compatibility with community thinking and functional initiatives.

Evaluating the options for surge capability

When considering the surge facility options available to a health care organization, it is important to start at the neighborhood level and work outward. Can any closed wards be opened? Does the organization have a satellite outpatient facility that can be converted to inpatient use to increase hospital capacity? What are the closest available large-capacity venues, such as veterinary hospitals, exhibition halls, or schools that could be used to expand capacity?

Mobile medical facilities and portable surgical units can also be attractive candidates to serve as surge facilities; however, a disadvantage of using these facilities is their considerable cost. Cash-strapped hospitals and other health care organizations may find it difficult to dedicate huge sums of money for infrastructure changes that may rarely, if ever, be used. For this reason, many organizations are looking at ways to retrofit their existing buildings to add surge capacity while controlling costs.

Design considerations for dual use in existing buildings

Health care facilities that have one purpose, such as a surgery suite in nonemergency circumstances, but which can be converted to increase surge capacity in an emergency, are called dual-use facilities. Hospitals themselves can be equipped for dual use during a crisis, but the cost of retrofitting a hospital for dual use is prohibitive for many organizations. The Joint Commission encourages health care organizations undertaking new construction to build for dual use (see Sidebar 2 on page 5 for information about building considerations for dual use facilities). Health care leaders should also consider becoming involved in the construction and planning of new structures, such as libraries, civic centers, or community centers so that these buildings can incorporate dual-use concepts into their construction plans.

Sidebar 2. Building code variances

Disaster planning highlights the need for changes in building code requirements to meet the demand for high-volume patient care. Most of these recommendations could also apply to the new construction of schools, libraries, hotels, and other buildings in a community. Some of the variances that health care organizations need to consider include the following:

- Wide hallways and stairwells to allow stretchers to pass each other
- Redundant power, such as a second generator or a duplicate electrical system that serves as a backup for the primary system
- "Clean" rooms that contain self-decontaminating surfaces, negative pressure air-handling systems, and controlled pressure, temperature, and humidity
- Horizontal construction with larger and faster elevators to avoid bottlenecks when moving patients to different floors
- Multiple patient drop-off entrances to prevent traffic jams
- HEPA filter systems that trap biological agents in incoming air and expose them to ultraviolet light to render them harmless
- Storage for medical equipment which protects supplies from biological and radiological threats
- Docking stations to accomodate 18-wheeler response vans that meet all standards of care

---

Coordinating efforts with local, state, and federal emergency management planners

Hurricanes Katrina and Rita illustrated that state and local preparedness is a key factor in a successful response during the first 24–28 hours after a disaster. The relationships and agreements established before a disaster occurs are critical to an effective emergency response.

Health care organization leaders should evaluate their surge capacity outside of their own institution in the context of their local communities as well as at the regional level (see Sidebar 3 for a list of issues that leaders should consider regarding collaborating with other health care organizations during emergencies).

Sidebar 3. Leadership issues for collaborating with proximate health care organizations

- What health care organizations are geographically proximate (all types, whether offering similar services or not)?
- What proximate health care organizations offer similar services?
- What resources (such as supplies, beds, and staff) might be shared or pooled in an emergency response?
- What might our organization be able to provide for proximate health care organizations? What provisions can we make to offer such services/supplies in the event of a disaster or emergency?
- What in-kind or reciprocal agreements might we make with each organization?
- How will we communicate with proximate health care organizations? Who should be contacted at each organization?
- If care recipients must be evacuated from our organization, which neighboring organization could receive transferred individuals?
- What suppliers/vendors does each proximate organization rely on for materials that might be needed in an emergency? What are their back-up plans for supplies in case

> of an emergency? Are all of the region's health care organizations relying on the same vendors?
>
> Source: Joint Commission on Accreditation of Healthcare Organizations: *Guide to Emergency Management Planning in Health Care.* Oakbrook Terrace, IL: Joint Commission Resources, 2002.

The catastrophe in New Orleans showed the nation nothing if not the reality that disasters can cripple entire regions. Institutions must put cooperative agreements in place with state and regional partners and also work with federal representatives who can ensure that sufficient resources are available to handle a widespread emergency.

Certain locations in the country are already doing this. For example, New York City understands, because of its recent history and proximity to other states, that a disaster that occurs inside the city could also impact New York State, New Jersey, and Pennsylvania if the city's ability to respond to the emergency is overwhelmed by the severity of the disaster. As a consequence, a significant amount of regional planning occurs in that city.

Obtaining needed personnel and supplies

One of the key components of an effective health and medical care response is ensuring an adequate number of qualified health care providers who are available and willing to serve in a mass casualty event. Having sufficient supplies, pharmaceuticals, and equipment is also critical.

Obtaining a sufficient number of staff members

A model for determining the number of staff needed for a surge facility is the Modular Emergency Medical Stem (MEMS) designed by the U.S. Department of Defense. The system is based on the incident command system, which is commonly used by the emergency medical services community. The system sets up a network used to access patient care personnel through neighborhood emergency help centers and acute care centers. Activities that can help in the search for additional qualified personnel in a time of need include the following:

- Recruiting from retired or currently unemployed but qualified volunteer providers within the community and state
- Making use of reserve military medical and nursing providers and other responders, as well as an expanded group of providers, such as veterinarians, dentists and dental auxiliary providers, pharmacists, and health professional students
- Reallocating providers from nonemergency care and nonemergency sites to emergency response assignments and from unaffected regions to affected regions (this will involve identifying skill sets of each practitioner group [such as paramedics and nurse midwives], so as to optimize reassignment potential)
- Creating and training a pool of nonmedical responders to support health and medical care operations
- Making adequate provisions to protect providers (and their families) who serve in mass casualty event situations to ensure their willingness to respond

Perhaps the best known source of supplementary medical personnel is the Medical Reserve Corps (MRC) Program, which organizes the services of more than 27,000 practicing and retired physicians, nurses, and other health professionals as well as ordinary citizens who wish to volunteer in community public health efforts and help during large-scale emergencies. Founded by President George W. Bush in 2002 in cooperation with the USA Freedom Corps, the MRC specializes in identifying, training, and organizing volunteer medical and public health professionals.

Two additional resources exist for the recruitment of medical staff in a worst-case scenario. The first is the National Disaster Medical System (NDMS), established in the 1980s by the U.S. Departments of Health and Human Services and Veterans Affairs and the Federal

Emergency Management Agency. NDMS organizes 7000 health care volunteers in locally sponsored specialty teams that become federalized upon activation. The second resource is the Public Health Service Commissioned Corps headed by the surgeon general. The corps consists of roughly 6000 physicians, nurses, pharmacists, allied health care workers, dentists, scientists, computer specialists, and other officers available to offer health care—related expertise in times of war or national emergencies.

Local medical, nursing, and allied health care students can also help provide care in times of need. In addition, the American Red Cross, temporary medical staffing agencies, and volunteer programs, such as AmeriCorps and SeniorCorps, provide medical personnel and volunteers to health care organizations during emergencies.

Education of the existing hospital staff is also important and involves the following areas: better disaster-response awareness, improved skills, an understanding of roles and responsibilities, more effective communication, and experience in cooperating with other staff members as well as personnel from outside agencies and organizations during emergencies. Strengthening emergency training programs fortifies preparedness, but the skills most valuable during a disaster are those practiced by staff every day.

Medical supplies and equipment

A number of options exist to acquire the needed beds, medical supplies, and equipment in a time of crisis. The Strategic National Stockpile, a program of the Centers for Disease Control and Prevention (CDC), maintains large quantities of medications and medical supplies, such as airway maintenance, IV maintenance, and medical surgical items to be used in public health emergencies including infectious disease outbreaks, natural disasters, and manmade disasters. Needed medicines and supplies can be delivered free of charge to any state as part of this program. Each state is then responsible for distributing supplies to local communities. To respond to this additional need, the medical center may need to consider equipment rental or leasing options.

The experience of the medical teams that set up the surge hospitals in Louisiana and Texas following the hurricanes was that the Strategic National Stockpile may not be able to deliver needed medical goods for several days during emergencies of extreme magnitude. In such emergencies, hospitals and medical centers may have to order equipment from local suppliers or request donated items from physician offices, medical schools, local armories, medical supply houses, and other sources. This fact underscores the value of establishing partnerships with such organizations in advance to accelerate the procurement of supplies in an emergency.

Surge facility pharmaceutical procurement can be more problematic than that of disposable equipment and supplies because of the legal requirements surrounding the prescription, storage, and preparation of medications. Ordering drugs could pose a problem if the surge facility does not have preexisting contracts with pharmaceutical suppliers. One way of handling this problem is to have a sponsoring hospital or other health care organization order medications for the surge hospital. Another option is for a hospital to establish an advance contract with a pharmaceutical distributor that would be implemented only in an emergency. If possible, the number of supplies held in inventory at the surge hospital should be sufficient to last at least three days per patient.

Leaders in charge of establishing and operating surge hospitals

It is vital that the leaders who have integral roles in establishing and maintaining surge hospitals are visible within the community and ensure consistency in the way surge hospitals operate. The intent of setting up the surge hospital is to demonstrate to stricken communities that the medical community will continue to take care of the ill and injured. In this role, the leaders of the state are key. Advance planning for emergency events is crucial in enabling them to project consistency and to protect and enhance the public trust. To promote visibility, officials must maintain communications with the public through personal visits to the hospital site as well as through media interviews and appearances.

Disasters happen locally, requiring a local response. As such, the states within the U.S. have various designated government officials who possess the authority to call for the establishment of surge hospitals. In Texas, for example, the country judge has the power to order the creation of a surge hospital. However, if it becomes clear that the emergency will have a statewide effect, the governor takes charge of the effort and delegates the establishment of surge hospitals to the senior medical officer in the state, usually the commissioner of health or director of the public health department. This is what occurred as Texas prepared for Hurricane Rita.

The state's senior medical officer's role in surge hospitals

The senior medical officer in the state appoints a medical director of the surge hospital, who then assembles a set-up team. Sometimes the person recommended to oversee the creation of a surge hospital is a physician who has developed a relationship with state officials and has become a trusted advisor. This is the way Raymond Swienton, M.D., FACEP, was given the authority to recommend the sites for and supervise the opening of the surge hospitals at Louisiana State University and at an empty former retail store a few blocks from the Earl K. Long Medical Center in Baton Rouge. Swienton is the co-director of Emergency Management Services of the Disaster Medicine and Homeland Security Section, and associate professor, Division of Emergency Medicine in the Department of Surgery at the University of Texas Southwestern Medical Center at Dallas. In addition, Swienton served as a senior advisor to the State of Louisiana's Secretary of Health as well as the State Health Officer and staff. Over the previous two years, he has become well known to the senior state health care leadership by providing disaster preparedness education and training programs and helping establish these programs statewide.

Effective communication in and with surge hospitals

Communication is often the weakest link in mass casualty incident responses [3]. This fact is borne out by the experience of those who worked in the post-Katrina surge hospitals in Louisiana and Texas. The surge hospital at the empty former retail store site was no exception to this rule. Cellular access was sporadic at best and often not available for an hour or more. Radio communication with arriving buses or emergency services vehicles was essentially nonexistent. Inside the facility itself, communication posed a separate challenge because of the size and acoustic environment of the facility.

A redundant communications system that includes two telephone systems, two-way radios, more reliable paging systems, and better satellite communications needs to be explored to mitigate the negative effects of poor communication on patient care.

Other issues to consider
Sufficiency of care

Ideally, the goal of the surge facility is to maintain high standards of care. In practice, however, medical treatment in a surge hospital may reach only the level of sufficiency of care because of the challenging circumstances under which the facility must operate (see Figure H.1 for an illustration of the difference between the standard of care and sufficiency of care).

In a sufficiency-of-care facility, the medical staff faces challenges such as limited privacy for patient assessments, crowded conditions, limited access to medical records, and inadequate access to testing capabilities. For example, of all the surge hospitals set up after Hurricane Katrina, the empty former retail store veered the furthest from the accepted standard of care—but it still delivered sufficient care. The goal of any sufficiency-of-care-facility is to treat each patient and then transfer him or her to a facility with full capability to treat patients at an

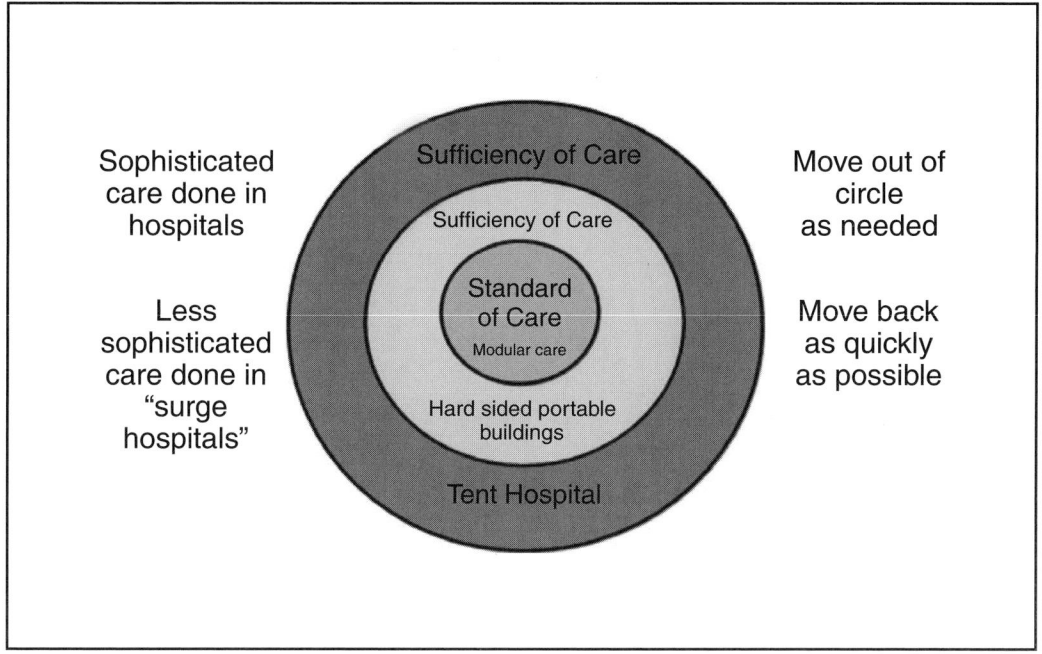

Figure H.1 Standard of care vs. sufficiency of care. The concept of sufficiency of care—medical care that may not be of the same quality as that delivered under nonemergency conditions, but is sufficient for need—is often the reality of surge hospitals because of the difficult circumstances in which care is provided.

ideal level of care. Again, this is what occurred at the empty former retail store site, which remained open for only five days.

The veterinary hospital in College Station, Texas, was able to deliver a higher quality of care because, although it was intended for use as an animal hospital, it contained most of the equipment and supplies necessary to treat human patients. In addition, electrical power, the water supply, and the telephone system were all in working order and it had backup power systems, access to medical gases, and a high standard of cleanliness.

Any plan for a surge hospital that is envisioned as a sufficiency-of-care site should be part of a community response network. This way, all invasive procedures, deliveries, or surgical needs can be transferred to a standard-of-care-based hospital unless emergent intervention is needed to save a life. To handle such emergent cases, advanced airway equipment, ventilator support, portable dialysis units, and monitoring capabilities should be available on site.

Legal and reimbursement issues

Anytime health care workers perform volunteer services, they expose themselves to the risk of having claims filed against them by patients who believe they have been harmed during the delivery of care. The state and federal governments have methods by which the law can be changed to provide some liability protection. During the crisis in the Gulf Coast, for example, the governor of Louisiana waived the state of Louisiana licensing restrictions to allow access to all licensed providers throughout the U.S. The federal government also set aside certain national laws so that health care workers responding in an emergency could act as their professional judgment dictated while delivering care without fear of medical liability. For example, the U.S. Department of Health & Human Services afforded liability protection to health care workers who volunteered to treat hurricane victims.

The Emergency Medical Treatment and Active Labor Act (EMTALA), which states that emergency rooms must diagnose, treat, and stabilize a patient before being able to transfer him or her, was also waived because, during an emergency, transfer may be the most expedient action. By prearranged cooperative agreement, particular medical centers in a community may be designated to accept certain types of patients, such as burn or trauma victims. Therefore, if a burn victim arrived at a surge facility during an emergency, the patient would immediately be transferred to the preselected hospital.

A number of recent laws and agreements have made it easier for medical personnel from other regions to provide health care assistance to affected areas. The need to make the best possible use of volunteer health workers in an emergency led to the development of the Emergency System for Advance Registration of Health Professions Volunteers (ESARHPV) [4]. This act, still in its developmental stages, will enable each state and U.S. territory to set up a standardized, volunteer registration system for medical workers. Each state's system is designed to contain up-to-date information about a volunteer's identity, licensing, credentialing, accreditation, and privileging in hospitals or other medical organizations. Such a system will allow each state to rapidly identify professional health care volunteers during mass casualty events and will enable states to share these preregistered and already credentialed health care workers nationwide.

The Emergency Management Assistance Compact (EMAC), enacted by Congress in 1996, also facilitates mutual aid between 49 U.S. states, the District of Columbia, Puerto Rico, and the Virgin Islands in times of crisis. EMAC, which is administered by the National Emergency Management Association, is not an agency of the federal government, but is instead an agreement among the states to provide aid across state lines when any type of disaster occurs. The governor of the affected state must first declare a state of emergency, and then the state can request the assistance it needs. This appeal then activates the response from other EMAC-member states, putting the EMAC system of coordination and deployment in motion. EMAC garnered national attention in 2004 when four major hurricanes hit the U.S. in a six-week period, triggering what was then the largest use to date of state-to-state mutual aid in U.S. history.

Under the compact, licensed physicians or other health care workers who travel to any of the EMAC member states or territories (once the conditions for providing assistance have been met) will have their credentials honored across states lines. EMAC provisions addressing liability and workers compensation issues for these personnel alleviate the financial and legal burdens of the responding states.

EMAC enabled a massive deployment of medical personnel and resources in response to Hurricanes Katrina and Rita. More than 31,000 workers, including medical personnel, search and rescue staff, law enforcement officers, waste management experts, and fire fighters were dispatched from dozens of states to Louisiana and Mississippi.

Reimbursement is another issue that the federal government would need to examine so that certain provisions of reimbursement for Medicare and Medicaid might be relieved in a disaster situation. Some of these federal requirements involve certifying the quality of the facility, the privileging of its staff, and the upkeep of medical records to secure reimbursement from the federal government. Many of these requirements would have to be set aside so that the health care system does not end up with two disasters—one caused by the event itself, and the other caused by the loss of revenue to the health care organizations involved in providing care.

Ensuring that long-term surge hospitals offer safe care

All surge facilities must ensure that the care they provide is safe. In addition, certain quality assurance processes must be followed in surge hospitals so that, for example, patients are identified and drug errors do not occur. The longer a facility remains operational, the more demands must be made on both its environment of care and the process of care delivery to make sure they are in line with high standards of care. These demands can ensure that, while expedient care may be given, substandard care is never allowed.

The possibility of surge hospitals operating on a long-term basis adds a third dimension to the concept of the emergency event itself. Health care organizations are used to thinking about emergency events on two levels of magnitude, each with its own response. The first level of emergency can be called the major incident. Examples include a school bus accident with multiple casualties, or an industrial explosion producing numerous burn victims. The local hospital needs to respond by activating its emergency management plan in order to have enough staff available to manage the situation; however, this type of event is usually short-lived—lasting perhaps 24 hours—and the community and its hospital both remain intact.

The second type of emergency event can be characterized as the disaster. For example, Hurricane Katrina was a disaster in Gulf Port and Biloxi, Mississippi, because the health care infrastructure was damaged as was the infrastructure of the community. The disaster presents as a community-wide problem that can extend for many weeks or months and may need extensive state and federal resources to ameliorate the situation.

The third level of emergency, virtually unvisited by health care planners until recent events thrust it into view, can be described as the catastrophe: a series of disasters occurring to the same community in a short period of time. What happened in New Orleans after the levees broke was a catastrophe. First, the hurricane hit, causing serious but manageable damage. Then the levees broke, flooding the city. As a consequence, the community's entire infrastructure broke down: sewer, water, and electrical power were all disabled. The ability of health care and emergency medical services to respond was totally disrupted. Finally, civil disturbance occurred as desperate people fought to survive. This event was unprecedented in recent U.S. history and can only be compared to the San Francisco earthquake and fire of 1906, which ranks as one of the most serious natural disasters of all time.

What happened in New Orleans has forced health care organizations to think about how surge hospitals can be used on a long-term basis to supply needed medical care. Most pointedly, Charity Hospital, which was significantly damaged in the disasters, has prompted the need for patients who would normally be treated at the hospital to instead seek care at surge hospitals in the area. The surge hospital that was initially established in this area (and which will be developed further in two additional phases) could be used by the Federal Emergency Management Agency (FEMA) as a model for the nation.

The initial stage of the surge hospital that was set up after Charity Hospital was severely damaged was the tent hospital established on October 8, 2005, in the parking lot of the old Charity Hospital. This surge hospital remained in place when this publication went to press. The next phase being considered is a hard-sided shelter system with individual rooms, each with its own bathroom.

Louisiana State University (LSU), which operated Charity Hospital, expects to set up a modular component structure over the next six months that has been used nationwide and meets all Joint Commission standards. Such a structure may represent a permanent solution to the problem of a replacement for hospitals that must be rebuilt due to extensive damage from a disaster. This type of premanufactured component construction is assembled on site and is built to last for years. Alternatively, the permanent facility might evolve into a site that has a main hospital downtown with eight satellite offices that could accommodate outpatient surgery suites or clinics. These satellites could be converted into surge hospital space within hours. Other options were being considered as this paper went to press.

Possible development of Joint Commission standards for surge hospitals

In the aftermath of the hurricanes that caused significant damage to health care organizations on the Gulf Coast, the Joint Commission is considering the development of a set of standards with which surge hospitals would need to comply. These standards would assure the public that the care received in a given surge hospital—or in the health care system as a whole—is safe. If the development of these standards moves forward, the Joint Commission will work with health care organizations that are developing plans for surge facilities so that these standards can be implemented quickly and with minimal cost.

Case studies

This section examines several surge hospitals that were set up after Hurricanes Katrina and Rita devastated the Gulf Coast. They illustrate the variety of forms the concept can take as well as the variety of responses medical personnel were able to coordinate in response to the recent disasters.

Case Study 1: "Katrina Clinic," Houston, Texas

The Houston Astrodome served as a shelter for more than 25,000 of the people who fled the levee breaches that followed Hurricane Katrina's destruction in New Orleans. In response to this onslaught of evacuees in crisis, many of whom had lived in appalling conditions for days, Baylor College of Medicine (BCM) in Houston set up "Katrina Clinic" in Reliant Arena, a building adjacent to the Houston Astrodome.

Three days after the storm hit, Harris Country, Texas Judge Robert Eckels and Houston Mayor Bill White asked George Masi, chief operating officer of the Harris Country Hospital District, to coordinate a facility that could manage the health needs of the arriving multitudes. The Houston Astrodome in Reliant Park, in ordinary times used as a livestock exhibition hall, had been long designated a shelter by local officials involved in disaster planning. The team from Baylor College of Medicine had roughly 15 hours to prepare before the first busload of patients arrived.

The set-up team employed stored rods and curtains used for exhibitions to separate rooms into spaces that could be used for patient registration, triage, exam rooms, and a pharmacy. Tables, computers, photocopiers, and telephones were gathered from around the site and brought to the clinic, which had the benefit of full electrical power, working toilets, and potable running water. The team acquired a number of donated X-ray machines from a national medical supply corporation and a major pharmaceutical company sent a mobile laboratory on an 18-wheeler truck. Two national drug store chains set up pharmacies at the site, one housed in two mobile homes. Many local businesses donated medical supplies and the Red Cross provided cots. For the most part, the 100,000-square-foot clinic was prepared to provide care to patients by midnight.

Supervised by medical director Thomas Gavagan, M.D., MPH, vice chair for community health in the Department of Family and Community Medicine at BCM, the clinic processed 150 patients per hour over 15 days—or a total of more than 10,000 people.

Originally equipped with 20 examination rooms, the clinic quickly ballooned to 65 exam rooms. The medical staff members worked 36 hours straight after the clinic opened, and were finally relieved after a call for medical volunteers produced about 2,700 responders. For the rest of the time, 25 physicians were assigned to work per each 12-hour shift. The staff administered thousands of immunizations—10,000 tetanus shots alone—and filled a similar number of prescriptions. The site remained an outpatient facility; acutely ill patients were sent to local hospitals for treatment.

Paul Sirbaugh, M.D., Director of Prehospital Medicine at Texas Children's Hospital, oversaw a special pediatric clinic at the Astrodome so that children could be seen by a physician without having to be separated from their parents. Mental health needs were seen as crucial to the care of hurricane survivors, so psychiatric staff from BCM stepped in to provide mental health counseling.

The clinic's medical staff treated patients with broken bones, chest pain, and withdrawal from drug addiction, but most of the patients had chronic conditions, such as asthma, diabetes, and high blood pressure. One patient presented with a gunshot wound to the arm. On the fourth day of operation, physicians began to see quite a few pediatric patients with some type of gastrointestinal infection that caused diarrhea and vomiting, presumably from exposure to the contaminated water in New Orleans. The infection was transmitted to several hundred people before physicians identified the cause as the Norwalk virus and promptly provided treatment. As the number of acute care cases decreased, evacuees at the Astrodome began requesting assistance for more mundane medical needs, such as prescription eyeglasses or other minor complaints for which they could not seek care in New Orleans because of a lack of health insurance.

As patients continued to pour into Katrina Clinic, Houston's mayor requested that a second clinic be opened at the George R. Brown Convention Center. Physicians from the University of Texas Health Science Center in Houston staffed this site. It processed 500 to 700 evacuees each day, for a total of more than 9,000 patients.

Katrina Clinic remained open for 2½ weeks at a cost of $4.1 million. After it closed down, the Red Cross established an outpost at the site to deliver first aid to evacuees.

Thomas Gavagan, M.D., MPH served as the primary source of information for this case study.

Case Study 2: Dallas Convention Center

Physicians, employees, and students from the University of Texas (UT) Southwestern Medical Center at Dallas began gearing up their relief efforts even before Hurricane Katrina evacuees started pouring into Dallas. They established a medical command center at the Dallas Convention Center, where they set up a surge facility. The site for the facility was chosen by officials from the City of Dallas Office of Emergency Management and the city fire marshal's office, Dallas Fire-Rescue.

In Dallas, faculty and employees from UT Southwestern volunteered in large numbers, working at Reunion Arena and the Dallas Convention Center to help with the relief effort. Volunteers included physicians as well as nurses, pharmacists, respiratory therapists, and allied health care workers.

Kathy J. Rinnert, M.D., MPH, assistant professor of emergency medicine at UT Southwestern Medical Center in Dallas and attending physician at Parkland Health and Hospital Systems and Raymond Fowler, M.D., associate professor of emergency medicine at UT Southwestern Medical Center and deputy medical director for operations and quality assurance for the Dallas Area Bio Tel (EMS) System, both served as medical directors of the site. More than one hundred physicians from UT Southwestern as well as medical staff from Parkland Health and Hospital Systems, Children's Medical Center of Dallas, Methodist Hospital of Dallas, Medical City Hospital, and Baylor Medical Center worked up to 20-hour days to care for the sick and injured. The site was staffed locally with no support from out-of-state medical volunteers. Facilities included an 11-bed urgent care center and a 20-bed chronic care center.

The 8,200-square-foot surge facility was open from September 1 through September 16. Faculty, staff, residents, and medical students treated more than 4,000 evacuees during the first week alone, and a total of roughly 8,600 patients over the 16 days of operation. The medical staff treated not only patients from the shelter set up at the site, but also those from other shelters and hotels in Dallas. Wounds were the principle injuries seen during the first three days, followed by gastrointestinal disorders, and then acute exacerbations of chronic medical conditions such as asthma, diabetes, and cardiovascular problems.

Located one sub-basement level down from the main floor, the facility shared space with an evacuee shelter ringed by a variety of social service agencies, such as the Red Cross, the Salvation Army, and the Texas State Child Protective Services Agency. Medical equipment, supplies, and pharmaceuticals came from the local medical community, primarily Children's Medical Center and Parkland Health and Hospital Systems, the largest contributor. Telephones, copiers, fax machines, and other office equipment were provided by the City of Dallas.

According to Rinnert, the main advantages of a surge facility site such as a convention center include the flexibility of the space, which can be cordoned off as circumstances dictate, and the availability of air conditioning in a climate that normally averages more than 100° Fahrenheit in September. Several disadvantages were the austere appearance of the site, which had bare concrete floors and harsh fluorescent lighting, and the absence of showering facilities. Overall, however, the convention center proved to be a satisfactory environment for a surge facility.

Kathy J. Rinnert, M.D., MPH, served as the primary source of information for this case study.

Case Study 3: Basketball arena and field house at Louisiana State University, Baton Rouge

Planning for the surge hospital

When Jimmy Guidry, M.D., the state health officer of Louisiana and medical director for the Louisiana Department of Health & Hospitals (DHH), heard that large numbers of patients had not been evacuated from New Orleans hospitals and nursing homes before Hurricane Katrina hit, he decided that the state needed to have an additional acute care facility in place in Baton Rouge, knowing that existing hospitals would be inundated with patients. Raymond Swienton, M.D., served as an advisor to Guidry to aid in the selection of the site for this surge hospital. Because of a longstanding relationship between the DHH and Louisiana State University (LSU), Guidry selected Chris Trevino, M.D., director of emergency medicine at St. Elizabeth's Hospital in Gonzales, Louisiana, and medical director of emergency medical services for the state of Louisiana, to oversee the establishment of a surge hospital at the university. Guidry then chose the LSU Pete Maravich Assembly Center (PMAC), a basketball arena, as the site of the surge hospital and LSU's Carl Maddox Field House, located next door, as a special needs shelter. The two sites were chosen because of their size and the availability of medical staff from LSU.

Guidry selected Walter Cain, M.D., medical director of LSU's Fire and Emergency Training Institute and attending physician at Earl K. Long Hospital, a part of LSU's Health Care Services Division, to set up the special needs shelter. Cain then asked Stephen Barr, assistant technical director of the LSU Theater, to help convert the field house into a special-needs hospital, primarily for nursing home patients.

Setting up the surge hospital

The PMAC began as a medical triage facility, but was soon transformed into a surge hospital. The 800-bed facility at the PMAC became the largest acute care field hospital to be established in the U.S. since the Civil War.

The LSU administration drew on its student government to take charge of the volunteer efforts of the students, faculty, and staff. The student leaders set up a volunteer hotline and Web site for volunteer registration. They handled more than 1,000 calls per day from people at LSU who wanted to volunteer or provide lodging to displaced persons or emergency personnel. Student volunteers staffed 80 to 90 people per shift to work in both hospitals. After the schedules were finalized, the students called volunteers back to give them their shift assignments. The student leaders managed nonmedical volunteers both at the field house and at the PMAC. Eighty-five nonmedical volunteers worked 12-hour shifts daily. Student volunteers also helped set up the surge facilities by moving boxes, setting up shelves and tables, and performing other nonmedical tasks. LSU Chancellor Sean O'Keefe met with medical staff daily to assess their most pressing needs.

A significant number of health care providers arrived from out of state. For example, the Illinois Medical Emergency Response Team assisted teams from medical centers in Texas as well as local medical volunteers from Baton Rouge, especially those from St Elizabeth's Hospital.

The special-needs hospital at the field house took only approximately two days to establish because the state had experience in creating back-up special-needs facilities for nursing home patients who have to be evacuated because of power outages and other similar problems. Setting up the PMAC had to proceed rapidly because patient arrival was imminent, so the emergency room at the PMAC was up and running in eight or nine hours. Electricity was in good working order and generator backup was available.

The DHH, through one of its components, the Bureau of Emergency Medical Services, was intimately involved in the emergency room's set up, providing both paramedics and supplies. Two years before, Guidry and the rest of the medical leadership in the state had evaluated what it would take to set up a field hospital and had purchased supplies and equipment through a grant from the U.S. Department of Homeland Security. As a result, the state already had a 200-bed hospital and all the supplies associated with it in storage. Training had also been in place. In fact, just a week before, the state held a disaster exercise to prepare for a fictional storm named "Hurricane Pam."

Private emergency medical service companies lent volunteers and equipment. Trevino also obtained assistance from the nursing, respiratory therapy, and other professional staff at St. Elizabeth's Hospital to set up and staff the PMAC emergency room. During the first 48 hours of operation, the medical and professional staff worked straight through, without leaving the facility, perhaps sleeping for an hour or two at a time. After the third day, hundreds more volunteers from other local hospitals arrived to lend a hand, but the huge volume of patients continued to demand 12-hour shifts or more.

Large sports arenas typically have sizeable entry ports where trucks can easily bring equipment into the site. The medical team chose one of the larger of these ports as a triage center. They set up tables in the port, where physicians and nurses could examine the patients coming in by ambulance or bus and then send them into the arena on foot or by wheelchair or stretcher. At times, convoys of up to 15 ambulances, each carrying four patients, would arrive at once. Busloads of 50 patients would also arrive; sometimes, only a few on each bus were ill. Healthy passengers who had traveled 60 miles from New Orleans wanted to exit the bus, use the bathroom, and have something to eat or drink before getting back on the bus to be transferred elsewhere. Patients coming in by helicopter entered at a different port and then were triaged. In total, both hospitals treated or housed roughly 6,000 patients in addition to the people who simply used the facility as a stopover before being bused to a shelter. Counting those people, both facilities served 15,000 to 20,000 people.

Areas of the PMAC were reserved for laboratory, X-ray, electrocardiogram, and ultrasound services. The staff also arranged for dialysis patients to be transported to a local dialysis center for treatment. The hospital even had 80 beds equipped with a cardiac monitoring system. As for meals, one of the larger local church groups called Trevino and announced they could provide up to 16,000 cooked meals a day for both the PMAC basketball arena and the special-needs field house next door. LSU volunteers also donated food. Meals were provided four times per day so that staff and volunteers could eat during night shifts.

Security was initially provided by the LSU security force and was later supplemented by SWAT teams and the National Guard. Neither site had a major security incident, although a potential security threat occurred when healthy individuals arriving in buses were originally told they could not leave the bus unless they were sick. This problem was resolved by allowing everyone off the bus to freshen up and have some food and drink. After the riders understood that the facility was a hospital and not a shelter, they returned to their seats on the bus.

Treating patients

As patients poured into the facilities at LSU, they quickly filled the basketball arena's emergency room to capacity and spilled over into the field house for four to five days. The initial surge of patients was from hospitals and nursing homes, but buses full of evacuees soon transported a population of all ages to the facilities. The principal condition treated was the exacerbation of chronic medical conditions such as diabetes or asthma because of dehydration and because patients had not been able to take their prescribed medications for several days. Another issue was the fact that some patients could not recall the names of the medications they had been taking. The staff also saw some cases of trauma and delivered several babies who needed resuscitation. At one point, the hospital had 14 ventilatory patients. Because the patients arrived so early after the disaster, only a few cases of infectious disease, such as abscesses and cellulitis, were seen.

When the patients came in such waves, the primary goal of the medical team was to treat them as quickly as possible. After the first day, the documentation process began to take shape and by the third day, the site had a full medical records system in place.

As soon as it became apparent that large numbers of new patients were no longer arriving from New Orleans, Trevino began to close the PMAC facility down, recognizing that, as functional as the facility was, it was not optimal for patient care; however, as of this writing, the LSU field house remains open as a special-needs shelter for nursing home patients.

Some disadvantages

As a university with more than 30,000 students, LSU presents some disadvantages as a surge hospital site. For example, housing a medical facility at a university can be disruptive to student life. Imagine seeing Blackhawk helicopters full of evacuated patients landing on the quad. Secondly, sheltering sick patients and medical personnel on a university campus holds the potential for transmission of disease. Operationally, it is problematic to expect a university to essentially shut down its educational function and take over disaster relief in an emergency. Other venues, such as an exposition center similar to the Houston Astrodome or other multiuse facilities, can more easily cancel events to gear up for an emergency situation while maintaining logistical and infrastructure support.

Chris Trevino, M.D., served as the primary source of information for this case study.

Case Study 4: Empty former retail store in Baton Rouge, Louisiana
Establishing the surge hospital

Physicians from the University of Texas (UT) Southwestern University Hospitals took leadership positions in providing emergency care and mental health services in the state of Louisiana after Hurricane Katrina struck the Gulf Coast. UT Southwestern's Raymond Swienton, M.D., and William M. Cassidy, M. D., associate professor of medicine at Louisiana State University Medical Center (LSU), chose to locate one of the temporary field hospitals in a building that had formerly housed a large retail store in Baton Rouge, Louisiana. They chose the site because it was located just one half block from LSU's Earl K. Long Medical Center and because LSU had been in the process of purchasing the property, which was to be torn down to make space for the construction of new clinics. The location proved to be desirable in terms of management of emergencies, medical staffing, and supplies.

Cassidy served as medical director of the facility, but he gave responsibility for the actual set up to Steven Winkler, MHA, former senior director of risk management at Baton Rouge General Medical Center, and Monica Nijoka, MHA, BSN, R.N., former vice president of patient care services at the same medical center. The team first arrived at the site at 4:30 P.M. on Thursday, September 2, 2005. By 7:00 P.M. the next day, they were ready to provide care to patients.

The neglected site was daunting. The floor was greasy and layers of dust covered everything. There was virtually no lighting, the telephones were out of order, and only one toilet functioned. The inside temperature reached 100° Fahrenheit. Over 400 volunteers worked to clean the site, remove trash, fix the plumbing, and install electrical outlets and emergency power. Winkler and Nijoka designed the layout of the surge facility and developed a staffing plan for the professional staff. They supervised information systems personnel who installed a computer system that would allow medical staff to document information in computerized patient records.

At the Louisiana Department of Health and Hospitals, urgent contracting deals were made with national vendors to acquire medical supplies, medications, beds, and other equipment. These expensive acquisitions were needed because the state stockpiles had already been deployed at the LSU campus sites. The team obtained the rest of its materials by way of donations from local supply houses, physicians' offices, and hospitals. Intravenous (IV) poles never appeared, so the staff made do by stringing rope along the ceiling and then using metal chips to hang the intravenous bags from the rope. They set up the pharmacy in the area where the store's pharmacy had originally been.

Treating patients

Most patients were assessed at the centralized triage station at the PMAC Center on the LSU campus and then transported to the surge hospital by emergency medical services or bus.

Staffing at the site consisted of physicians, nurses, technicians, social service workers, and other health care workers from local hospitals, home health care agencies, and physicians' offices. Disaster medical assistance teams (DMATs) from all parts of the U.S. also descended on the site, with particular assistance from the DMAT in Iowa. Most of the professional staff worked in 12-hour shifts, while nonmedical volunteers put in shifts that lasted from one to 36 hours.

Volunteer medical workers fulfilled a number of vital roles, including nursing, pharmacy, registration, central supply, social service, mental health, discharge planning, waste handling, respiratory therapy, and food service. In addition, a number of local restaurants, caterers, and church groups sent cooked meals to the site. Several volunteers were dedicated to the scheduling of professional and nonprofessional staff and also assisted in the credentialing of the professional staff. Many local volunteers also sorted and distributed the donated clothing and toys brought to the site.

The team decided to locate the triage area in what had been the oil-change department inside the store's automotive service center because it afforded a wide space that could accommodate incoming buses and ambulances. Triage was divided into two areas: decontamination/security and registration/medical triage. The local fire department set up portable showers outside of the building where patients showered and were given clean clothing before entering the building. Most of the clothing worn by patients had to be destroyed because of contamination from the polluted water that had flowed into New Orleans. After being scanned for weapons by hand-held security wands, patients proceeded through registration and into medical triage, where physicians, nurses, and paramedics assessed their vital signs and general condition. The state police, National Guard, and a private security guard firm maintained security at the site.

The surge hospital served about 250 patients over the course of three days. Like the other post-hurricane surge hospitals, this facility mainly saw patients whose chronic conditions were made worse by the loss of their prescribed drugs. Although the medical staff saw some rashes and infections from exposure to contaminated water, their main task was to stabilize the patients and get them back on their prescribed medications. The staff maintained paper records and computer files on all patients that included information about where they were transferred or discharged.

Lessons learned

In the confusion that occurred after Hurricane Katrina hit, communications seemed to be the weakest link at the site. The telephone system took a long time to be installed and cellular phones were inoperable most of the time. When communications did get through, the information was often incorrect. For example, the hospital team was told that the location would be used heavily to free up space at the two surge facilities set up at LSU. However, the site was closed after three days while the field house at the university remained operational for weeks after the event. Twice word came that many more patients would soon be arriving, but additional patients never arrived. In fact, the hospital could have handled many more patients. As a result, the staff viewed the facility as sound but underutilized.

Overall, the strongest factor was the spirit of volunteerism among the workers. When asked to perform, volunteers and local suppliers could not do enough, according to Winkler and Nijoka. Only two suppliers refused to send needed provisions, because the hospital could not issue purchase order numbers, and had no means to ensure payment.

Steven Winkler, MHA, and Monica Nijoka, MHA, BSN, R.N., served as the primary sources of information for this case study.

Case Study 5: A veterinary hospital in College Station, Texas

Hurricane Rita also produced an unlikely site for a surge facility: the Large-Animal Hospital at the College of Veterinary Medicine and Biomedical Sciences at Texas A&M University. The university transformed the veterinary hospital into a special needs shelter that cared for 320 patients—primarily geriatric nursing home patients, pediatric burn victims, physically handicapped children, and home health care patients—from Houston and Galveston. University staff emptied the hospital of all of its animals (including 20 horses), then cleaned and sterilized the building and made it ready for use in less than a day under the direction of William Moyer, D.V.M., head of the Department of Large Animal Clinical Sciences. At its peak on the night before the hurricane hit, the facility housed about 650 people, including patients, families, and caregivers. The transfers of high acuity patients from less sophisticated shelters into this facility and free transfers back and forth between the surge hospital and St. Joseph Hospital, the largest hospital in the area, allowed St. Joseph Hospital to never exceed 80% occupancy. This enabled the standard of care to be met despite transfers of large numbers of patients with critical medical needs.

Paul Carlton, M.D., of the Texas A&M University System Health Science Center (HSC), served as the medical director of this surge hospital. Carlton, a former surgeon general of the U.S. Air Force, worked with HSC staff as well as representatives of the CDC, Public Health Service, and FEMA to establish the facility. The volunteers set up the first 600 bed component before the arrival of any outside help, and an additional 500 beds from the CDC were added before the storm hit. Thus, the 1,100 bed surge facility was prepared to provide care prior to Hurricane Rita's assault. The staff included physicians, nurses, medical and veterinary students, and many volunteers. Only one medical procedure had to be done, which was to treat an abscess. At one point, Evelyn Castiglioni, Ph.D., head of the university's Department of Veterinary Anatomy and Public Health and an accomplished harpist, calmed patients with an impromptu concert. The hospital remained open for six days.

Lessons learned

The main advantage of converting veterinary hospitals into surge hospitals is their state of readiness. The state-of-the-art facility was a fully equipped hospital, so no building issues had to be dealt with. The power system had an emergency generator for continuous power if commercial power was lost and the building was plumbed with medical gases and suction so that portable equipment did not have to be used. Use of this site shows that a veterinary hospital can be an ideal model for the surge hospital in a catastrophic situation.

Closing Comment

Advance planning, coordination of resources, effective communication, and visible leadership are critical to ensuring that surge hospitals can be set up quickly and can provide care to patients during emergencies. Health care organizations must prepare for the possibility that their buildings could be too damaged to function during as well as after a disaster, necessitating the use of surge hospitals—some of which may need to operate for months or years until permanent health care organization facilities can be rebuilt. As the Joint Commission considers the need for standards to ensure the quality of care being provided at surge hospitals, health care planners at all levels must familiarize themselves with the challenges associated with surge hospitals and must develop thorough plans for their use in emergencies.

References

1. Agency for Healthcare Research and Quality: Surge Capacity—Education and Training for a Qualified Workforce. *Issue Brief No. 7*, Oct. 2004. http://www.ahrq.gov/news/ulp/btbriefs/btbrief7.pdf (accessed Nov. 3, 2005).
2. M. Romano. At capacity and beyond. *Modern Healthcare* p. 16, Sept. 2005.
3. B. E. Hayes et al. A prehospital approach to multiple-victim incidents. *Ann Emerg Med* 15:458–462, Apr. 1986.
4. Public Law 107–188, 107th Cong., *Public Health Security and Bioterrorism Preparedness and Response Act of 2002*, Section 107.

Appendix I Medical-Surgical Supply Formulary by Disaster Scenario

Background

The following is a proposed starting point for planning and coordinating medical/surgical supplies for hospitals throughout the United States during a large scale CBRNE (Chemical, Biological, Radiological, Nuclear, and Explosive) or Natural disaster. These supply formularies were created based on feed-back and input from multiple hospitals and healthcare systems and have been reviewed by AHRMM members, their clinical representatives, and members of HIDA. The lists are intended only as starting points for preparedness efforts and should be modified to fit each hospital according to its individual needs and feedback from its clinicians.

"Large scale" refers to events that will produce casualties beyond that which can be planned for by a single hospital. By definition, the event will not impact a single facility but will affect communities and regions. These events will require planning beyond the individual hospital and will include all segments of supply and points of care in a region. Hospitals must be self-reliant until Federal aid arrives, within 24–72 hours after Federal Emergency Management Agency (FEMA) has been contacted and the event has been declared a Federal disaster.

Medical/Surgical Supply Formularies

Under this plan, medical/surgical supplies are separated into seven formularies and a staff formulary. It is important to note that these formularies are for medical/surgical supplies and do not include products for Radiology or Pharmacy. The Core Formulary has the basic supplies needed for each adult casualty in any type of disaster scenario. The Pediatrics Formulary includes the basic supplies needed for each pediatric casualty regardless of type of disaster. The remaining five specialty formularies are supplemental to the Core or Pediatric Formulary and include only the supplies specific to each type of disaster listed in (Figure I.1). In addition to patient formularies, the Staff Formulary contains the supplies needed for each hospital staff person.

Considerations for Materials Management Professionals

Hospital's Internal Supply Chain

Included in each hospital's plan should be the ability to redirect supplies already within the hospital's supply chain to the areas first impacted. Step one for Materials Management is to examine the hospital's internal supply chain. With clinical experts, the hospital units/departments should be identified that might be closed in the event of a large-scale disaster.

Materials Management should identify the supplies that might be diverted from these areas and routed to the first response areas. Also, stretchers from these areas should be identified, as many of the events will produce casualties beyond a single hospital's ability to provide available beds.

Working with Suppliers and Others

Materials Management must determine the amount of supplies to keep on hand until replenishment

---

Presented by the Association for Healthcare Resource & Materials Management (AHRMM), the Health Industry Distributors Association (HIDA), and the Health Industry Group Purchasing Association (HIGPA).

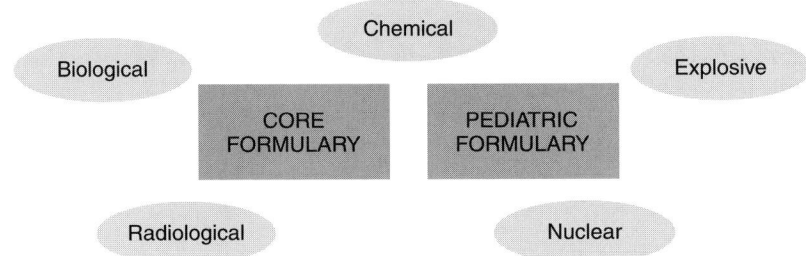

Figure I.1

arrives. Each facility's disaster readiness team must investigate the best means for having quality supplies that are readily available. This determination is individual to each facility.

When working with suppliers, Materials Management should determine the length of time needed for delivery from the time of the first call. Additionally, the clinicians will need to determine the maximum number of casualties the hospital will be able to treat during this period of time. Based on the maximum number of casualties before suppliers' replenishments arrive and the amount of supplies that could be diverted from other areas of the hospital, Materials Management will be able to determine how much additional product must be kept on hand.

Essential to this plan is working with suppliers and establishing pre-event orders that can be activated with a single phone call or email. Each order will be specific to the individual hospital's needs by type of disaster using the supply formulary model. This preplanning also will help the suppliers maintain adequate inventory, which will assure that the pre-order can be delivered at any time with complete fill levels.

Other Critical Components

Since disaster scenarios of this size will exceed the hospital's ability to support casualties, it demands a community response plan. Work with local agencies, including fire fighters, public health department, Civil Defense, any offices of Emergency Preparedness, and other members participating in the Metropolitan Medical Response System as well as with other hospitals and healthcare providers that service the community. Cooperative agreements should be drafted among all the hospitals and healthcare providers for mutual support.

A single source of communication should be identified for the entire community, and each hospital should use this source to request additional supplies and to coordinate the flow of supplies to the areas most in need. With the possibility that every hospital is placing demands on supply sources, this coordination is imperative to prevent chaos.

This plan should be practiced with the community and community agencies to identify where the plan might need to be revised or strengthened. It is essential that the preparedness plan(s) be in place and tested soon. The real danger is not to plan for the unthinkable.

Table I.1 Disaster supply formularies

CORE FORMULARY

Instruments/Equipment
BP Cuffs, Disposable
BP Manometer
Batteries-AA, AAA, D, C,
  1 gross per incident
Artificial Resuscitator Bag,
  10% child, 5% infant

Sharps: NDL/Syringes
10cc Needless Syringes
60cc Needless Syringes
3cc 23G1″ Safety Syringes
3cc 22G11/2″ Safety Syringes
TB Syringes
Insulin Syringes
Blunt Plastic Cannula
Lever Lock Cannula
18G 11/2″ Safety Needles
20G 1″ Safety Needles
Sharps Container
20G IV Start Catheter
18G IV Start Catheter
Winged Infusion Set 23GA & 25GA

Irrigation Solutions
Normal Saline Irrigation Solution 2000cc
Sterile Water Irrigation Solution 2000cc

IV Access/Supplies
IV Start Kits
Micro Drip Tubing
Adult Drip Tubing
Blood Admin. Tubing
Disposable IV Pressure Bag
Metri Set Tubing
Arterial Line Tubing

IV Solutions
LR 1000cc
NS 1000cc
Central Vein Catheter Kit
Multi Lumen Central Catheter Kit
Long Arm Board
Short Arm Board
Stopcock

Linen
Disposable Sheets
Disposable Pillows
Disposable Pillow Covers

Hand Hygiene
Providine/Iodine Scrub Brushes
PCMX Scrub Brushes (1 box per 100 casualties)

Patient Personal Care Supplies
Bath Basin
Emesis Basin
Facial Tissues
Bedpan
Urinal
Belonging Bag
Regular Soap
Mouth Care Supplies

Miscellaneous
Sterile Lubricant
Alcohol Wipes
PVP Wipes
Tongue Depressors
5 in 1 Connectors
Garbage Liners
Blood Glucose Testing Supplies
Waterproof Markers
Body Bag (25 per 100 casualties)
Blank Labels/Tags
Individual Bottled Drinking Water

PEDIATRIC FORMULARY

Instruments/Equipment
Disposable BP Cuffs-Neonatal, Infant, Child, Small Adult
Artificial Resuscitator Bag Masks: Ped, Infant

Patient Personal Care Supplies
Bath Basin
Cotton Swabs
Facial Tissues
Diapers
Pacifier
Belonging Bag
Cotton Balls

Respiratory System Supplies
Nasal Airways
Oral Airways
Oxygen Cannulas
Oxygen Masks

ER/Trauma/Surgical Supplies
Scalpel #11
Sutures (to be ordered individually by box)
General Instruments Tray
Facial Suture Tray
Chest Drainage System
Buretol Tubing 60 drops

Thoracostomy Tray
Chest Tubes (8, 10, 12, 24, 32)
Thorastic Catheter with Tubing and Container
Sterile Towels
Sterile Sheets
Small Sterile Basins
Electrodes
Monitoring Electrodes

Dressings
Bandage Scissors
2 × 2 Dressings
4 × 4 Dressings
Adhesive IV Dressing
4″ Bandage Rolls
1″ Paper Tape
Adhesive Bandages

Linen
Disposable Sheets
Disposable Pillows
Disposable Pillow Covers

Muscle/Skeletal Supplies
Limb Restraints

GI System Supplies
Anti-Reflux Valve (10, 12, 14)
Feeding Tubes (5, 8)

Sharps: NDL/Syringes
Bulb Syringes
Safety Syringes (21, 25)
Filter Needles
Catheter Tip Syringe 60cc
Sharps Container
Luer Lock Syringes 20cc, 60cc
Syringes 1, 3, 5, 10cc

IV Access/Supplies
IV Start Kits
Stopcock
T-Connector
IV Start Catheter (18, 20, 22, 24)
Arm Boards – Infant, Child
Blood Administration Tubing
IV Filters (.22 micron, 1.2 micron)
Syringe Pump Tubing
Micro Drip Tubing

IV Solutions
Glucose Water
NS 10cc
NS 1000cc

Table I.1 (*Continued*)

Irrigation Solutions
Normal Saline Irrigation Solution 2000cc
Sterile Water Irrigation Solution 2000cc

Miscellaneous
Sterile Lubricant
Alcohol Wipes

CHEMICAL

Respiratory System Supplies
ABG Kits
Nasal Airways (6.5, 7.0, 7.5, 8.0) 1 box per 100
Oral Airways (3, 4, 6) 1 box per 100
Oxygen Cannulas
Oxygen Masks
Yankauer Suction Tips
Connecting Tubing
Suction Kit/Cup 14F × 22

GU System Supplies
Urine Multi-Stix
Foley Catheter Trays
Urometers

Irrigation Solution
Sterile Water Irrigation Solution 3000cc

Miscellaneous
Disposable Sheet
Balanced Salt Solution

BIOLOGICAL

GU System Supplies
Urine Multi-Stix
Foley Catheter Trays
Urometers

Miscellaneous
50 Micron Mask
Stomach Tube

RADIOLOGICAL

GU System Supplies
Urine Multi-Stix
Foley Catheter Trays
Urometers

Irrigation Solution
Sterile Water Irrigation Solution 3000cc

Miscellaneous
Disposable Sheet
Balanced Salt Solution

NUCLEAR

GU System Supplies
Urine Multi-Stix
Foley Catheter Trays
Urometers

Alcohol Swab Sticks
Tongue Blades
Heel Warmers
Tape Measure
Body Bag
Disposable Linen Savers

Irrigation Solution
Sterile Water Irrigation Solution 3000cc

Miscellaneous
Disposable Sheet
Balanced Salt Solution

EXPLOSIVE

GU System Supplies
Urine Multi-Stix
Foley Catheter Trays w/Bags
Urometers

ER/Trauma/Surgical Supplies
Scalpel Blade Holder (#3, #4)
Scalpel Blades (#10, #11, #15, #20)
Disposable Safety Scalpel (#15)
Suture Sets
Silk & Gut Sutures (ordered in bulk by facility)
Thoracostomy Tray
Peritoneal Lavage Tray
Chest Tubes (12, 24, 28, 36)
Chest Drainage Tube with Container
Sterile Towels
Sterile Sheets
Large Sterile Basin
Small Sterile Basin
Trocar Chest Tube
Skin Stapler
Electrodes
Tracheotomy Kit

Dressings
Bandage Scissors
Impregnated Dressing
3″ Dressing
ABD Pads
4 × 4 Dressings
Self Adhering Dressing
4 × 4 Sponges
4″ Bandage Rolls
3″ Elastic Bandage
4″ Elastic Bandage
6″ Elastic Bandage
Sterile Cotton Applicators
2″ Porous First Aid Tape
3″ Porous First Aid Tape
Adhesive Bandages
1″ Paper Tape

Safety Pins
Povodine Iodine Swab Sticks
Povodine Iodine Wipes
Hydrogen Peroxide
Individual Bottled Drinking Waters

GI System Supplies
Piston Irrigation Sets
Gastric Lavage Kits
Anti-Reflux Valve (8, 12, 18)

Irrigation Solutions
Normal Saline Irrigation Solution 2000cc
Sterile Water Irrigation Solution 2000cc

Muscle/Skeletal Supplies
Medium Slings
Large Slings
Small Cervical Collars
Universal Cervical Collars
Knee Immobilizers
Wrist Restraints
Restraint Belts
OCL Splints Plaster
Plaster Impregnated Gauze Roll 4″

STAFF

Hand Hygiene
Personal Hand Foam Sanitizer

Protective Gear
Sterile Gloves, All Sizes (1 box per 100 casualties)
Exam Gloves, Medium (1 box per 25 casualties)
Latex Free Gloves, Medium (1 box per 200 casualties)
Fluid Resistant Gowns
Masks
Goggles
Shields
Balanced Salt Solution for Eye Wash
Isolation Gown (4 per staff member)
Fluid Resistant Gowns (1 per staff member)
Hair Cover
Liquid Scrub Soap
Individual Bottled Drinking Water

Index

Aberration detection:
  algorithms, 43
  challenges in hospital-based, 45
  control chart usage, 43–4
  issues, 45
Absorption chiller, 230, 231, 232
Acetaminophen, 58, 59
Acetylcholinesterase, 75, 151, 152
Aconitine, 17, 22
  see also Poison bullets
Acute Care Hospital, 267, 268, 274, 276, 281
Acute radiation sickness (ARS), 63, 133
Acute respiratory distress syndrome (ARDS), 52, 282
Acute stress disorder (ASD), 162, 164, 198
Advanced Practice Registered Nurses (APRNs), 135
Aerosol, 23, 49, 51, 52, 56, 58, 59, 68, 74, 91, 95, 96
Aerosolization, 91, 129
Agency for Healthcare Research and Quality (AHRQ), 10
Al Qaeda, 27, 62
ALL-CLEAR™, 90
Amateur radio:
  Amateur Radio Emergency Services (ARES), 190
  Amateur Radio Relay League (ARRL), 219
  external hospital communications, 220–2
  Federal Emergency Management Agency (FEMA), 220
  hams, 220
  hospital disaster plan, 224
  Radio Amateur Civil Emergency Service (RACES), 220
  redundant systems and pathways, 222–3
  resources, 223–4
Amateur television, 224
Ambulance, 108, 109, 125, 138, 242
American College of Obstetricians and Gynecologists, 179
American Hospital Association, 5
American Psychiatric Association, 157, 164
American Red Cross, 169, 211
American Society of Heath System Pharmacists (ASHP), 201
Amnesia, 164
Analgesics, 55, 86
Anorexia, 55
Anthrax:
  causative agent, 49
  clinical description, 49
  diagnosis, 49
  differential diagnosis, 49
  medical management, 49–50
Antibiotic resistant infections, 37
Antitoxin, 50, 151, 179
Anxiety, 126, 141, 154, 165, 171, 174, 198, 272, 288, 291
Apnea, 76, 77, 78, 81, 130, 131
Arenaviruses, 54
Armed Forces Radiobiology Research Institute, 63, 70
Arms Control and Disarmament Agency, 27
Arthralgia, 55, 57

Aspirin, 55
Association for the Advancement of Medical Instrumentation, 238
Association of American Medical Colleges, 10
Asthma, 77, 260
Ataxia, 59, 65
Aum Shinrikyo, 25
Australian Department of Defense, 27
Authority having jurisdiction (AHJ), 229
Avian influenza (H5N1) virus, 282

Bacillus globigii, 22, 24, 91
Behavioral Health Disaster, 143, 168, 169
Behavioral Health Regional Crisis Response Information System (BHRCRIS), 170
Bereavement, 160, 164
Biokombinat, 29
Biological contamination:
  food, 19
  water supplies, 19
Biological weapons, 17–31
  Arthashastra, 18
  plague, 17, 18, 22, 28
  smallpox, 52, 56, 91, 150, 178, 187, 189, 194
  zoonoses, 17
Biological Weapons Anti-Terrorism Act, 26
Biological Weapons Convention, 23, 24
Biomedical Engineering, 207
Biomedpreparat, 29
Biopreparat, 23
Bioterrorism and nurses/nursing:
  bioterror agent exposure, 193–4
  hospital expansion, 196–8
  triage, 195–6
  vulnerable groups, 194–5
Bioterrorism and obstetrics:
  Bacillus anthracis (anthrax), 179
  Brucellosis, 180
  Clostridium botulinum (botulism), 179
  Francisella tularensis (tularemia), 179
  management of the exposed pregnant woman, 178
  Q fever, 180
  staff training, 177
  Variola virus (smallpox), 178–9
  Viral hemorrhagic fever, 179–80
  Yersinia pestis (plague), 179
Bioterrorism and psychiatry:
  acute and repeated exposure to traumatic stress, 159–60
  acute crisis response effort with ongoing care, 167
  acute traumatic stress and grief reactions in patients and staff, 161–2
  critical incident stress management with hospital staff and first responders, 166–7
  mitigating the second disaster, 163
  preventive interventions with high risk individuals and families, 163–4
  psychological first aid, 162–3

Bioterrorism and psychiatry: (*Continued*)
  psychological impact of real or potential biological contamination, 157–8
  psychotherapeutic and psychopharmacologic treatments for post-traumatic disorders, 171
  reversing the invisibility and violation of terrorism, 159
  September 11 incident, 168–70
  traumatic grief, 160
  triage and acute psychosocial and psychopharmacological treatment, 164–6
  uncontrollability, 158
  unique effects on first responders and their families, 161
  unpredictability, 158
Blister agents *see* Vesicants
Bolivian hemorrhagic fever, 23
Botulism intoxication:
  causative agent, 50
  clinical description, 50
  diagnosis, 50
  differential diagnosis, 50
  medical management, 50–1
Bradyarrhythmias, 77
Bradycardia, 75, 77, 153
Brain stem infarction, 50
Bronchopneumonia, 56, 86
Broselow-Luten system, 147
Brucellosis:
  causative agent, 55
  clinical description, 55
  diagnosis, 55
  differential diagnosis, 55
  medical management, 55
Bucharest Institute of Bacteriology and Pathology, 20
Burns, 62, 64, 86, 87, 145, 152, 162, 164, 165
Butyrylcholinesterase, 75

Center for Genetic Engineering and Biotechnology, 27
Center for Mental Health Services (CMHS), 163, 164, 168
Center for Substance Abuse Prevention (CSAP), 168
Center for Substance Abuse Treatment (CSAT), 168
Center for Trauma Response, Recovery, and Preparedness (CTRP), 168
Certified Registered Nurse Anesthetists (CRNAs), 184
Chemical Agent Monitor (CAM), 91
Chemical warfare agents, 20, 73, 151, 153
CHEMPACK containers, 202–3
  emergency medical service (EMS) container, 202
  hospital container, 202
Chickenpox, 52, 150
Chikungunya, 25
Childbirth, 165
Children, 49, 51–2, 143–54
  botulinum toxin, 25, 27, 28, 29, 31, 50, 148, 151
  radiation, 59, 62, 63–4, 153–4
  vulnerabilities, 143,148, 169,169, 183, 201, 238, 270
  see also Pediatrics
Chills, 26, 51, 53, 55
Cholera, 28, 29
Cholinergic receptor, 75
Civil War, 19, 161
Clinical engineering department – emergency preparedness:
  business resumption planning, 215
  communications, 209–10
  departmental preparedness, 211
  departmental response, 215–17
  departmental staff care, 210–11
  incident command system, 209
  individual preparedness, 211
  lessons learned, 208–9
  medical technology, 211–14
  priorities, 209
  vendor preparedness, 214–15
Clothing, 18, 19, 59, 62, 64, 75, 76, 77, 89, 98, 103, 104, 106, 112, 129, 133
Cold zone, 92, 103, 123
Coma, 64, 81, 152
Community-acquired pneumonia (CAP), 281, 282
Community outreach, 169
Community preparedness, 205
Conjunctivitis, 58
Connecticut Capitol Region Council of Governments, 124
Contact dermatitis, 52
Contamination reduction zone, 123
Continuing Medical Education activities (CMEs), 135
Control charts, 43–4
Crew Resource Management, 247–8
  mannequin, 249
  moulage, 249
Crisis resource management (CRM), 249
Critical care, 186, 229–32
  HVAC system, 229, 230
  power failures, 4, 238
Critical Incident Stress Debriefing (CISD), 126, 137
Critical thinking, 243, 244, 245
Crowd control, 190
CT scanners, 209, 214
Cumulative Summation (CUSUM) charts, 45
Cyanide:
  history, 79–80
  mechanism of toxicity, 80–1
  medical management, 81–2
  minimal to mild exposure, 81
  physical characteristics, 80
  severe exposure, 81
Cyanosis, 51, 57

Decontamination and personal protection:
  certification of decontamination, 94–5
  patient identification, 92–4
  personal protection equipment, 95–7
  removal of clothing, 89
  site layout, 92
  site security, 92
  skin contamination, 89–91
  skin protection, 97–9
  surgical wound decontamination, 91–2
Defense Department's Domestic Preparedness Program, 2
Defense Research and Development Establishment (DRDE), 28
Dehydration, 145, 194
DeKon139, 90
Demron™, 98
Dengue, 54
Department of Children and Families (DCF), 168
Department of Defense, 27, 196
Department of Environmental Protection (DEP), 140

Department of Health and Human Services, 2, 3, 270
Department of Mental Health and Addiction Services (DMHAS), 168
Department of Public Health (DPH), 139, 140, 277
Department of State, 27
Department of Veteran's Affairs, 168
Depersonalization, 164
Depression, 159, 161, 171
Device simulators, 257
Diagnostic and Statistical Manual, 157
Diaphoresis, 49, 151
Diarrhea, 38, 85
Diphtheria, 49
Disaster Cart, 211, 213, 214
Disaster Kit, 211, 217
Disaster lists, 185
Disaster Medical Assistance Teams (DMAT), 139, 223
Disaster plan, 224
Disaster Response, 9, 168, 169
Disinfection, 285
Disseminated intravascular coagulation, 54
Dry decontamination, 9
Dysarthria, 50
Dysentery, 27
Dysesthesias, 59
Dysphagia, 50
Dysphonia, 50
Dyspnea, 49, 57, 84, 85, 87

E-SARS Registry, 289, 290
Early transient incapacitation (ETI), 64
Eastern (EEE) and Western equine encephalitis (WEE), 25
Eastern equine encephalitis, 27
EasyDECON™, 90
Ebola, 23, 25, 54, 151, 179
Edgewood Chemical Biological Center (ECBC), 91
Electromagnetic interference (EMI):
  backup systems, 237–8
  e-bombs, 235
  filters and shielding, 237
  grounding, 237
  intentional, 235
  mitigation, 235
  overview, 233–5
  security approach, 238
  testing, 238
Electronic Surveillance System for the Early Notification of Community-based Epidemics (ESSENCE) system, 11
ELISA, 53, 57, 58
Emergency Department Preparation – bioterror:
  decontamination, 140–1
  notification and preparation to receive patients, 138–9
  patient flow, 136–7
  planning, 136
  post incident return to normal operations, 141–2
  preparation, 135–6
  security, 137–8
Emergency Management standards, 6, 267
  Emergency Management plan (EMP), 268, 278
  hazard vulnerability analysis, 229
Emergency Medical Service (EMS), 10, 119–33
  800 MHz, 221
  Hospital Emergency Administrative Radio (HEAR), 221
  UHF, 221, 224
  VHF, 54–5, 179–80, 221, 259–60
Emergency Medical Services Authority, 10
Emergency preparedness plans, 2
  business resumption planning, 215
  emergency communications, 219
  Incident Command System (ICS), 209
  Lessons Learned, 18, 208
EMS preparation for terrorist events:
  patient decontamination, 122–4
  patient transportation, 125–6
  personnel and training, 120–1
  planning, 124–5
  preparation, 119
  return to service, 126–7
  treatment protocols, 122
  urban vs. rural preparation, 119–20
Environmental Protection Agency (EPA), 3, 96, 268
Epidemic, 3, 18, 21, 24, 39, 178
Epistaxis, 70, 84
Erythema, 54, 83, 85
Erythema multiforme, 52
Ethyl lactate, 95
Ethylene glycol monomethyl ether, 90
Ethylene oxide, 230
Exponentially Weighted Moving Averages (EWMA), 45
External contamination and injury, 64–6

Facilities Management Team (FMT), 285, 291
Faith-based organizations, 160
Fear, 19, 21, 136, 157, 164, 272
Federal Communications Commission (FCC), 219, 220
First responders, 161, 166, 270
Foot and mouth disease, 22

Glanders:
  causative agent, 55–6
  clinical description, 56
  diagnosis, 56
  medical management, 56
  prophylaxis, 56
Glaucoma, 84
Granulocyte-macrophage colony-stimulating factor (GM-CSF), 69, 87
Green zone *see* Cold zone
Grief, 160, 161, 173
Guillain-Barré syndrome, 50

Hams, 219, 220
Hazard Vulnerability analysis Matrix, 268
Hazardous Materials Incidents, 120
HAZMAT, 91, 109, 114, 140
Head injuries, 145
Headache, 26, 51, 52, 54, 71, 76, 81
Health Maintenance Organization (HMO), 41
Health Resource Services Administration (HRSA), 202
Hematopoietic, 54, 64
Hematuria, 54
Hemolysis, 149
Hemolytic uremic syndrome, 54
Hemorrhagic conjunctivitis virus, 28
HEPA, 91, 97, 110, 187, 189, 274, 286
Hepatitis, 22, 54, 57

High altitude detonation of a nuclear weapon (HEMP), 233, 235
High-fidelity mannequin simulation, 241
Homeland Security Grant Program8A, 3
Hospital Authority Head Office (HAHO), 281, 291
   Infection Control Enforcement Team (ICET), 291
Hospital disaster drill, 276
Hospital Drill Planning, 268
Hospital Emergency Area Radio network, 4
Hospital Emergency Department data, 40–1
   acquisition and presentation, 43
   confirmatory clinical data, 41
   control chart usage, 44–5
   data analysis, 43
   non-traditional health indicator data, 42
   pre-diagnostic clinical data, 41–2
Hospital Emergency Incident Command System (HEICS), 6, 10, 184, 223, 272, 274
Hospital large-scale drills:
   decontamination, 274–6
   drills, 276
   examples, 276–7
   hospital drill planning, 268–74
Hospital power:
   alternate cooling strategies, 231–2
   code required systems, 229–30
   commissioning, 232
   emergency generator coordination, 232
   HVAC system impact on generator size, 230–1
   loss of normal power, 231
   recommended systems, 230
Hospitals:
   challenges and constraints, 1–2
   communications, 4, 7–8
   decontamination, 5, 9–10
   design and conduct, 6–7
   exercises, 11–12
   observations, 4
   requirements, 2–3
   security, 4–5, 8–9
   staff protection, 6, 10–11
   staff training, 5–6, 10
Hot zone, 25, 123
Hurricane, 139, 160, 208, 219, 220
HVAC equipment, 187
Hydration, 116
Hydrocyanic acid (HCN), 80
Hydrogen cyanide, 80, 81
Hydroxycobalamin (vitamin B_{12a}), 82
Hyperesthesia, 54, 55
Hyperglycemia, 75
Hypertension, 78
Hypoallergenic, 95
Hyponatremia, 149
Hypotension, 50, 54, 66
Hypothermia, 145, 151
Hypoxia, 77, 81

Ice storm, 4, 208
Immune system, 145, 178, 180
Immunization, 6, 11, 18, 24
Intelligence agencies, 61, 201
Interdepartmental communications, 190

Internal contamination, 67–8
International Code of Diseases (ICD) Clinical Modifications, 38
International Electrotechnical Commission, 233
Internet, 41, 169, 190, 211, 222, 235
Iraqi Intelligence Service, 28
Iroquois Indians, 19
Irradiation, 62, 63
Islamic terrorists, 61
Isolation, 23, 55, 56, 95, 169
Isolation rooms, 282
Israel Institute of Biological Research (IIBR), 28

JCAHO Accreditation Manual, 267
Joint Commission for the Accreditation of Healthcare Organizations (JCAHO):
   Center for Medicaid and Medicare Services (CMS), 267
   Emergency Management standards, 6, 267
   Health Insurance Portability and Accountability Act of 1996 (HIPAA), 2, 41
   see also JCAHO Accreditation Manual
JumpSTART system, 146

Katrina, 220

Lambert-Eaton myasthenic syndrome, 50
Laryngitis, 57
Lassa Fever, 180
Lay healers, 160
LD_{50}, 84, 87
Leadership, 23, 120–1, 135, 141, 177, 184, 244
Leprosy, 19, 23
Leptospirosis, 54
Leukemia, 54
Leukopenia, 54, 56
Lobar pneumonia, 56
Local Emergency Planning Committees (LEPCs), 124
Low Earth Orbit Satellites (LEOS), 235

Malaria, 19, 53, 54
Mass casualties, 3, 61, 183–90
   Departmental Plan, 184
   Patient Flow, 136, 187
Mass Casualty Board Game, 120
Mass Casualty Incident (MCI), 139, 223
Mass Casualty Plan, 184
Maxwell's Laws, 233
MDF-200™, 90
Measles, 52
Medical Effects of Ionizing Radiation Course, 62–3
Medical gasses, 187, 213
Medical Management of Radiological Casualties, 63
Men, 17, 19, 160, 170
Meningitis, 49, 51
Mental health providers, 163, 164
Metropolitan Medical Response System (MMRS), 2, 11, 197
Mission Oriented Protective Posture (MOPP), 96
Mock Bioterrorism Drill, 245
Modular Emergency Medical System (MEMS), 196
   Acute Care Center (ACC), 196
   Neighborhood Emergency Help Centers (NEHCS), 196
Monkeypox, 52
Mononucleosis, 53, 57

Motor symptoms, 50
Mouse-neutralization assay, 50
MRI, 217

Naples Campaign of 1494, 18
National Center for Biotechnology, 29
National Center for Health Statistics, 41
National Disaster Medical System (NDMS), 139, 223
National Electric Code, 229
National Fire Protection Association, 10, 209, 268
National Incident Management System (NIMS), 6, 209, 223
National Traffic System (NTS), 219
Nerve agents:
 cardiovascular effects, 77
 central nervous system (CNS), 77
 dermal and skeletal muscle effects, 77
 gastrointestinal effects, 76
 history, 73–4
 mechanism of toxicity, 75
 medical management, 77–9
 minimal to mild vapor exposure, 77
 moderate vapor or liquid exposure, 77
 ocular, nasal and airway effects, 75–6
 physical characteristics, 74–5
 severe vapor or liquid exposure, 77
Neupogen®, 69
New Weapons and Equipment Development Committee, 27
North American Emergency Response Guidebook, 122, 123
Nursing *see* Bioterrorism and nurses/nursing

Obstetrics *see* Bioterrorism and obstetrics
Office of Emergency Medical Services (OEMS), 197
Operating room preparation – mass casualties:
 capacity expansion, 187
 communications, 190
 departmental plan, 184–7
 individual preparation, 183–4
 patient flow and infectious considerations, 187–9
 security/crowd control, 190
 training drills, 189–90
Operating systems, 215
Organophosphate poisoning, 50, 152

Pandemic Influenza, 268
Papules, 52
P-charts, 44
Pediatric Disaster Assistance Tool (PDAT), 147
Pediatrics – bioterror:
 anthrax, 148–50
 biological agents, 148
 botulinum toxin, 151
 chemical agents, 151
 cyanide, 152–3
 mental health considerations, 154
 nerve agents, 151–2
 plague, 150–1
 pulmonary agents, 152
 radiation, 153
 riot control agents, 153
 smallpox, 150
 special vulnerabilities, 143–8
 tularemia, 151
 vesicants, 152
 viral hemorrhagic fever, 151
Penicillin, 49, 50
Personal protection equipment:
 Level A, 96
 Level B, 11, 96
 Level C, 11, 96, 99, 110
 Level D, 97
Pharmacy – emergency preparedness:
 antidotes, 202–3
 staffing concerns in a crisis, 204–5
 strategic national stockpile, 203–4
 training and participation of the pharmacy staff in community preparedness efforts, 205
Pharmacy and Therapeutics Committee, 202
Photophobia, 54, 56
Plague:
 causative agent, 51
 clinical description, 51
 diagnosis, 51
 differential diagnosis, 51
 medical management, 51–2
Plant toxins, 17
Pneumonia, 49, 51, 53, 56, 57, 85, 283
Pneumonic plague, 49, 51
Poison bullets, 22
Poisson distribution, 44
Polio, 50
Post Anesthesia Care Unit (PACU), 184, 216
Post Traumatic Stress Disorder (PTSD), 170–1
Powered Air Purifying Respirator (PAPR), 98, 110, 275
Protopam chloride *see* Pralidoxime chloride
Psittacosis, 27
Psychiatry *see* bioterrorism and psychiatry
Psychological first aid (PFA), 162–3
Psychological trauma, 157, 159, 160, 171
Pulmonary edema, 24, 57–8
Purpura, 54
Pustules, 52

Q Fever:
 causative agent, 56
 clinical description, 56–7
 diagnosis, 57
 differential diagnosis, 57
 prophylaxis, 57
 treatment, 57

R400 bombs, 28
Radiation Emergency Assistance Center/Training Site (REAC/TS), 67
Radiation poisoning, 63
Radio frequency identification tags (RFID), 137
Radiological Dispersion Devices (RDDs), 61, 91
Radiological warfare, 2, 61
Radiology, 213–14, 224
Rajneeshees, 25–6
Reactive Skin Decontamination Lotion (RSDL), 90
Red Cross, 141, 161, 169, 211
Red Cross Disaster Mental Health Services, 163
Red zone *see* Hot zone
Regression modeling, 45
Revolutionary War, 18

Ricin intoxication:
    causative agent, 57
    clinical description, 57
    diagnosis, 57
    differential diagnosis, 58
    treatment, 58
Rita, 220

S charts, 44
Salmonella typhimurium, 25–6
Salvation Army, 161
Sandia National Laboratorics, 90
Saranex®, 96
Sargramostim (Leukine®), 69
Sarin, 25,73–4, 77, 95, 157, 159
SARS – prototype for bioterrorism:
    Infection Control Measures, 284–9
    outbreak resolution, 292
    recognition of outbreak in Hong Kong, 281–2
    recognition of the outbreak in PYNEH, 282–3
    response at emergency room level, 283
    response at HAHO level, 291–2
    response at hospital management level, 289–91
    response at ward and department levels, 283–4
Scientific Center for Quarantine and Zoonotic Infections (SCQZI), 29
Scientific Research Agricultural Institute (SRAI), 29
Scorpions, 17, 20
Second aid, 162
Serratia marcescens, 22
Shigella, 26
Shock, 49, 54, 58–9, 160–1, 165, 166
    see also Bioterrorism and psychiatry
Simulation:
    adaptation to medicine, 243–4
    crew resource management, 247–9
    drills for bioterrorism, 250–1
    elements of simulation education, 244–6
    history, 241–3
    medical professionals, 249
    moulage vs. mannequin training, 249
    post-simulation period, 246–7
    preparing for biodisasters, 255–65
Smallpox:
    causative agent, 52
    clinical description, 52
    diagnosis, 52
    differential diagnosis, 52
    medical management, 52
    vaccine/prophylaxis, 52–3
Smoke control systems, 229
Snake toxins, 17, 20
Social services, 157–8, 160–1, 163, 169, 172
    see also Bioterrorism and psychiatry
Sociovocational functioning, 164
Solon of Athens, 19
Soviet biological weapons program, 23–4
Staphylococcal enterotoxin B intoxication:
    causative agent, 58
    clinical description, 58
    diagnosis, 58
    differential diagnosis, 58
    medical management, 58–9

Strategic National Stockpile (SNS), 11, 202–203
    12 Hour Push Pack, 203, 204
    CHEMPACK, 202, 203
    points of dispensing (POD's), 204
    Vendor Managed Inventory (VMI), 204
Stress management, 159, 165–6
Suicidality, 161, 171
Sulfur mustard (HD), 82, 83–7
Syndromic surveillance systems, 37–8

Tabun, 73–4, 130, 202
Thrips palmi, 27
Thyroid, 67–8, 70, 153
TOPOFF exercise, 5, 120
Toxin weapons, 19–20, 24
Trauma screening questionnaire, 164
Triage, 12, 41, 103, 137, 164–7, 177, 185, 195–6, 207, 248, 258
Trichothecene mycotoxin (T2) intoxication:
    causative agent, 59
    clinical description, 59
    diagnosis, 59
    differential diagnosis, 59
    medical management, 59
Tropical Storm Allison, 208
Tularemia:
    causative agent, 53
    clinical description, 53
    diagnosis, 53
    differential diagnosis, 53–4
    medical management, 54
Tyvek®, 94, 112, 276

U-charts, 44
Unwanted memories, 160, 164
U.S. Army General Order No. 100, 19
U.S. Army Medical Research Institute of Infectious Diseases (USAMRIID), 24
U.S. biological weapons program, 24–5
U.S. Centers for Disease Control and Protection, 19

Vaccination, 178–9, 196, 201, 204
Vaccinia immune globulin, 53, 178
Varicella *see* Chickenpox
Variola *see* Smallpox
Venezuelan equine encephalitis, 23, 31
Venomous insects, 19–20
Ventilators, 108, 187, 189, 203, 212–13
Vesicants:
    airways, 85
    arsenical vesicants, 83
    bone marrow, 86
    British-Anti-Lewisite (BAL), 83
    central nervous system, 85–6
    death, 86
    eyes, 84–5
    gastrointestinal tract, 85
    history, 83
    mechanism of toxicity, 83–4
    medical management, 86–7
    mustard, 20, 81, 82, 85, 152
    phosgene oxime (CX), 83

Vesicants: (*Continued*)
    physical characteristics, 83
    skin, 85
Vesicles *see* Smallpox
Vibrio cholerae, 21
Viral hemorrhagic fever:
    causative agent, 54
    clinical description, 54
    diagnosis, 54
    differential diagnosis, 54
    medical management, 55
Viral syndrome, 38
Volunteers, 205, 211, 219–20, 273, 289
VOM, 211
VX, 74–5, 80, 90–1, 130, 202

Warm zone, 93, 123
Water supplies, 19, 21, 78, 119–20
Weaponized chemicals, 151–2
    cyanide, 79–82, 131, 132, 152
    nerve agents, 73–9, 81, 130–1, 151–2
    pulmonary agents, 130, 132, 152
    riot control agents, 130, 132, 151, 153
    vesicants, 82–3, 85, 90, 131, 145, 152
Weapons of mass destruction (WMDs) – countries thought to possess:
    Afghanistan, 23, 27, 61
    Australia, 27
    Brazil, 27
    Canada, 27, 164, 276, 289
    China, 27, 160, 235, 242, 282
    Cuba, 27
    Democratic People's Republic of North Korea, 29
    Egypt, 28
    France, 20, 22, 28, 82
    India, 17, 28
    Iran, 27, 28, 79, 83
    Iraq, 27, 28, 29, 74, 83
    Israel, 28, 159
    Kazakhstan, 23, 29
    Libya, 27, 29
    Pakistan, 29, 235
    Saudi Arabia, 29
    South Africa, 29
    South Korea, 29
    Sudan, 27, 29
    Syria, 27, 29, 31, 79
    Taiwan, 27, 31
    United Kingdom, 31, 73, 276, 289
    Uzbekistan, 31
Wells *see* water supplies
Wheezing, 59, 77, 115, 242, 248–9
Wideband RF, 233
Wood's ultraviolet lamp, 95
Working Group on Civilian Biodefense, 179
World Trade Center, 26, 40
World Trade Organization (WTO), 208
World War I, (WWI) 17, 21, 22, 32, 73, 79
    Germany, 20
    United States of America, 21
World War II, (WWII), 17, 21, 22
    Germany, 20, 22, 73
    Japan, 21
    post-WWII to modern era, 23
    United States of America, 24, 143, 148, 150
World War III (WW III), 257
Wrist band, hospital, 92
Wyeth Calf Lymph Vaccine, 52
Wyeth Dryvax Variola Major vaccine, 150

X-bar, 44
Xenophobia, 169
X-rays, 63, 235

Yellow fever, 19, 22, 27, 29, 54, 151
Yellow rain, 23, 59
Yellow zone *see* Warm zone
Yersinia pestis, 21, 29, 51, 57, 91, 150, 179
Yom Kippur War, 28

Zyklon B, 79